BMA

D1345695

Operating Room Leadership and Perioperative Practice Management

Operating Room Leadership and Perioperative Practice Management

Second Edition

Edited by

Alan David Kaye MD, PhD
Louisiana State University Health Science Center, New Orleans, LA

Richard D. Urman MD, MBA
Brigham and Women's Hospital, Harvard Medical School, Boston, MA

Charles J. Fox, III MD
Louisiana State University Health Sciences Center, Shreveport, LA

Managing Editor:
Elyse M. Cornett, PhD
LSU Health Shreveport, Shreveport, LA, USA

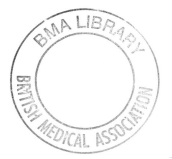

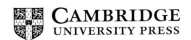
CAMBRIDGE
UNIVERSITY PRESS

CAMBRIDGE
UNIVERSITY PRESS

University Printing House, Cambridge CB2 8BS, United Kingdom

One Liberty Plaza, 20th Floor, New York, NY 10006, USA

477 Williamstown Road, Port Melbourne, VIC 3207, Australia

314–321, 3rd Floor, Plot 3, Splendor Forum, Jasola District Centre, New Delhi – 110025, India

79 Anson Road, #06-04/06, Singapore 079906

Cambridge University Press is part of the University of Cambridge.

It furthers the University's mission by disseminating knowledge in the pursuit of education, learning, and research at the highest international levels of excellence.

www.cambridge.org
Information on this title: www.cambridge.org/9781107197367
DOI: 10.1017/9781108178402

© Cambridge University Press 2012, 2019

First published 2012 by Cambridge University Press
This edition published 2019

Printed in the United Kingdom by TJ International Ltd. Padstow Cornwall

A catalogue record for this publication is available from the British Library.

ISBN 978-1-107-19736-7 Hardback

Cambridge University Press has no responsibility for the persistence or accuracy of URLs for external or third-party internet websites referred to in this publication and does not guarantee that any content on such websites is, or will remain, accurate or appropriate.

....

Every effort has been made in preparing this book to provide accurate and up-to-date information that is in accord with accepted standards and practice at the time of publication. Although case histories are drawn from actual cases, every effort has been made to disguise the identities of the individuals involved. Nevertheless, the authors, editors, and publishers can make no warranties that the information contained herein is totally free from error, not least because clinical standards are constantly changing through research and regulation. The authors, editors, and publishers therefore disclaim all liability for direct or consequential damages resulting from the use of material contained in this book. Readers are strongly advised to pay careful attention to information provided by the manufacturer of any drugs or equipment that they plan to use.

I dedicate this book to my wife, Dr. Kim Kaye, my son, Aaron Joshua Kaye, my daughter, Rachel Jane Kaye, and my many colleagues at LSU School of Medicine and Tulane School of Medicine in New Orleans. I am honored to be a part of your lives.

A. D. K.

I dedicate this book to my wife, Dr. Zina Matlyuk-Urman, my parents, and our daughters, Abigail Rose and Isabelle Grace; to my colleagues among physicians, nurses, and administrators at Harvard who supported my efforts in writing this book; and to my patients who I hope will be the ultimate beneficiaries of this work.

R. D. U.

I dedicate this book to my wife, Mary Beth, for her selfless devotion to our family, and to our kids, Chris, Mary Elise, Patrick, Julia, Claire, and Margaret, who enrich our lives more than we ever imagined.

C. J. F.

Contents

Section 1 — Leadership and Strategy

Section 2 — Economic Considerations, Efficiency, and Design

Section 3 — Surgical and Anesthesia Practice Management

Contributors

Bret D. Alvis, MD
Nashville Veterans Affairs Medical Center, Nashville, TN, USA

Steven D. Boggs, MD, MBA
The University of Tennessee College of Medicine, Memphis, TN, USA

Todd Brown, RN, MBA
Director Alvarez & Marsal/Adjunct Professor at IUPUI, Indianapolis, IN

Ann Bui, MD
Oakland Medical Center, Department of Anesthesiology, 2nd Floor, 3600 Broadway Oakland, CA, USA

Blas Catalani, MD, MPH
University of Tennessee Health Science Center, Memphis, TN, USA

Debbie Chandler, MD
LSU Health Shreveport, Shreveport, LA, USA

Seth Christian, MD, MBA
Perioperative Management Fellow, Department of Anesthesiology, Tulane University School of Medicine, New Orleans, LA, USA

Jill Cooley, MD
University of Tennessee Health Sciences Center, Department of Anesthesiology, Memphis, TN, USA

Elyse M. Cornett, PhD
LSU Health Shreveport, Shreveport, LA, USA

Judith S. Dahle, MS, MSG, RN
Senior Clinical Director – Perioperative Services, OR Efficiencies Perioperative Consulting Team, OR Efficiencies LLC, Naples, FL

Franklin Dexter, MD, PhD
University of Iowa, Iowa City, IA, USA

Dietrich Doll, MD, PhD
St. Marienhospital Vechta, Vechta, Germany

Christoph Egger, MD, MBA, FACHE
Klinik Beau-Site, Bern, Switzerland

Jesse M. Ehrenfeld, MD, MPH
Vanderbilt University Medical Center, Nashville, TN, USA

Richard H. Epstein, MD, CPHIMS
University of Miami, Coral Gables, FL, USA

Jonathan P. Eskander, MD, MBA
Department of Anesthesiology, LSU Health Shreveport, Shreveport, LA, USA

Charles J. Fox, MD
Louisiana State University Health Sciences Center, Shreveport, LA, USA

William R. Furman, MD, MMHC
Surveyer, The Joint Commission, Oakbrook Terrace, IL, USA

Aiden Feng, MD, MBA
Brigham and Women's Hospital, Boston, MA, USA

Omar A. Gafur, MD
Instructor of Anesthesiology, Boston University School of Medicine

Brenda A. Gentz, MD
University of Arizona, Tucson, AZ, USA

Peter A. Gold, MD
Northwell Health Orthopedic Institute, Great Neck, NY, USA

Ori Gottlieb, MD, FASA
Associate Professor of Anesthesia & Critical Care, Department of Anestheisa & Critical Care, University of Chicago, Chicago, IL

Michael Green, DO
Drexel University College of Medicine,
Philadelphia, PA, USA

Michael R. Hicks, MD, MBA, MHCM, FACHE
University of North Texas Health Science Center,
Fort Worth, TX, USA

Mark R. Jones, MD
Beth Israel Deaconess Medical Center, Boston,
MA, USA

Zeev Kain, MD, MBA
University of California School of Medicine,
Irvine, CA, USA

Alicia G. Kalamas, MD
Medical Director, Preoperative Clinic and Associate
Clinical Professor, Department of Anesthesia and
Perioperative Care, University of California, San
Francisco, CA, USA

Alan David Kaye, MD, PhD
Louisiana State University Health Science Center,
New Orleans, LA, USA

Adam B. King, MD
Nashville Veterans Affairs Medical Center, Nashville,
TN, USA

Kyle R. Kirkham, MD, FRCPC
University of Toronto, ON, Canada

Lyubov Kozmenko, BSN
LSU School of Nursing Faculty, Acting Director
of the Simulation Center, LSU School of Medicine,
New Orleans, LA, USA

Valeriy Kozmenko, MD
Department of Anesthesiology, LSU School
of Medicine, New Orleans, LA, USA

Henry Liu, MD
Drexel University College of Medicine,
Philadelphia, PA, USA

Jody Locke, MA
Anesthesia Business Consultants,
Jackson, MI, USA

Markus M. Luedi, MD, MBA
Bern University Hospital Inselspital, Bern,
Switzerland

Alex Macario, MD, MBA
Stanford University School of Medicine,
Stanford, CA, USA

Matthew D. McEvoy, MD
Nashville Veterans Affairs Medical Center,
Nashville, TN, USA

Ross Musumeci, MD, MBA
Anaesthesia Associates of MA, Assistant Professor
of Anesthesia, Boston University School of Medicine,
Boston, MA, USA

Matthew B. Novitch, BS
Medical College of Wisconsin, Wausau, WI, USA

Juhan Paiste, MD, MBA
University of Alabama at Birmingham School of
Medicine, Birmingham, AL, USA

Shilpadevi Patil, MD
LSU Health Shreveport, Shreveport, LA, USA

Pat Patterson, BA
Editor, OR Manager Newsletter, Rockville, MD, USA

Sonya Pease, MD, MBA
Chief Medical Officer, TeamHealth Anesthesia,
Knoxville, TN, USA

Cory Roberts, BS
Medical Student, Tulane Schoool of Medicine,
New Orleans, LA

Nigel N. Robertson, MB, ChB, FANZCA
Staff Specialist Anesthesiologist, Auckland
City Hospital, Auckland, New Zealand

Keith J. Ruskin, MD
Professor of Anesthesiology and Neurosurgery,
Yale University School of Medicine,
New Haven, CT, USA

Laurie Saletnik, RN, DNP
Johns Hopkins Hospital, Baltimore, MD, USA

Elie Sarraf, MD
University of Vermont College of Medicine,
Burlington, VT, USA

John Schlitt, MD
Capitol Anesthesiology Association,
Austin, TX, USA

Jonas Schnider, MD, MBA
Bern University Hospital Inselspital, Bern, Switzerland

Chris Sharp, MD
University of Tennessee Health Sciences Center, Department of Anesthesiology, Tennessee TN

Thomas J. Sieber, MD, MBA
Kantonsspital Graubuenden, Chur, Switzerland

David S. Silver, BS
Medical Student, Tulane School of Medicine, New Orleans, LA

Douglas P. Slakey, MD, MPH
Regents Professor and Chairman of Surgery, Department of Surgery, Section of General Surgery, Tulane Medical Center Surgery & GI Clinic, New Orleans, LA

Devona Slater, CHC, CMCP, CHA
ACE President & Sr. Compliance Auditor, Anesthesia & Pain Management Compliance Auditors, KS, USA

Brian C. Spence, MD, MHCDS
Dartmouth Geisel School of Medicine, Lebanon, NH, USA

Frank Stueber, MD
Bern University Hospital Inselspital, Bern, Switzerland

Ezekiel B. Tayler, DO
Main Line HealthCare ICU Intensive Medicine, Philadelphia, PA, USA

Terrence L. Trentman, MD
Mayo Clinic, Phoenix, AZ, USA

John M. Trummel, MD
Dartmouth Geisel School of Medicine, Lebanon, NH, USA

Mitchell H. Tsai, MD, MMM
University of Vermont College of Medicine, Burlington, VT, USA

Richard D. Urman, MD, MBA
Brigham and Women's Hospital, Harvard Medical School, Boston, MA, USA

Shermeen B. Vakharia, MD, MBA
University of California School of Medicine, Irvine, CA, USA

Thomas R. Vetter, MD, MPH
Dell Medical School at the University of Texas at Austin, Austin, TX, USA

Sanjana Vig, MD, MBA
University of California, San Diego, CA, USA

Steven Waldman, MD, JD
Clinical Professor of Anesthesiology, University of Missouri at Kansas City School of Medicine, Kansas City, MO, USA

John J. Wellik, CPA, MBA
Senior Vice President, Chief Administrative Officer, United Surgical Partners International, Inc., Addison, TX, USA

Michael R. Williams, DO, MD, MBA
Chief Executive Officer, Hill Country Memorial, Fredericksburg, TX, USA; Executive Vice President, AnesthesiaCare, an EmCare Affiliate, Dallas, TX, USA

Melvin Wyche III, MD
Director of Simulation and Assistant Professor, Department of Anesthesia, LSU School of Medicine, New Orleans, LA, USA

Longqiu Yang, MD
Huangshi Central Hospital, Huangshi Shi, Hubei Province, China

Foreword 1

Evolution describes our past. Revolution defines our future. Surgical services are in a period of revolutionary change, and financial and operational efficiency will remain important. However, it is no longer sufficient to simply refine our current processes. We must reengineer our models, designing toward our future of bundled care, shared risk, and value-based payments to determine our success.

We must also look outside of our traditional temporal and geographic boundaries. The days when a surgical encounter is viewed as an event in isolation must be put behind us. To maximize the value provided to our patients, we will include preconditioning efforts prior to surgery, and examine the longer-term outcomes and effects of our actions during the perioperative and recovery periods. Through integrating multidisciplinary teams into the entire care process, we will draw on the unique talents and knowledge of each group, maximizing safety, efficacy, and patient satisfaction.

Expanding our geography will ensure that our patients receive care in the most convenient and cost-effective location. Ambulatory, office-based, and nontraditional procedural locations such as radiology and gastroenterology suites are experiencing increasing demands for service. Applying the knowledge held by experts in OR suite management will be critical for the success of these areas.

This textbook highlights processes, techniques, and expert knowledge to prepare today's and tomorrow's leaders for these challenges. Only through exemplary leadership will we be able to realize the success which is critical for our sustained vision of providing excellence to the patients we serve.

Paul St. Jacques, MD
President, Association of Anesthesia Clinical Directors (AACD)
Quality and Patient Safety Director,
Department of Anesthesiology,
Vanderbilt University Medical Center,
The Vanderbilt Clinic,
Nashville, TN

Foreword 2

Healthcare delivery, surgery, anesthesia, and operating rooms (ORs) have all undergone astonishing changes in the past decades. Coupled with scientific advancement, all areas of medicine now recognize the importance of providing cost-effective care. For this reason, it is somewhat surprising that a standardized curriculum has not been developed for anesthesia residents and anesthesiologists who are interested in leading and managing operating suites. Individuals wanting to assume leadership in these areas must have specialized knowledge over unique areas of finance, operations, management, legal issues, and electronic records. This second edition of *Operating Room Leadership and Perioperative Practice Management* by Drs. Kaye, Fox, and Urman goes a long way in bridging this gap. The standardization of an essential corpus of knowledge that should be mastered for OR leadership will be another step in this process. The International Consortium on OR Management, Education and Training (iCORMET) fully supports such steps and commends the authors of this volume.

Steven D. Boggs, MD, MBA
President, iCORMET,

Steven Dale Boggs, MD, FASA, MBA
Professor and Chair
Department of Anesthesiology
The University of Tennessee College of Medicine
Memphis, TN

Preface to the Second Edition

With the operating room (OR) and practice management science constantly evolving, we undertook a laborious task of writing a second edition to this already popular textbook. We changed the title of the book to reflect the inclusion of topics related to perioperative practice management, adding topics that are important for anesthesiologists, surgeons, nurses, and administrators. Thus this new edition is now entitled *Operating Room Leadership and Perioperative Practice Management*. We hope that you find the additional topics useful in your daily clinical practice or administrative activities, especially given the constantly evolving regulatory and payer environments and published research. We have significantly updated and expanded each section of the book, with an emphasis on areas such as leadership training, teamwork, and OR culture change; perioperative surgical home; non-OR locations; efficiency, scheduling, and budgeting; anesthesia practice management and post-anesthesia care unit. Three chapters speak exclusively about nursing, education, and checklists.

We believe that our book currently represents the only up-to-date, evidence-based text that encompasses the "A to Z" of OR management: metrics, scheduling, human resource management, leadership principles, economics, quality assurance, recovery, information technology, ambulatory practice, and topics specific to surgeons, anesthesiologists, and pain service providers.

Years ago, the OR stood alone, and little attention was given to the perioperative period. This is because until the 1980s the OR generated large profits, despite its inefficiencies. Thus, hospital administrators allowed it a great deal of autonomy. However, today's administrators realize that, although the OR is typically one of the biggest sources of revenue for a hospital, it is also one of the largest areas of expense. This, coupled with increasing requirements for cost containment in healthcare and a demand for accountability to the federal and state governments, insurance companies, hospital administrators, surgeons, and patients, has magnified the need for an effective and efficient perioperative process. While there was little centralized leadership in the perioperative period of the past, perioperative management is now a critical feature of successful hospitals.

As mentioned above, today's perioperative practice of medicine has evolved significantly and is now influenced by a vast array of factors, both medical and administrative. Because of this, knowledge of hospital economics and administration, OR mechanics and metrics, preoperative patient optimization strategies, human resources, financial planning, governmental policy and procedures, and clinical perioperative management is necessary in order to succeed. A good management team must bring together these diverse components to maximize productivity. Today there are more regulations, quality measures, and outcome expectations, which push innovation and result in additional burdens and challenges for hospitals. The need for this expensive technology, to compete with other hospitals, forces reform and new thoughts for traditional ways of the past. Staffing ratios, preoperative visits, and postoperative care will be highly scrutinized financially, while clinical and administrative "multitasking" is now expected. Putting an emphasis on quality data definition and collection, leadership style, simulation, and OR design will lead to the creation of a more productive and efficient perioperative process.

We should not lose sight of the fact that the OR is where miracles happen every single day through teamwork, natural talent, hard work, and empathy. From all of this, we create game-changing and life-altering experiences for patients. Without effective and efficient leadership from all areas – nursing, administration, surgery, and anesthesia services – we are doomed to fail. Let us also remember that all of us will be patients one day, and so let us strive to make a first-class OR in the best interests of everyone.

As we have observed from our real-life experiences collectively accumulated over the past three decades, the science of perioperative patient care is constantly evolving. This speaks to the enormous complexities in all aspects of management and development of a winning OR. We applaud all the authors for their hard work and dedication. Their chapters give a practical insight into creating a successful perioperative program.

We all face challenges in the OR environment. We hope the ideas and practical solutions discussed in this expanded second edition will benefit any stakeholder in administration, surgery, anesthesia, or nursing services, as we all do our best to move forward into the future.

Alan D. Kaye, MD, PhD
New Orleans, LA

Richard D. Urman, MD, MBA
Boston, MA

Charles J. Fox III, MD
Shreveport, LA

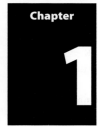

Chapter

1

Leadership Principles

Christoph Egger and Alex Macario

Contents

Evolution of Leadership

What Is Leadership?

As individuals move up within an organization and accept more responsibility, their interest in leadership rises as they have more people reporting to them. Leadership is about leading people, or the *capacity to lead*, and specifically the behavior of an individual when directing the activities of a group towards a shared goal [1]. Akin to a conductor of an orchestra, a leader has a capacity to direct and motivate multiple professionals to perform to their peak ability while minimizing uncoordinated activity.

In our own experience, leadership is about making sure everyone in the organization (1) shares vision and purpose, (2) is engaged in the future outcome of the organization, and therefore (3) favors collaboration over pursuing their own agenda. Among many other responsibilities, leaders are role models for the values of the organization, set the optimal course, and establish priorities. Making people connect and collaborate, as well as finding the appropriate style and amount of communication, are formidable challenges, but central tasks for healthcare leaders.

Just because a person is in a leadership position doesn't make him or her a leader [2].

The goals of this chapter are to review what is known from the published literature about leadership in general and in the context of healthcare organizations to illustrate the operating room (OR) suite as a challenging workplace, where different parties must cooperate or thwart each other, and to identify the challenges inherent to an OR leadership position.

Predispositions for Leaders

Trait theory, which suggests that leadership abilities depend on the personal qualities of the leader, is controversial. However, some traits are related to leadership emergence and effectiveness. Leadership emergence refers to whether and to what degree an individual is viewed as a leader by others within a work group. On the other hand, leadership effectiveness is a phenomenon affecting interactions between groups, and refers to a leader's performance in influencing and guiding the activities of his or her unit toward achievement of its goals.

Five dimensions can be used to describe the most prominent aspects of personality: neuroticism, extraversion, openness to experience, agreeableness, and conscientiousness. This five-factor model of personality was also shown to be a reasonable basis for examining dispositional predictors of leadership [3]. Extraversion and conscientiousness are the most important traits of leaders, and these dimensions are more strongly related to leadership emergence than to leadership effectiveness.

The following traits are associated with successful leaders [4]: humility, courage, integrity, vigilance and passion, inspiration, sense of duty and dedication, compassion, discipline, generosity, dedication to continuous learning, collaborative approach, and competitiveness.

Appendix A has a checklist that may be a way for leaders to self-assess some of their own strengths and weaknesses as leader. In addition, it could be used by people working in a surgical suite to evaluate the OR director.

Leadership Styles

Multiple differing leadership styles have been described. Some aspects of each leadership style definition overlap with one another [5–8] (Box 1.1).

The mix of the healthcare workforce and the complexity of the medical workplace demand a team approach to problem solving. This requires a leader who is comfortable "sharing power" by empowering

---

Box 1.1. Leadership Styles

Authoritarian (coercive, commanding) leaders employ coercive tactics to enforce rules and to manipulate people and decision making.

- Derived from the Prussian military, the command-and-control model is the primary management strategy.
- Believe in a top-down, line-and-staff organizational chart with clear levels of authority and reporting processes.
- Demand immediate compliance to orders and accomplish tasks by bullying and sometimes demeaning the followers.
- Used in situations where the company or group requires a complete turnaround.
- May be effective during catastrophes or dealing with underperforming employees, as a last resort.

Pacesetting leaders set high performance standards for themselves and their followers and exemplify the behaviors they are seeking from other group members.

- Give little or no feedback on how the followers are doing except to jump in to take over when the followers lag.
- Work best when followers are self-motivated and highly skilled.
- May be effective to get quick results from a highly motivated and competent team.

Transactional leaders balance and integrate the organizational goals and expectations with the needs of the people doing the work.

- Work through creating well-defined structures, clear goals, and distinct rewards for following orders.
- Motivate workers by offering rewards for what the leaders need to be done.
- Offer the appeal of employment and security in return for collaboration and assistance.

Authoritative (visionary) leaders mobilize people toward a compelling vision.

- Most effective when a new vision is needed, or when the path to that vision is not always clear.
- Though the leader is considered an authority, this type of leader allows followers to figure out the best way to accomplish their goals.
- May be effective when changes require a new vision, or when a clear direction is needed.

Coaching leaders are genuinely interested in helping others succeed and hence develop people for the future.

- Help employees identify both their strengths and weaknesses, and provide feedback to their subordinates on their performance.
- By delegating tasks they give employees challenging assignments.
- May be effective to help employees improve their performance or develop long-term strengths.

Democratic (participative) leaders build consensus through participation.

- Give members of the work group a vote or a say in nearly every decision the team makes.
- A collaborative process brings a family atmosphere to the workplace and creates respect for the contributions made by each member.
- When used effectively, the democratic leader builds flexibility and responsibility. This helps identify new ways to do things with fresh ideas.
- The level of involvement required by this approach (e.g., decision making) can be time consuming.
- Appropriate for building buy-in or consensus, or for receiving input from valuable employees.

Affiliative leaders often are more sensitive to the value of people than reaching goals.

- Pride themselves on their ability to keep employees happy, and create a harmonious work environment.
- Attempt to build strong emotional bonds with those being led, with the hope that these relationships will bring about a strong sense of loyalty in their followers.
- May be appropriate to resolve tensions in a team or to motivate people in difficult situations.

Authentic leaders use a deep self-awareness to engage followers, to shape organizational environments, and

---

eventually allow the organization to achieve persistently high performance.

- Authenticity involves both owning one's personal experiences (values, preferences, thoughts, emotions, and beliefs) and acting in accordance with one's true self.
- The ability of a leader to behave authentically as a person (authenticity of the person) positively affects his or her leadership efficacy (leadership multiplier).

Transformational leaders care about human understanding – they transform and motivate followers through their idealized influence (or *charisma*) and role model, intellectual stimulation, and individual consideration.

- Aim at creating an environment where every person is empowered and motivated to fulfill his or her highest needs.
- Each member becomes a part of a collective identity and productive learning community of the organization.
- See themselves as servants to others and guide them in creating and embracing a vision for the organization. This inspires and brings forth top performance and creates a belief system of integrity. Servant leadership demands that a leader places company goals and values first, the management team and employees second, and the leader's own welfare third. In this paradigm, leaders exist to permit production and to obliterate obstacles, not acquire power, glory, wealth, or fame.

people and is able to make decisions with a balance of idealism and pragmatism – a leadership concept described as "leading from behind" [9]. This type of leader understands how to create an environment or culture in which other people are willing and able to lead. For example, the image of the shepherd behind his herd is based on Nelson Mandela's autobiography *Long Walk to Freedom* and acknowledgment that leadership is a collective activity in which different people act at a different time.

This image of leadership is backed by the idea of Theory Y people, as described in McGregor's *The Human Side of Enterprise* [10, 11]. According to McGregor, people can be divided into the two groups, Theory X and Theory Y. Theory X assumptions are:

- People are inherently lazy and will avoid work if they can.
- Most people have little desire for responsibility and prefer to be directed.
- People must be coerced, controlled, or threatened with punishment to get them to perform.

On the other hand, Theory Y postulates that:

- Work is as natural as play and rest.
- People are ambitious, self-motivated, and will readily accept greater responsibility.
- People will use their creativity, ingenuity, and imagination to solve problems.

In reality, a person's beliefs will fall somewhere between Theory X and Theory Y. Whereas Theory X leaders enforce the rules of behavior and punish those who violate the standards, Theory Y leaders function as "coaches," encouraging their team. They focus on developing and facilitating the team through nurturing, encouragement, support, and positive reinforcement.

Situational Leadership

Goleman suggests that successful leaders employ multiple leadership styles and should be able to move between leadership styles according to a specific situation (situational leadership) [6]. OR leadership requires this adaptive style because of the personalities encountered in a highly trained and demanding workplace. For example, during a cardiac resuscitation, an authoritarian or coercive leadership style may be appropriate to make sure all Code team members receive clear instructions. In contrast, an affiliate style may be appropriate to resolve a conflict between two surgeons disputing over a certain OR time slot.

Goleman's situational leadership model suggests that although leaders may have a preferred style, they must identify and select the appropriate mix of various leadership behaviors in a given situation.

"Emotional intelligence" (EI) may be a better predictor and attribute of leadership effectiveness than intellectual intelligence (IQ) or technical skills [12]. EI is a person's ability to be aware of and being able to manage and use emotions appropriately in dealing with people under various situations (Box 1.2). Experienced leaders with well-developed EI competencies may be more effective and have more satisfied and committed staff members, who better attend to patient care needs.

Box 1.2. Five Main Components of EI

Self-awareness	Understand one's own emotions, strengths, weaknesses, needs, drives, and their effect on others.
Self-regulation	The ability to control and manage feelings and moods so they are appropriate.
Motivation	A passion to work for reasons that goes beyond money and status; persistence and confidence.
Empathy	The ability to understand the emotional makeup of other people; sensitivity to others' needs and emotions.
Social skill	Proficiency in managing relationship and building strong collaborative networks; ability to influence and lead people.

Difference between Management and Leadership

An often heard concept is that managers are people busy with operational tasks (command and control), whereas leaders engage in strategic endeavors (vision and mission, change management). To quote Naylor, most persons have worked "with leaders who were not particularly skilled at management, but who had an ability to win loyalty and carry others with them through their clarity of vision, generosity of spirit, and 'people skills'. Ironically, then, leadership may be most obviously exerted when others follow a person who has no direct authority over them, and may be less important in strictly hierarchical organizations where managerial discipline prevails" [13].

The differences between managers and leaders then may simply be attributed to different leadership styles (e.g., transactional and transformational) or different leader positions (top executive versus middle management).

Significance of Leadership for Healthcare Organizations

Governments around the globe are increasingly searching for cost containment practices to counter mounting healthcare expenditures. This has led to declining reimbursement for physician and hospital services, the replacement of fee-for-service payments

with bundled prospective payment systems (PPS) using case-based lump sums based on diagnoses-related groups (DRG), and capitation and other compensation systems that shift financial risk from the payer to the service providers. For example, one of the major goals of the Patient Protection and Affordable Care Act (PPACA), a US federal statute signed into law in 2010, is to reduce healthcare costs. Specifically, structural changes in the healthcare system made by the PPACA aim to shift the healthcare system from paying-for-quantity to paying-for-quality (value-based care [VBC]).

Such profound transformation with reimbursement, technological, policy, and procedural and structural changes intensifies the need for and challenges of healthcare leadership [14].

There are unique leadership challenges inherent to healthcare [15]:

- Healthcare leaders face inconsistent or conflicting dynamic demands from external stakeholders (e.g., patients, regulatory, institutional and market forces, and others).
- As a "human" service rendered directly by providers, healthcare is prone to natural variability.
- Healthcare is a technology-intensive sector with a high frequency of innovation. Such advances exacerbate tensions in balancing cost, quality, and access to healthcare services.
- Healthcare leaders must interact with powerful and dominating professionals (e.g., physicians) who may not be employees of the organization.

Leadership in the Healthcare Literature

In 2002, a review of 6,628 articles revealed that most of the healthcare and business literature on leadership consisted of anecdotal or theoretical discussion [16]. Only a few articles include correlations of qualities or styles of leadership with measurable outcomes such as positive changes in organizations. It is still unclear what leadership attributes are important in improving either patient care outcomes or team and organizational outcomes.

There are, however, some specific studies of leadership in healthcare that are noteworthy [15]. Transformational leadership style is more likely to be used by leaders in not-for-profit organizations than by leaders in for-profit organizations. In the hospital setting, transformational leadership style has been shown to be positively and significantly associated with staff satisfaction, extra effort from staff, perceived unit performance, and staff retention. Some weak evidence indicates that leadership matters more for nonprofessionals (e.g., nursing assistants, clerks, secretaries) than professionals.

Managers with higher ranks demonstrate more transformational behavior than those lower in the hierarchy. Of note, healthcare leaders may perceive the use of rewards as transformational leader behavior. In contrast, surveys of leaders in industries outside healthcare indicate the use of such reward systems as linked to a transactional leadership style. Physician executives with management degrees were more likely to provide transformational leadership than those without training [17]. Despite evidence that supports transformational leadership theory for the healthcare setting, leadership style is but one important factor in successful organizational change. Organizational structure and culture matter just as much. Participative and person-focused leadership styles are positively associated with nursing staff's job satisfaction, retention, and organizational commitment.

In the healthcare and hospital setting, leaders must take into account their followers' expectations and understand how and why professionals respond (or not) to different leadership styles.

The Healthcare Leadership Alliance (HLA) has developed the HLA Competency Directory as an instrument for healthcare executives to use in assessing their expertise in critical areas of healthcare management [18]. Within the HLA Competency Directory, the competencies are categorized into five critical domains and, within each domain, 3–4 clusters of competencies (Table 1.1).

Managers with advanced education may be more effective in leadership roles. Junior nurse managers value clinical and communications skills compared to senior managers who value negotiation skills and business knowledge more [15].

A systematic review of articles related to physician leadership and EI showed that many authors from a broad range of medical specialties recommend cultivating physician leadership, including EI training, at an executive level in all medical institutions. Although evidence supports the association of EI with business outcomes outside of healthcare, there is a paucity of scientific research examining the benefits of EI in healthcare. A gap has been described between advocacy for EI as an essential training competency in

Table 1.1 HLA Competency Directory

Competency domain	Competency cluster
Communication and relationship management	• Relationship management • Communication skills • Facilitation and negotiation
Leadership	• Leadership skills and behavior • Organizational climate and culture • Communicating vision • Managing change
Professionalism	• Personal and professional accountability • Professional development and lifelong learning • Contributions to the community and profession
Knowledge of the healthcare environment	• Healthcare systems and organizations • Healthcare personnel • The patient's perspective • The community and the environment
Business skills and knowledge	• General management • Financial management • Human resource management • Organizational dynamics and governance • Strategic planning and marketing • Information management • Risk management • Quality improvement

healthcare and the critical need for further rigorous study of the issue [19].

Physician Leadership

Hospitals with the greatest clinician participation in management scored about 50 percent higher on important drivers of performance than compared to hospitals with low levels of clinical leadership [20]. Doctors in physician-led organizations seem to be leading in the areas of quality, service, and cost [21]. Physicians have to have enough power and authority to affect change – to determine how quality is defined, what protocols will be developed, and how to hold each other accountable for meeting objectives [22]. In the perioperative setting, strong physician leadership is required for compliance with surgical checklists and site marking to prevent wrong-site surgery. On matters of clinical medicine and practice, physicians listen to respected peers. A well-trained and accepted physician leader may better inspire, convince, and influence their colleagues. It is critical for this person to serve as a change agent to manage and influence clinical practice patterns and adherence to guidelines.

However, a common myth is that a physician successful in clinical practice can easily transfer to leading an organization [23]. In fact, being a medical expert does not guarantee being a good leader. It is challenging to hire physician leaders who will end up being successful as it is difficult to assess candidates for leadership positions. Deegan et al. point out that "as a consequence of the way … physicians have been selected, educated, and socialized during their training many are highly competitive, relatively independent practitioners. They often eschew teamwork and collaboration and other affiliative behaviors" [24]. When assessing physician leader candidates, the use of a structured decision-making process for assessment and selection should be considered. Physicians aspiring to be leaders actively reflect and internalize the results of feedback and link this information directly to a formal plan of study to gain the competencies needed for their future leadership roles. Physicians in the midst of the transition between clinical and managerial/leadership positions start to realize the substantial differences between clinical and managerial/leadership positions, and that the behaviors that serve them well in their clinical workspace (such as the OR) may be the exact opposite of what they need as executive leaders in hospitals (Table 1.2).

Various barriers exist for physicians to take leadership roles [25]:

- Identity linked to leadership roles may threaten the physicians' view of themselves as clinical professionals.
- Deep-rooted skepticism about the value of spending time on leadership.
- Lack of career development or financial incentives.
- Lack of leadership and management training.
- Risk of losing credibility with clinical colleagues and others.
- The greater risk of unemployment as a leader/manager than as a clinician.
- A loss of popularity due to making tough decisions.
- The need to learn to being accountable to their organization as opposed to their colleagues.

Table 1.2 Differences between Clinicians and Manager/Leader

Clinician	Manager/leader
Clinical competence	Interpersonal competence
1:1 interaction	1:N interaction
Doers	Planners
Value autonomy	Value collaboration
Reactive	Proactive
Identification with profession	Identification with company
Patient advocate	Organization advocate
Lay IT/IS skills	IT/IS power user
Informal communication	Formal communication
Leadership skills optional	Leadership skills essential
Member of "brotherhood/sisterhood"	Member of the "dark side"
Micromanaging a must	Overmanaging a sure way to fail
Independent	Adaptation to a boss
Pursuit of self-interest	Trustworthiness

- A need to overcome an us-versus-them mentality between physicians and health administrators.

For newly appointed physician leaders, a robust onboarding and specific leadership program is critical. Onboarding may include coaching, which can be driven by another leader from within the organization who has more leadership experience, or by an external coach. In the past, healthcare has been slow to adopt systematic organizationally based leadership development programs. Instead, responsibility for leadership development has often been left to individuals and the profession.

Leadership Is Critical in the Management of Perioperative Services

The OR suite is a complex working environment, with different groups of individuals involved in a coordinated effort to perform highly skilled interventions. This is analogous to high-reliability organizations, such as aviation, the military, and nuclear industries, where the importance of a wide variety of factors for development of a favorable outcome has been long stressed [26]. These include ergonomic factors such as the quality of interface design, team coordination and leadership, organizational culture, and quality of decision making.

The role of a leader and manager is central to forming high-performance interprofessional teams.

Underlying key principles for successful team building are a shared vision and mission. To align the goals of employees and physicians, the leader must convey the vision and strategies [27].

The following factors contribute to the growing need for a dedicated professional as a perioperative leader:

- Growing surgical caseload, exceeding regular workday shift-hours.
- Medical consumables included in case-based lump-sum payment, which cannot be charged separately to the payer.
- Multiple lines of authority causing a lack of continuity and ownership for decisions.
- Large variety of professionals working in the OR suite.
- Difficulties in recruiting and retaining healthcare professionals.
- Increasing number of ORs and creation of different OR suites within the same facility.
- Increasing number of nonsurgical interventions outside the surgical suite with growing need for hospital-wide provider scheduling.
- Lack of physician involvement in OR leadership.

Challenges in OR Leadership

Organizational Structures of OR Leadership

Hospitals have always been in search of the optimal OR leadership structure. The need for leadership training was recognized more than 60 years ago. For example, in the English literature of the 1950s, a textbook contained descriptions of the ideal OR governance structure and recommended that "the administration of the surgical department shall be under the direction of a competent registered nurse who has executive ability and who is specially trained in operating-room management" [28]. In 1983, an article about OR management delineated eight managerial measures to improve OR management efficiency and effectiveness. One of these measures was the identification of a clear line of authority and appointment of an individual with far-reaching responsibilities, including policy making, running the daily schedule, and managing staff stepping out of line [29]. The article pointed out that this person would not only have to be a senior physician with institutional authority but also be formally recognized as being in charge.

There is no perfect organizational structure. The organizational structure of an OR suite must be individually tailored to its internal and external needs.

Small organizations often feature a flat hierarchy and do not require many formal organizational structures. These organizations benefit from close relationships between people. This allows for quick and informal problem solving. An OR charge nurse or nursing director as the sole formal leader may be sufficient in small OR suites since ad hoc problem-solving groups form spontaneously and dissolve naturally.

Large organizations, on the other hand, with several surgical subspecialties require a more complex organizational and leadership structure because cooperation and coordination of tasks among departments is challenging. OR suites of large medical centers often feature several complementary leadership structures (Box 1.3).

Outside of the United States, OR management is a relatively young science, and knowing the leadership literature is also a recent phenomenon. In Germany, OR management first appeared in the scientific literature in 1999. The reason this topic produced interest much later than it did in the United States may be the introduction of the German DRG reimbursement, a PPS for inpatient hospital services in 2003. In the United States, PPS was introduced in the 1980s. With the introduction of government-mandated healthcare cost containment measures such as PPS, hospital revenues declined and hospital and physician executives aimed to find innovative ways to increase OR efficiency (see Franklin Dexter's chapter).

Lonely at the Top

Leaders are often alone with their thoughts because they need to keep an emotional distance and avoid conflict of interests in their professional environment [33]. Leaders are able to develop relationships with people based on respect, not on friendship [34]. In addition, leaders are often surrounded by people with opposite opinions on certain topics for valid reasons. Making decisions that are unpopular with some stakeholders and being attacked for those decisions may increase isolation for the leader. Decision making in uncertainty is a task that exacerbates the leader's loneliness.

One of the interesting observations by leaders is how streams of information suddenly dry up when that person becomes the head of an organization or a group. People hesitate to speak freely with a leader and so adopt a more formal tone while

Box 1.3. Leadership Positions and Structures for the Surgical Suite

Physician OR leadership position (e.g., OR medical director): May be a facilitator, mediator, and negotiator position to balance the priorities of each group in the OR (surgeons, anesthesiologists, nurses, hospital administrators, etc.).

Alternatively, the **OR medical director** may be positioned to be a distinct authority: A position frequently recommended by the German OR management literature ("OR manager") [30, 31]. This may be explained by the fact that in Germany, as in many other European countries, most physicians are employed by the hospital. Where there are many independent, powerful physicians (especially surgeons), a tall or centralized organization with a top decision-making leader may be an ineffective leadership structure.

A **standing OR committee** with strategic and oversight responsibilities (e.g., "OR oversight committee," "OR board"): This committee may consist of the chairs of surgical services and/or departments, the chief of the anesthesia department and nurse managers of the perioperative area, and representatives of the hospital administration. The role of this committee is to provide fair and balanced OR governance [32].

Additional **smaller OR management teams** may be formed with operational responsibilities (e.g., OR executive committee): A typical formation includes a senior surgeon and anesthesiologist (who may be medical co-directors of the OR suite), the director of surgical services, and a senior hospital executive.

Administrative executive physician: This position may be labeled Chief Medical Officer or Vice President of Medical Affairs, and refers to a position often used as a third-party mediator to facilitate finding solutions between two conflicting parties (e.g., between different surgical departments or between the hospital administration and anesthesia department).

communicating. The challenge for a leader then is to find and develop other methods for figuring out what is really going on. A leader in the surgical suite needs to work hard to get people to share their views, and must proactively develop positive relationships so that colleagues feel comfortable and provide their honest opinions.

Culture and Informal Organization

Understanding the organizational culture of the OR suite is key to successful and effective leadership. For example, change management and implementing patient safety initiatives are hard to accomplish without understanding the values, assumptions, preferences, unwritten rules, and behaviors of a certain workplace. If leaders are not conscious of the culture in which they are embedded, those cultures will manage them [35]. The leader needs to perceive the functional and dysfunctional elements of the existing culture and to manage cultural evolution and change in such a way that the group can thrive.

Organizational culture is the essence of the informal organization [36].

In 1976, Hall developed the iceberg analogy of culture [37]. If the culture of a society was an iceberg, some aspects of culture would be easy to see and understand, above the surface. On the other hand, below the water, there is a larger portion of culture hidden beneath the surface that is related to the beliefs, existing relationships, and values of a society. This underwater part of the iceberg culture is difficult for the new leader to understand and includes elements such as the definition of sin, concept of justice, work ethic, definition of insanity, approaches to problem solving, fiscal expression, and approaches to interpersonal relationships. Hall suggests that the only way to learn the invisible bulk of the culture below the surface is by actively participating in the culture. Similarly, organizational culture comprises the visible values and behaviors within an organization, shaped by employee perks and benefits, policies and procedures, and the company brand [38]. It often turns out that the majority of what drives the behaviors within the organization is unseen and inaccessible to leaders unless they actively seek that information, far below the surface. This culture includes the history of the institution, the existing relationships among people and departments, the incentive system and the unintended consequences of the incentive system, and relationships with various stakeholders. "The way things get done around here" is a one working definition within the hidden part of organizational culture. If leaders are unaware of these aspects of corporate culture, they may feel frustrated at not being able to get things accomplished.

In addition to the formal relationships depicted on organizational charts, in every OR suite, there are also information relationships. There may be an informal network, coalitions of people, and even hierarchy. For example, a powerful surgeon may be able to exert his or her influence on the scheduling process and circumvent official scheduling rules. These informal affiliations shape the organization's culture, and they can either facilitate or impede change. An important aspect of perioperative leadership is understanding and accepting these relationships, managing the informal chain of command, and even leveraging these affiliations.

People Alignment and Change

Tensions between the different professional groups working in the OR probably existed ever since the first surgeries were performed. A nursing report from Australia from the early twentieth century noted that the "disaccord between nurses and physicians often led to troubles in the OR because the physicians would never announce the beginning of surgeries in a timely fashion, but would then suddenly appear in the OR where they would have to wait for the nurses to be finished with their preparatory work" [39].

A core issue for leaders of the OR suite is that the goals of the various professions are not well aligned with those of the hospital and the OR suite. This dilemma is known in economics as "principal–agent problem," where difficulties arise under conditions of incomplete and asymmetric information when a principal hires and motivates an agent to act on behalf of the principal [40]. Getting people to move in the same direction is a crucial leadership activity. People alignment involves communicating the organization's direction to those whose cooperation may be needed to create coalitions that help people understand the overall vision and stay committed to its achievement [41]. One of various managerial mechanisms that may be used to align the interests of the agent in solidarity with those of the principal is performance measurement. In the OR environment, well-designed reporting systems must define relevant performance measures (key performance indicators). This feedback is provided to those owning the critical processes and should be gauged in relation to the OR suite's goals and its most important stakeholders. The OR environment with conflicting goals requires a strong leadership to enforce hospital and OR suite strategies. In US hospitals, the shift toward employment of physicians continues to grow, becoming an important focus of alignment.

Another core leadership activity involves establishing the organization's direction, i.e., producing change and transformation. Reasons for organizations to initiate change include barriers to collaboration due to silos, insufficient innovation, and unpreparedness to excel in the future. Change rarely happens in a linear fashion. Instead, it more often is a cyclical process. Kotter's cyclical accelerator model involves eight key components [42]:

1. Create and sustain a sense of urgency: Top leaders describe an opportunity that will appeal to individuals.
2. Build and maintain a guiding coalition of effective, volunteer employees who role-models the change.
3. Formulate a strategic vision and develop initiatives designed and executed fast and well enough to make the vision reality.
4. Enlist a volunteer group of employees who buy in to the envisioned goals and share a commitment toward making the change.
5. Enable action and empowerment across employees by removing barriers such as inefficient processes or hierarchies.
6. Generate and communicate short-term wins to provide proof that the change created actual results.
7. Sustain acceleration: Adapt quickly to shifting business environments in order to maintain speed and enhance competitiveness.
8. Institute change: Individuals must understand the importance of agility and speed for the organization's success.

Various change initiatives in the perioperative setting have been described following Kotter's model [43–45].

How can a leader assess his or her individual impact? Covey encouraged leaders to work within their smaller *circle of influence*, wherein they will be able to make a difference, as opposed to spending time in their *circle of concern*, whereby they have very little to contribute [46]. For example, our circle of concern may include the broader issues of politics and the reforming and uncertain future of healthcare, such as PPACA. Covey recommended that the energy of leaders be focused on their circle of influence, i.e., on the issues they have influence over, such as the adoption of lean management system into day-to-day hospital operations.

Effective leaders recognize two primary types of change: from the *outside-in* (structural) and from the *inside-out* (cultural/behavioral). A focus on cultural change is a core to sustaining structural change. It is cultural change – the change of the collective behavior of individuals within the organization – that will make possible a structural change at the organization and administrative levels. And it is changing people from within which makes organizational change so difficult. For example, in a complex clinical environment like a quaternary care hospital's OR, the culture may need to be fundamentally addressed before structural changes, such as checklists and other patient safety measures, can be successfully implemented [47].

However, it is hard for leaders to simultaneously tackle all "soft" issues (such as culture and motivation) that are necessary for transforming organizations. Sirkin et al. have found that focusing on these issues alone may not bring about change because organizations also need to consider the hard factors such as the time they take to complete a change initiative, the number of people required to execute it, etc. [48]. There is a consistent correlation between the outcomes of change programs (success versus failure) and the following four variables:

D The **duration** of time until the change program is completed; for change program, this refers to the amount of time between reviews of milestones.

I The project team's performance **integrity**; that is, the capabilities of project teams.

C The **commitment** of senior executives and staff to change.

E The **effort** over and above the usual work that the change initiative demands of employees.

The DICE framework comprises a set of simple questions that help executives score their projects on each of the four factors. Organizations can use DICE assessments to force conversations about projects, to gauge whether projects are on track or in trouble, and to manage project portfolios.

Social Capital

Waisel described social capital as an overall indicator of the quality of the relationships within a community and applied it to the OR suite [49]. Increasing social capital improves communication and trust that, in turn, improves most cooperative undertakings. In the OR suite, the social capital benefits of expectations of trust, robust norms, and better communication help to achieve community goals.

The norm should be that medical professionals seek flawless behavior, particularly in regard to interacting with others and respecting operational guidelines. Other than in the case of small teams, large groups of people are less likely to have developed personal histories of successful interactions. In the absence of a personal history of trust, the expectation of trust from social capital permits individuals who enter into negotiations to assume that they will be treated in a fair, appropriate, and civil manner. Functional operational guidelines help to develop trust in the organization. Improved behavior and successful interactions increase trust and communication, which, in turn, improves the OR working environment and increases the success of cooperative ventures, such as having more efficient ORs.

Importance of Building Trust on Survival of Coalitions

Dialogue promotes understanding between parties in conflict, and the resulting relationship promotes trust between diverse entities [50]. This trust is based on the fact that there is respect for one another's opinion and that team members are willing to listen and share viewpoints openly. If and when leaders promote an environment in which they are comfortable taking on the challenging dialogues (i.e., productive conflict), they can effectively lead change and build respect in the perioperative setting. This leads to a stronger team and better adherence to patient safety measures. A common example is OR nurses speaking up prior to a wrong-site surgery.

The Impact of Leadership on Patient Safety and Quality Initiatives

Many have stated that the magic ingredient to success in patient safety is leadership [2]. Communication and leadership failure are two of the most frequent causes of adverse events [51]. Previous studies have identified that teamwork, communication, and situation awareness are most important to work safely and effectively in a surgical environment and for minimizing technical errors [52, 53].

How is a leader able to move the team to the next level of safety culture? Before a change can be successfully implemented, the leader must first assess and understand the culture. Only a deep awareness of the organization's culture allows the leader to set off effective change.

In the UK in 1997, the concept of "clinical governance" relating to a comprehensive framework to improve the quality of care was introduced into the National Health Service (NHS). Clinical governance is defined as a framework through which NHS organizations are accountable for continuously improving the quality of their services and safeguarding standards of care by creating an environment in which excellence in clinical care can flourish. Leadership, teamwork, effective communication, ownership, and systems awareness are the foundations of clinical governance [54].

Successful centers are more likely to have a shared sense of purpose, leaders with a hands-on leadership style, and clear accountability structures [55, 56].

Leaders may have a direct impact on the behaviors of the employees, by taking part in the execution of the strategy and clarifying the expected results and aligning the rewards system. The leader must identify the right person for the right role, and with execution as part of the expected behavior, it becomes part of the culture [57].

There is evidence that prevention of harm to patients and transformation to a higher state of sustainable reliability are directly related to governance board engagement and administrative execution [58]. Risk-adjusted mortality rates have been shown to be significantly lower for hospitals whose governing boards have a quality committee as compared to those who don't. Hospital boards seem to be more successful when they set specific aims to reduce harm and make a public commitment to quality improvement that is measurable [59].

There exists evidence that greater engagement of hospital leadership at the board and executive level is associated with better quality outcomes, as measured by the *CareScience Quality Index* – a single quality measure that embraces risk-adjusted rates of adverse outcomes of mortality, morbidity, and complications [60].

Studies on seven dimensions of culture by one of the major patient safety organizations in the United States, the National Quality Forum (NQF), revealed the importance of the following [4]:

- Communication: High-performing organizations have clear communication channels within their structures and systems and excellent linkages with outside organizations.

- Underlying values: Leaders drive values, values drive behaviors, and the collective behaviors of individuals in an organization define the corporate cultures that drive performance.
- Leadership: The success of high-performing organizations revolves completely around leaders at every level, and the structures and systems they put in place enable expressions of group values.
- Teamwork: High-performing organizations have invested in knowledge and skill development to build great teams.
- Unity and trust: Unity around a constancy of purpose cannot happen without trust.
- Reliability: High-performing organizations have formally or informally adopted the characteristics of high-reliability organizations (e.g., Six Sigma).
- Energy state: cultures that are transforming or constantly improving have a capacity for extra effort over and above that needed to deliver basic care.

However, efforts for improving healthcare quality and patient safety haven't yet achieved the desired optimal state. Katz et al. have identified that conflicting messages about the relative value of productivity and safety may be one essential obstacle in healthcare organizations [61]. While the usual official mission of a healthcare organization includes high-quality patient safety, maintaining these tenets often entails working at a slower pace and exerting extra effort, conflicting with the organization's other goals – optimizing productivity and economic efficiency.

As an example, despite national efforts to prevent wrong-site surgeries, these remain prevalent. These "never events" likely occur in part because of production pressures. Changing hospital culture and ensuring that physicians collaborate and follow standardized protocols is continual work of the hospital leader. Senior hospital leaders need to ensure that the time and resources that are needed to improve broken processes are made available [62].

Game Theory in the OR Context

The OR Suite's Stakeholder

A stakeholder is any group or individual who can affect or is affected by the achievement of an organization's purpose [63]. For the perioperative leader, it is important to identify the relevant stakeholders and their specific needs, expectations, and preferences.

This will allow the leader to drive the various parties toward meeting common goals and to give priority to competing stakeholder interests and claims (stakeholder salience). Various individuals or groups have a specific interest in the OR suite, with the action of each stakeholder directly affecting the other:

- Patient: suffers from sickness or injury and expects high-quality medical services at no additional risk to safety.
- Surgeons: expect maximum convenience and service, easy and fast access to OR time (especially for add-on and emergency cases), and state-of-the-art equipment. They are powerful stakeholders since they assign the medical priority, which determines the urgency of a case.
- Anesthesiologists: the OR provides a place to practice; they prefer little down time and predictable finish times.
- Nurses: expect predictable working hours and an enjoyable workplace, without disruptive behavior or harassment.
- Suppliers: surgical support services and housekeeping; the OR must consider the concerns of its suppliers.
- Executives/Administrators: want efficient use of OR time, high utilization and low staffing cost, and limited capital expenditures in equipment.
- Owners: want to maximize the quality and reputation of their healthcare organization, as well as their return on investment as applicable.

Understanding the stakeholders' needs and expectations allows a leader to better manage them. The tools required to manage stakeholder expectations include good communication, active listening, trust building, and negotiating skills, addressing concerns, and quickly resolving issues. They will, as the common refrain goes, not be able to make everybody happy. An OR leader will have to make some decisions which will satisfy one or more parties and others less so. Depending on the combination of power,[1] legitimacy, and urgency, the OR leader will assign priority to a specific stakeholder (stakeholder salience) [64]. Urgency is directly related to the medical priority of a case, which is usually determined by the surgeon. Independent of whether the information about urgency is reliable, high urgency of a case combined with the surgeon's power will benefit the surgeon with decision making in case scheduling. Each stakeholder may attempt to manipulate the priorities of the manager. It is helpful to the manager to have policies that establish principles to maintain order and fairness.

Game Theory Concepts

Leaders in the perioperative setting should understand essential game theory concepts to influence the interactions between individuals and groups as well as to achieve a cohesive team with mutual goal-oriented benefits. Game theory was developed gradually in the twentieth century by mathematicians, economists, and other scientists and yielded more than ten Nobel Prizes to date [65, 66].

Game theory is a method used in economics and business for modeling behaviors of interacting parties. Parties can be team players (same goals) or opponents (different or opposing goals) [67]. Players in a game can choose to either cooperate or fail ("defect"), but none of the players is aware of the other's choice. If every player chooses to cooperate, all can gain. However, if one chooses to defect, that person's individual gains are usually much bigger. If all defect, everybody loses, or gains very little.

There are several dilemmas that hinder participants from cooperating:

- Prisoner's dilemma: A situation in which two parties would each gain more by cooperating with each other. Instead, they each act independently and "defect," betraying the other party. This ultimately results in a lesser gain for each of them. It also undermines any momentum toward an alliance.
- Tragedy of the commons: A situation similar to the prisoner's dilemma, except that it involves more than two parties.
- Free rider: A situation that can lead to the loss of shared resources. Individuals may be able to enjoy a community resource without paying for it. But if no one voluntarily pays and everyone chooses instead to be a free rider, the resources will soon be exhausted.
- Stag hunt: In this situation, a group can win a massive reward if all the members cooperate with

---

[1] In this context, power is defined as the ability to bring about the desired outcomes; legitimacy as a generalized perception that actions taken are desirable, proper, or appropriate within some socially constructed system of values and beliefs; and urgency as the degree to which stakeholder claims call for immediate attention.

each other. However, members may elect to defect to chase smaller but surer individual rewards.

Several outcomes of games can be observed. The zero-sum game, also known as win–lose game, reflects a situation where a fixed pie must be divided among participants. In this situation, the "payoff," or reward to one player is charged to his or her opponent; thus the sum of the reward and loss is zero. In other words, if one of the participants gets more of the pie, the other loses by an according amount. In non–zero-sum games, cooperative behavior leads to a net increase in the value of the system.

Rewards and punishments depend on whether both cooperate, both choose to betray, or one player cooperates and the other betrays. The greatest reward is given to a player who betrays his or her opponent when the opponent chooses cooperation. If both players cooperate, the individual rewards are lessened. Reward diminishes further if both players defect and is least for the player who cooperates when his or her opponent defects. If one player cooperates and one defects, the combined reward for both players is less than if they had both cooperated. No player can reliably predict what his opponent will do, and both will have to play the game again.

In various sciences, game theory is used to model tactical situations (games), in which an individual's success in making choices depends on the choices of others. Game theory provides a way to understand various kinds of confrontation and offers an explanation why cooperation may be the ideal response in some situations. Individuals and groups can avoid some traps in game theory by cooperating, instead of allowing destructive competition.

Game Theory Applied to the OR Suite

All parties working in the OR generally share common goals (such as maximizing care for the patient), although conflicting goals may occur. In the OR, iterative prisoner dilemmas may be observed – a series of games in which one participant may choose to either cooperate or defect with another participant [49].

Understanding the types of interactions (games) would help the participants to better predict outcome and adapt their own behavior to optimize that outcome. Types of games seen in the OR suite include the following [68, 69]:

- Zero-sum (win–lose) game: For example, OR time for a surgeon is often allocated from a fixed amount of staffed OR time. If surgeon A is allotted more OR time, this amount of time must be deducted from the time allotted to one or more of his colleagues.
- Non–zero-sum game: For example, cooperative interaction and synergies between surgeons, anesthesiologists, OR nursing staff, and the hospital administration can improve efficiency, throughput, and, hence, productivity.

There are many examples of selfish actions in the OR suite:

- Anesthesiologists being inflexible in the preoperative evaluations, unreasonably limiting their work hours, unnecessarily canceling or delaying cases, obstructing the OR schedule, inconveniencing patients, or taking a passive role in the turnover and flow of cases.
- Surgeons making unreasonable demands on access, providing inaccurate information about the case (e.g., estimated duration, medical information, urgency, etc.), demanding immediate compliance with their wishes, and defecting through disruptive behavior, or gaming to get their cases done at night.
- Hospital administration not providing adequate support personnel and space (e.g., concentrating on short-term budget issues).

A poorly run OR will see "mutual defection," as illustrated by comments from staff such as "Why should I do this-or-that when so-and-so won't do his job?" Such a situation may be caused when staff members cooperate until one party deviates from the common rules and then 'defect' forever. Alternatively, staff members may deduce that in a finite series of interactions, the one strategy that miniminzes unfair gain by others if for all players to 'defect'. For salaried employees, working quickly in an OR may be 'punished' by being assigned additional cases, for no increase in compensation, and once observed, may result in a person not working as efficiently as before. A good leader gathers the best players to win the game cooperatively and makes OR nurses understand that it is their job to help the surgical team, such as for example by helping to make sure there are no retained sponges [70]. Understanding game theory would help a leader to recognize the interdependence of all players in the game, the need to become allocentric, and the need to think ahead, considering all possible consequences.

Conclusion

Leadership in a medical environment may be different than that in a corporation as the optimal combination of leadership styles is likely to be different between the two. For example, an OR chief needs to be wary of an authoritative style because the OR environment is a collegial place with people having a collective responsibility and ownership. Being professional and steady-mannered while having the courage to take criticism openly and accept personal weaknesses in a very dynamic environment is crucial to becoming a leader in OR management.

Appendix

Characteristics of Leadership

Integrity: Core to Building Trust

- Promptly takes ownership of difficult situations
- Perceived as direct, truthful
- Can present unvarnished truth in an appropriate and helpful manner
- Keeps confidences
- Not afraid of failure
- Admits mistakes
- Doesn't misrepresent for personal gain

Vision and Purpose

- Communicates an inspired vision or sense of core purpose
- Dissatisfied with the status quo
- Talks beyond today and about possibilities
- Shoulders blame rather than searching for excuses
- Optimistic
- Creates milestones and symbols to rally support
- Makes the vision sharable by everyone
- Inspires and motivates the entire unit

Political Savvy

- Can maneuver through complex political situations
- Sensitive to how people and organizations function
- Anticipates where difficulties/barriers are and plans approach accordingly
- Views politics as a part of organizational life and has a willingness to adjust

Decision Making

- Makes decisions based on a mixture of analysis, wisdom, experience, and judgment
- Most solutions and suggestions will be judged as outstanding when appraised over time
- Most sought after by others for advice and guidance
- Resists being hypnotized by complexity

Negotiating

- Prepares well before entering a negotiation
- Knows the best and the worst parts of a negotiated agreement
- Manages the tension between claiming and creating value
- Is in control of emotions during the negotiation process
- Probes behind positions and explores underlying, deeper interests
- Overcomes barriers to cooperation and engages in joint problem solving
- Understands difficult situations and develops tactics to deal with them
- Attempts to reach a mutually satisfactory agreement (consensus, as opposed to compromise)

Motivating Others

- Creates a climate in which people want to do their best
- Possesses knowledge and skills to recognize and develop talent
- Motivates many kinds of direct reports and team or project members
- Pushes tasks and decisions down
- Drives continuous process improvement
- Empowers others
- Invites inputs and shares ownership and visibility
- Makes each individual feel their work is important
- Involves being a person people like working for and with

References

1. Merriam Webster online dictionary. 2011. www .merriam-webster.com (accessed November 4, 2016).

2. C. R. Denham. May I have the envelope please? *J Patient Saf* 2008; 4: 119–23.

3. T. A. Judge, J. E. Bono, R. Ilies et al. Personality and leadership: A qualitative and quantitative review. *J Appl Psychol* 2002; 87: 765–80.

4. C. R. Denham. Values genetics: Who are the real smartest guys in the room? *J Patient Saf* 2007; 3: 214–26.

5. J. Hoyle. *Leadership styles*. Thousand Oaks, CA: Sage, 2006.

6. D. Goleman. Leadership that gets results. *Harv Bus Rev* 2000; 78: 78–90.

7. W. L. Gardner, B. J. Avolio, F. O. Walumbwa. *Authentic leadership theory and practice: Origins, effects and development*. Amsterdam, Oxford: Elsevier JAI, 2005.

8. D. Goleman, R. Boyatizis, A. McKee. *Primal leadership. Realizing the power of emotional intelligence*. Boston: Harvard Business School Press, 2002.

9. L. A. Hill. Where will we find tomorrow's leaders? *Harv Bus Rev* 2008; 86: 123–9, 38.

10. D. McGregor. *The human side of enterprise*. New York: McGraw-Hill, 1960.

11. D. McGregor, J. Cutcher-Gershenfeld. *The human side of enterprise*. Annotated edn. New York: McGraw-Hill, 2006.

12. D. Goleman. What makes a leader? *Clin Lab Manag Rev* 1999; 13: 123–31.

13. C. D. Naylor. Leadership in academic medicine: Reflections from administrative exile. *Clin Med* 2006; 6: 488–92.

14. L. R. Herald, J. A. Alexander, I. Fraser et al. Review: How do hospital organizational structure and processes affect quality of care? A critical review of research methods. *Med Care Res Rev* 2008; 65: 259–99.

15. M. J. Gilmartin, T. A. D'Aunno. Chapter 8: Leadership research in healthcare. *Acad Manag Ann* 2007; 1: 387–438.

16. C. Vance, E. Larson. Leadership research in business and health care. *J Nurs Scholarsh* 2002; 34: 165–71.

17. S. Xirasagar, M. E. Samuels, T. F. Curtin. Management training of physician executives, their leadership style, and care management performance: An empirical study. *Am J Manag Care* 2006; 12: 101–8.

18. Healthcare Leadership Alliance. 2013. www.healthcare leadershipalliance.org (accessed November 4, 2016).

19. L. J. Mintz, J. K. Stoller. A systematic review of physician leadership and emotional intelligence. *J Grad Med Educ* 2014; 6: 21–31.

20. J. W. Mountford, C. When clinicians lead. *McKinsey Quarterly* 2009.

21. D. Liu. 2013. www.davisliumd.com/why-health-care-reform-wont-happen-without-physician-leadership/ (accessed November 4, 2016).

22. S. Rodak. 2012. www.beckershospitalreview.com/ hospital-key-specialties/7-strategies-to-develop-a-clinical-integration-network.html. (accessed October 28, 2016).

23. A. M. Desai, R. A. Trillo, Jr., A. Macario. Should I get a Master of Business Administration? The anesthesiologist with education training: Training options and professional opportunities. *Curr Opin Anaesthesiol* 2009; 22: 191–8.

24. M. J. Deegan. 2002. www.researchgate.net/publication/ 228644480_EMOTIONAL_INTELLIGENCE_ COMPETENCIES_IN_PHYSICIAN_LEADERS_ AN_EXPLORATORY_STUDY (accessed October 28, 2016).

25. C. Carruthers, J. Swettenham. Physician leadership: Necessary and in need of nurturing – Now. *Healthc Q* 2011; 14: 6–8.

26. R. Aggarwal, S. Undre, K. Moorthy et al. The simulated operating theatre: Comprehensive training for surgical teams. *Qual Saf Health Care* 2004; 13 Suppl 1: i27–32.

27. R. Cullen, S. Nicholls, A. Halligan. Reviewing a service – Discovering the unwritten rules. *Clin Perform Qual Health Care* 2000; 8: 233–9.

28. M. T. MacEachern. *Hospital organization and management*. Chicago: Physicians' Record Co., 1957.

29. W. F. Hejna, C. M. Gutmann. The management of surgical facilities in hospitals. *Health Care Manage Rev* 1983; 8: 51–5.

30. A. Baumgart, G. Schupfer, A. Welker et al. Status quo and current trends of operating room management in Germany. *Curr Opin Anaesthesiol* 2010; 23: 193–200.

31. G. Schüpfer, M. Bauer. Wer ist zum OP-Manager geeignet? *Anaesthesist* 2011; 60: 251–6.

32. P. Patterson. Is your OR's governing structure up to today's intense demands? *OR Manager* 2008; 24: 1, 6–7.

33. M. Bauer, J. Hinz, A. Klockgether-Radke. Göttinger Leitfaden für OP-manager. *Anaesthesist* 2010; 59: 69–79.

34. S. Birk. The 10 most common myths about leadership. *Healthc Exec* 2010; 25: 30–2, 4–6, 8.

35. E. H. Schein. *Organizational culture and leadership*. San Francisco: Jossey-Bass, 2010.

36. D. J. Teece. Firm organization, industrial structure, and technological innovation. *J Econ Behav Organ* 1996; 31: 193–224.

37. E. T. Hall. *Beyond culture*. Garden City, NY: Anchor Books, 1976.

38. A. Rius. GothamCulture. 2015. http://gothamculture .com/2015/04/30/iceberg-organizational-culture-change-infographic/ (accessed November 4, 2016).

39. E. P. Evans. Nursing in Australia. *Int Nurs Rev* 1938; 12: 261.

40. K. M. Eisenhardt. Agency theory: An assessment and review. *Acad Manag Rev* 1989; 14: 57–74.

41. J. P. Kotter. *Force for change: How leadership differs from management.* New York: Free Press, 1990.

42. J. P. Kotter. *The heart of change: Real-life stories of how people change their organizations.* Boston, MA: Harvard Business Review Press, 2012.

43. B. A. Simon, S. L. Muret-Wagstaff. Leading departmental change to advance perioperative quality. *Anesthesiology* 2014; 120: 807–9.

44. K. Donahue, B. Mets. A move to universal OR start times. A case study of leading change in an academic anesthesia department. *Physician Executive* 2008; 34: 24–7.

45. T. Braungardt, S. G. Fought. Leading change during an inpatient critical care unit expansion. *J Nurs Adm* 2008; 38: 461–7.

46. S. R. Covey, K. A. Gulledge. Principle-centered leadership and change. *J Qual Participat* 1994; 17: 10.

47. C. J. Lockwood. Contemporary OB/GYN. 2010. http://contemporaryobgyn.modernmedicine.com/ contemporary-obgyn/news/modernmedicine/modern-medicine-now/implementing-checklists-may-require-cultu?page=full (accessed November 4, 2016).

48. H. L. Sirkin, P. Keenan, A. Jackson. The hard side of change management. *Harv Bus Rev* 2005; 83: 108–18, 58.

49. D. B. Waisel. Developing social capital in the operating room: The use of population-based techniques. *Anesthesiology* 2005; 103: 1305–10.

50. M. M. Chadwick. Creating order out of chaos: A leadership approach. *Aorn J* 2010; 91: 154–70.

51. The Joint Commission. *Improving America's hospitals: The Joint Commission's report on quality and safety 2007*: Oak Brook, IL: The Joint Commission, 2007: 45–8.

52. M. Leonard, S. Graham, D. Bonacum. The human factor: The critical importance of effective teamwork and communication in providing safe care. *Qual Saf Health Care* 2004; 13 Suppl 1: i85–90.

53. S. Yule, R. Flin, S. Paterson-Brown et al. Non-technical skills for surgeons in the operating room: A review of the literature. *Surgery* 2006; 139: 140–9.

54. M. E. Braine. Clinical governance: Applying theory to practice. *Nurs Stand* 2006; 20: 56–65; quiz 6.

55. A. S. Frankel, M. W. Leonard, C. R. Denham. Fair and just culture, team behavior, and leadership engagement: The tools to achieve high reliability. *Health Serv Res* 2006; 41: 1690–709.

56. M. A. Keroack, B. J. Youngberg, J. L. Cerese et al. Organizational factors associated with high performance in quality and safety in academic medical centers. *Acad Med* 2007; 82: 1178–86.

57. J. Collins. Level 5 leadership. The triumph of humility and fierce resolve. *Harv Bus Rev* 2001; 79: 66–76, 175.

58. H. J. Jiang, C. Lockee, K. Bass et al. Board engagement in quality: Findings of a survey of hospital and system leaders. *J Healthc Manag* 2008; 53: 121–34; discussion 35.

59. J. Conway. Getting boards on board: Engaging governing boards in quality and safety. *Jt Comm J Qual Patient Saf* 2008; 34: 214–20.

60. T. Vaughn, M. Koepke, E. Kroch et al. Engagement of leadership in quality improvement initiatives: Executive quality improvement survey results. *J Patient Saf* 2006; 2: 2–9.

61. T. Katz-Navon, E. Naveh, Z. Stern. The moderate success of quality of care improvement efforts: Three observations on the situation. *Int J Qual Health Care* 2007; 19: 4–7.

62. R. L. Kane, G. Mosser. The challenge of explaining why quality improvement has not done better. *Int J Qual Health Care* 2007; 19: 8–10.

63. R. E. Freeman. *Strategic management: A stakeholder approach.* Boston: Pitman, 1984.

64. R. K. Mitchell, B. R. Agle, D. J. Wood. Toward a theory of stakeholder identification and salience: Defining the principle of who and what really counts. *Acad Manag Rev* 1997; 22: 853–86.

65. Wikipedia, the free encyclopedia. https://en.wikipedia.org/wiki/Game_theory (accessed November 4, 2016).

66. Nobel Media. www.nobelprize.org/nobel_prizes/ economic-sciences/laureates/index.html (accessed November 4, 2016).

67. L. Fisher. *Rock, paper, scissors: Game theory in everyday life.* London: Hay House, 2008.

68. A. P. Marco. Game theoretic approaches to operating room management. *Am Surg* 2002; 68: 454–62.

69. A. P. Marco. Game theory in the operating room environment. *Am Surg* 2001; 67: 92–6.

70. S. B. Dowd, A. Root. The hospital manager and game theory: Chess master, poker player, or cooperative game player? *Health Care Manag (Frederick)* 2003; 22: 305–10.

Chapter

2

The Path to a Successful Operating Room Environment

Ross Musumeci, Alan David Kaye, Omar A. Gafur, Charles J. Fox, and Richard D. Urman

The operating room (OR) typically has a fast paced, high stress environment with complex professional interactions. Clinical competence is a basic requirement for work in the OR, but to excel it is necessary to manage those interactions successfully. A firm understanding of human behavior and important leadership skills make this task much easier. There are over a dozen subgroups of workers who must act as a cohesive team to achieve optimal performance and provide excellent patient care (Figure 2.1).

A Closer Look at the OR Manager/Director

There are at least four distinct stakeholders in the OR: hospital administration, nursing, anesthesiology, and surgery. Each of these stakeholders has their own interests that may not coincide, and the OR manager/director must be able to balance the needs of these different groups in order to maximize productivity and minimize conflict. The key characteristics of an effective OR manager/director are listed in Box 2.1.

A more detailed job description of the OR manager/director can be found on the website of the American Association of Clinical Directors at www.aacdhq.org.

Anesthesiologists who have the characteristics listed in Box 2.1 are particularly qualified to fill the OR manager/director position because they typically have a constant presence in the OR without the need for office hours, and they usually have a clear understanding of OR processes. Hospital administrators may prefer anesthesiologists or nurses for the OR manager/director position, because their economic interests are often directly aligned with those of the hospital.

A successful OR manager/director must have the support of the hospital Chief Executive Officer and the chairpersons of the departments of surgery, nursing, and anesthesiology. It is necessary for all departments to give up some of their own authority and control so that the OR manager/director can run the OR in a manner that benefits everyone. The OR manager/director must also have the support of his or her own specialty group, because the position will require time that could otherwise be spent on their own specialty group activities. For this reason, and also to emphasize the neutrality of the OR manager/director position among all departments, the OR manager/director and/or the manager/director's practice should be compensated by the hospital.

Psychology in the OR

An understanding of fundamental psychology is extremely valuable in any professional setting, but this is particularly true in the stressful and emotionally charged environment of the OR. Understanding psychological insights quickly can significantly improve the quality of communication. Indeed, for leaders

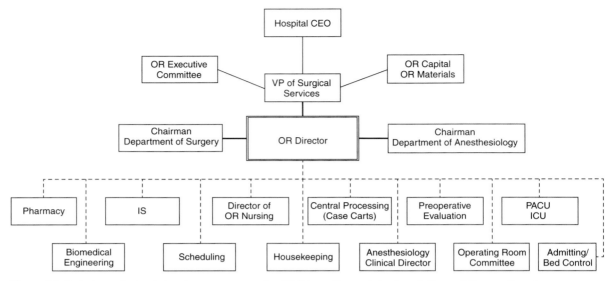

Figure 2.1 Typical organizational chart for management of an OR. Taken with permission from R. Urman, S. Eappen. Operating room management: Core principles. In: C. A. Vacanti, P. K. Sikka, R. D. Urman, M. Dershwitz, B. S. Segal. *Essential Clinical Anesthesia*, 1st edn, Cambridge University Press, 2011.

Box 2.1. Characteristics of an Effective OR Manager/Director

Strong problem solving and organizational skills
Even-tempered
Ability to commit significant amount of nonclinical time
Strong clinician garnering respect of other clinicians
Strong interpersonal and negotiation skills
Ability to understand business/financial concerns of institution and physicians
Understanding of perioperative processes
Understanding of scheduling systems and information technology
Good understanding of organizational dynamics; ability to understand divergent needs and concerns of different stakeholders and bring them together
Commitment to overall performance of OR suite rather than individual department

in the OR, recruiting staff members who possess strong psychological insights can make a significant contribution to the success of the group. Moreover, members of surgical, nursing, and anesthesia teams who are effective leaders typically possess these valuable abilities.

Interpersonal difficulties are common in the OR, and those that achieve the greatest success and respect in that setting are able to communicate effectively and overcome situational problems.

Emotional Intelligence

One aspect of psychology that is particularly relevant to the practice of medicine, and the OR environment in particular, is emotional intelligence (EI). It is a set of skills that enables people to recognize their own and others' emotions, and to use that information in ways that improve their interpersonal interactions. EI is a topic that is relatively unknown in medicine, but it is well known in the business community. This section will discuss the components of EI, ways to measure it, its relevance to practice management, and its application to the practice of medicine in general. This subject presents readers with a huge opportunity for self-improvement on both a personal and professional level. The only requirements are an open mind and a motivation.

Weschsler first referred to the collection of skills that comprise EI when he noted the difference between "intrapersonal and interpersonal" intelligence in the 1940s. However, the term *emotional intelligence* was coined by Leuner in 1966. The first models of EI were introduced in the late 1980s and early 1990s by Greenspan, and Salovey and Meyer. The concept was fully popularized in the business community through a series of articles and books published by Daniel

Goleman starting in the late 1990s. Dr. Goleman presented the topic in a simple fashion and made a compelling argument for the importance of EI as a leadership skill. Subsequently, many others have published on the topic with variations in the style and structure that they use to present the topic.

As it is a relatively new concept, it is no surprise that there is some controversy surrounding the nature of EI and the validity of it as a psychological construct. Arguments exist about whether it is an ability that is learned, a trait that is inherited, or some combination of the two. Some psychologists argue that tests for measuring EI are collectively quantifying other individual abilities for which proven testing already exists, and that EI adds nothing new. Dr. Goleman has also attracted his share of critics who say that he uses proprietary data that are unavailable for outside review to support his claims of the value of EI as a leadership skill.

Despite all the controversy, there is evidence supporting the worth of EI in professional interactions, with increasing value at higher levels of leadership. The popularity of Dr. Goleman's writing over the past decade indicates that his way of presenting the concept of EI has struck a chord among those in the business world. Leadership is a somewhat nebulous concept that is difficult to define accurately, and identifying the core elements necessary for high-quality leadership is even harder. Whether EI is a new concept or not, it appears that the way it has recently been presented has made its utility as a leadership skill more obvious and easier to understand, thereby making it more accessible for those of us who are not psychologists.

Emotional Pathways

If we dramatically simplify the human emotional reaction to outside stimuli, there are two main pathways through which we respond. There is a relatively fast and unconscious pathway that travels through the amygdala, and a slower, more deliberative pathway that travels through the prefrontal cortex. It is the faster pathway through the amygdala that Goleman refers to as the "low road," which is responsible for some of the more interesting and problematic emotional responses humans have.

It is this pathway that is responsible for the phenomenon of "emotional contagion." If a human subject is asked to look at pictures of the face of another individual with emotional expressions, the subject will eventually begin to take on the emotional state,

and even the physiologic response of the person in the pictures. This happens without any conscious action on the part of the subject and happens without their knowledge. It is as if the individual "feels" rather than sees the emotion in the pictures. Scientists now understand that the human limbic system functions as an "open loop," meaning that human emotions are responsive to the emotions of others around them. If two individuals that are monitored engage in a conversation, their moods and their vital signs tend to converge to a similar state within a period of 15 min. An understanding of this phenomenon helps to explain why people who work together over long periods of time seem to take on similar emotional states. It follows that the leaders of an anesthesia department, or a medical group, must be particularly careful about the emotional state they project, as everyone usually watches "the boss."

If reactions through this unconscious, faster pathway are to be managed for better outcomes in our interpersonal interactions, it is necessary to anticipate how we are likely to behave in difficult situations. It makes sense that a little self-education on how to anticipate and be proactive in managing our own emotional responses might be useful, as the logic provided by the slow-moving prefrontal cortex is going to arrive too late to prevent the low road from reacting!

The Components of EI

The components of EI differ slightly depending on which author one reads, but the differences are minor. Goleman divides the four components of EI into the categories of "personal competence" and "social competence." Under each category, the components include awareness and management.

Personal competence
1. Self-awareness
2. Self-management
Social competence
3. Social awareness
4. Relationship management

The names of all of the components of EI make their descriptions self-evident, but there is more to them than the names imply. Self-awareness means that one needs to be able to read one's own emotions, and many of us are probably already fairly good at that. However, if one makes an effort to pay attention to one's own emotional state, there is probably more that can be learned. More important than knowing how we feel at

19

any given time is learning how those feelings affect our behavior. Learning how feelings affect our behavior is much less obvious to the individual than it is to the observers around them. For example, learning that you are particularly prone to having a short temper when you become stressed or easily distracted from details when you are angered would be valuable information the next time you find yourself experiencing those emotions.

Individuals with high levels of self-awareness are confident. They have already made an accurate and realistic self-assessment, so they know their strengths and weaknesses, and they are able to use their assessment to guide their decisions. They know where they are headed and why. Because they are well grounded, they do not feel compelled to act impulsively, but instead are reflective and thoughtful. When they do act, it is with conviction and genuineness.

Self-management involves the ability to maintain control over your emotions, and requires that you have already attained an adequate level of self-awareness, because you cannot control what you cannot perceive. Similarly, you cannot hope to control the emotions of others until you can control your own, making self-management an essential skill for leadership. Individuals who are skilled in self-management tend to be honest and transparent, and act only in ways that are consistent with their own values rather than following the crowd. They are driven to an inner standard of excellence and are able to maintain discipline and motivation in pursuing it. Because their inner emotional turmoil is minimized, they are able to cope with external uncertainties more effectively. This makes them adaptable, optimistic and ready to seize opportunities when they present themselves.

Social awareness includes empathy, or the ability to sense others' emotions and to understand their perspective. This is true both at an individual and an organizational level. Individuals skilled in social awareness are able to sense the emotional currents, the politics, and the decision-making networks within an organization. They are able to sense the requirements for effective communication in a given situation and to determine what is needed to motivate people.

Relationship management requires individuals to use their social awareness to guide communication in a positive way. Leaders with good relationship management skills are able to guide followers with a compelling vision. To do this, they utilize a range of tactics for persuasion. They take an interest in developing others as a means of both improving the health of the organization and developing a sense of support and community among the group. They also realize the importance of workplace relationships, and understand that nothing important is completed alone. They seek common ground, and work on building a network. Their communication and persuasion skills allow them to act as change catalysts or conflict managers, and they are effective at teamwork and collaboration.

Measuring EI

Several tests are available for measuring EI, and quantifying EI may be useful in certain circumstances. Some of the better-known tests for EI are:

- the Mayer–Salovey–Caruso Emotional Intelligence Test
- the Emotional Competency Inventory
- the Emotional and Social Competency Inventory
- the Bar-On Emotional Quotient Inventory
- the Trait Emotional Intelligence Questionnaire

There are also testing services that are available online for both self-evaluation and 360-degree evaluations. A full discussion of the characteristics and individual merits of the available tests is beyond the scope of this chapter.

Resonant and Dissonant Leadership

Leaders with high levels of EI are able to provide "resonant" leadership. The term "resonance" refers to the reinforcement of sound through synchronous vibration, and individuals in a resonant group "vibrate" with the leader's enthusiastic energy. Resonant leaders are attuned to group emotions and are able to communicate in a way that connects with those they seek to persuade. They can sense the mood of a crowd and modify their communication style to suit the immediate needs of their audience. They speak enthusiastically and authentically and drive group emotions in a positive direction.

Dissonant leadership represents the other end of the spectrum. Dissonance refers to an unpleasant sound due to a lack of harmony. Individuals in a dissonant group are out of sync, and beset with negative emotions, which distract them from important tasks in the workplace. Dissonant leaders are out of touch with group emotions, and as a result tend to drive group emotions in a negative direction.

The Importance of EI and Resonant Leadership

Daniel Goleman has investigated the characteristics that distinguish truly successful leaders from others. He found that individuals with high levels of intelligence and training do not always make the best leaders. They may have a wealth of good ideas, but without the ability to motivate others to execute them, the ideas themselves are worth little. Goleman found that while adequate training and intelligence are entry level requirements for leadership, it is an individual's EI that determines whether he or she excels, and the importance of EI increases at higher levels of leadership.

A quote from the first lines of Goleman's book, *Primal Leadership*, explains why this might be so: "Great leaders move us. They ignite our passions and inspire the best in us. When we try to explain why they are so effective, we speak of strategy, vision or powerful ideas. But the reality is so much more primal: Great leadership works through the emotions."

Intelligence, training, and a well-reasoned argument are not always enough to inspire people to follow. The way to achieve an action on something is to get people emotionally involved and inspired. They must be motivated, not just convinced.

This is true in the OR. Anesthesiologists, nurses, and surgeons work in a high-pressure environment that demands self-control and teamwork. Furthermore, anesthesiologists, nurses, and surgeons work alongside hospital administrators and others, all of whom have motivations that do not fully coincide. The organizational dynamics of the hospital are complex. In this setting, a resonant leader can have a significant impact on the workplace environment. Resonant leaders are skilled in conflict resolution and persuasion, and are able to successfully navigate the complex political landscape of the OR. They are inspirational leaders whose optimism and motivation serve to increase teamwork and efficiency. They have a positive impact on the job satisfaction of department employees and may also be able to improve the group's relationship with hospital administration and the security of their hospital contract. People who have spent time in more than one anesthesia, nursing, or surgery department can readily attest to the fact that there are significant differences in the workplace environment between departments and that those differences can have a big impact on how much they enjoy their work. Such differences are largely due to the effect that the group's leader has on department employees.

Traditional medical school training does not include EI, which is somewhat curious given the high level of EI that medical practice requires. This is especially true for anesthesiologists, who have approximately 5–10 min to reassure their nervous patients during the preoperative interview. A study in the *Journal of the American Medical Association* that examined differences between physicians with fewer than or more than two lifetime malpractice claims showed that the physicians with fewer claims spent more time with their patients, used more humor in their patient interactions, and spent more time eliciting their patients' questions and concerns. This supports the contention that EI-related skills are important in reducing the likelihood of malpractice claims. In the author's personal experience, it is also true that anesthesiologists who have previously established good relationships with nurses and surgeons are more likely to be perceived positively and supported by them in the event of a bad outcome and a subsequent malpractice case. Within the anesthesia practice, good relationships among partners are invaluable to the long-term health of the group. Groups consisting of individuals with higher levels of EI are less likely to have significant conflict that goes unresolved.

A meta-analysis of EI published in the *Journal of the Royal Society of Medicine* examined available data on the subject in 2007 [1]. Analysts found that EI is a valid construct that is worthy of further research, and that it is a valuable predictor of performance in the workplace. It correlates well with academic success, and is a better predictor of job performance and satisfaction than traditional personality measures. However, there are few studies specifically related to EI and healthcare. Most of the existing studies contain unsubstantiated claims of its importance, and make the assumption that it is a quality that can be altered or changed. Although there is evidence of the value of EI in the business world, the same is not yet been demonstrated in healthcare, and the positive impact of resonant leadership that is discussed in this chapter is extrapolated from results in the business world, not proven through rigorous, scientific study. Areas that are cited by the study for future research include medical student selection and training, its impact on quality of care, and its impact on the job satisfaction and burnout rate of healthcare workers.

Improving EI

The first step for those who are interested in improving their EI is to recognize the potential benefits. Habits and behaviors that have been ingrained for many years are not readily amenable to change, so a significant degree of motivation is necessary to succeed. Unless the potential benefits of improved EI are understood and internalized, it is unlikely that one will have sufficient motivation for this undertaking. It is also important to realize that attention to EI skills is an ongoing effort, not a time-limited process.

Further reading and self-education are also advisable. Although the basic concepts of EI are amenable to this brief description, there is much more to the topic that should be well understood before embarking on an attempt at improvement. The books on this subject are filled with illustrative stories that help to solidify the concepts of EI, and to clarify what is needed to improve.

There are differing opinions on specific means for improving EI skills, and on whether it is even possible to do so. The process is complex, but the basic steps are straightforward. An initial self-assessment should determine areas of strength and potential areas for improvement. Testing may be helpful. Using your self-assessment, a comparison with the existing reality, and the desired future provides a roadmap for change. It is an iterative process of self-observation and attempts at behavior modification in which individuals debrief themselves after an encounter in which they are either satisfied or unsatisfied and then make a plan for their next encounter.

Although this topic may seem straightforward, many find it to be compelling. We deal with human emotions every day, and they become such a routine part of our daily lives that we take them for granted. The construct of EI brings them back into focus and emphasizes their importance in our professional lives. The process of paying closer attention to how we interact with others almost invariably provides information that is actionable and potentially valuable.

Psychology in the OR: Transactional Analysis

Transactional analysis is a method to rapidly analyze and understand behavior. In short, it allows one to focus on elements of one's personality that are flawed, allowing one to respond better to others without conflict. In *Born to Win*, the defining book on transactional analysis, a description of "winners" is presented: winners are not helpless, they are authentic. They are not isolated, and they work for the greater good of the situation. Their timing is right with responses appropriate to the situation, making the other person involved feel dignified and worthwhile [2].

Transactional analysis provides a method to achieve awareness and self-responsibility on a daily basis. It involves four types of analysis. Structural analysis is the analysis of individual personality; transactional analysis is the analysis of what people do and say to each other; game analysis is the analysis of ulterior transactions leading to a payoff; and script analysis is the analysis of specific life dramas that a person compulsively plays out [2].

One Example, Structural Analysis

Structural analysis involves gaining an understanding of another person's thoughts, feelings, and behaviors [2]. A multitude of factors, which can originate from previous experiences in a person's lifetime, can dictate how that person communicates. The thoughts, feelings, and behaviors of an individual are identified as "ego states," which are described as "parent," "adult," and "child."

Parent ego state reflects behaviors and attitudes incorporated from external sources, usually one's parents [2]. An example of the parent ego state in the OR is someone criticizing a hairstyle, the color of the OR, nurturing feelings, or critically commenting on the fact that someone was injured because he or she were out late. Anytime people behave like their parents, they are in the parent ego [2].

The adult ego state reflects objective information gathering, rational thinking, and problem solving. The adult ego state calculates and responds in a dispassionate manner, much like a computer [2]. For example, when someone is asked what eight plus three equals, the adult ego would respond after calculation with the answer 11. If the surgeon asks the anesthesia provider what the blood pressure is at the moment, communicating the current blood pressure would be an adult ego state response.

The child ego state reflects all the natural impulses from childhood. An example in an OR is an anesthesiologist saying that surgeon X scares him, or that he wishes he could take time off to have fun. Anytime you act or feel as when you were a child – including joy, laughter, rebellion, and sorrow – you are in a child ego state [2].

Complementary Transactions

In a complementary transaction, an inquiry from one particular ego state is met with a response from the same ego state [3]. Complementary transactions can occur between any of the ego states. Figure 2.2 gives an example of a complementary transaction.

Crossed Transactions

A crossed transaction occurs when an inquiry from one particular ego state is met with a response from a different ego state. The results of a crossed transaction can rapidly escalate into an argument, friction, withdrawal between two people, hostility, emotional pain, and other destructive consequences. Figure 2.3 gives an example of a crossed transaction.

The successful OR worker must master the art of communication and identify pathological interactions in others. The ability to understand pathological forms of communication in others gives you the opportunity to make accommodations for them and rescue an otherwise failed interaction.

Transactional analysis is one tool available to improve communications and to attempt to insure a well-functioning workplace. As might be expected, pathological behaviors can be clearly and rapidly identified and proper responses taught to any individual. The many concepts described within transactional analysis include practical lessons well suited for the OR.

Below is a summary of items to consider when trying to improve self-awareness and management of emotions, or to develop effective communication skills.

What time did you administer the antibiotics?   At 6:00 PM

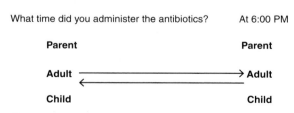

Figure 2.2 An example of a complementary transaction.

What time is it?   Crazy surgeon, you are always in such a hurry!

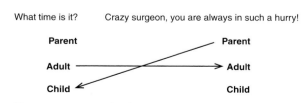

Figure 2.3 An example of a crossed transaction.

To Develop High Self-Awareness

- Reflect on the encounter *when you are calm* and engage in an inner dialogue
- Seek input from others and be honest with yourself
- Make accurate appraisals of what is going on
- Get in touch with your feelings
- Pay attention to your actions/observe their impact
- Learn what your intentions/goals are each day

To Manage Your Emotions

- Take charge of your thoughts
- Don't overgeneralize
- Stay away from destructive labeling/avoid mind reading
- Don't have rules about how others should act
- Don't inflate the significance of an event

To Develop Effective Communication Skills

- Use sensitivity
- Use self-disclosure
- Acknowledge ownership of your statements
- Use assertiveness
- Use dynamic listening

The Role of the Human Resource Department

A hospital's human resource (HR) department has become crucial to the success of today's hospital. Healthcare institutions are under enormous pressure to control costs and improve quality, and for most institutions this involves reducing personnel. This reduction in human capital has forced new responsibilities on the doctors, nurses, technicians, and administrators working in the hospital setting. Effectively managing this scenario requires managers to take a more active role in developing very accurate job descriptions and protecting these "multitaskers" from burnout by creating a work culture that is enjoyable and fair. The HR department plays an important role by ensuring a safe and fair workplace environment, by managing employee benefits in a way that makes employees feel valued, and by delicately handling a difficult situation in the event that an employee's contract must be terminated. The success or failure of the HR department can profoundly affect the hospital's culture and patient outcomes.

Successful hospitals create a culture of accountability. The current national culture, which shuns personal responsibility, makes it more difficult for hospitals to do this. The HR department, in many instances, must educate its workers on accountability and explain how this will improve patient outcome and personal satisfaction. OR committees have limited means to deal with dysfunctional workers who happen to play important roles as nurses, anesthesiologists, or surgeons. Educational seminars on team training and EI training (discussed earlier in this chapter) involve case presentations and "role-playing." Team training involves active participation and illustrates the importance of every job if excellent patient outcomes are to be achieved.

The diversity of our nation has changed dramatically in the last 20 years and will continue to evolve. Because of this, hospitals must remain diverse and culturally sensitive by reflecting the community in which they reside. Hospital HR departments should insist on culturally diverse employment for all segments working within the hospital. Excellent patient outcomes can only be achieved if cultural beliefs and needs are understood. According to Anderson et al., there are six HUMANE steps that healthcare institutions can take to become culturally competent: *h*ire a diverse workforce [4]; *u*nderstand the community in which the hospital exists [5]; *m*ake cultural competency a business priority [6]; *a*dopt cultural and communication capabilities that reflect the community [7]; *n*urture the community's culture by engaging leaders and staff in outreach programs [8]; and constantly *e*valuate and continue to develop programs that encourage community involvement [9].

Disruptive behavior is a major issue for hospital HR departments. Although disruption can occur within any segment of the hospital workforce, the majority of recent work deals with the disruptive physician. Recent changes in healthcare have resulted in a loss of physician autonomy, which has caused an increase in frustration and disruptive behavior. Most recent research links workforce safety and patient outcomes with teamwork. Physicians act as the leader of the team, so the effectiveness of their communication with team members directly affects many aspects of patient care.

Disruptive behavior by one team member can negatively impact a whole department. Hospital policy and medical staff by-laws must exist and clearly state a course of action to deal with these individuals. An aggressive, zero-tolerance stance toward disruptive behavior is advisable for a productive and patient-centered work environment. From an educational standpoint, case studies vignettes and workshops on improving communication skills among team members are important ways to reinforce or instruct team members on how to conduct themselves properly.

Team Training

In 1999, *To Err Is Human* revealed that approximately 98,000 deaths occur annually as a result of medical errors. This resulted in a public outcry for patient safety. The federal government, through the Agency for Healthcare Research and Quality (AHRQ) and the Department of Defense (DoD), has served as the leader in this movement. They have implemented a team approach to patient safety and initially put their program in place, through the DoD, within military treatment facilities and casualty combat care arenas. The initial results show promising results, so the Joint Commission and the Accreditation for Graduate Medical Education moved quickly to laud the importance of teamwork in patient safety.

The program initiated by the DoD and the AHRQ is called the TeamSTEPPS program. Success in the military arena and subsequent requests from healthcare institutions for a similar program has accelerated the push for the establishment of a national program through the AHRQ. Currently, the AHRQ is developing the infrastructure necessary for national implementation of a TeamSTEPPS program. The program consists of three phases.

Phase I, the assessment phase, evaluates the organizational readiness of your institution and identifies potential leaders that will make up the institutional change team. This stage also identifies barriers to this change and whether sufficient resources are in place to support the proposed change. The AHRQ offers an assessment tool that aids healthcare organizations in a site appraisal. It provides direct feedback on: assessing awareness about safety issues; evaluating specific patient safety interventions; tracking change in patient safety over time; setting internal and external benchmarks; and fulfilling regulatory requirements or directives.

Phase II involves the planning, training, and implementation of the TeamSTEPPS program. In this phase, the change team must complete a 2.5-day train-the-trainer program. Provided in this session is the TeamSTEPPS curriculum, which includes case studies, scenarios, multimedia, and simulation. Each department involved in the change will take part in a 4-h session aimed at developing a plan tailored to fit its unique situation. Peer and instructor feedback helps the participants fully understand the mission and crystallize learning objectives. Once the learning objectives are understood, the plan can be adapted easily to numerous situations.

The goal of phase III is to sustain and spread the advances achieved through teamwork performance, clinical practices, and outcomes. During this phase, participants integrate teamwork skills and tools into their daily practice and monitor the ongoing effectiveness of the TeamSTEPPS intervention. They develop an approach for continuous improvement and spread the intervention throughout the organization. This ongoing process is managed by the change team and involves continual training of the core curriculum through refresher courses and new employee orientation.

Summary

The nature of the OR environment makes an understanding of psychological concepts extremely valuable. The high level of stress that exists in the OR tends to magnify existing, undesirable personality traits, and to make effective communication more difficult. Without effective communication, it is challenging to navigate successfully the complex organizational dynamics and politics that exist in the OR. Developing a better understanding of the nature of human interactions, and improving one's skills in this area, is not easy but is worth the time and effort. Multiple conceptual frameworks exist, and users should choose one that resonates with them, because motivation is the key to success. EI, transactional analysis, and other available models provide a framework for readers to take routine skills of personal interaction that they take for granted, and turn them into potent tools that can enhance their professional performance. Attention to this area of performance, along with the assistance of a good HR department to insure a healthy workplace environment, can have a profoundly positive impact on teamwork, job satisfaction, and patient care.

References

1. YF Birks, IS Watt. Emotional intelligence and patient-centred care. *J R Soc Med* 2007; 100: 368–74.

2. M James, D Jongeward. *Born to Win*. Boston: Addison-Wesley, 1971, pp. 2–20.

3. FS Perls. *Gestalt Therapy Verbatim*. Boulder, CO: Real People Press, 1969, pp. 121.

4. D Goleman. What makes a leader? *Harv Bus Rev* 1998.

5. D Goleman, R Boyatzis, A McKee. *Primal Leadership, Learning to Lead with Emotional Intelligence*. Boston: Harvard Business Press, 2002.

6. H Weisinger. *Emotional Intelligence at Work*. San Francisco: Jossey-Bass, 1998.

7. DL Van Rooy, C Viswesvaran. Emotional intelligence: A meta-analytic investigation of predictive validity and nomological net. *J Vocat Behav* 2004; 65: 71–95.

8. W Levinson, DL Roter, JP Mullooly, VT Dull, RM Frankel. Physician – patient communication. The relationship with malpractice claims among primary care physicians and surgeons. *JAMA* 1997; 277: 553–9.

9. D Goleman. *Social Intelligence, The New Science of Human Relationships*. New York: Bantam Books, 2006.

Suggested Reading

A Alonso, D Baker, R Day, et al. Reducing medical error in the military health system: How can team training help? *Hum Resour Manage Rev* 2006; 16: 396–415.

American Organization of Nurse Executives. 2006. AONE guiding principles for excellence in nurse/physician relationships. http://net.acpe.org/services/AONE/Index.html (accessed January 21, 2012).

LM Anderson, C Shinn, MT Fullilove, et al.; Task Force on Community Preventive Services. The effectiveness of early childhood development programs. A systematic review. *Am J Prev Med* 2003; 24(3 Suppl): 68–79.

DP Baker, JM Beaubien, AK Holtzman. *DoD Medical Team Training Programs: An Independent Case Study Analysis*. Washington, DC: American Institutes for Research, 2003.

SR Covey. *The 7 Habits of Highly Effective People*, 3rd edn. New York: Free Press, 2004.

LT Kohn, JM Corrigan, MS Donaldson. *To Err Is Human*. Washington, DC: National Academies Press, 1999.

J Longo. Combating disruptive behaviors: Strategies to promote a healthy work environment. *OJIN* 2010; 15(1).

G Porto, R Lauve. 2006. Disruptive clinician behavior: A persistent threat to patient safety. *PSQH*. www.psqh.com/julaug06/disruptive.html (accessed January 21, 2012).

EM Rogers. *Diffusion of Innovations*, 5th edn. New York: Free Press, 2003.

Chapter 3

Strategic Planning

Michael R. Williams

Introduction

In his book *Sensemaking in Organizations*, Karl Weick describes the story of a small Hungarian military unit on maneuvers in the Alps of Switzerland [1]. It seems that the young lieutenant in charge dispatched a small group of men into the icy wilderness for a reconnaissance mission. After two days, the group had not returned, and the lieutenant feared he had sent these men to their death in an ill-fated mission. However, later that day the men suddenly appeared, marching back into camp unharmed. When he asked them how they found their way back to camp they simply explained that when they thought all was lost, one of the men found a crumpled map in his pack. They reviewed the map, checked their provisions, and devised a plan to return back to the base camp to join their fellow soldiers. As they were explaining this, the lieutenant asked to see the map and only then did anyone realize that the map was a map of the Pyrenees and not the Alps!

This story exemplifies the fact that you can have the wrong map, yet still get to your destination if you have a purpose and are willing to try. Most organizations become lost because they invest a great deal of time and effort on developing a map, but do little to understand their purpose. Other organizations begin with a defined purpose, but never take the time to design and build a map, providing a pathway to achieve the purpose. The union of purpose and planning leads to a strategic purpose for the organization. Design, implementation, and execution of strategic action plans ultimately leads to an organization that provides strategic performance. Organizations that achieve focused strategic performance year after year become highly successful, high-performing organizations. They are built upon a clear purpose, great planning, active execution of the plan, accountability for the goals and targets at all levels, and finally follow-through by leadership.

The focal subject of this book is the development and enhancement of operating room (OR) leadership and management. In every imaginable modern healthcare structure the OR exists as a subunit of a larger organization, whether a hospital, ambulatory surgery center, office-based surgical suite, or even a military field unit surgical suite. They all exist within a much larger organizational structure. It will be important for operating leadership to understand how the strategic planning and purpose of the OR must support the strategic planning and purpose of the larger organization it serves. This chapter will focus on the steps required to assess purposeful planning for the larger organization. However, the OR's strategic planning process can follow the same steps, as described below. These steps include discussions of the organization's mission, vision, and values statements. These are key corporate documents, which create the foundational structure for a corporate purpose, and in turn build the necessary foundation needed to begin a strategic planning process. Collectively, these define the reason to exist and the behaviors by which those in the organization's community agree to live to achieve the defined purpose. Once purpose is better defined with some clarity, a map must be developed in order to clearly delineate the pathway to follow to achieve the purpose. We will call the map the "strategic plan." Strategic planning has an inherent process that will be described in more detail below.

Development of Purpose

To fully develop the reason this organization has to exist, and the value it adds, three statements should be developed. These statements, which by their very formation will aid in clarification of the purpose, are the "mission statement," the "vision statement," and the "statement of values."

Mission Statement

The mission statement is probably the most important piece of the organization's overall development of purpose. Great leaders in history have not been remembered and respected because of their charisma or their image, but rather because of the mission they pursued and believed in could be easily understood and agreed with by their followers and admirers. For this reason, the mission statement must be objective and easily understood so that everyone is clear on how his or her individual role drives the overall mission. Peter Drucker, considered by many to be the father of modern management, once stated "One of our most common mistakes is to make the mission statement into a kind of hero sandwich of good intentions. It has to be simple and clear" [2].

A well-written mission statement should have at least three parts. First, be aware of needs that exist in your market area or your area of expertise. Do these needs translate into opportunities for the organization? If so, can the organization perform these and perform them well in a way that makes a difference? Second, take a look at what the organization truly believes in. If there are strong beliefs, these can often be transformed into strong actions that have real meaning. The third important aspect speaks to team and organizational commitment to the stated mission. Do those who must deliver on the stated mission truly believe in it? If the entire community can commit to the tenets of the mission statement, it has a much higher chance of being successful. Drucker discusses the story of the Ford Edsel car, which failed miserably on the market. As Drucker describes it, the Edsel did not fail as a result of poor planning or engineering. In fact, it is considered one of the best-engineered and researched automobiles in history. However, no one at Ford truly believed in it or fully committed to it [3]. Although an organization can set audacious goals, the goals must have the commitment of the entire populace of the organization. In conclusion, before writing the mission statement, be sure you understand the needs of the industry, market, and customers served; next, validate that the organization has the competencies and capacities to deliver on these needs; and finally, check the team commitment to this mission.

The first mistake many groups make when building an organizational mission statement is being too verbose. Lengthy mission statements quickly lose meaning and clarity. In order to be effective, a mission statement must be easy to read and understand, while being meaningful to all members of the organization's stakeholder group. It must be concrete and direct in message. It must answer the question "How do we intend to be the absolute best in this industry in delivering our specific mission?" [3].

The mission statement should balance what we know to be possible and within our limits with the stretch goals that appear to be unobtainable. Planners must always consider the organization's strengths, weaknesses, resources, and people skills among other qualities. According to Drucker, "It should be a precise statement of purpose, not a slogan, and should fit on a T-shirt" [4]. The words it contains must be carefully selected for clarity and meaning. The power of the statement will be found in its brevity and simplicity. Finally, the most senior leaders should be writing the mission statement in the organization – the people who are ultimately responsible for achieving it. Once the mission statement is developed, the vision and values statements can be constructed. From that point forward, all of the organization's decisions must be linked to the mission.

Vision Statement

Many people confuse vision statements with mission statements and often mix the distinct purpose of each statement. These two statements are very different in content and purpose, yet must work to support each other in parallel. Therefore, it is important to have one of each before beginning a strategic planning process. Like the mission statement, the vision statement must be concise, clear, and vivid in language. It should be inspiring and challenging, and it should avoid use of complicated concepts.

Most vision statements reveal a compelling idea of what ultimate desired outcome might be achievable in 5–10 years or longer. The idea is to create a mental picture that stirs emotions, inspires the team, and calls everyone to action. Vision statements are not built around goals, but rather describe the ultimate outcome of the organization's goals and do not come with any expectation of measurability. They simply describe the best possible outcome and do not provide any form of a measurement of success. This is the function of the organization's goals and objectives. They must inspire, motivate, and stimulate a "what if" form of creativity. Vision statements, like mission statements, should be developed by the most senior leaders. These leaders will create the inspiring vision as the best possible outcome achievable via the mission statement, goals, and objectives.

Although knowledge from the mission statement, goals, and objectives allows one to see things as they are, imagination stimulated by the vision statement allows one to see what is possible. It is important to open up all the possibilities in the visioning process in order to release a tremendous source of creativity, passion, and energy. Two examples of corporate vision statements include those of Toyota and Amazon. Toyota's Global Vision Statement is "Toyota will lead the way to the future of mobility, enriching lives around the world with the safest and most responsible ways of moving people. Through our commitment to quality, constant innovation and respect for the planet, we aim to exceed expectations and be rewarded with a smile. We will meet challenging goals by engaging the talent and passion of people, who believe there is always a better way" [5]. In comparison, Amazon's corporate vision statement is "Our vision is to be earth's most consumer centric company; to build a place where people can come to find and discover anything they might want to buy online" [6]. Be creative, audacious, brief, and inspiring. Take a long forward view and the power of the vision statement will be unleashed.

Values Statement

The potential power of the statement of values for the organization is often greatly underestimated. Organizational values must be direct reflections of the character values believed and lived each day by the organizational membership. When writing the values statement the leaders must allow the frontline staff to open their inner selves, expressing what they truly believe in a very honest, open manner. Values provide the compass when we are lost, the principles we must depend upon, and the behaviors that define how the organizational culture will act in good times and bad [7]. In short, values reflect our personal and organizational "line in the sand" and are our defined "guardrails" along our journey.

Values should align with the mission and vision statements. They should be empowering, and help to provide clarity for each individual in the organization or department. Properly constructed value statements should easily drive employee engagement and a commitment to the mission of the organization or department. In writing the values it is important to be clear and direct. The language used should be very simple. The stated list of values is unique in that it should be constructed with input from everyone in the organization. Leaders must avoid dictating values. Rather, leaders should clearly express the values they personally believe in, and then work to become knowledgeable of the values the organizational community believes in. The combination of these two lists will begin to build a values statement that the entire organization can believe in and honor with their daily actions.

Strategic Planning

Properly executed strategic planning is often the first step in any organization's journey to become a high-performing organization. This process draws the map that the organization will follow to achieve its stated mission. This is a process that must be performed by the organization's highest-level leaders, with oversight by the organization's governing body. Poor planning leads to poor performance. The planning must be carried out with a serious focus on gaining answers to many questions. What is occurring in our industry currently and what trends are expected over the next three to five years? What is our understanding of our competitors and their capabilities? What are our capabilities? What can we execute better than anyone else?

The following information will discuss the process in more specific detail.

Timeline

Many organizations have a strategic planning process in place that works well for their annual calendar. However, for those that do not we will present a suggested timeline example for a calendar year–based organization to follow. The OR leadership will need to understand and honor the planning timeline followed by the larger organization. However, the OR leadership will be responsible for developing a more focused plan that is specific with regard to OR goals, objectives, measures, and targets, while assuring that the OR plan directly supports the organizational plan. Timing for the OR plan will need to begin after completion of the larger organizational plan. However, it will be clear that there is much information gathering needed before beginning the focused planning process.

For a calendar year–based organization, the final approved strategic plan must be ready to become actionable by January 1 of each year. The specific timeline chosen is dependent upon factors unique to each organization. These include the size of the planning team, capabilities of the team, access to necessary data, frequency of planning meetings, and the hierarchy of who must give input to the developing plan.

A sample calendar year–based planning cycle is shown in Box 3.1.

SWOT Analysis

The SWOT (strengths, weaknesses, opportunities, and threats) analysis should be one of the earliest actions completed so that the leadership can assess the current positioning of the organization.

The entire planning team should participate in this self-analysis. Input should be sought from many stakeholders. Once the information is gathered it can be edited, clarified, simplified, and then prioritized. The four parts of the assessment – the departmental or organizational strengths, weaknesses, opportunities, and threats – are equally important, and with adequate input from different perspectives inside the organization, the SWOT analysis will achieve its full potential.

The SWOT analysis always begins with an assessment of the organization's strengths. "Strengths" refers to the capabilities of an organization, an operation, or a department. The assessment should focus on an understood ability to make improvements in or perform certain activities or functions. If they are lacking or become diminished, the organization or department will suffer in some way.

Next is an assessment of the organizational and/or departmental weaknesses. This assessment is a close, focused look at the existing shortage in capabilities, lack of competencies, and lack of resources within the organization. The weaknesses part of the assessment can be very insightful. However, in many organizations where honesty is not a part of the culture, the weaknesses portion of the assessment may be understated.

The opportunities section requires a more forward-looking view of the organizational and departmental potential, both in the external and internal environments. This section of the assessment requires consideration of industry trends, customer needs, stakeholder needs, team member skill development,

Box 3.1. An Example of a Calendar Year–Based Planning Cycle

February 2013	Begin strategic planning process for 2014
May 2013	Present draft of leadership plan to governing body
June–August 2013	Move draft leadership plan to final form
August 2013	Present final leadership plan to governing body
September 2013	Begin taking plan to support departments
October 2013	Develop departmental action plans
November 2013	Finalize full organizational plan
January 2014	Full organizational plan becomes actionable

and possible competitive advantages that should be given attention in the future in order to gain a competitive advantage.

Finally, the threats include those factors that alone, or in combination, could cause the business to fail, lose market share, or become weaker at the least. Threats have the potential to cause permanent damage to the organization, or at least stop the forward progress of the organization. Threats should be considered as permanent injuries, not temporary "bumps in the road."

Competitive Analysis

The basic origin of the word "strategy" comes from a military application for planning a specific action in order to obtain a certain goal. Even with the nonmilitary use of the word "strategy," there is an implied need for the understanding of the organization's competitors, and the need to position the organization in the competitive environment before building a plan to obtain the set goals. Competitive analysis becomes an integral requirement of any strategic planning process. The strategy of an organization or department should focus on the unique qualities and abilities that separate the organization from all its competitors. What sets this organization apart? What makes it unique? The SWOT analysis should help with this understanding. The competitive analysis can take many forms; however, the best is "Porter's five competitive forces that shape strategy" [8].

The five forces include the "threat of entry," the "power of the buyers," the "threat of substitute products or services," the "power of the suppliers," and the "rivalry among existing competitors." In addition to an understanding of each of the five competitive forces, an understanding of industry analysis is also very important. The scope of this chapter does not allow for a full in-depth discussion of these forces: a brief discussion of each is described below; for further understanding the reader is directed to the book *On Competition* by Michael E. Porter [8].

The threat of entry focuses on the issues created by a new competitor entering the organization's market with new capabilities, new capacities, different pricing structure, lower costs, and an immediate ability to take away market share and affect the profitability of the organization. In the case of threat of entry, it is important for the organization/department to be aware of their industry on a national, state, and local level. Leadership should always be aware of growing industry trends that might attract the attention of possible new entrants to the market. For an OR, this might be a new ambulatory surgery center, a new surgeon opening an office-based surgical suite, or an industry trend that is moving certain procedures from the OR to the physician's office.

The power of buyers represents the power of the customer and can create competitive forces by forcing down prices, demanding higher quality, and/or demanding other new services. Buyers can gain large amounts of power in industries where the prominent products are relatively standardized and undifferentiated. This allows the buyers to leverage one organization against the other. Nongovernmental, commercially insured buyers of healthcare services are now more price sensitive than previously as insurance deductibles and copays are much larger. Governmentally insured (i.e., Medicaid, Medicare, etc.) buyers who have small to nonexistent deductibles remain much less sensitive to pricing. An example of this might be the impact that low-priced, cash-based imaging centers have had on hospital-based imaging departments. To clearly understand the competitive power of buyers the organization/department must clearly understand the needs and wants of their customers as well as the ability of the customer population to shop around for services.

The threat of substitutes is of concern when new services, technologies, or procedures are being created that will remove the need for these same services and procedures to be performed in the OR. Substitutes could occur downstream or upstream of the OR.

For example, for many years ORs performed large numbers of gastric ulcer operations. Several years ago acid-blocking medications were created that reduced the incidence of gastric ulcers, which in turn greatly reduced the need for these surgeries. Substitutes can cause permanent negative impact on the profitability of the organization and OR, especially if the substitute attacks a high-frequency procedure for the OR. Another example is the impact cardiac stents and cardiac angioplasty has had on the number of open heart procedures performed.

The power of suppliers focuses on the competitive threat of all those sources of resources required for the organization or OR to function. In the case of the OR, suppliers include surgeons who bring the patients, primary care physicians and mid-level providers who refer patients to surgeons, and equipment and supply vendors who provide the necessary supplies for the surgeries to occur. Vendor suppliers can gain power and pricing strength when the number of vendors is concentrated and there are no substitutes for what they provide. Vendors can also increase prices and power when their supplies are in high demand, when the vendors do not depend upon the organization or industry for much of their revenue, when the cost of switching to other vendors is high, and when products among vendors are well differentiated. Referring physicians can gain power as suppliers by limiting the flow of patients to the OR and the organization.

Rivalry among existing competitors is the most obvious source for competitive threats and is usually the one organizations focus on the most. This focus on known competitors can be accurate or can create a distraction from the other sources of competitive threats when the existing competitors do not present much competition.

It is important to be aware of this rivalry when certain situations exist, including when there are numerous competitors in the same market of the same size and power offering the same list of services, when barriers to exit from the industry are high, and when the overall industry growth rate is slow. This rivalry of existing competitors is most destructive when it leads to pricing competition, and can greatly impact profitability. This is especially harmful when fixed costs of the organization are high and pricing decreases start to drive margins closer to the total cost levels.

Industry analysis is heavily based upon the understanding of Porter's five competitive forces. The five forces reveal the drivers of the industry competition, the attractiveness of an industry at a given time, and allow better understanding of the positioning of the organization in the industry. This focus on competitive forces and gaining a better understanding of the industry allows the organization to direct energy on driving improved economic value. The organizational strategic plan can then be designed with a much better understanding of where the competitive strengths and weaknesses exist. Better focus on decision making should be the result of this effort.

Goals, Objectives, Measures, Actions, and Targets

When the organization begins the actual process of strategic planning, it is important that a leadership team focused on the planning process be identified. This team can begin communication with members of the governing body to gain alignment on the organizational goals before initiating the planning process. For the strategic plan to be effective and easier to execute, the number of goals should be limited to one for each of the major focus areas of the organization or department, and no more than five to six in total. Most healthcare organizations will have focus areas such as people, growth, finance, community, quality, and service. A common mistake is to have too many goals, making it difficult for the resources of the organization to be focused and applied where needed.

Once the goals are clearly stated, one to two objectives per goal are agreed to. The objectives must describe brief action statements that will lead to accomplishment of the stated goal they support. Goals drive the overall strategic direction of the organization and become extremely important. Planning groups and members of the governing body should give ample time to clearly state the organizational goals. Goals and objectives must be clear, "high level" in focus, and achievable. The objectives must be clearly measurable with achievable targets. Also, supporting departments such as the OR must be able to develop their action plans consistent with the organizational objectives and goals.

Each stated objective must be measurable in a way that is available in the organization's data, easily understood, and in units of measure that clearly signify their importance to the organization. Therefore, when measures are established for each objective, it is important that team members, at all levels, are able to easily interpret what the individual measure indicates

and what the directional trends in the measures indicate. As departments begin to develop their individual supporting strategic documents, it is important that they have their own measures that provide direction and accountability for the department staff. Action plans are developed for each objective at all levels of the organization. These action plans must be specific, easy to place into action, and flexible as progress with the strategic plan moves forward or action plans become irrelevant.

Targets for each measurable objective need to be achievable and clearly driven by the action plan. Targets should be established at levels that require effort to reach, but are not unobtainable. Unobtainable targets quickly become irrelevant to the organizational teams. Targets must be kept real and attainable, but not so low that they are too easy to reach.

Monitoring

Every well-designed strategic plan will become actionable and measurable with carefully conceived targets to attain. In order to hold the organizational team accountable for performance on the strategic plan, there must be a way to monitor incremental achievements as the strategic plan year progresses. Active monitoring of the plan allows the organizational team to "keep score" as progress on the plan is made or not made throughout the year.

The best monitoring tool is the Balanced Scorecard, developed by Dr. Robert Kaplan and Dr. David Norton in the early 1990s [9]. The balanced scorecard provides several advantages for monitoring the strategic plan. First, it provides a single-page summary of current status on the key issues/targets of the strategic plan. Second, it provides focus and clarity for any teams within the organization/department that might be working on different aspects of the strategic plan at the same time. Third, it allows for fixed periodic measured results to be published, which allows mid-year course corrections as needed with the strategic plan. Last, it has been shown to enhance other improvement programs in existence in the organization, such as activity-based costing, Six Sigma, Lean, etc. Other attributes of the balanced scorecard include the ability to better balance financial and nonfinancial measures, balance long- and short-term measures, and balance lead indicators with lag indicators so that you can look at outcomes of decisions as well as predictors of certain interventions. This discussion only serves as a brief introduction to the balanced scorecard as a tool.

Summary

Proper strategic planning is one of the most important processes an organization can use to drive higher levels of performance. It is also a process that requires a willingness to work through multiple steps in the process and understanding that the more effort the team makes to understand strategic plan the better the end product. Strategic planning forces the organizational leadership to revisit the organization's mission, vision, and values. Also, an annual strategic assessment, in the form of a SWOT analysis, is healthy at least on an annual basis if not more often. Focused energies on the organization's strategic initiatives will produce better performance with clear measures and open sources of reporting and scoring by using the chosen monitoring tool. Highly successful organizations are focused, strategic organizations that master the art of planning with purpose. Also, they complete the execution loop of strategy execution, accountability of clear measures, and follow-through with ongoing monitoring of the organization's results. These are the organizations that succeed year after year.

References

1. K. E. Weick. *Sensemaking in Organizations*. London: Sage, 1995, pp. 54–5.

2. P. F. Drucker. *Managing the Nonprofit Organization*. New York: Harper, 1990, p. 5, 7.

3. J. Welch, S. Welch. *Winning*. New York: HarperCollins, 2005, p. 14.

4. E. H. Edersheim. *The Definitive Drucker*. New York: McGraw-Hill, 2007, p. 170.

5. The Toyota Global Vision. 2011. www.toyota-global .com/company/vision_philosophy (accessed April 29, 2012).

6. The Amazon.com Vision Statement. 2011. http://phx .corporate-ir.net/phoenix.zhtml?c=97664&p=irol-faq (accessed April 29, 2012).

7. J. Kouzes, B. Posner. *The Leadership Challenge*, 4th edn. San Francisco: John Wiley, 2007, p. 52.

8. M. E. Porter. *On Competition*, updated and expanded edn. Boston: Harvard Business School, 2008, pp. 3–24.

9. R. Kaplan, D. Norton. *The Balanced Scorecard: Translating Strategy into Action*. Boston: Harvard Business Press, 1996.

Chapter

4

Decision Making
The Art and the Science

Michael R. Williams

Contents

In any moment of decision the best thing you can do is
the right thing, the next best thing is the wrong thing,
and the worst thing you can do is nothing.

– Theodore Roosevelt

Introduction

Decisions are a part of our daily life. We are confronted
with choices every day and in most cases must make
decisions with limited information. Many of these
daily decisions have a minor impact on our lives; however, some of them carry great impact. This impact
may be focused only on our individual lives or may
also impact the lives of many other people. How we
make decisions is extremely important; however, most
of us do not consider or take time to understand the
best ways to make decisions. The question is often
"Why did that individual or those people make such
a bad decision?" When we are not included in the
decision process, we often feel frustration and waning
support for the decision. The leadership of the operating room (OR) or surgical services department of
every hospital is faced with decisions on a daily basis.
Sometimes such decisions have focused impact on
certain stakeholder groups, such as physicians, surgical technicians, anesthesia personnel, nursing staff,
and patients and their families. At other times such
decisions impact the lives of only a few individuals.
This chapter will focus on helping leaders better
understand how to avoid making poor choices, how to
structure a decision-making process that will engage
the talents and perspectives of the entire team, frame
the decision in the proper context, evaluate all appropriate alternatives using different analytical tools, be
aware of possible decision biases, and finally move to
make the decision and implement it.

Building the Decision Team

The first step of a successful decision-making process is the building of an informed, thoughtful, and
focused team. Arguably, this step could be considered
the most important in the process. The right team will
move the decision process a great distance toward
the goal of making the best decision. This step in the
overall process must be approached by the leader
with a clear understanding of both how a team
functions, and those qualities important to have on
a high-performing team. In Patrick Lencioni's book,
The Five Dysfunctions of a Team, he clearly describes
those qualities [1]. The five dysfunctions that must be
avoided are: the "absence of trust," "fear of conflict,"
"lack of commitment," "lack of accountability," and
"inattention to results." Trust forms the foundation
needed for the other team functions to work.

Begin by gathering individuals who trust each other. If this is not possible, trust must be established as quickly as possible in order to move through the decision-making process quickly. The absence of trust allows the team to move forward with a foundational flaw and leads to future failure. The higher the level of trust, the faster the team can move on the work ahead of it. Everyone must be willing to share mistakes and weaknesses in order to show they can be vulnerable to others on the team.

Without trust it will become impossible to avoid the second dysfunction: fear of conflict. When fear of conflict exists, team members remain guarded in discussion and are incapable of engaging in an open exchange of ideas. This results in the suppression of their true feelings on most issues and therefore prevents the team from adequately exploring all alternatives presented in the decision-making process. When the team has lack of trust and fear of conflict they begin to feel as if the team meetings are not worth the time needed and begin to demonstrate a lack of commitment to the team's assigned work.

Lack of commitment to the team is the third dysfunction. In meetings these individuals never air their true feelings on the matters being considered. They never buy in to the process or the final decision, yet they often act as if they are in full agreement with the team at meetings, only to express lack of support for the team and the decision when outside the team. This lack of commitment leads to the fourth dysfunction: the avoidance of accountability.

When individuals are not trusting, fear conflict, and/or lack commitment to the team, they begin to hesitate to hold team members accountable to the work of the team. Because they do not believe in the team or its work, they will choose to avoid accountability. When accountability is absent, the focus on results and the measurement of results ultimately cause the team to fail, and decisions they make will fail or at least never reach their full potential.

The final dysfunction, inattention to results, allows individual team members to focus on their personal needs and interests. This focus on individual needs always overshadows any concern or focus on the needs or work of the team. Therefore, most decisions made by such a team will fail, and ultimately the team will fail.

The team should be constructed with a focus on avoiding these dysfunctions and looking to build a team with the desirable qualities enhanced. Other important considerations include finding people with full authority to allocate necessary resources to the final decision and the authority to implement the final decision. Key stakeholder groups should be represented either directly or indirectly. Both proponents and opponents of the decision at the start of the process should be included. These different perspectives add value and a rich quality to the discussion and final decision. Outside opinions should also be sought as necessary from consultants with an expertise in the areas being evaluated for the decision [2]. Keep the size of the team manageable and consider the meeting environment and location of meetings so that open discussion and trust can be fostered and developed. Last, consider any positional hierarchy on the team so that meetings can be held in an open environment. Even the setting of the meeting can give way to a sense that only one or two individuals will make the decision: for example, a table in a boardroom with only one chair at the head of the table. There will need to be a team leader; however, the role of the leader should be focused on facilitation of open discussion, and not decision making, in the team meetings.

Framing the Decision

Framing is the second step in the decision-making process and is equally important to the first step of assembling the team. If framed incorrectly, the right decision may not even be considered, much less reached as the final outcome. However, proper framing will set the direction of discussions and can often speed the process on the proper path. Framing is the responsibility of the team leader, as he or she will also facilitate the discussions and insure that the focus stays inside the proper frame. Alan Rowe describes frames as "the prisms through which we view the world . . . they determine both what we see and how we interpret it" [3].

Avoid framing with current assumptions only or intuitive guesses by team members as to the meaning of the decision. When set, the frame will guide all future team discussions, options considered, alternatives developed, and certainly final decisions made. The team leader must be vigilant for team members attempting to frame the decision from an individual perspective. Those individuals who understand framing will also know the power of the frame in leading to the final decision. Indeed, as Jeffrey Pfeffer states in *Managing with Power*, "Establishing the framework within which issues will be viewed and decided is often tantamount to determining the result" [4].

The leader should make sure to encourage and direct the framing to remain focused on the course that most benefits the organization. Don't allow the team to automatically accept an initial framing. Ask for many different team opinions and perspectives before making any decisions. Look for personal and individual biases. Also, uncover and challenge any assumptions that might exist under a dominant member's presence and opinions. Lastly, ask the leader to place him or herself in the perspective of other members to clearly look at different angles to the frame [2]. This deliberate attempt to find the best frame for the benefit of the organization and the team sets the frame and moves the process forward. The team will appreciate the sincere attempt by the leader not to dominate the framing of the issue. At the end of the process, the decision will have better support by the entire team and will be more easily implemented across the entire OR. Finally, do not hesitate to adjust the frame or reframe the decision if issues or alternatives develop that significantly change the direction of the decision from the organization's perspective.

Develop and Evaluate Possible Alternatives

All good decision makers should seek multiple possible alternatives before making a decision. Finding, selecting, and evaluating alternatives will allow the best possible decision to be found and chosen by the team. The team should seek to avoid a simple yes or no decision, which is what occurs in the absence of alternative choices. The team leader must encourage a search for varied alternatives that look from several different perspectives and angles represented by the members of the team. If the leader does not seek alternatives, the risk will exist that the team will develop a single focus, leading to a single, untested decision. This atmosphere prevents innovative thought and appropriate vetting of the eventual decision.

In order to encourage development and discussion of alternatives, the leader should encourage outside opinions at the team meetings, look at other like companies in order to benchmark how they have addressed similar questions, ask team members to step out of their traditional job roles and think from a different perspective, ask probing questions, allow views and discussions different from that of their own, revisit abandoned alternatives from time to time in order to reevaluate their relevancy, and consider hybrid alternatives as well [2].

Also, the team leader must establish some rules for the group to follow in order to encourage the development of alternative thoughts. Such rules should allow for and encourage active listening, equal respect for all team members, acknowledgement of failures without judgment, and tolerance of conflicting views. The leader must keep the discussion focused on the issues and alternatives and not on the individuals presenting their thoughts, while keeping the atmosphere in the room as light and unthreatening as possible.

According to David Matheson and Jim Matheson in *The Smart Organization*, the best alternatives have certain characteristics, given below.

- They are broadly constructed and not only a simple variation of another alternative or concept. They should offer a broad range of options.
- They are true alternatives and not just "straw men" presented to make another choice appear superior and reasonable. False choices must be avoided.
- They are feasible choices given the organization's resources, capabilities, and capacities. It is important to remain realistic regarding what the organization can do. The team can build a feasibility test that each alternative must be able to pass. It is important not to waste the team's valuable time on alternatives that can never become a reality for the organization.
- They are sufficiently numerous to represent a true choice. However, be mindful that each selected alternative must be fully evaluated, so be selective in the process [5].

The next step in the decision-making process is to take each alternative and analyze it using a varied set of analytical tools. These are discussed below.

Evaluation of Alternatives and Use of Analytical Tools

Most likely, each alternative will need to be fully evaluated from a variety of perspectives using different analytical tools. It is important for the team to enumerate those variables important to the final decision and therefore create a screen or filter by which each alternative can be evaluated. Such variables might include *time* to implement, *benefits* to the organization if chosen and implemented, the *ethics* of the decision and whether there are any ethical or *legal issues*, what are the required *resources* to complete implementation, *how feasible* is the alternative and what are the possible obstacles to implementation. Additional variables could include the *overall risk* of the alternative, the *financial impact* of the alternative at maturity, what *intangibles* might be affected by the alternative, and lastly the *costs* to implement and use the alternative on a long-term basis.

As the decision team filters each alternative for all the variables listed above they will need to be aware of the further analysis necessary for each choice. Analytical tools are available to assess the financial impact of each possible choice, the probability of a particular alternative succeeding or failing, the development of further details that exist inside each alternative and how each alternative performs in a "trade off" against other alternatives, and prioritization of each choice as to how it best addresses the key objectives of the overall decision.

From a financial analysis perspective there are several commonly used analytical tools. These include the return on investment (ROI), net present value (NPV), internal rate of return (IRR), break-even analysis, and sensitivity analysis. These will be described below as to their individual benefits and the process involved in completing each. Other tools such as the prioritization matrix and the decision tree will also be discussed below. Any discussion of advanced decision support computer software or related enterprise-level software is beyond the intended scope of this chapter.

The ROI is a calculation of the percentage return from the chosen investment that can then be compared to other investment returns that might be expected from alternative investments using the same capital dollars. The net return of an investment is simply the subtraction of the total costs of the project from the total cash benefits. Then the ROI is calculated by dividing the net return by the total investment amount. For example, let's assume that an item of imaging equipment is being evaluated with an upfront cost of $400,000 and with an expected annual return of $100,000 per year over 5 years. The total return would be $500,000 and the net return would be $500,000 minus the total cost of $400,000

($500,000–$400,000 = $100,000). The net investment return of $100,000 is then divided by the total investment cost of $400,000 ($100,000/$400,000 = 0.25), resulting in a healthy ROI of 25 percent.

The NPV takes into consideration the fact of using today's dollars and adjusting future values for the time value of money and the fact that future dollars are never worth more than present dollars. When cash flows can be predicted, the best predictive financial tool to use is the calculation of the NPV. The NPV takes into consideration the future cash flows, the ongoing cost of capital or risk, and the initial investment cost to start the project. In the end, the NPV gives an accurate assessment of the present value of the decision today while using future dollars in the calculation. It can be a complicated calculation; however, most financial calculators and computer spreadsheet programs can perform the actual calculations, and they will not be discussed here. It is most important for the decision team to estimate future cash flows from the possible investment and alternate investments being evaluated. It is also important for the team to determine the discount rate or the rate of return if the same dollars were placed into an alternative investment with similar risk. The future cash flows are then discounted by the discount rate and the sum of these discounted cash flows results in a total present value. Total investment costs of the project are then subtracted from the total present value to give the NPV. This NPV can then be compared to similar NPV calculations of other investment alternatives under consideration. A possible example of the use of this might be if a surgical department was considering expanding to include a new service line not currently provided.

The IRR is similar to the NPV calculation. It is defined as the discount rate that will cause the NPV to be equal to zero. Then, when comparing alternative decisions, the one with the higher IRR will be the best from a financial return perspective. In most cases, the IRR of a given decision alternative should be higher than the risk-free treasury bond rate and higher than the organization's hurdle rate or internal discount rate.

The break-even analysis is useful when evaluating an investment that will allow new revenue generation or enhanced revenue from an existing service. An example might be the addition of a specific spinal surgical procedure to an existing spine program in a hospital not currently performing these procedures.

The break-even analysis would help the team determine how many of these procedures at a given unit value would need to be completed in order to reach a break-even state with the total investment costs of the program. The variables to be considered would include the unit contribution amount, unit variable costs, and total fixed costs. The unit contribution amount is the "contribution margin" of each procedure – that is, the procedural revenue minus the variable cost of each procedure. The total fixed costs are then divided by the unit contribution of one procedure with the resulting quotient being equal to the number of units needed for a break-even volume. This is the total number of these procedures needed to cover the fixed costs of this alternative. The team must then decide if this volume is achievable – and if so, over what time frame – and what resources exist or are needed to support such an endeavor.

Sensitivity analysis is a tool that allows the decision team to take the previously calculated NPV amount and then assess the probability of specific variables required in the alternative actually occurring. After the probability of a single variable is changed, the NPV can be recalculated using a computer spreadsheet. This analysis allows individual items to be changed to determine the overall impact on the program's financial outcome.

For a more complete review of these financial analytical tools with examples of the needed calculations, consult any business finance text or similar searches on the web. As to other types of nonfinancial analysis, consider the prioritization matrix and the decision tree. These will both be discussed in more detail below.

The prioritization matrix is a useful tool to analyze the nonfinancial value of a particular alternative. With this tool, the team must develop a clear list of expected objectives that would be achieved if the program alternative were successful. Each objective is then prioritized and weighted accordingly. Also, each alternative being analyzed is assigned a probability (using a scale of 1–10, with 10 being the best) of achieving each selected objective. A total score is then calculated and the alternative with the highest score is the better choice (see Figure 4.1).

In Figure 4.1, alternative B would be the better alternative given this set of probabilities and weighted objectives.

The decision tree tool builds a "roadmap" of possible decisions inside a single alternative with assigned probabilities to each decision pathway. To provide the most accurate assessment of the given alternative using the decision tree, the decision team must ask each member, and outsiders as needed, for individual estimates of probabilities in order to develop a final probability set for each decision node. For the sake of completeness, each member of the team should also estimate financial values with each probability if possible. Decision trees work best when the team can accurately predict probabilities and financial outcomes of the separate parts of the given alternative (see Figure 4.2) [2].

For a more detailed discussion on using and constructing more complex decision tree tools, refer to the web as well as statistical texts and decision theory business texts.

Role of Bias in Decision Making

Despite best efforts on the part of decision team members, it is normal for specific types of decision biases to enter into the decision-making process. It is best for all members of the team to be frequently reminded by the team leader and other members how they can be aware of and guard against the several forms of cognitive decision biases.

Alternative	Lower costs (4)	Higher revenues (3)	Short implementation (2)	Patient satisfaction (1)	Total score
A	$5 \times 4 = 20$	$1 \times 3 = 3$	$10 \times 2 = 20$	$10 \times 1 = 10$	53
B	$8 \times 4 = 32$	$1 \times 3 = 3$	$8 \times 2 = 16$	$6 \times 1 = 6$	57

Figure 4.1 A prioritization matrix.

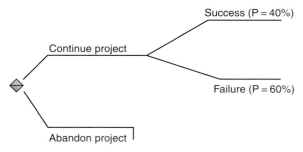

Figure 4.2 A decision tree – basic form.

The first form of bias is the "overconfidence bias." People by nature are overconfident in their personal decisions and judgments; they are also overly optimistic in these decisions and judgments. The combination of overconfidence and optimism can lead to faulty decisions. The second form of bias is the "sunk-cost effect." The sunk-cost effect describes how humans will invariably commit to decisions in which they have already invested a large amount of time, money, or other personal resources. These previous investments of resources in one alternative investment prevent individuals from making a clear alternative decision that might be better. Third is the "recency effect," also known as an example of the "availability bias." This bias is in effect when those making the decision place too much emphasis on information that is readily available when faced with the decision. They focus on recent events they think are similar to the decision facing them. The fourth bias is the "confirmation bias," which causes humans to gather information that confirms their existing views about a decision, and causes them to devalue any information that does not support their preconceived ideas about the decision. Fifth is the "anchoring bias," whereby the decision evaluation is begun from an arbitrary reference point, which if improperly placed, or anchored, will skew the final decision to a faulty conclusion. There are several other cognitive biases; however, those mentioned above are the most common. So how can the decision team diminish the effects of these biases? Mainly by keeping a high level of awareness in the team so that they can recognize if these start to appear in the decision process. Also by looking for forms of measurable feedback once the decision is made in order to retrospectively review how the decision was made and if any bias impacted the final decision.

Make the Decision and Begin Implementation

After the team has agreed on an amount of time to complete its assessment of the decision and alternatives, the leader must move the team to a close. Even with disagreement between team members, the team leader must move to get the decision finalized. First, he or she must keep the team's focus on the previously agreed upon common goal. Also, the team might agree to briefly revisit and reexamine all alternatives and related summary assumptions. If the process begins to drag on, the leader will need to set a clear time deadline. The leader may need to remind the entire team that if a consensus decision cannot be reached, a majority vote will carry the final decision. Both deciding too early and too late in the process can be problematic; therefore a vote may be needed to reach the deadline. After the decision is made, the team should agree to come out of the final meeting in unity behind the final decision despite the voting results.

Next the decision will need to be explained to those in the organization who will be affected by it or expected to carry out the implementation. Explain how the process worked and why the final alternative was chosen. Clearly describe the implementation process and timeline while recognizing all those who participated in the decision process. Lastly, ask for feedback and allow the postdecision process to be a time of learning for the future. This also allows others to be heard and valued even though they were not directly involved in the process.

Summary

High-reliability organizations allow the formation of a well-tested process for decision making. There is a proven process described that, when followed, will allow the best decision team to be selected, a clear process to be defined, and alternative decisions to be developed and analyzed individually and in comparison with each other. Also, the team will engage in open discussion, the avoidance of cognitive biases, and ultimately reach the best alternative of those considered. Finally, the decision will be reached, and clearly communicated, and then the implementation process will begin. Those organizations that are best at decision making will always use every opportunity to learn from each decision made, in order to improve in the future. Whether in the surgical suite or in the organization as a whole, those leaders who have a better understanding of decision making will always be in the best position to lead others in easy and difficult times alike.

Decision making is a leadership skill that is worthy of the time required to develop it further. Few leaders are fully competent at it or work to become competent at it.

References

1.   P. Lencioni. *The Five Dysfunctions of a Team*. San Francisco, CA: Josey-Bass, 2002, pp. 188–9.

2.   R. Luecke. *Decision Making, Five Steps to Better Results*. Boston, MA: Harvard Business Press, 2006, pp. 13, 27–8, 54–5, 57–8.

3.   A. J. Rowe. *Creative Intelligence*. Upper Saddle River, NJ: Prentice Hall, 2004, p. 68.

4.   J. Pfeffer. *Managing with Power*. Boston, MA: Harvard Business Press, 1992, pp. 63–4.

5.   D. Matheson, J. Matheson. *The Smart Organization*. Boston, MA: Harvard Business Press, 1998, pp. 42–3.

Chapter

Implications of Emotional Intelligence and Collaboration for Operating Room Leadership and Management

Markus M. Luedi, Jonas Schnider, and Frank Stueber

Clients do not come first. If you take care of your employees, they will take care of the clients.

– Sir Richard Branson

In 1989, Donald Berwick called for continuous improvement as an ideal in healthcare [1]. The physician from the Harvard Community Health Plan asked the New England Journal of Medicine's readers to visualize two industrial assembly lines supervised by two different foremen:

> "Foreman 1 walks the line, watching carefully. 'I can see you all,' he warns. 'I have the means to measure your work, and I will do so. I will find those among you who are unprepared or unwilling to do your jobs, and when I do there will be consequences. There are many workers available for these jobs, and you can be replaced'" [1].

> "Foreman 2 walks a different line, and he too watches. 'I am here to help you if I can,' he says. 'We are in this together for the long haul. You and I have a common interest in a job well done. I know that most of you are trying very hard, but sometimes things can go wrong. My job is to notice opportunities for improvement – skills that could be shared, lessons from the past, or experiments to try together – and to give you the means to do your work even better than you do now. I want to help the average ones among you, not just the exceptional few at either end of the spectrum of competence'" [1].

Asking the readers which leadership approach works better and by which "foreman" they wanted to be supervised is rhetorical. It has become established wisdom that leadership is not simply the capacity to master situations, but is the embodiment of emotional and social intelligence towards self-management,

influence, developing others, inspiration, teamwork, and organizational awareness [2]. The basis for achieving such behavior as a leader depends on emotional intelligence, including the psychological dimensions of self-awareness, self-regulation, motivation, empathy, and social skills [3]. Yet managers, especially young managers, often lack empathy. Experience and reflection cannot be substituted, but personal development and feedback can be institutionalized. Bunker et al. pointed out that successful leadership must not give any team member the impression that emotional competencies are optional [4].

An appropriate metric for evaluating perioperative performance is not only the immediate medical result but also the entire process of care [5]. For the evaluation to be meaningful, feedback must be provided, and a means must exist for implementing recommendations. Feedback is institutionalized in training [6], but as we know from other fields such as sports or music, expert performance, too, is enhanced through feedback [7]. However, a culture of constructive feedback can only be established with the willingness to explore the self-in-group, mandating awareness for personal characteristics unknown to self and unknown to others [8]. Feedback should be based on direct observation [9] rather than on one's performance in general [10], and the content of the critique must be completely separated from any personal judgement [11]. Operating room (OR) leadership must implement and cultivate a vivid, proactive feedback culture towards a positive change of individuals and the organization.

Daniel Goleman pointed out that emotionally competent leaders understand their impact on others, and he described a simple notion as *the* hidden driver of great performance: "Don't be a CEO, be a doctor" [12]. Dimensions of emotional and social intelligence can be found in the competencies promulgated by the Accreditation Council for Graduate Medical Education [13].

Medicine is a team activity and extensively involves emotional intelligence. Recently, we called for efforts to be made to institutionalize patient centered dialogues within medical specialties but also, specifically, between of them [14]. For example, whereas risk–benefit discussions between two clinicians, presented as pro–con debates, are popular in all branches of medicine, physicians must learn to focus on their patients' needs. This is especially true for acute care physicians such as anesthesiologists and surgeons, who must begin aiming for an "internal action logic" towards "collaboration and intense focus on truth" as a fundamental leadership quality described in management sciences [14, 15]. However, leaders must remember that a group of emotionally intelligent people does not necessarily result in an emotionally intelligent group. Moreover, Gratton described "that the greater the proportion of experts a team had, the more likely it was to disintegrate into nonproductive conflict or stalemate" [16]. Like dialogues with patients, dialogues with colleagues can be learnt and improved. While task related competencies are high among experts, we assume that behavior aiming to improve relationships may lead to an improvement in this regard. As Vanessa Urch Druskat pointed out, team members must feel that they work better together than individually. Therefore, leadership must build trust, a sense of group identity, and establish rules to support awareness and manage emotions within and outside the team [17]. Specifically, in the hectic of daily clinical work, overemphasizing on task accomplishment, rather than relationship-building behaviors, can be detrimental for team work. The makeup of the team is a critical component of delivering safe and high-quality patient care. In acute care situations such as perioperative medicine, failure to consider relevant personality characteristics poses a significant risk for wrongly identifying and choosing "successful" staff for the team.

Social media platforms such as Facebook, LinkedIn, WhatsApp and Twitter represent tremendous achievements of the twenty-first century, and offer opportunities for real-time and asynchronous dialogues with patients and within and between medical specialties. Such dialogues can provide an avenue towards patient centered collaboration. In a milestone publication, Andrew P. McAfee described opportunities accruing from social software platforms in areas such as broadcasting, networking, collective intelligence, and self-organization for enterprises [18]. These are opportunities that could benefit OR management for both formal and informal networking towards collaboration. John Abele described a way to build community toward a vision by convincing workforces who don't necessarily need to work together directly to, nonetheless, do so: "Inspiring them with a vision of change that is beyond any of their powers to bring about individually, convincing them that the other collaborators are vital to the effort and preventing any one party from benefiting so much that the others feel being exploited" [19]. Herminia Ibarra called leaders to link different "social worlds," ideas, and (human) resources across departments to those inside. A crucial component in this effort is an authentic leader, who provides a capable role model at top [20].

From management science we know that it is of utmost importance to instill an atmosphere of trust, to create an environment where individuals' spheres of influence overlap and where collaboration is rewarded. It is essential to define a purpose that guides people at all levels to achieve together; it is important to instill a culture of contribution in which people are encouraged to go beyond their specific roles [21]. Acting both as contributing team members and effective leaders is essentials for surgeons and anesthesiologists to foster full potential of effective teamwork in the OR [22]. Figure 5.1 displays a way in which engaging and inspiring people outside one's formal control toward a common goal can be visualized and understood.

A leader should aim to "hire civility," i.e., to choose team members for competencies such as listening and keeping promises, and within the team to further implement "civility" and group norms toward a common base that rewards positive behavior and penalizes rudeness [23]. Anticipating the evolution of anesthesiology and acute care medicine, we expect that emotionally intelligent physicians will be likely to become successful anesthesiologists. Considering that emotional intelligence can be learned, it appears of utmost priority for OR leaders to raise awareness of this human quality. We support career-long training of anesthesiologists in emotional intelligence and leadership competencies [24]. Beyond ensuring OR efficiency and patient safety, choosing team members

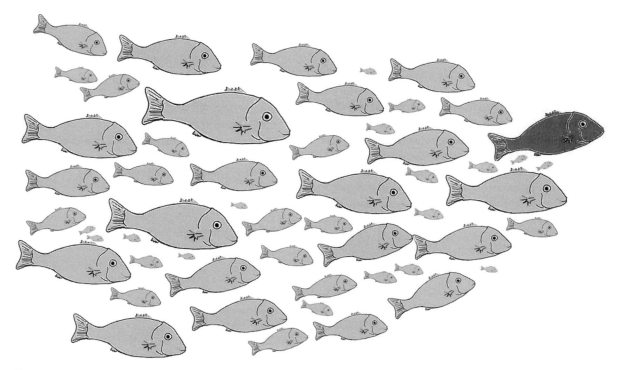

Figure 5.1 Engaging and inspiring people outside one's formal control toward a common goal: Decades of management science research have taught us that leadership is not about mastering situations but rather about emotional intelligence embracing dimensions such as self-management, influential social interaction, and inspiring/developing others. Such behavior is individually achieved by self-awareness, self-regulation, motivation, empathy, and social skills. Since experience and reflection cannot be substituted, personal development and feedback must be institutionalized, any team member must know that emotional competencies are mandatory, not optional.

is "probably *the* critical task of leadership" in OR leadership and management [25]. From a managerial point of view, patients do not necessarily come first; because, "if you take care of your employees, they will take care of the clients."

References

1. Berwick DM. Continuous improvement as an ideal in health care. *N Engl J Med* 1989; 320: 53–6.

2. Goleman D, Boyatzis R. Social intelligence and the biology of leadership. *Harv Bus Rev* 2008; 86: 74–81.

3. Goleman D. What makes a leader? *Harv Bus Rev* 2004; 82: 82–91.

4. Bunker KA, Kram KE, Ting S. The young and the clueless. *Harv Bus Rev* 2002; 80: 80–7.

5. Norcini JJ. Work based assessment. *BMJ* 2003; 326: 753–5.

6. Norcini J, Burch V. Workplace-based assessment as an educational tool: AMEE Guide No. 31. *Med Teach* 2007; 29: 855–71.

7. Ericsson KA. Deliberate practice and acquisition of expert performance: A general overview. *Acad Emerg Med* 2008; 15: 988–94.

8. Ingham H, Luft J. The Johari window: a graphic model of interpersonal awareness. Proceedings of the Western Training Laboratory in Group Development, University of California, Los Angeles, 1955.

9. Ramani S, Krackov SK. Twelve tips for giving feedback effectively in the clinical environment. *Med Teach* 2012; 34: 787–91.

10. Cantillon P, Sargeant J. Giving feedback in clinical settings. *BMJ* 2008; 337: a1961.

11. van der Leeuw RM, Slootweg IA. Twelve tips for making the best use of feedback. *Med Teach* 2013; 35: 348–51.

12. Goleman D, Boyatzis R, McKee A. Primal leadership: The hidden driver of great performance. *Harv Bus Rev* 2001; 79: 42–53.

13. Arora S, Ashrafian H, Davis R, et al. Emotional intelligence in medicine: A systematic review through the context of the ACGME competencies. *Med Educ* 2010; 44: 749–64.

14. Luedi MM, Doll D. In dialogue. *Anesth Analg* 2016; 123: 1339–40.

15. Rooke D, Torbert WR. Seven transformations of leadership. *Harv Bus Rev* 2005; 83: 66–76.

16. Erickson TJ, Gratton L. Eight ways to build collaborative teams. *Harv Bus Rev* 2007; 11: 1–11.

17. Druskat VU, Wolff SB. Building the emotional intelligence of groups. *Harv Bus Rev* 2001; 79: 80–91.

18. McAfee AP. Shattering the myths about Enterprise 2.0. *IT Management Select* 2009; 15: 28.

19. Abele J. Bringing minds together. *Harv Bus Rev* 2010; 89: 86–93, 164.

20. Ibarra H, Hansen MT. Are you a collaborative leader? *Harv Bus Rev* 2011; 89: 68–74.

21. Adler P, Heckscher C, Prusak L. Building a collaborative enterprise. *Harv Bus Rev* 2011; 89: 94–101.

22. Giddings A, Williamson C. *The Leadership and Management of Surgical Teams.* The Royal College of Surgeons of England, 2007.

23. Porath C, Pearson C. The price of incivility. *Harv Bus Rev* 2013; 91: 114–21.

24. Luedi MM, Doll D., Boggs SD, et al Successful personalities in anesthesiology and acute care medicine – Are we selecting, training, and supporting the best? *Anesth Analg* 2017; 124: 359–61.

25. Luedi MM, Boggs SD, Doll D, et al. On patient safety, teams and psychologically disturbed pilots. *Eur J Anaesthesiol* 2016; 33: 226–7.

Chapter

6

Operating Room Culture Change

Shilpadevi Patil, Debbie Chandler, Elyse M. Cornett, and Charles J. Fox

Introduction

Operating room (OR) culture is defined as interpersonal, social and organizational factors that affect healthcare environment and patient care. The OR is a very complex, dynamic, and high-stakes environment that relies on contributions from team members from multiple disciplines. To make changes that will improve OR culture and lead to better patient outcomes, a multimodal approach should be adopted and should include all team members. Training residents to recognize the importance of OR culture in various ways and most importantly through quality improvement projects is an essential part of producing lasting changes. Current trainees are the ones who will go on to establish standards for their future practice.

In 2000, the Institute of Medicine report "To Err is Human" discussed the concept of medical error and has influenced public and professional consciousness by highlighting the importance of building a culture of safety as a prerequisite for reducing patient harm and improving healthcare quality. The dominant refrain by ensuing patient safety movement has been the call for a culture change: to move healthcare from a blame and a shame response to error toward a high reliability response that confronts, reports and learns from error. We have to strive to create a safety-conscious culture in healthcare. Errors should be used as opportunities to learn and improve. We must educate team members and reframe events as systems failures rather than fatalistic accidents. As we strive for a culture change, interventions are required to foster a collective approach to responsibility. Efforts at culture change must address the tendency to ensure that institutional disclosure policies are equitably followed for all patients [1].

The presence of autocratic leadership with an inflexible work hierarchy can suppress effective communication and lead to poor teamwork. Traditional hierarchy, which is the norm for surgeons in the OR, creates an environment of monologue, that is, telling and informing rather than a dialogue that constitutes asking, conversing, and debating. This type of practice can compromise patient safety. Poor communication and understanding are the most important human factors that are associated with healthcare errors. Hence, effective communication and collaborative teamwork can avoid crisis situations in the OR.

The goals of this chapter are to understand the need for culture change and how patient safety outcomes can be improved. Some of the ways this can be done are through education to improve teamwork, teamwork communication skills, attitudes and values towards teamwork, change from conventional multiprofessional teamwork to interprofessional teamwork. All these can in turn create a positive OR environment change, ultimately translating into behavioral change, defining a safety culture. Improved clinical teamwork has been shown to have a strong correlation in lowering patient mortality and increasing work morale. Any introduction of a protocol or culture change should aim at patient safety principles of democracy, teamwork, collaboration and respect and practices (briefing, debriefing and close call reporting). Other than teamwork and good management for patient safety, OR personnel safe working conditions, with stress recognition and job satisfaction are also important aspects of OR culture. Checklists not only improve communication but also teamwork and safety.

Concept and Role of a Medical Director

Leadership is essential in guiding employees to do a better job and to improve an organization so it continually meets the needs of the patients it serves. An effective leader is an individual who possesses management skills and guidance skills that that are consistently present in the OR.

The medical director in the OR plays a leadership role to an array of medical professionals including physicians, nurses, technicians, aides, business leaders, and information experts. The medical director's job purpose is to ensure the best possible care for patients in that facility. The medical director should possess and articulate a clear vision for OR organization and a commitment to serving patients. The director is responsible for creating an environment that fosters changes that may be required to achieve that commitment. It is important for the director to consistently spread knowledge and understanding of the institutional goals to the employees. The medical director should also demonstrate the value of teamwork, continuous learning, honesty, integrity and ethical behavior, and respect to individuals.

The medical director should also lead or be an integral part of OR committee and/or departmental meetings. The meetings should focus on key issues and the implementation of policies that govern the OR. The issues presented by the medical director are better received by the staff if they are data driven.

The OR can be a high-stress environment where professionals from diverse background come together to work with different work commitments, pay grades, and views on trying to work together as a team. Conflicts are bound to happen in this stressful environment. Conflict management and resolution with redirection to emphasize workplace goals is another critical role of a medical director.

In addition, the medical director should be a part of the search committee for nursing and support personnel of the OR. To ensure a very good OR nursing leadership, the medical director should also work on an evaluation process and job descriptions of the administrative positions. Thus medical directors should have an active role in the human resources

division of their department as well. They should then work on building a strong working relationship by supporting those chosen for those roles. They should also try to understand and assist the business manager or administrator to help manage the departmental budget and available resources without compromising patient care. They should also assist in managing various data of the ORs at every level of patient care.

In summary, for medical directors, aiming for the highest standards of patient care quality with available resources should be the goal, but boosting morale of the working environment and staff in the ORs should also be a major priority. Creating an environment where everyone would like to work and be treated as a patient should be the ultimate goal [2].

Bridging Gaps with Communication

Communication errors can lead to adverse events in various domains of healthcare. Communication has been identified as primary point of vulnerability for patient safety and efficiency in the OR. Hierarchy in the OR among surgeons, anesthesiologists, residents, nurses, scrub technicians, assistants and aides may restrain communication. In turn, this can negatively affect the efforts to improve OR culture to promote patient safety. Communication is also a powerful tool that will facilitate the steps in OR culture change. Consequently, the OR manager should promote communication among care team members, and between providers and patients.

Providers must keep close contact with patients by continuously assessing and evaluating the patient. In all aspects of patient care including preoperative, intraoperative, and postoperative, communication with the patient is paramount. In the preoperative phase, the charge staff for scheduling will learn about the patients' needs and wants, along with their preferences that must be taken seriously. For example, some patients, by religious conviction, will not accept a blood infusion during surgery, some will not agree to have surgery on some specific holidays, some will opt for special days of the week to have surgery, some will refuse to be anesthetized by trainees. All of these needs should be scrupulously analyzed in order to provide the patient with the maximum safety, confidence, and comfort.

Communication with the patient by the preoperative staff is vital, as the patient needs to be reassured that this is not the last second of his life. To keep high his level of confidence, some short expressions that just require a nod from the patient will be helpful at reducing stress: Are you cold? Do you feel comfortable? Are you okay? Do you have any questions? These questions demonstrate empathy and care to the patients which can help the healthcare team be prepared for the patient and the patient to feel comfortable and secure.

Communication is also the key that will open the path to the most efficient performance in the OR. Open, direct, and honest communication among anesthesiologists/anesthesia providers, surgeons, surgical staff, and nurses results in a successful surgery. One strategy to improve communication includes a time-out before surgery to have an open discussion about the strategy and plan for the procedure. Once in the OR, verbal communication might be not recommended as a silent space plays an important role in OR, but nonverbal or body language communication might be used as ways to ensure communication between the sender and receiver. To prevent any miscommunication, the choice of the communication method should be discussed between the OR manager and other care givers before surgery to ensure that everyone is on the same page.

Furthermore, in the OR all differences should be put aside and every team member should showcase constructive and patient-oriented behavior, regardless of others' attitudes. The OR manager should be a role model and should demonstrate calm control and a positive attitude even when dealing with the worst-case scenario. Full cooperation with colleagues drives a successful performance in the OR. Those repeated successful performances have major impacts on improved workplace productivity and income.

Communication continues after surgery during recovery time. Communicating in a kind and gentle manner until the patient has full awareness and complete anesthetic recovery is invaluable. The healthcare team that consistently practices empathy, compassion, and understanding to their patients will ultimately be the most successful. The Centers for Medicare and Medicaid Services use a value-based purchasing program and have incorporated Hospital Consumer Assessment of Healthcare Providers and Services scores, also known as Patient Satisfaction Scores, into their inpatient prospective payment system. Therefore, physician and healthcare institution reimbursement are now directly affected by the patient experience. All healthcare teams should strive to ensure the best possible experience for their patients [3].

In summary, communication in the OR can be in different forms at various levels such as pre-, peri-, and postoperative patient care, check-backs, call-outs, hand-offs [4]. And while optimal strategies for improving surgical culture remain uncertain, identifying and assessing the most common domains of OR culture is critical. Once identified, interventions to improve OR culture and measuring the outcomes of that change in terms of efficiency and better healthcare are important. Communication along with teamwork and safety climate have been the key domains of OR surgical culture. Multiple studies have shown that improvement in these domains is associated with better patient outcomes by reducing postoperative complications and lowering postoperative mortality (with absolute risk reduction by 1.7%). Other studies have also shown decreases in OR delays and improved healthcare efficiencies.

Managing Diversity among Staff

The ongoing diverse workforce naturally leads to the emergence of a diverse teamwork in facilities, and the OR team is not an exception. Indeed, the OR team – consisting of the surgeons, anesthesiologists, surgical technicians, and nurses – is inherently diverse with regard to multiple medical specialties and training. In addition, the team is also diverse in terms of religion, race, gender, ageism, and affectional orientation. All of these differences may trigger behavioral barriers that could impede collegiality and cooperation among team members. Hence, the OR manager must find adequate strategies to bring all team members together as a team committed to OR safety and maximum satisfaction to patients and care givers, while also increasing workplace productivity and motivation [5]. Some strategies available to the OR manager include awareness training, two-way communication, and constructive behavior evaluation [6]. These are resources that will allow the OR manager to minimize the negative consequences of diversity problems at work while maximizing the benefits.

The OR manager should also make an effort to be aware of each team member's diversity. The OR manager should be the junction that reconciles patient and healthcare team member's differences. The healthcare staff employee records and patient records are available onsite and should include this kind of helpful information. In addition to the OR manager, it is also important that all members of the healthcare team be aware of each other's differences, while acknowledging that they must cooperate as a team. What should matter are the medical credentials, the ability to team up, the dedication and commitment, and the cultural and language skills as required by the workplace, not skin color, religion, race or ethnicity. Workers are expected to respect, accept, and value each other, and work as a care team that shares one common goal, to always provide a new patient with the chance to survive a complicated health problem. Finally, in the workplace the interests of the patient should be (and are) of paramount importance and should remain the focus of the team members at all times.

Creating a Culture of Safety

Patients should remain safe and have high satisfaction after surgery. Therefore, some strategies such as time-outs, turn over times, safety measures check, and checklists should be applied to increase patient's safety.

Time-out is a very necessary tool that will help in preventing adverse events. It is important that one member of the team is reading patient's information while the rest of the team quietly listens attentively. All team members, anesthesia provider, surgeon, and circulating nurse should comply with the time-out. Time-outs are mandated by the Joint Commission and all hospitals should ensure that they are being performed. Based on the Joint Commission, the content of a time-out should include verifying the correct patient, the correct site, the correct side, and patient positioning during surgery. Some institutions even include antibiotics and venous thromboembolism prophylaxis in their time-outs.

Safety measure checks should be performed by the entire healthcare team and not be limited to the OR nurses. No one should assume it is the other's responsibility. It is the responsibility of the team (anesthesiologist, surgeon, supportive staff, and nurse) to verify that safety measures are being applied, such as proper positioning and proper padding of a patient during surgery.

Another way to reinforce the culture of safety is to create standard checklist [7]. A well-designed and consistently implemented checklist can be lifesaving. A standard checklist can improve clinical outcomes, prevent mistakes, and help prepare the OR for surgery in a timely fashion. Examples of checklists include a surgical safety checklist, a preoperative checklist, and an OR cleaning checklist. See Box 6.1.

Box 6.1. Preanesthesia Induction Checklist

Patient has had no food or drink for the appropriate time period

Patient drug allergies and drug interactions are noted

Suction is working

Upper airway status has been evaluated

Anesthesia workstation can provide ventilation with 100 percent oxygen under positive pressure

Audible and visual alarms are set appropriately

Emergency drugs are present in the room

Drugs are drawn up into labelled syringes

Anesthetic vaporizers are connected

Intravenous access is functional

Sterile needles and syringes are on hand

Laryngoscope, tracheal tubes, and suction apparatus are on hand

Monitors are functioning with appropriate waveforms

NPO status and aspiration risk confirmed

Source: Date from [8].

Promotion and Hiring

Promotion and hiring are two ways to select an OR manager. Whether recruiting an OR manager from the outside or promoting an inside staff member, there are advantages and disadvantages to both. When choosing an OR manager, some types of administration opt for outsourcing. Their reasoning is that someone new to the site might bring new experiences and sometimes more credentials; moreover, the outsourced staff could at first be more respected by employees who expected some positive change from the actual administration. However, such an option can drive a negative reaction from staff members who may have career leadership aspirations. They might perceive this as an obstacle to advancement opportunities and, as a result, might quit in an effort to find a better place where their career leadership goal can be fulfilled.

Promotion, however, seems like the most natural approach for filling a leadership position. First, new OR managers who are former employees know the system well. They know how to get things done well without taking a long time to learn workplace procedures. Second, their strengths and weaknesses are well known by staff members who have already worked with them. Third, the staff knows about the new manager's characteristic dedication, professionalism, reliability, and cooperation at work. Fourth, an inside promotion can stimulate other employees who will perceive the leader as a role model. As a result, they may perform better at work to try and follow the leader's steps in an administrative role.

Simulation Training for Safety and Team Building

Many errors in the OR have been caused by failure in nontechnical skills and teamwork. As discussed earlier, unintended harm to patients has been a major cause of poor outcomes for surgical patients and often reflects failure of teamwork. Multiple groups of providers such as nurses, surgeons, and anesthesiologists, each with their own training and group philosophy, may limit effective team building. In addition to technical skills, cognitive and interpersonal communication skills, teamwork is currently considered an integral part of patient safety and efficiency in the OR.

Simulation has been used successfully for teaching and improving technical skills across all disciplines of medicine. Likewise, and most recently, multidisciplinary simulation has been used for training team skills. The multidisciplinary approach adds realism to patient case scenarios and prompts realistic responses. Many studies on multidisciplinary onsite simulation training to improve teamwork in the OR have shown more effective teamwork and communication, leading to improved culture [3, 4]. This type of training has also increased situational awareness, leadership skills, and decision making resulting in increased patient–staff satisfaction [9]. Multidisciplinary training can take place in the simulation center, at the point of care (or off-site) and may employ high- and low-fidelity equipment. Simulation is an attempt to recreate the OR atmosphere in which training is most likely to be transferable to the clinical setting. Feedback to the employees who have undergone simulation training is a very important feature of simulation training. It can be in the form of video recordings or verbal feedback but regardless of the format used, educating the team members is the overall goal. The scenarios used for team training should be tailored to the conditions and experiences of that specific healthcare institution. Simulation training has also been used to identify errors during the implementation of new technology and techniques. Improved clinical teamwork has a strong correlation with lowered patient mortality and increased work morale [4, 10, 11].

Conclusion

It is not only the diverse skill sets of the team members who are important to OR function but also the ways in which these team members work together. It is important that the team members value working together with a positive attitude that is sustained over time. The OR director or manager plays an instrumental role in the maintenance of employee attitudes, motivation, and productivity. Educational intervention is the most important step to improve teamwork, communication skills, and patient care. OR directors and managers must strive to guide the attitudes of the team members toward cohesive work and help them understand the importance of the working team concept and its sustainability. Diversity is an important component of every workplace, including the OR. It is crucial for leaders and coworkers to be aware of their fellow coworker's diversity and potential diverse needs. The leaders of healthcare teams have an opportunity to create an accepting and empathetic environment that fosters the uniqueness of each employee, while at the same time encouraging everyone to work together as a team regardless of differences. If employees are able to put differences aside and focus on patient care, the team will produce better outcomes, both for patient satisfaction and for employee satisfaction.

References

1. A. Bleakley, J. Allard, A. Hobbs, "Towards culture change in the operating theatre: Embedding a complex educational intervention to improve teamwork climate," *Med. Teach.*, vol. 34, no. 9, pp. e635–e640, Sep. 2012.

2. C. Dodge, "The role of the medical director," *Ambul. Surg.*, vol. 12, no. 1, pp. 7–9, May 2005.

3. T. C. Tsai, E. J. Orav, and A. K. Jha, "Patient satisfaction and quality of surgical care in US hospitals," *Ann. Surg.*, vol. 261, no. 1, p. 2, Jan. 2015.

4. G. D. Sacks, E. M. Shannon, A. J. Dawes, et al. "Teamwork, communication and safety climate: A systematic review of interventions to improve surgical culture," *BMJ Qual. Saf.*, vol. 24, no. 7, pp. 458–67, Jul. 2015.

5. L. Picco, Q. Yuan, J. A. Vaingankar, et al. "Positive mental health among health professionals working at a psychiatric hospital," *PLoS One*, vol. 12, no. 6, p. e0178359, 2017.

6. J. Sorensen, M. Norredam, N. Dogra, M.-L. Essink-Bot, J. Suurmond, A. Krasnik, "Enhancing cultural

competence in medical education," *Int. J. Med. Educ.*, vol. 8, pp. 28–30, Jan. 2017.

7. A. S. Al-Qahtani, "The surgical safety checklist: Results of implementation in otorhinolaryngology," *Oman Med. J.*, vol. 32, no. 1, pp. 27–30, Jan. 2017.

8. D. Wetmore, A. Goldberg, N. Gandhi, J. Spivack, P. McCormick, S. DeMaria, "An embedded checklist in the Anesthesia Information Management System improves pre-anaesthetic induction setup: A randomised controlled trial in a simulation setting," *BMJ Qual. Saf.*, vol. 25, no. 10, pp. 739–46, Oct. 2016.

9. N. E. Epstein, "Multidisciplinary in-hospital teams improve patient outcomes: A review," *Surg. Neurol. Int.*, vol. 5, no. 7, pp. S295–303, 2014.

10. S. Espin, W. Levinson, G. Regehr, G. R. Baker, L. Lingard, "Error or 'act of God'? A study of patients' and operating room team members' perceptions of error definition, reporting, and disclosure," *Surgery*, vol. 139, no. 1, pp. 6–14, Jan. 2006.

11. S. B. Tan, G. Pena, M. Altree, G. J. Maddern, "Multidisciplinary team simulation for the operating theatre: A review of the literature," *ANZ J. Surg.*, vol. 84, no. 7–8, pp. 515–22, Jul. 2014.

Chapter

7

Disruptions in Surgery

David S. Silver and Douglas P. Slakey

Introduction

Medical errors continue to be a significant cause of injury and death. In the United States, it is estimated that medical errors result in 44,000–98,000 unnecessary deaths each year and over one million unintentional injuries [1]. Sentinel events are unanticipated outcomes resulting in death or serious physical or psychological harm, unrelated to the presenting disease. While sentinel events are the errors that make the headlines, such as wrong site or wrong patient surgery, the majority of medical errors are less dramatic, may even escape notice, and do not always translate directly into an adverse outcome [2, 3]. These small errors are frequently the result of system errors and deficiencies rather the mistakes of individuals. The Institute of Medicine's reports on quality in healthcare delivery, *To Err Is Human* and *Crossing the Quality Chasm*, describe designing systems with an emphasis on human factors and safety [3, 4]. These principles have been the center of many recent research efforts. The focus of error prevention continues to shift away from individual mistakes to systemic failures and system inadequacies.

In a complex setting such as the operating room (OR), gathering meaningful data for quality improvement is a challenge. Recently, surgical flow disruptions (SFD) have been used as a proxy measurement to understand better how to improve current systems. The goals of this chapter are to summarize how human factors apply in the context of surgery, to define and describe previous research into SFD, and to offer strategies to start to manage disruptions in the OR.

Human Factors in Surgery

Human factors is a discipline that explores the interface between humans and the systems in which they work. The field includes the study, design, implementation, and testing of environments and processes to ensure safe, effective, and efficient use to accomplish an intended goal. Concerning healthcare, human factors research focuses on maximizing human performance and efficiency, to promote health, safety, comfort, and quality of life for not only patients but also practitioners [5]. There are three fundamental principles to keep in mind when evaluating systems based approaches to medical errors: (1) human error is unavoidable, (2) defective systems allow human error to cause harm to the patient, and (3) systems can be designed to prevent or detect failure before actual harm to the patient occurs [6]. With these principles in mind, there have been many different frameworks and strategies established to build and improve on existing systems. One widely applied and cited model that helps to conceptualize a complex system is Reason's Swiss Cheese Model.

British psychologist James Reason pioneered the modern field of systems analysis with his famous and widely studied "Swiss Cheese" model. Reason presented this model an explanation of preventable error. The model explains that every step in a process has the potential to contribute to systemic failure. The slices represent multiple layers of defense while the holes that make up Swiss cheese are systemic shortcomings. An error, when the holes in different layers align, perfectly penetrates all defensive layers. In summary, most accidents or adverse outcomes result from the combined effect of many smaller errors due to underlying system flaws that when aligned lead to disastrous consequences [7, 8]. A major aspect to understand in this model is that the holes (errors) will always exist; therefore, it is important to provide multiple layers of defense to decrease the chance of alignment, allowing individual errors to amass and result in an adverse outcome. This model also relates to the idea of failure mode and effects analysis.

The Swiss Cheese Model has been extended to include the concepts of active and latent failures. Active failures are unsafe acts committed by humans, typically by accident, with an immediate negative impact [9]. An example of an active failure in surgery would be an unintentional ligation of an artery. A latent failure is the result of circumstances, deficiencies, or holes in the system. An example of a latent factor could be improper labeling of a medication vial that eventually leads to incorrect dose administration. What makes latent failures particularly dangerous is that the impact may not be immediately apparent. A latent failure may only become apparent once an adverse outcome has occurred and is recognized. The OR provides an environment and opportunity to study latent failures due to the inherent complexity and acuity of activity that routinely takes place.

Despite representing only 1.9–3.6 percent of all hospitalizations, surgery represents 46–65 percent of all adverse events [10, 11]. ORs are complex, high-stress environments that challenge systems design for many reasons. First, each OR has a different personnel dynamic with multiple care teams such as nursing, anesthesia, and surgery. Further complicating this is the fact that each individual member of the team has different training, varying immediate goals, different measures of productivity and success, and yet all members are expected to work seamlessly in a tight setting [12]. In addition to diverse team members in the OR during a single procedure, the hospital operating area likely houses multiple specialties. High patient volume and turnover with many different specialties, each with their unique configurations, and confounded by personnel frequently coming in and out of the OR, create a complex daily environment.

In addition to personnel complexities, the actual working environmental plays a role in surgery performance and outcomes. For example, Spaghetti syndrome, a term used to describe the congestion created by wires, cables, and lines is a typical scenario first described in the intensive care unit [13]. An environment with complex technical equipment that is often not be well organized illustrates an accident waiting to happen. In addition, clutter, noise, temperature, and lighting have all been demonstrated to play a role in surgical outcomes.

It is self-evident that the OR has the potential to be an incredibly high-stress environment. There is clear evidence that excessive levels of stress have an effect on outcomes in surgical performance. Quantitative and qualitative studies have recognized stress as an essential component of surgical performance [14]. In addition to environment, communication, and team dynamics, interruptions and distractions are frequently a factor in surgical systems failure.

Both active and latent errors occur in the OR. Active failures usually are identified quickly as they become evident and are typically straightforward to measure. In contrast, investigators and quality improvement teams are challenged with how to measure, characterize, and quantify systemic issues and potential latent errors. In order to properly measure latent errors, teams often utilize proxy measurements that operationalize different hard to measure components of systems, such as SFD.

Flow Disruptions

Mihaly Csikszentmihalyi first described the concept of flow. Csikszentmihalyi wrote that flow is that state of optimal experience when individuals or groups are fully immersed in the task in front of them, leading to optimal production in that particular situation [15]. Individuals are so absorbed that nothing outside seems to matter [15, 16]. This state is colloquially known as being "in the zone," and the theory describes that performance is at its peak when the state of flow is reached. When in the state of flow, individuals operate at their personal capacity [16]. To reach a state of flow, there must be a balance between the task, the skill of the individual or team, and the environment. Flow has been tied to performance and is explained by improved concentration and intrinsic motivation. Although not explicitly stated, the idea of flow can also be connected to mindfulness or being fully present and attentive in the task or moment. Practices that emphasize being fully present and reaching one's "flow" have been linked to better clinical decision making, with due attention to present moment, improved clinician mental health, and reduced burnout.

As a complex activity, surgery possesses natural flow when procedures progress with ease and fluidity.

Csikszentmihalyi even mentions the field of surgery specifically in his writing about how performers involved in demanding tasks with critical implications can reach flow [17]. Wiegmann et al. defines SFD as deviations from this natural fluidity of a procedure that can thereby potentially compromise the safety of the operation [18]. Flow disruptions provide a proxy measurement for quality and safety by operationalizing latent errors. Also, application of the previous concepts show that flow disruptions represent barriers to optimal performance and can lead to increased intraoperative stress and increased mental workload. Individual flow disruptions may not lead to an adverse outcome, but the accumulation of disruptions may highlight the process and system holes that could lead to error.

The significance of flow disruptions and their relationship to quality has been explored. Some studies have looked at the nature and frequency of SFD. In 2006 Healey et al. looked to quantify flow disruptions in urology procedures. A trained observer recorded a mean of .45 event per minute and found most of the distractions to be related to team communication, equipment or environmental issues, and procedural challenges. This study also found disruptions relating to outside or case irrelevant conversations, work environment issues, telephone calls, and equipment failures. Healey found discussions to be the most frequent and severe interruptions in their observed procedures [19]. Healey and colleagues later examined distractions and interruptions during fifty general surgical procedures. They defined disruptions as a break in attention, evidenced by observed behavior. The interruptions were characterized by a rating system from least severe or potentially distracting (1) to a completion interruption (9). The team recorded phone calls, beepers, communications with external staff and other noise of varying volumes that may have influenced teamwork in OR and outcomes [20].

In 2007, Wiegmann and team also explored disruptions in surgical flow. The team also recorded errors and disruptions in flow during 31 cardiac procedures. These recordings were classified and analyzed by a team of human factors experts. Similar to Healey's findings, Wiegmann found the flow disruptions to be mostly related to communication or communication breakdown. In fact, 52 percent of the disruptions were related to teamwork or communication, and the number of disruptions was the strongest predictor of error. An example of communication breakdown provided in this study was "surgeon was under the impression that the patient had been given x when x had not been given." Wiegmann found that there was a correlation between rate of errors and SFD. Specifically, the relationship was significant for disruptions classified under teamwork or communication errors. This was one of the earlier studies to present the empirical link between flow disruptions and OR errors [18].

Building on the previous work, in 2010 Parker and her team developed and validated a tool to categorize latent errors that may lead to adverse outcomes. The tool provides a tested framework to categorize "precursor events" and help teams to design their own interventions to reduce error through system diagnosis and improvement. The tool was validated and demonstrated to be simple and clear for observers of diverse academic backgrounds to use [21].

Catchpole expanded the scope of the topic to look outside the OR and to include trauma patients and handoffs [22]. They found that for trauma patients, the most common flow disruptions were coordination issues and communication failures, which is consistent with previous studies. They analyzed flow disruptions during care transitions that patients experience during trauma care. By studying 181 trauma patients, they found that 42 percent experienced at least one disruption during the transition of care and 53 percent of the disruptions were related to poor coordination of care. Disruptions included: patient taken to the incorrect room, critical team members missing, and imaging equipment occupied, all resulting in a delay of care. One important finding presented in this study was that the sicker, more acute patients had less standardized handoffs, and more flow disruptions, despite not having an increased number of handoffs [22].

One gap in the current literature is the question of to what extent individual OR team members recognize and perceive OR flow disruptions. Silver et al. performed a survey of over 100 staff members from three academic institutions using the validated tools described. Sixty-five percent of respondents acknowledged that flow disruptions happen either several times a day or every procedure and 40 percent of respondents ranked poor communication between teams to be the most frequent cause of SFD. Finally, respondents felt that staff burnout, patient safety, and economic consequences were the most significant consequences of repeated flow disruptions [23]. Consistently throughout the literature, authors note that flow disruptions in surgery are common and in and of themselves do not indicate a failure. Furthermore, flow disruptions may or may not be significant in causing adverse outcomes due to an overwhelming number of variables within an OR. The challenge for researchers and those charged with improving outcomes effectiveness is accurately measuring and categorizing flow disruptions to further understand where individual processes may have holes.

Opportunities for Leadership and Improvement

Understanding the concept of SFD provides an opportunity for improvement when applied with the goal to improving OR systems. The first step is to quantify and categorize SFD with the validated tools previously mentioned. The information gathered with these tools can be used to help improve operations and also provide a foundation for understanding factors leading latent failures and adverse events [21].

In addition to measurement, one strategy that has been explored to decrease SFD is an approach borrowed from aviation called "sterile cockpit." In commercial aviation, the sterile cockpit is that time from 0 to 10,000 feet and vice versa. A sterile cockpit protocol is activated when critical periods of a procedure are occurring. The sterile cockpit concept ensures that during critical times, all communication or movement is restricted to essential information. Once the critical period is over, everything else can resume. This has been explored by teams in cardiothoracic operating. In contrast to aviation, there is generally no discrete period, such as takeoff or landing, during a surgical operation; therefore, to successfully implement a sterile cockpit protocol, the OR team would have to identify high risk or high mental workload tasks, or critical time intervals [24]. To achieve this, communication and training are essential.

Team huddles, briefings, and debriefs are opportunities to look at one or multiple cases for a particular team and have a discussion as a unit. The huddle can be used in the OR to improve situational awareness, to bring up potential issues or high-risk factors, to identified factors which could contribute to error or adverse outcomes, and to initiate actions for future procedures. A daily huddle has been shown to improve team satisfaction and decrease interruptions and delays [25].

Conclusion

Strengthening systems to support people working within the OR environment is essential if meaningful and sustainable improvements in outcomes and effectiveness are to be achieved. Transient, "feel good" fixes do little to address underlying causes of error and adverse outcomes, but are typically the focus of management because they are easy. Understanding *SFD* and the relationship to *latent and active errors* assists teams responsible for systems change to characterize, measure, and assess the existing work environment and proposed and implemented systems changes. The next decade is sure to witness dramatic advancements in systems engineering in complex healthcare delivery environments such as the OR. The application of artificial intelligence to this field will make error and outcome analysis, including analysis of SFD, more powerful than ever, resulting in systems that better support the people working to ensure patient outcomes are the best possible.

References

1. Weingart SN, Wilson RM, Gibberd RW, Harrison B. Epidemiology of medical error. *BMJ*. 2000;320: 774–7.

2. Leape LL. Error in medicine. *JAMA*. 1994;272:1851–7.

3. Kohn LT, Corrigan JM, Molla S. To err is human. *Medicine (Baltimore)*. 1999;126:312.

4. Institute of Medicine (US) Committee on Quality of Health Care in America. *Crossing the Quality Chasm. A New Health System for the 21st Century*. Washington, DC: National Academies Press, 2001.

5. Sanders MS, McCormick EJ. Human error, accidents, and safety. *Hum. Factors Eng. Des.* 1993:655–95.

6. Etchells E, O'Neill C, Bernstein M. Patient safety in surgery: Error detection and prevention. *World J. Surg.* 2003:936–41.

7. Reason J. Human error – Models and management. *BMJ*. 2000;320:768–70.

8. Reason J. *Human Error*. Cambridge: Cambridge University Press, 1990, 1056–7.

9. Wiegmann DA, Shappell SAS. A human error analysis of commercial aviation accidents using the Human Factors Analysis and Classification System (HFACS). *Aviat. Space Environ. Med.* 2001;72:1–17.

10. Zegers M, de Bruijne MC, de Keizer B, et al. The incidence, root-causes, and outcomes of adverse events in surgical units: implication for potential prevention strategies. *Patient Saf. Surg.* 2011;5:13.

11. Gawande AA, Thomas EJ, Zinner MJ, Brennan TA. The incidence and nature of surgical adverse events in Colorado and Utah in 1992. *Surgery*. 1999;126:66–75.

12. Catchpole K, Mishra A, Handa A, McCulloch P. Teamwork and error in the operating room: Analysis of skills and roles. *Ann Surg*. 2008;247:699–706.

13. Cesarano FL, Piergeorge AR. The Spaghetti syndrome. A new clinical entity. *Crit. Care Med*. 1979;7:182–3.

14. Arora S, Sevdalis N, Nestel D, Woloshynowych M, Darzi A, Kneebone R. The impact of stress on surgical performance: A systematic review of the literature. *Surgery*. 2010;318–30.

15. Csikszentmihalyi M. *Flow: The Psychology of Optimal Experience*. New York: Harper & Row, 1990.

16. Mirvis PH. Flow: The psychology of optimal experience. *Acad. Manag. Rev*. 1991;16:636–40.

17. Nakamura J, Csikszentmihalyi M. The concept of flow. *Posit. Psychol. Collect. Work*. 2014: 239–63.

18. Wiegmann DA, ElBardissi AW, Dearani JA, Daly RC, Sundt TM. Disruptions in surgical flow and their relationship to surgical errors: An exploratory investigation. *Surgery*. 2007;142:658–65.

19. Healey AN, Sevdalis N, Vincent CA. Measuring intra-operative interference from distraction and interruption observed in the operating theatre. *Ergonomics*. 2006;49:589.

20. Healey AN, Olsen S, Davis R, Vincent CA. A method for measuring work interference in surgical teams. *Cogn. Technol. Work*. 2008;10:305–12.

21. Parker SEH, Laviana AA, Wadhera RK, Wiegmann DA, Sundt TM. Development and evaluation of an observational tool for assessing surgical flow disruptions and their impact on surgical performance. *World J. Surg*. 2010;34:353–61.

22. Catchpole KR, Gangi A, Blocker RC, et al. Flow disruptions in trauma care handoffs. *J. Surg. Res*. 2013;184:586–91.

23. Silver D, Kaye A, Cornett E, Fox C, Slakey D. Disruptions in surgical workflow: Perceptions and implications. Poster presentation. *J. Am. Coll. Surg.*, 2017;225:108.

24. Wadhera RK, Parker SH, Burkhart HM, et al. Is the "sterile cockpit" concept applicable to cardiovascular surgery critical intervals or critical events? The impact of protocol-driven communication during cardiopulmonary bypass. *J. Thorac. Cardiovasc. Surg*. 2010;139:312–9.

25. Jain AL, Jones KC, Simon J, Patterson MD. The impact of a daily pre-operative surgical huddle on interruptions, delays, and surgeon satisfaction in an orthopedic operating room: a prospective study. *Patient Saf. Surg*. 2015;9:8.

Chapter

8

Influence of Operating Room Staffing and Scheduling on Operating Room Productivity

Franklin Dexter and Richard H. Epstein

Definitions

Vocabulary is an important part of understanding research in operating room (OR) management [1]. Paradoxically, it is not possible to search the OR management literature successfully using PubMed without first knowing the corresponding vocabulary [1]. When people refer to "efficiency," but what they really mean is "make more money," then their search will not find the papers about what they truly care about [1]. Precise vocabulary matters, just like for drug names and anatomy [1].

Staff Scheduling and Assignment

Staff scheduling is the process of deciding which nurses, anesthesia providers, and other personnel work each shift on each day. Staff scheduling for a future date usually is performed before the surgical cases to be performed on that date have been scheduled.

For example, the OR nurses create their work schedule two months in advance. Ms. Jamison and Mr. Green are scheduled to work 8 a.m. to 4 p.m. on March 8.

Staffed hours are the hours into which cases are scheduled (e.g., 7 a.m. to 3 p.m.).

Staff assignment is the process of deciding who will take care of patients in a given location on a specific day. Most assignments are typically made on the workday prior to the date of surgery.

For example, tomorrow, Dr. Waters will be supervising two Certified Registered Nurse Anesthetists (CRNAs) in ORs 9 and 10.

Elective, Urgent, and Emergent Cases

We are not aware of any one best answer as to what constitutes an elective, urgent, or emergent case [2]. Still, differentiating among such cases is necessary to plan staffing. The following is a set of reasonable definitions that provide for different operational decisions.

An *elective case* can be defined as one for which the patients can wait at least 3 days for surgery without sustaining additional morbidity [3]. The choice of 3 days corresponds to patients waiting from Friday to Monday. At a facility with patients scheduled for elective surgery on Saturdays, two days would be used as the threshold.

For example, shoulder arthroplasty and breast biopsy cases are elective.

An *emergent case* can be defined as one for which the patient is likely to sustain additional morbidity and/or mortality unless the surgical care is started in less time than needed for a team to be called in from home. In this context, "likely" to have a worse outcome means based on scientific studies, such as published observational studies. Through the use of this evidence-based definition, the appropriateness of the relevant staffing decision can be made by reviewing data on prior emergent cases [3].

For example, cesarean sections because of a prolapsed umbilical cord or placental abruption are emergent.

An *urgent case* is defined as one for which the safe waiting time lies between that of an emergency and an elective case [3]. Almost all nonelective cases are urgent cases.

For example, appendectomy is an urgent case. The procedure is not an emergency, because the patient can wait long enough for an OR team to come to the hospital from home. A cadaveric renal transplant would also be urgent, not emergent for the same reason.

From a practical viewpoint, sufficient staff need to be present in-house to deal with emergent cases, whereas providing staff who take calls from home to cover urgent cases that cannot be covered by the in-house call team is a viable approach. The cost differential between having sufficient staff in-house to handle urgent cases vs. having them taking calls from home can be considerable [3, 4]. Planning sufficient staffing for the urgent cases is important. Surgical procedures for patients who are inpatients preoperatively generally represent urgent cases. Delaying surgery and thereby increasing hospital length of stay is counterproductive [5, 6].

Definitions Related to Service-Specific Staffing

Surgical service refers to a group of surgeons who share allocated OR time (i.e., service-specific staffing). An individual surgeon, a group, a specialty, or a department can function as a surgical service, depending on how OR time is allocated. *Service* simply refers to the unit of OR allocation.

For example, two ORs are allocated to the urological surgeons practicing at a hospital, any of whom can schedule cases in these rooms daily. Then, "Urology" is a service.

For example, two general surgeons are partners in General Surgical Associates (GSA), one of two independent general surgery groups that practice at a hospital. If these two general surgeons are together allocated OR time, then they represent a service, "GSA."

For example, a busy orthopedic surgeon, Dr. Bones, is personally allocated 8 h of OR time every Tuesday. Then, from the perspective of allocating OR time and scheduling cases on Tuesdays, that "Dr. Bones" represents a surgical service, even though there may also be an "Ortho" service. The service-specific staffing is that one OR for 8 h every Tuesday.

Even when a surgical suite does not have a formal organizational plan for allocating ORs (i.e., "block schedule"), there can be service-specific staffing (i.e., OR allocations). In this regard, "services" need not be specific clinical subspecialties in the medical staff organizational structure. Rather, they reflect the activities of individuals or groups of surgeons who use the OR facilities and thus require organized staffing to support those activities. In some circumstances, several disparate subspecialties (e.g., "oral surgery" and "plastic surgery") may share allocated OR time and thus function as a service.

For example, an 8-OR surgical suite has the official policy that all of its cases are scheduled on a first-scheduled, first-served basis. However, in reality, cases of the same specialty usually are scheduled into the same ORs, since this simplifies the distribution of resources (e.g., surgical equipment, video towers) and assignment of nursing and anesthesia teams who specialize in the area of surgical practice. Some nurses preferentially care for patients undergoing neurosurgery and otolaryngology cases, some mostly gynecology or general surgery, and so forth. In this case, the services correspond to the specialty teams.

Allocated OR time is the interval of OR time with a specified start and end time on a specified day of the week that is assigned by the facility to a surgical service for scheduling cases (Figure 8.1). Allocated OR time is effectively the same thing as staffed hours, but often the phrase "staffed hours" is used to refer to the sum of multiple services' allocated OR time. Some facilities have OR time that is staffed and available for cases, but not allocated to a specific service. Such OR time has been allocated to a "pseudo-service," variably named the "Open," "Unblocked," "First-Scheduled, First-Served," or "Other" service. Knowing the allocated time for a service on a day of the week quantitatively describes the minimum anesthesia and nursing capacity for the surgeons. This is in contrast to "block time" that effectively predicts whether a surgeon will have many hours of cases on some future data.

For example, Urology is allocated OR time in two rooms from 7 a.m. to 4 p.m. on Monday to Friday. This does not mean that the department's surgeons are limited to scheduling cases only if they can be completed by 4 p.m. Instead, it means that staffing has been *planned* for the department's surgeons between 7 a.m. and 4 p.m. The definition applies whether or not at that hospital it happens that the department's surgeons actually finish by 4 p.m. If the urology service's cases run past 4 p.m., and if nursing and anesthesia teams were to plan its staff scheduling to match the allocated OR time, then they would need to work beyond the end of regularly scheduled hours.

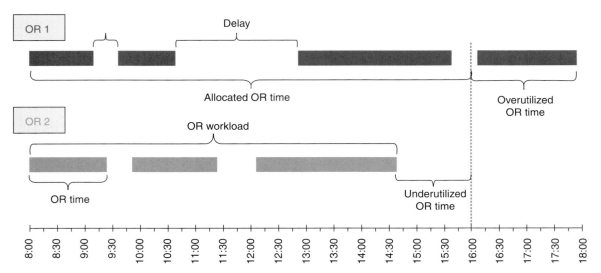

Figure 8.1 An example of an OR schedule.

OR time of a case is defined as the interval from when a patient enters an OR until that patient leaves the OR (i.e., "wheels-in" to "wheels-out"). This definition is used often because these events are unequivocal and thus have good interrater reliability. The use of anesthesia information management systems to provide such data automatically can make OR management easier [7].

Turnover time is the time from when one patient exits an OR until the next patient on that day's OR schedule enters the same OR [8, 9]. Separating turnover time from the OR time of a case permits the two to be studied statistically as separate processes (see "Impact of Reducing Surgical and Turnover Times"). Cleanup times and setup time characteristically are recorded separately from OR times, and then combined. In part, this is because it is hard to define when cleanup has ceased and setup has begun for the next case, and these activities may overlap. Turnover times include cleanup times and setup times, but should exclude planned or unplanned delays between cases (e.g., when a to-follow surgeon is given a scheduled 12:30 p.m. start time and the prior case in the OR ended at 11:00 a.m., or if the second of third cases in an OR cancels and the third patient is not available; see Figure 8.1). Hospital surgical suites may consider times between cases that are longer than a defined interval (e.g., 90 min) to represent delays, not turnovers, when computing turnover times to focus statistics on the latter cleanup and setup times [8].

This is because it is difficult to determine retrospectively the cause of such outliers, and these are usually unrelated to the process of room setup and cleanup. It is common for hospital analysts to ignore this distinction, resulting in invalid estimates of the actual turnover time and its variance.

For example, staffing is planned from 7 a.m. to 3 p.m. A patient arrived at the holding area at 7:45 a.m., her intravenous catheter was placed at 7:50 a.m., she entered the OR at 7:59 a.m., the trachea was intubated at 8:12 a.m., the operative site was prepared at 8:15 a.m., and the incision was made at 8:23 a.m. The patient left the OR at 10:59 a.m. From the perspective of OR scheduling, the case started at 7:59 a.m. The OR time of the case was 3 h.

For example, a surgeon is scheduled to perform a hepatic resection. However, soon after incision, the patient is found, unexpectedly, to have widespread peritoneal metastases and the incision is closed without performing the planned procedure. The patient exits from his OR 2.5 h earlier than planned. Including a planned 0.5-h turnover, the second case of the day could start 3 h earlier than planned. However, the second case of the day in that OR will be performed by a different surgeon. He is unavailable, caring for patients in his outpatient office. The result is a delay of 3 h. That delay should not contribute to the calculation of turnover times.

OR workload for a service is its total hours of cases including turnover times (Figure 8.1). This excludes the urgent cases for that service if separate OR time is allocated for urgent cases performed by all services. Turnover times are applied, by convention, to the service performing the prior case in the OR. Thus, there is no turnover time for the last case of the day in the OR.

Underutilized OR time = [allocated OR time] – [OR workload], or zero if this value is negative (Figure 8.1) [10]. This means that underutilized OR time equals the allocated OR time minus the OR workload, provided the allocated OR time is larger than the OR workload. Otherwise, the underutilized OR time is 0 h. Thus, underutilized OR time represents the time for which staffing was planned, but no work was performed. This equation applies only when the allocated OR time is calculated based on minimizing the inefficiency of use of OR time, defined several paragraphs below.

Adjusted utilization = 100% × (1 – [underutilized OR time] ÷ [allocated OR time]) [9]

For example, staffing is planned from 8 a.m. to 4 p.m. An OR's last case of the day ends at 2 p.m. The OR workload is 6 h. There are 2 h of underutilized OR time. The adjusted utilization is 75 percent, where 75% = 100% × (1–2 h / 8 h) [9]. The maximum value of "adjusted utilization" is 100 percent.

Overutilized OR time = [OR workload] – [allocated OR time], or zero if this value is negative (Figure 8.1) [10]. Thus, overutilized OR time represents the time during which work was performed, but staffing was not planned in advance. The adjusted utilization ignores overutilized OR time, which is one of the reasons why utilization is not a useful metric for facilities that typically do not finish the OR schedule prior to the end of allocated OR time. This equation applies only when the allocated OR time is calculated based on minimizing the inefficiency of use of OR time.

For example, an OR is staffed from 8:30 a.m. to 6 p.m. The last case of the day in the OR ends at 8 p.m. Then, there are 2 hours of overutilized OR time.

Inefficiency of use of OR time = [(cost per hour of underutilized OR time) × (hours of underutilized OR time)] + [(cost per hour of overutilized OR time) × (hours of overutilized OR time)] [10–12]. The cost of an hour of overutilized OR time is always more expensive than the cost of an hour of underutilized OR time. This equation, the one for underutilized OR time, and the one for overutilized OR time collectively are the three simultaneous equations defining OR efficiency.

OR efficiency is the value that is maximized when the inefficiency of use of OR time has been minimized [10].

"Efficiency" is characteristically thought of as the ratio of an output to the necessary input. For example, in a factory producing widgets, efficiency can be the number of widgets produced divided by the labor cost of producing those widgets. Thus, efficiency could be increased by producing more widgets with the same number of workers, or the same number of widgets with fewer workers. In the OR setting, when surgeons and patients are provided open access to OR time on any future workday, the output (e.g., number of cases performed) is a constant (see "Tactical versus Operational OR Management Decisions"). One cannot "manufacture" more cases on the day of surgery. Maximizing "efficiency" then is achieved by minimizing the input. That occurs when service-specific staffing and case scheduling are so good that there are both 0 h of underutilized OR time and 0 h of overutilized OR time. In practice, this is an unachievable goal, due to variance in surgical times for identically scheduled cases. Thus, optimizing OR efficiency requires a managerial objective to minimize the total cost of the underutilized and overutilized OR time.

For example, Vascular Surgery is allocated two ORs every Friday. Why was this decision made? If the department's surgeons were allocated three ORs, then much of the OR time would be underutilized. That would reduce OR efficiency. If the department had been allocated one OR, then the surgeons would have been working late to finish their cases, resulting in much overutilized OR time. That would reduce OR efficiency. The choice of two ORs provided the best balance.

In our experience, this example provides what most facilities consider the objective of OR allocation, providing the right amount of OR time to get the cases done (i.e., not too much or too little). That is the essence of operational OR management decision making. This objective must be differentiated from the longer-term tactical stage of OR allocation, wherein an increase or reduction in allocated OR time is expected to result in a change in OR workload [13].

The example also shows why good operational decisions cannot be made based on OR utilization. True, OR allocation would not be three ORs, based on either OR efficiency or OR utilization, because there would be many hours of underutilized OR time. However, the choice of one or two ORs would not be clear based on OR utilization because the resulting hours of overutilized OR time are not included in the calculation of utilization (which, by definition, cannot be higher than 100%). In contrast, decision making based on OR efficiency considers both the expected underutilized and overutilized OR time. At facilities where there is substantial overutilized OR time, basing allocations on utilization statistics will have a large negative impact on OR efficiency.

For example, Dr. Sato is an orthopedic surgeon in a solo practice. She is allocated OR 1 on Mondays and Wednesdays for 10 h, from 7 a.m. to 5 p.m. Dr. Ho is another orthopedic surgeon in a solo practice. He is allocated OR 1 on Tuesdays and Thursdays for 10 h, also from 7 a.m. to 5 p.m. Both Drs. Sato and Ho consistently perform slightly less than 10 h of cases in their allocated OR time, virtually never more. Both perform spinal surgery cases. However, Dr. Sato tends to perform one more case of the same type as Dr. Ho within the allocated OR time because Dr. Sato operates much more quickly than Dr. Ho. OR efficiency is identical and unaffected by how quickly Dr. Sato operates (see continuation of the example at the end of this section).

Managerial Cost Accounting

Labor cost equals the sum of two products: staff scheduled hours multiplied by the cost per hour of staff scheduled hours and hours worked late multiplied by the cost per hour of hours worked late [14, 15]. More complicated managerial accounting models generally are not needed for purposes of OR allocation and case scheduling. Labor cost can generally be estimated as the sum of the allocated OR time multiplied by the cost per hour of staffed hours and the hours of overutilized OR time multiplied by the cost per hour of overutilized OR time.

OR productivity equals the OR workload divided by the labor costs [14].

For example, the only anesthesia service that a group provides at an outpatient surgery facility is OR anesthesia. Staffing is planned for five ORs from 7 a.m. to 5 p.m. There is virtually never any overutilized OR time. Then, each increase in OR workload (i.e., the cases performed) results in an increase in OR and anesthesia group productivity.

For example, a hospital has substantial underutilized OR time and substantial overutilized OR time. Recent increases in elective OR workload have resulted in cases finishing in the early evenings, resulting in increased overutilized OR time. The increase in OR workload could be reducing

OR productivity. That would be happening if the cost per hour of overutilized OR time is much higher than the cost per hour of regularly staffed hours.

Although it may seem good to make operational OR management decisions based on increasing OR productivity, we recommend against the approach. Instead, make operational OR management decisions to maximize OR efficiency. Usually the decisions will be the same, but not always [14].

We recommend decision making based on OR efficiency, for two reasons [2, 16]. First, whereas decisions based on OR efficiency are invariant to the perspective of the cost assessment, decisions based on labor cost are not. There is no one best answer as to whose labor costs should be used to make decisions. For example, although from the perspective of the anesthesia group, the ideal would be to make the decisions based on its labor costs, other reasonable options include the labor cost of the hospital or society. Second, labor costs vary depending on staff scheduling and staff assignment, whereas OR efficiency does not. If labor costs were used, distributed decision making would no longer be consistent depending on the perspective of who makes the decision. For example, if one CRNA works overtime to cover for another CRNA who has called in sick, that would affect decisions based on labor costs but would not affect decisions based on OR efficiency.

Revenue is the money received from third parties in return for having provided care for a specific patient.

Variable costs are costs that increase proportionate to the volume of patients receiving care [17].

For example, the amount of anesthetic medications used will vary with the number of patients who receive anesthesia care. Hence, pharmacy costs are variable costs.

Fixed costs are those costs that are not related to the volume of patients receiving care.

For example, the surgical tables cost the same regardless of how often they are used. Surgical tables are a fixed cost. For example, a new eight-OR ambulatory surgery center has virtually no overutilized OR time but considerable underutilized OR time. On a short-term basis, labor costs can be viewed as fixed. Even if OR workload increased moderately, all the cases would still be completed within allocated OR time. The number of OR nurses needed to staff the ORs would be unchanged. However, on a longer-term basis, labor costs could be reduced by closing an OR if the OR workload does not increase sufficiently.

Contribution margin equals revenue minus the variable costs for providing care to those patients. These include revenue and variable costs associated both with the current case and those related to subsequent care due to complications.

For example, consider the calculation of contribution margin for a colon resection in which the wound becomes infected. Revenue and variable costs need to be included due to the original surgery as well as the full hospitalization including three trips back to the OR to wash out the wound.

Profit equals revenue minus the sum of fixed and variable costs. This is the same as contribution margin minus fixed costs.

For example, let us return to the orthopedic surgeons, Drs. Sato and Ho, who were described previously. Dr. Sato performs one extra spinal surgery case in the same number of hours of OR time than does Dr. Ho. For the anesthesia group, Dr. Sato is more profitable than is Dr. Ho, because the anesthesia group gets more revenue for the same fixed costs of staffing the OR. However, the implants that Dr. Sato chooses cost 80 percent of the revenue while those that Dr. Ho chooses cost 50 percent of the revenue. Thus, for the hospital, Dr. Sato is less profitable than Dr. Ho [18]. Both still have a positive contribution margin, but only slightly so for Dr. Sato.

OR Efficiency on the Day of Surgery

OR efficiency is maximized by choosing staffing and scheduling cases to minimize the inefficiency of use of OR time, the latter being the [(cost per hour of underutilized OR time) × (hours of underutilized OR time)] + [(cost per hour of overutilized OR time) × (hours of overutilized OR time)]. If one considers the cost of one hour of overutilized time to one hour of underutilized time to be the fixed ratio, R (typically 1.5–2.0), the value to be minimized can be expressed in terms of hours: (hours of underutilized OR time) + R × (hours of overutilized OR time). This relationship is further simplified on the day of surgery.

At most surgical facilities, OR nurses are full-time hourly or salaried employees. Thus, on the day of surgery, the increment in nursing labor cost from 1 h of underutilized OR time is negligible relative to the cost from 1 h of overutilized OR time. Finishing cases early, but still before the end of staffed hours, reduces labor costs negligibly versus the labor cost that would result from a reduction in overutilized OR time. The

same applies to CRNAs and/or anesthesiologists who are employees of the surgical facility or corresponding anesthesia group.

Few anesthesiologists and CRNAs in private practice can earn enough money to cover the cost of their salary plus benefits unless they are scheduled to care for whatever patients may need urgent surgery (i.e., who are inpatient preoperatively [5, 6]), along with patients having elective, scheduled surgery. Thus, the incremental revenue lost on the day of surgery by having 1 h of underutilized OR time is negligible relative to the indirect/intangible costs from working late unexpectedly (i.e., the opportunity cost of being idle is effectively zero) [19, 20].

Consequently, on the day of surgery, the cost per hour of underutilized OR time is negligible relative to the cost per hour of overutilized OR time [2, 21]. Thus, on the day of surgery, minimizing the inefficiency of use of OR time (see "Definitions") requires only that management minimize the hours of overutilized OR time, since the cost per hour of this time is a constant [2, 21]. As explained below, "minimizing" on the day of surgery includes case and staff assignment decisions, as all cases are performed unless patient safety would be affected.

Case scheduling to maximize OR efficiency minimizes hours of overutilized OR time, as previously reported for surgical suites [22]. The following two scenarios illustrate the implications of the results.

For example, an anesthesiologist is assigned to an OR staffed from 7 a.m. to 3 p.m., but with one expected hour of overutilized OR time. The anesthesiologist works quickly. She places every intravenous catheter and arterial cannula on the first attempt and performs a fiber optic intubation in 10 min. Because of her rapid work, the cases finish at 3 p.m., preventing 1 h of overutilized OR time. Thus, the anesthesiologist increased OR efficiency [21].

A different anesthesiologist is assigned to another OR staffed from 7 a.m. to 3 p.m., but with 7 h of scheduled cases. The anesthesiologist works equally quickly, resulting in cases finishing at 2 p.m. instead of at 3 p.m. Because overutilized OR time was not reduced, the anesthesiologist did *not* increase OR efficiency [21].

These scenarios show that "working fast" is *not* synonymous with increasing OR efficiency. The last scenario of the preceding section showed that working fast is not synonymous with maximizing profit, either. Analogously, "working slowly" is *not* synonymous with decreasing OR efficiency. Sometimes, "working fast" may increase OR efficiency, and "working slowly" may decrease OR efficiency [2, 23]. But this will be entirely dependent on the circumstances.

For example, a different anesthesiologist is supervising resident physicians in two ORs. Staffing is planned from 8 a.m. to 4 p.m. The anesthesiologist needs to decide which of the two ORs to start first. One OR is scheduled with two cases from 8 a.m. to 6 p.m., the other with five cases from 8 a.m. to 3 p.m. To maximize OR efficiency, the anesthesiologist should first start the OR expected to have 2 h of overutilized OR time [21].

By following this simple principle, individual and collective decision making can be closely linked to enhancing OR efficiency. Without understanding the principles of OR efficiency, the anesthesiologist is likely to have made the opposite decision because there are more cases in the other OR.

The same principles and use of scenarios can be applied to housekeepers, OR nurses, managers, postanesthesia care unit nurses, etc. [2, 7, 12]. In essence, all decision making on the day of surgery that has "improving efficiency" as the goal revolves around this concept of reducing overutilized time. Again, working faster per se does *not* increase OR efficiency; rather, OR efficiency is increased only when working faster reduces overutilized time.

For example, staffing is planned from 7 a.m. to 3 p.m. Recently the hospital hired a new OR nurse. On Monday, she assisted in OR 12, resulting in cases finishing at 2 p.m. instead of 3 p.m. On Tuesday, she assisted in OR 14, resulting in cases finishing at 4 p.m. instead of 5 p.m. She increased OR efficiency more on Tuesday than Monday, because reducing 1 h of overutilized OR time increases OR efficiency more than does reducing 1 h of underutilized OR time.

Tactical versus Operational OR Management Decisions

Consider a common OR management problem: staffing is planned from 7 a.m. to 3 p.m. A surgeon has been allocated 8 h of OR time every Wednesday for years, and the hospital has an "official" policy that elective cases may only be scheduled into allocated time. The surgeon has always underestimated the OR times of his cases in order to bypass this constraint. He has never finished before 6 p.m. and usually ends between 7 and 8 p.m.

The anesthesiologists and OR nurses may complain about working late every Monday because the surgeon is being allowed to "overbook" his schedule. They may lobby to have a committee meet to rectify the situation. Simultaneously, the administrators may discuss the surgeons' lack of respect for rules and hospital resources. Nevertheless, physicians who refer their patients to the surgeon reward him by continuing to send him work because their patients are pleased with his expeditious service.

The fundamental issue is the surgeon's frequent misrepresentation of the estimated OR times of his cases, in order to get them onto the OR schedule [24]. The merits of the tactical issue (i.e., whether this is overall good or bad practice) have little relevance to OR productivity. The relevant operational decision is clear: managers should change staffing to match the reality of the existing workload [15]. Doing so neither increases nor reduces OR capacity or convenience for the surgeon and his or her patients. What it does is to reduce labor costs by reducing the hours worked late, since staff scheduling is adjusted based on staffed hours [14]. From the surgeon's perspective, the only thing that will change is that he can provide more realistic estimated OR times, since there will no longer be a need to "adjust" the times in order to get the cases running past the end of the regular workday on the schedule. From the perspective of the anesthesiologists and the OR nurses, complaints about working "late" will disappear, as the regular hours in the surgeon's OR now extend to 12 h, and staff working in that OR can expect to work for this period of time.

For example, when an anesthesiologist was hired, the job description said that work hours were 7 a.m. to 5 p.m., and he accepted a salary based on this assumption. Yet, every Wednesday for the past 5 years, the anesthesiologist has finished working between 7 p.m. and 8 p.m. Staffing is subsequently changed to be to 8 p.m. because that is the reality of the existing OR workload. Planning the staffing to 8 p.m. does not change the workload. Rather, it results in the work being planned long in advance.

In the two preceding scenarios, the surgeon and patient are choosing the day of surgery. Cases are not being turned away, provided they can be done safely, even if they will likely be performed in overutilized OR time [25]. Subject to that priority, OR time can be allocated based on maximizing OR efficiency. To describe operational reality, mathematics needs to be based on the surgeon and patient having open access to OR time on the workday of their choosing.

For example, all ORs are allocated at a hospital for 8 h. The adjusted utilizations range from 75 to 85 percent among the surgical services. Thus, there is essentially only underutilized OR time. At this hospital, allocating OR time based on OR efficiency would give precisely the same result as allocating OR time based on adjusted utilization. This is because virtually no OR ever finishes late. A zero has been substituted for the hours of overutilized OR time in the equation for the inefficiency of use of OR time (see "Inefficiency of Use of OR Time"). The surgeons can be considered to have open access to OR time on the workday of their choosing, and they have chosen to perform cases only when they can be completed within allocated hours.

The two preceding scenarios demonstrate that service-specific staffing can be considered for any facility when decisions are made based on OR efficiency and on surgeon and patient open access to OR time on any future workday. The next scenario shows that the assumption of fixed hours applies only to a minority of surgical suites [11].

For example, an ambulatory surgical center has a policy that OR time is allocated based on OR utilization. Staffing is planned from 7 a.m. to 3 p.m. This policy is enforced strictly. A surgeon asks to book a case to start at 1 p.m., with an expected (realistic) OR time for the case of 2.5 h. He is told "No," that would be unacceptable, because the case will likely end at 3:30 p.m.

The preceding scenario will seem unreal to most clinicians in the United States. That is the point. Only scheduling cases if they can reasonably be expected to finish by the end of allocated OR time is not the reality of short-term operational decision making at many facilities. Although considering a facility to have fixed hours of OR time is an accurate and practical model from a tactical perspective, it is not realistic for day-to-day decision making for all surgeons at a surgical suite [2, 25–27].

We return to the first scenario of this section, which describes persistent overutilized OR time. Should the surgeon be encouraged to continue to schedule cases beyond the hours that have been allocated? That is a reasonable tactical question, which includes consideration of the financial impact of the surgeon's cases versus the long-term effects on hiring and retention of OR nurses and anesthesia providers [13]. The tactical decision can, and probably should, be considered from multiple perspectives, including societal. However, the operational decision making focuses on the reality of the existing workload. Operational decisions, specifically service-specific staffing, are what most managers can control.

Truly not having fixed hours of OR time, despite an official policy against overbooking elective cases, is particularly common at hospitals at which surgeons mischaracterize cases as "urgent" to get them onto the OR schedule.

For example, an academic department is allocated three ORs from 8 a.m. to 4 p.m. on all workdays. No elective case is scheduled unless it will fit into the 8 h based on mean historical OR time data from the OR information system. The service schedules 20 percent of its OR hours as urgent cases. The patients are inpatient preoperatively [5, 6]. Many of these patients likely could have waited safely for several days for surgery. Thus, these were elective cases. However, having the cases wait for surgery would be counterproductive economically. The surgeons reasonably called the cases "urgent" to achieve open access to OR time and thus bypass the policy against overbooking. OR efficiency would have been greater had more OR time been allocated originally. This would have allowed the cases to be performed in allocated, rather than in overutilized, OR time.

Suppose that on a long-term (tactical) basis, the behavior of the academic surgeons was considered so bad that penalties were applied. Then, there would be very little overutilized OR time. The methods described in this chapter would be valid and appropriate, but not necessarily a useful improvement. Consequently, there is reason to consider whether the behavior of the above surgeons is inherently bad.

From the societal, hospital, and surgeons' perspective, likely the behavior is good, or at least not bad enough to penalize the surgeons. They are serving as their patients' advocates, assuring timely surgery. Among patients who are inpatient preoperatively, the surgeons are reducing hospital lengths of stay. Among patients who are outpatient preoperatively, most patients only have two preoperative visits with the surgeon, making surgeon flexibility to schedule initial consultations very important to growth in surgical practices [28]. Further, in some healthcare systems, including that in the United States, the more cases that the surgeons perform, the higher are hospital and physician contribution margins.

Hospitals receiving fee-for-service reimbursement achieve an overall positive contribution margin for the elective cases of almost all surgeons, [13, 26, 29] because a large percentage of OR costs are fixed (e.g., surgical robots, video equipment for minimally invasive surgical suites, and anesthesia machines). If professional revenues for the anesthesia providers and surgeons were also considered in the calculation of contribution margin, then every surgeon would provide an overall positive contribution margin for his or her elective cases. The implication, then, is that if a case can be performed safely, it is economically irrational not to perform the case [13, 26, 30].

The rationale for providing surgeons with open access to OR time, provided a case can be performed safely, makes particular sense for hospitals with ICUs that often are full. For patients needing such care, the ICU is a frequent bottleneck that results in delays or cancellations of surgical cases. There are two ways to approach this problem, other than simply providing and staffing more ICU beds.

One strategy to reduce the risk of delays or cancellations is to adjust the days that services are scheduled to perform surgery [31, 32]. Although such techniques can be implemented practically [31, 32], the incremental benefit to hospitals may be small. If most surgeons schedule patients for ICU admission on the same days of the week, usually the cause of case cancellations is visible to the surgeons. The surgeons generally suffer more, financially, from case cancellations and delays than do hospitals and anesthesiologists. In this situation, the hands-on facilitation of a local OR manager or an expert in managing organizational conflict can help, with tabular and graphical summaries of the impact of decisions on cancellations [32]. Such interventions are valuable and important [33]. However, they are not commonly decisions made by anesthesia group managers or OR nursing directors, although they can facilitate such processes.

The second of the two strategies is to provide surgeons with flexibility on the days when they have OR time. Cases should get onto the OR schedule to assure that the expensive bottleneck (the ICU) is always full. For example, although 90 percent of patients may have ICU lengths of stay <2 days following coronary artery bypass graft, there can be marked variability in length of stay [32, 34, 35]. Consequently, predictions can be inaccurate for the number of open ICU beds available daily as a result of patient transfers from the unit.

When the bottleneck to doing surgery is downstream from ORs and the service time for that downstream process is highly variable, then flexibility in scheduling the OR cases is needed to maximize throughput. This does present some inconvenience to surgeons and patients in that they do not know with certainty the date when the procedure will be performed until very close to the day of surgery, but is preferable to having the case cancelled on the day of surgery due to inadequate ICU resources.

The same logic applies to expensive capital equipment (e.g., intraoperative magnetic resonance imaging), that, like the ICUs, is a fixed cost that is best kept as fully utilized as possible. In the future, more ORs will include more technologically advanced equipment, resulting in even higher capital costs. The percentage of hospital costs for surgery that are attributed to labor likely will decrease as capital costs increase to support these and other expensive technologies. To maximize use of that equipment, surgeons should have open access to OR time to do a case on whatever future workday they are available, provided the case can be performed safely using existing equipment. For example, if two surgical services have allocated time on the same day of the week and are vying for the one operative robot, providing the services the ability to book elective cases on days other than on the date of their surgical block will increase the utilization of this expensive resource.

The caveat of allowing open access to OR time "provided the case can be performed safely" is of strikingly large importance. Safety includes access not only to specialized surgical equipment, but also to limited ICU beds, hospital ward beds, postanesthesia care unit beds, nonfatigued staff, etc. What can be done safely limits how much work can be done in a surgical suite on any given day [2, 12, 13, 32, 36]. Characteristically, tactical decision making limits what can be done safely. Then, operational decision making functions within these boundaries.

Based on these arguments, realistic operational decision making needs to function within a structure that allows the surgeon and patient to choose the day of surgery. The reason why this is so important is that surgeons are not the individuals primarily responsible for OR efficiency through their filling of the OR time allocated to them. Rather, the parties primarily responsible for OR efficiency are the nursing and anesthesia group managers who choose the OR allocations to match staffing to the surgeons' workloads. The latter refers almost entirely to the durations of the hours in each OR into which cases are scheduled, numbers of ORs usually only being numbers of flexible rooms to facilitate turnovers and urgent cases, etc.

For example, for 1 week each year, most of the otolaryngologists are away at a conference. There is substantial underutilized OR time, resulting in poor OR efficiency. This is an example of poor OR management. The managers should have increased OR efficiency by adjusting staffing to match the surgeons' and patients' hours (e.g., by encouraging months in advance for some nurses and anesthesia providers specializing in this area of care to use some of their accrued vacation).

Planning Service-Specific Staffing and Scheduling Cases Based on Increasing OR Efficiency

Allocating OR time (i.e., planning service-specific staffing) and scheduling cases based on OR efficiency can increase OR productivity by reducing labor costs.

Performing Calculations Using Complete Enumeration

In practice, OR allocations that are calculated based on OR efficiency are done by service and day of the week. That is because day of the week is the best predictor of a service's workload [11, 37]. Calculating an OR allocation means determining how many ORs should be staffed daily for each service and, for each of these ORs, how many hours of staffing should be planned (e.g., 8, 10, or 13 h) [11, 37]. Calculations of optimal allocations can be done by complete enumeration [23]. Specifically, all possible staffing solutions are considered, starting with 0 h and progressively increasing staffed hours until additional increases in the staffed hours cause the efficiency of use of OR time to decrease for that service [37]. If shifts of 8, 10, and 13 h are considered, then the successive choices are 0, 8, 10, 13, 16, 18 h, etc. Increasing the staffed hours causes the efficiency of use of OR time to increase progressively to a maximum, after which it decreases [11]. The complete enumeration can be constructed such that every series of cases performed by the same surgeon on the same day would be performed in its original sequence and take the same amount of OR time [23]. The only change is in the start times.

For example, a surgeon is currently allocated 8 h of OR time individually on Tuesdays. The surgeon historically has done 9 h of cases every Tuesday. The hospital calculates that the expense of one hour of overutilized time is twice that of one hour of underutilized time; inefficiency is expressed in terms of the number of equivalent underutilized hours. Candidate allocations are 0, 8, 10, and 13 h. The inefficiency of use of OR time for each potential allocation is determined from the cost of the underutilized and overutilized hours that would have resulted. A 0-h allocation (A) would have resulted in 9 h of overutilized time, with an inefficiency of use of OR time proportional to 18 h. An 8-h allocation (B) would have resulted in 1 h of overutilized time, with an inefficiency proportional to 2 h. A 10-h allocation (C) would have resulted in one underutilized hour with an inefficiency proportional to 1 h. Finally, a 13-h allocation (D) would have resulted in 4 h of underutilized time with an inefficiency proportional to 4 h. Since the most efficient solution (i.e., smallest value of the inefficiency of use of OR time) was Allocation C, the surgeon should have been allocated 10 h of OR time in order to maximize the efficiency of use of OR time.

There is a unique solution to the choice of the OR allocation that will maximize OR efficiency if OR allocations can be of any duration (e.g., 9.27 h [11]), but not necessarily when fixed choices (e.g., 8, 10, 13 h) are considered. When two choices provide nearly the same inefficiency of use of OR time, the OR workload can be reviewed to consider which most closely matches how the surgeons in the service have historically been using their OR time.

For example, the cardiac surgeons perform an average of 14 h of cases each Tuesday, with a range of 12–15 h. Forecasted OR efficiency would be nearly identical whether 13 h of OR time were allocated in one OR or 8 h in each of two ORs. The cardiac surgeons have had two ORs (i.e., reliable first case of the day start times) for the past 6 years. They have consistently scheduled cases into those ORs such that there is only underutilized OR time, not overutilized OR time. Two ORs would be the most reasonable choice. In this example, planning OR allocation based on OR efficiency versus adjusted utilization results in the same decisions.

Maximizing OR efficiency is the same as minimizing the sum of underutilized hours and overutilized hours multiplied by the relative cost of overutilized to underutilized OR hours (see "Definitions" [11]). Thus, only the relative cost of overutilized to underutilized OR hours needs to be known, not the costs per se [11]. A commonly used [37] value for this ratio of costs is 1.75. This includes the direct costs of overtime at "time and a half" (1.50) and an increment (0.25) for indirect (intangible) costs of employee dissatisfaction, resignation, and recruitment and training [37]. Because of the marked effect of limiting consideration to common staff schedules (e.g., 8 or 13 h), the resulting inefficiency in use of OR time is characteristically highly insensitive to local experts' uncertainty in the choice of the value of this parameter [38].

For example, on three Wednesdays, a service performed 12, 7, and 15 h of cases, including turnover times. There are 8-h shifts, with overtime scheduled by rotation using a late list. The relative cost of overutilized to underutilized hours is considered 1.75. If the service were allocated 8 h of OR time each Wednesday, then the cost of the inefficiency of use of OR time would be proportional to 20.25 h, where 20.25 h = (0 underutilized + 1 underutilized + 0 underutilized + 1.75 × [4 overutilized + 0 overutilized + 7 overutilized]). If the allocation were two 8-h ORs each Wednesday, the cost would be proportional to 14 h, where 14 h = (4 underutilized + 9 underutilized + 1 underutilized). If the allocation were three 8-h ORs each Wednesday, the cost would be proportional to 38 h, where 38 h = (12 underutilized + 17 underutilized + 9 underutilized). Therefore, the service should be allocated two 8-h ORs to maximize OR efficiency.

There is only one answer to the question, "How close are current OR allocations to those that would maximize OR efficiency?" In contrast, there is no one answer to the question, "How close are current OR allocations to those that are optimal based on OR utilization?" The reason is that there is then the subsequent question of how to determine the optimal OR utilization. The best OR utilization varies among services because it is sensitive to many parameters, such as staffed hours, turnover times, day-to-day variability in OR workload, statistical distribution of OR times of cases, and so forth [25, 39]. Years of data can be required to estimate these parameter values sufficiently accurately to use them to decide on the OR utilization to use as the service's goal [40]. Allocating OR time based on OR efficiency simultaneously takes into account all of these issues. When a manager says "We allocate OR time based on OR efficiency," that is close to a sufficient statement to describe precisely

what happens in practice because the choice of the relative cost of overutilized to underutilized OR time is invariably close to 1.75 and insensitive to any differences. In contrast, when a manager says "We allocate OR time based on OR utilization," that alone says virtually nothing about what happens in practice at the surgical suite.

Calculated Staffing (OR Allocations) Differ from Those in Current Practice

OR managers' efforts to reduce labor costs must focus predominantly on OR allocation and case scheduling, because almost all of anesthesia providers' costs are labor costs. The viability of a surgical facility depends on the economics of the anesthesia providers. For 11 of 12 facilities studied, allocating OR time based on OR efficiency achieved significantly lower labor costs than the plans that were being used by the local managers [37, 41–43]. For 9 of the 11 facilities, the statistical method approach resulted in plans that reduced labor costs by at least 10 percent [37, 41–43]. The percentage increases in OR efficiency were, by definition, even more.

A common anecdote reveals how poorly many facilities plan service-specific staffing. Often OR nurses and anesthesia providers report that every OR finishes at least an hour or two late every day. To consider the irrationality [44] of the situation, suppose that the relative cost of overutilized to underutilized OR time were 2.0. Then, it would be twice as expensive to finish late versus early. With appropriate OR allocations, the odds for each service and OR to finish early should be approximately two chances in three. That is, if staffing decisions were made rationally, a given OR would finish early on 2 of every 3 days.

In practice, percentage reductions in labor costs are not proportional to the number of ORs [37, 41]. Even at facilities for which each allocation is for one room, but either for 8 or 10 h, savings are found [45]. Surgical suites at which many hours of OR time are allocated to services do not have the largest percentage improvements from applying the operations research to OR management. The explanation for this observation is that the principal challenge faced by managers is not the number of ORs to be allocated to services, but how to manage variability in OR workload from week to week. The fact that the OR allocation decision is stochastic is the conceptual problem in the practicing managers' decisions. The poor decisions are caused by cognitive biases that are observed for such decisions in other industries [44]. Implementation of improved decisions is not achieved by education alone, but rather by automating reliance on decision support software [44, 46].

For example, consider a service with OR workload averaging 6.5 h every Friday [47, 48]. Because there are no overutilized hours, allocation based on OR efficiency is identical to allocation based on OR utilization [45]. Once this principle is understood by managers, analysis is unneeded in the future. One analysis is sufficient. In contrast, suppose that the same facility has three of its eight ORs as unblocked, open, first-come, first-served "other" time. The surgical suite staffs in 8-, 10-, and 13-h shifts. Then, those three ORs could be allocated as 8/8/8, 8/8/10, 8/10/10, 10/10/10, 8/8/13, 8/13/13/, 13/13/13, 8/10/13, 10/10/13, and 10/13/13. Intuition will not help with this complex decision. The value of education is by increasing trust in relying on the statistical results [49, 50].

Hospitals generally should not artificially treat all ORs as having the same number of hours of cases [15]. The standard deviations among ORs in the daily total hours of cases including turnover times between 7:00 a.m. and 11:00 p.m. were estimated for 34 hospitals [51]. The hospitals did not have all ORs fully packed with the same end of the workday [12]. Many hospitals had standard deviations greater than 3 h [51]. Some ORs had underutilized OR time and other ORs had overutilized OR time; some ORs had 8 h allocations and other ORs had longer hours of allocated time; and/or some ORs finished before the end of an 8 h workday and other ORs were used for urgent cases, not finishing until late in the evening [2, 12].

Urgent Cases

Some hospitals have one or more ORs allocated for urgent cases during the regular workday. Typically, then, the appropriate number of ORs is chosen for such urgent cases by considering them to be performed by a pseudo-service, the "Urgent" service. The methods above are applied. At facilities not planning an OR for urgent cases, when calculating OR allocations for elective cases, each urgent case should be attributed to its surgical service.

The relative cost of overutilized to underutilized OR time may be appropriately higher for the urgent service than the other elective services, because the choice affects not just how often staff work late,

but also patient waiting time for urgent surgery. However, urgent cases often cannot start immediately (e.g., because the surgeon is not available), such that overutilized OR time would occur regardless of calculations. In practice, the use of the same relative cost for overutilized to underutilized OR time as above (e.g., a factor of 1.75) can provide answers that clinicians consider reasonable.

Amount of Data Required for Calculations

To assess how much data are required to produce acceptable results, a long series of data from a surgical suite was divided into training and testing datasets, with different training periods [16]. The complete enumeration was applied to the training data, and the expected labor costs that would have occurred during the subsequent testing period were calculated. Each increase in the number of months of data up to 9 months resulted in a statistically significant reduction in expected labor costs. There were large incremental benefits in using at least 7 months of data. For the studied hospital, there was no advantage to using more than 1 year of data.

The minimum amount of data needed for calculating OR allocations based on OR efficiency can be particularly important to managers at facilities purchasing a new OR information system, anesthesia information system, or anesthesia billing system. The minimum period of data indicates the time from installation of the system to when management changes based on resulting data can be implemented. Application of the statistical methods using as little as 30 workdays of system data provided better OR allocations to reduce labor costs than OR allocations established by the practicing managers with years of data [16].

Sources of Data

Data for analysis can come from an OR information system, an electronic anesthesia information management system, or anesthesia billing data [52]. OR information system data have the advantage of virtually always having necessary data fields completed. Anesthesia billing data have the advantage of accuracy, because billing errors can be costly or even lead to challenges of fraudulent behavior. When using anesthesia billing data, if the OR in which the case was performed is not available from the data, then the anesthesia provider (i.e., the person in the

OR delivering anesthesia care, not the supervising anesthesiologists) can be substituted for the OR field to calculate turnovers. Depending on the workflow among ORs, this substitution can be preferable.

Facilities with OR information systems that do not have data review at the time of data entry often have datasets that contain errors or omissions, including lack of knowledge of the actual ORs in which some cases were performed. This can occur if cases are moved during the day without correcting the corresponding information systems, or if the times of OR entry or exit are incorrectly entered. This manifests as the false appearance of two cases overlapping in the same OR at the same time. The typical fix is to change the recorded OR of each case that overlaps to a unique unknown OR. For example, suppose that one case is listed as being performed in OR 1 from 10 a.m. to 11 a.m. and another in OR 1 from 10:30 a.m. to 12 noon. Among all cases in the dataset, the latter case is the 139th for which the true OR is unknown. The second case can be considered to have been completed in the fictitious room "Unknown139." Making such a change affects calculated turnover times, since some turnovers between cases will be altered, and thus may affect OR allocations. Nonetheless, studies demonstrated that the impact of this adjustment on the labor costs that result from poor OR allocations is of negligible importance, for three reasons [53, 54]. First, OR allocations are based on each service's total hours of cases, a large number, plus total hours of turnover times, a much smaller number. Second, for cases in an OR that have a preceding case and a following case, two turnover times are lost. Yet, the turnover time between the remaining cases is increased between the two cases surrounding the reassigned case to the default maximum turnover time [53]. Third, the effect of allocating OR time only in fixed increments (e.g., 8 or 13 h) is of larger importance.

Assessing Trends, Seasonal Variation, and Data Errors

Use of complete enumeration assumes that there are no systematic differences among weeks in the expected OR workload (i.e., there are no trends or seasonal variation) [37]. National survey data show that these assumptions will hold for most facilities [55]. Raw data were reanalyzed from the 1994 to 1996 National Survey of Ambulatory Surgery. As a positive control, to assure that seasonal variation could be detected if present, the average number of myringotomy tubes inserted each day in ambulatory surgery centers of the United States was examined. As expected, myringotomy tube insertions peaked each winter, corresponding to the peak incidence of middle ear infections. Specifically, the average number of tubes inserted each day varied systematically among months for all 26 of the overlapping 11-month periods in the 36 months of the survey. In contrast, the average number of ambulatory surgery cases performed with an anesthesia provider each day in the United States per 10,000 persons was found not to vary systematically month to month on an 11-month basis.

Good routine practice is to test for statistically significant trends [56] or seasonality, to confirm that analysis is reasonable for each surgical suite. For example, the so-called *runs test* can be applied to the total labor cost over each consecutive 4-week period [37, 57]. Calculate the total labor cost for each 4-week period. Subtract the median from each value. Delete zero differences. Assign a "+" to positive differences and a "−" to negative differences. A "run" is defined as a series of one or more consecutive values that are the same. Finally, compare the number of runs of +'s and −'s to a critical value from appropriate statistical tables. For example, if over 10 weeks the values were + − 0 − − − + − + + there would be 5 runs (2 +, 1 + +, 1 − − −, and 2 −). At $P < 0.05$, the expected number of runs is between 2 and 10, so the null hypothesis that there is a trend would be rejected. This test, the Wald–Wolfowitz one-sample runs test, is available in most statistics packages.

In our experience, it is almost never necessary to incorporate methods appropriate for data with trends and seasonality into the analysis [12]. When the runs test detects trends or seasonality, characteristically this reflects a problem with the data or special conditions [56] that need to be modeled separately. For example, if a hospital opens a new three-room endovascular (interventional) suite in the middle of the data collection period, this may result in a positive trend in OR workload. Opening of a new surgery center may result in an abrupt decline in workload at the main facility [56].

In addition to using the runs test, plot each service's OR workload for the days of the week when the service is allocated OR time. The graphs are helpful to detect unrecognized errors in the data. For example, plotting OR workload for a service against time can show if a service had no cases listed for a day of the week for some part of the data period being used. This usually occurs when the data sent for analysis include one or more surgeons who recently left the facility and operated on the empty days.

Finally, look for the presence of many zero values in the histogram of OR workload for each combination of the day of the week and the service allocated OR time. This usually happens when the service's scheduling is characteristic of an individual surgeon rather than a group of surgeons. These "holes" often represent times when an individual surgeon is away (e.g., on vacation). These can be hard to identify in a graph of OR workload versus time. Such services may need to have their allocations of OR time combined with another service to achieve reliable staffing predictions.

Services with Low OR Workloads

Provided cases are scheduled sequentially into ORs, then services with average OR workloads that are consistently <8 h have no overutilized hours. Allocating OR time based on adjusted utilization does not differ from doing so based on OR efficiency. Many facilities appropriately apply a minimum adjusted utilization for OR allocations [58, 59]. For example, based on the relative cost ratio of 1.75 described above, if services' workloads were always the same each workday, then the optimal (minimum) value would be 68 percent [58, 59].

For example, a service's OR workload averages 6 h every Tuesday. The facility bases its decisions on the efficiency of use of OR time. The service's adjusted utilization is 75 percent. Thus, the service is allocated a single OR for 8 h. Because there are no overutilized hours, allocation based on OR efficiency is identical to allocation based on OR utilization. There are 0 h of underutilized time caused by OR allocation and case scheduling.

Each service not receiving an OR allocation on a given day (due to low historical workload) can be combined into an "OTHER" service (i.e., open, unblocked, first-scheduled, first-served time). At facilities without substantial cross-training of staff, there may be different "OTHER" services for different nursing teams. The calculations of the preceding sections are repeated for the "OTHER" service(s) on each workday.

Importantly, do not simply measure the average OR workload of a service, observe that it is too low for an allocation of an 8-h OR for the day, and then automatically pool it into "OTHER" service time. Apply the graphical methods of the preceding section to assure that the reason for a low OR workload reflects an actual low workload, not a service that operates every other week on the studied day of the week [12]. Likewise, assure that incomplete data or a trend in OR workload is not being observed.

Using Qualitative Information to Improve Forecasts

Qualitative information not available from information system data should be used when finalizing OR allocations.

For example, a surgeon operates at an outpatient surgery center on Fridays in her 8 h of allocated OR time. For years, she has consistently performed 7.0–7.5 h of cases at the surgery center in her OR time. The OR allocations are being updated for the next quarter. Based on historical data, she would, of course, be allocated 8 h of OR time on Fridays. However, she is 8 months pregnant and has requested 3 months of maternity leave. She should not be allocated OR time during the next quarter because it would be underutilized, thereby reducing OR efficiency. Even without personally allocated OR time, she would continue to have open access to OR time on any future workday, if she were to change her mind and work for a few days during her period of maternity leave. Note that if she were not provided open access to OR time, then there would be an adversarial relationship between the facility not wanting to plan a "block" for her versus her desire to keep some block time to provide herself and her patients some flexibility [44]. This highlights that providing open access to OR time on any future workday generally increases OR productivity.

While applying qualitative knowledge, though, focus on the cognitive bias that results in most of the inefficiency of use of anesthesia time, the bias being lack of use of the mathematics [44, 46]. The qualitative information should be used to update the *forecasts* of workload, not used to create an ad hoc process of converting from workload to OR allocations. We humans are good at forecasting changes in workload, not in making the mathematical conversions from mean workloads into appropriate OR allocations (staffing) [44].

Forecast Remaining Underutilized OR Time

A concern at some facilities is that underutilized OR time is needed for nonclinical, but nonetheless important activities. For example, equipment for the next day's cases may be set up by nurses whose ORs finish earlier than the end of their shift. The nursing supervisors at such facilities may express concern that changing OR allocations to increase OR efficiency will impair processes that function well by taking advantage of existing underutilized OR time.

Expected underutilized time can be estimated empirically after future OR allocations have been determined. Applying the allocations, each historical day's resulting total underutilized hours are calculated. The statistical distribution of each day's total hours of underutilized OR time can be described using histograms or percentiles.

Case Scheduling

Allocating OR time to increase OR efficiency is of little value unless cases are also scheduled into the OR time appropriately.

A series of thought experiments and computer simulations was performed to evaluate case scheduling based on maximizing OR efficiency [21]. The performances of different case scheduling heuristics were compared. The analyses showed that managers can achieve efficient OR scheduling while leaving case scheduling decisions to the convenience of surgeons and patients, provided three simple scheduling rules are followed. In other words, there are small differences in the resulting OR efficiency among different scheduling heuristics, with three exceptions.

The first of three scheduling rules is that a service should not schedule a case into another service's OR time if the case can be completed within its own allocated OR time [21].

For example, two thoracic surgeons are partners in a group that has been allocated 10 h of OR time on Tuesdays. One of the surgeons has scheduled 6 h of cases into the OR time, leaving 4 h of allocated but unscheduled OR time. A cardiac surgeon has scheduled 2 h of cases into his personally allocated 8 h of OR time. Nine days before the day of surgery, the second thoracic surgeon wants to schedule a new 2-h case. The available start time would be after her partner who has already scheduled cases. The case would not be scheduled into the cardiac surgeon's OR time, even if the second thoracic surgeon wants to start earlier. The reason is that the thoracic surgeons have available OR time for the case.

The reason for this result is that OR allocations are calculated based on expected OR workload on the day of surgery. Services fill their allocated OR time at different rates [60]. Some services have many patients who are inpatient preoperatively, and those cases typically would be booked in the OR scheduling system on the day before surgery [6]. Almost all facilities with allocated OR time follow the preceding scheduling rule. Thus, the importance of this finding was not that it showed a new way to schedule cases but that it showed that most facilities make decisions based on OR efficiency [21]. By definition, the decision would not represent a change in facility practice, but an unusual request of the second thoracic surgeon, because otherwise the thoracic surgeons would not have been allocated 10 h of OR time on Tuesdays.

The second of the three scheduling rules is that a case should not be scheduled into overutilized OR time if it can start earlier in another of the service's ORs [14, 22]. This applies to services allocated two or more ORs. Suppose that OR workload is 23 h. The expected hours of overutilized OR time would be slightly less if two OR were allocated for 13 h (total 26 h) versus three OR for 8 h (total 24 h). This result would be less reliable if case scheduling did not result in similar packing of the cases into the allocated OR time [14, 21, 61] Simulations show usually it does.

For example, a service has been allocated OR 3 and OR 5 from 7 a.m. to 3 p.m. One surgeon in the service has scheduled cases in OR 3 to finish around 2 p.m. OR 5 is empty. A second surgeon in the service wants an afternoon start. He asks to start an elective 3-h case at 2:30 p.m. in OR 3. Even though OR workload would be the same, scheduling the case into OR 3 would be expected to result in overutilized OR time and thereby reduce OR efficiency. His request should be denied. The surgeon should take the first case of the day, start in OR 5, or schedule the case on a different workday.

The preceding scenario matches what is done at most surgical suites. Cases are generally not scheduled into overutilized OR time when a service has another allocated OR that is empty. Consequently, as the first rule above, this rule shows that scheduling cases based on maximizing OR efficiency differs little from what is commonly done in practice [21]. Changes resulting from decision making based on OR efficiency generally do not affect case scheduling. Rather, they affect OR allocations (as above) and in the third rule regarding how OR time is released.

The third of the three scheduling rules is that if a service has already filled its allocated OR time, then, to maximize OR efficiency, its new case should be scheduled into another services' OR time instead of into overutilized OR time [21, 61].

For example, a service has filled its allocated OR time but has another elective case that it desires to schedule. If the OR time of another service were not released, the case would be performed in overutilized OR time. OR efficiency is greater by performing that case in the OR time allocated to another service that otherwise would be underutilized on the day of surgery.

For example, a surgeon appears to be subverting the case scheduling system for the "OTHER" service, which provides first-scheduled, first-served OR time. The surgeon seems to be creating fictitious patients to "hold" OR time for his cases (e.g., at the desirable 7 a.m. start time). At the OR Block Committee meeting, a manager suggests that there be the policy that when a case is cancelled, first access to cancelled OR time goes to other surgeons with waiting cases, not the surgeon canceling the case. That recommendation is not sound. When a service has filled its allocated OR time and has another case to schedule, OR efficiency is enhanced by releasing the OR time of the service expected to have the most underutilized OR time [60]. No cases should be waiting to be scheduled.

To evaluate which service should have its OR time released, simulations were performed scheduling new hypothetical cases into actual OR schedules. Services fill their allocated OR time at different rates. Thus, theoretically, the service that should have its OR time released for a new case should be the service that is predicted, at the time the new case is booked, to be the service that will have the most underutilized OR time on the scheduled day of surgery. In practice, performance is made only slightly worse (versus having perfect retrospective knowledge) by scheduling the case into the OR time of the service with the largest difference between allocated and scheduled OR time at the time when the new case is scheduled [60]. The latter is practically straightforward to implement.

In contrast, releasing the OR time of the service with the second most, instead of the service with the most, allocated but unscheduled OR time has a large negative effect on OR efficiency [60]. The reason is that usually a particular case can only be scheduled

into one or two services' OR time without resulting in overutilized OR time. The differences among those few services in their amount of expected open OR time often are large. This occurs because day-to-day variability in the OR workload of services on a day of the week generally exceeds variability due to the timing of how quickly different services filled their allocated OR time.

The timing of when allocated OR time should be released has been studied [62]. Potentially, the scheduling office could wait to release the allocated OR time until closer to the day of surgery, when data may be available on subsequently scheduled cases, in order to improve the quality of the decision. Slightly more than half of ORs have a change in one or more cases within 1 workday of surgery [6, 63]. However, simulation results were equivocal as to the benefit of such a decision [62]. Under two conditions, postponing the decision of which service had its OR time released for the new case until early the day before surgery had a negligible effect on resulting OR efficiency versus releasing the allocated OR time when the new case was scheduled [62]. First, this finding applied to an ambulatory surgery center with brief cases. At such facilities, typically there is only one good choice for the service to have its OR time released [60]. Thus, there is no good reason to wait in making the decision. Second, this finding often also applies to large surgical suites in which cases are scheduled as if there were many smaller suites. For example, at a 30-OR surgical suite, one nursing and anesthesia team may staff the six ORs used for general and vascular surgery. From the perspective of releasing OR time for a new general or vascular surgery case, only six ORs are available, not all 30 ORs.

For example, a hospital contains a team cross-trained in neurosurgery and otolaryngology. One week hence, on next Thursday, neurosurgery has been allocated one 10-h OR. Otolaryngology has been allocated one 10-h OR also. The otolaryngologists have scheduled 11 h of cases into their OR. A third otolaryngologist wants to schedule another 2-h case. The neurosurgeons have scheduled a case for 3 h from 7 a.m. to 10 a.m. The otolaryngologist with the new case can book the case because the surgeons have open access to OR time on whatever workday they choose. Provided the otolaryngologist is available at 10:30 a.m., then the neurosurgeons' OR time would be released. There is no advantage to waiting to schedule the case. Yet, if the neurosurgeon with the 7 a.m. to 10 a.m. case was to schedule another case, the scheduling office should contact the otolaryngologist and perhaps she would not mind starting her case later in the day.

Despite this consideration of how best to release allocated OR time, it is important to appreciate that results are *highly* sensitive to the OR time being allocated appropriately based on OR efficiency [14]. Issues of when to release allocated OR time vastly pale in practical importance to OR allocation and staffing [14]. The difference typically is less than one case between whether a 2 OR service has overall underutilized or overutilized time [23, 63]. This remarkable observation explains why the OR allocation decision is so important to reduce overutilized OR time, whereas the case scheduling decision is usually obvious (and, by corollary, absolute differences between scheduled and actual OR time generally can be neglected [2]). Although OR management problems are observed on the day of surgery, often the root cause and only practical way to fix the problem is to plan OR allocations and staffing properly several weeks or months before the day of surgery [14, 64]. The balance between the role of case scheduling versus OR allocations in causing inefficient use of OR time can be assessed for each facility by reviewing multiple examples as in this chapter and comparing each to the facility's current practices [65].

For example, OR information systems data are used to calculate OR allocations, which then are reviewed by the "block" committee. An ophthalmologist complains that his allocated OR time on Tuesdays has been "released" for 2 of the past 3 weeks. Each time, the otolaryngology service has filled its allocated 8 h of OR time and so has booked cases into his OR time. The ophthalmologist is upset that the schedulers are treating him unfairly by repeatedly releasing his allocated OR time. Although he schedules many cases a couple of days before the day of surgery, his OR workload is consistently at least 7 h each Tuesday. The ophthalmologist's concerns are well founded; this should not be happening. However, the problem is not that the schedulers are releasing his OR time. Rather, they are making the proper decision to maximize OR efficiency. The problem is that the otolaryngology service should be allocated more than 8 h of OR time. This is either a failure of statistical forecasting of the otolaryngology service's workload, which is uncommon, or a failure in appropriating allocating OR time based on the forecasted workload, which is more common [44]. At facilities with

frequent concerns about releasing of allocated OR time, be sure to focus on who is responsible for statistical calculations of the OR allocations and their use.

Although this chapter has focused on decision making before the day of surgery, the same principles apply to decisions made on the day of surgery [2, 23, 65, 66]. The principles described can also be used to decide how cases are moved on the day of surgery [65, 67], how staff members are assigned on the day of surgery [68], and how cases are sequenced in each OR [51, 69, 70].

Impact of Reducing Times on Productivity

Impact of Reducing Surgical and Turnover Times

The impact of interventions on labor costs can be forecast using each facility's own data, along with corresponding confidence intervals [12, 19]. For example, turnover times can be reduced between each case [12, 19]. Surgical times can be reduced to national average values for each procedure [20]. First case of the day starts can all be on-time [12, 59]. For all interventions, first the labor cost is calculated assuming that OR time is allocated and cases are scheduled based on OR efficiency. Second, the intervention is performed, thereby reducing OR workload by service. Third, using the revised workload values, OR time is reallocated based on OR efficiency and the new estimates for labor costs projected. Fourth, the differences are calculated. By analyzing the differences in 4-week periods, to prevent effects of variation by day of the week, confidence intervals can be calculated for the differences [19, 20, 37].

For example, consider a hospital that allocates 8 h of OR time to each of many small services, and each has an adjusted utilization less than 85 percent [20]. Cases are being scheduled based on OR efficiency (i.e., sequentially into ORs [21]). Reducing OR times cannot result in reduced overutilized hours because there are none. Labor costs will not be reduced (i.e., they are fixed to achievable reductions in OR times).

For example, a different hospital has few surgical services, most with more than one OR, and many ORs with workloads exceeding 8 h [20]. Then, reducing OR times can result in reductions in workload sufficient to reduce allocated OR time (e.g., an OR allocated for 10 h would now be allocated for 8 h). At this hospital, unlike the one in the preceding example, there would be financially important reductions in labor costs from reducing OR times.

Equivalent analyses can be performed at teaching facilities to calculate [20] the impact of longer OR times (due to factors such as teaching time and development of skills in trainees) [71, 72] on labor costs.

These examples show that, generally, cost reduction from reducing OR or turnover times can only be achieved provided OR allocations are reduced [12]. The initial impact of reductions in OR or turnover times may be increased underutilized OR time and/or reduced overutilized OR time. This initial step is evident to clinicians. The secondary step is revisions of OR allocations based on the new values of decreased OR workload. The latter step provides for the large reductions in labor cost.

Usually, reductions in labor costs from reducing turnover times tend to be small. At four academic tertiary hospitals studied, reductions in average turnover times of 3–9 min would result in 0.8–1.8 percent reductions in labor cost [19]. Reductions in average turnover times of 10–19 min would result in 2.5–4.0 percent reductions in labor costs [19]. These analyses can be fruitful in educating stakeholders that achievable reductions in the times to complete tasks often have less effect on OR efficiency than does good management decision making.

Impact of Not Changing Service-Specific Staffing

Some facilities do not make decisions systematically based on increasing OR efficiency and are unlikely to change their practices [44]. Then, the methodology above can be used to calculate the higher labor costs that the facility sustains from OR time not being allocated and cases not being scheduled based on OR efficiency [16, 37, 41].

For example, anesthesia group expenses exceed revenue at a facility. The calculation is performed using labor costs of anesthesia providers. The estimate of the resulting additional labor costs can be used by the anesthesia group and hospital when negotiating an appropriate administrative support agreement from the hospital [58, 73].

Development of administrative support agreements can also apply to negotiations with medical schools, ambulatory surgical facilities, or a multi-specialty group. At two academic medical centers,

estimated annual excess labor costs were $1.6 million and $1.0 million, respectively [41].

Impact of Not Reducing the Number of Allocated ORs

Some organizations aim to adjust their OR allocations to be as close as possible to those that are expected to maximize OR efficiency while not reducing the number of allocated ORs. This approach does not result in maximal OR efficiency. Instead, this approach reflects organizational support for opening as many ORs as are available for first case of the day starts (e.g., to achieve on-time starts for surgeons) [74, 75]. The mathematics can be weighted to allocate more ORs by repeating the analyses using a higher relative cost of overutilized to underutilized hours (e.g., 3:1). An increase in the relative cost gives an increase in how many ORs are allocated [12, 25]. The smallest value is chosen for which the allocated number of staffed ORs matches the desired, usually current, number of ORs. This analysis is run separately for each day of the week [25].

Increasing the number of allocated ORs results in a slightly smaller percentage increase in OR labor cost than in staffing [25]. The reason is that opening more ORs than are needed to maximize OR efficiency does not change OR workload. Thus, the increase in allocated OR hours increases underutilized OR time and reduces overutilized OR time. The cost per hour of overutilized OR time exceeds that of underutilized OR time. Consequently, the percentage reduction in OR efficiency is less than the percentage increase in allocated OR hours. The same argument applies to labor costs.

Forecasting the Time Remaining in Ongoing Cases

The preceding sections have focused almost entirely on decision making before the day of surgery, because good decision making *cannot* be done on the day of surgery unless the OR allocations chosen months ahead are appropriate. As considered in the section "OR Efficiency on the Day of Surgery," when there is consistent overutilized time on the day of surgery, first and foremost this is a failure months before in statistical forecasting of workload and managerial decision making [14]. However, to use those OR allocations in practice on the day of surgery, another set of data is needed: the forecasted time remaining in cases that are ongoing. In most hospital ORs, the cases running at the end of the day are those that took longer than scheduled [2]. Therefore, good decision making cannot be done in the late afternoon without estimating the time remaining in late running cases. The solution to this problem is not intuitive.

Forecasting the time remaining in cases is one of the most important determinants of decision making on the day of surgery, as it affects decisions such as calling for the next patient, moving cases, and staff relief. Even where there is no bias (i.e., systematic difference) between estimated OR times provided by surgeons and the actual durations from the OR information system (e.g., the average difference equals 0 min), there is substantial variance among historical OR times for the same surgeon and scheduled procedure or procedures that comprise a case [76].

Consider a laparoscopic small bowel resection scheduled for 2 h that has been in the OR for 0.5 h. The median expected time remaining is around 1.5 h. In contrast, suppose that the patient has been in the OR for 1.8 h. The median expected time remaining is not 0.2 h, but longer. The reason is that many of these resections took less than 1.8 h, so the median duration of the cases that took longer than 1.8 h is more than 2.0 h. The shorter duration cases have been excluded. For some of these longer cases, the laparoscopic approach may have been abandoned in favor of an open resection due to the presence of adhesions, or a complication ensued requiring additional time.

For any given combination of surgeon and procedure, there is considerable variation between the time when skin closure begins and when the patient leaves the OR (e.g., from 15 min to 90 min) [77, 78]. This "extra time" comprises the time for irrigation, inspection, and closure, for the patient to recover sufficiently from anesthesia to allow removal of the endotracheal tube, for monitors to be removed and intravenous lines secured, and for the patient to be transferred to the stretcher and transported out of the OR.

The time remaining in a case can be forecasted [77–80] using Bayesian methods by combining the scheduled OR time, historical case duration data, and elapsed times in the OR determined from real-time anesthesia information management system data. Practically, this requires computerization for two reasons. First, many cases running late at the end of the day include rare combinations of procedures with little or no historical data [76, 80–83]. These cases have a markedly

disproportionate impact on the overall variability in decisions involving case durations on the day of surgery [83]. Second, accurate predictions require data about how long cases have been underway and in which OR they are being performed. That can be inferred automatically based on the identifier of the anesthesia information system workstation transmitting pulse oximetry, electrocardiogram heart rate, and end tidal CO_2 partial pressures [84]. The method of automatic forecasting of the remaining time works well even in the absence of any historical data, and automatically incorporates predictive variability in case durations due to changes from the scheduled procedure [77].

Conclusions

OR allocation is a two-stage process [13]. During the initial tactical stage of allocating OR time, considering OR hours to be fixed is reasonable. For operational decision making on a shorter-term basis, such a conceptual model produces results markedly inconsistent with how surgical suites are and should be run. Instead, consider the workload to be fixed on a short-term basis. Provide staff flexibly to match the existing workload, not vice versa. Do so by making operational decisions based on maximizing OR efficiency, as this is an important step to maximizing OR productivity.

References

1. R. E. Wachtel, F. Dexter. Difficulties and challenges associated with literature searches in operating room management, complete with recommendations. *Anesth Analg* 2013; 117: 1460–79.

2. F. Dexter, R. H. Epstein, R. D. Traub, et al. Making management decisions on the day of surgery based on operating room efficiency and patient waiting times. *Anesthesiology* 2004; 101: 1444–53.

3. F. Dexter, L. O'Neill. Weekend operating room on-call staffing requirements. *AORN J* 2001; 74: 666–71.

4. F. Dexter, R. H. Epstein. Holiday and weekend operating room on-call staffing requirements. *Anesth Analg* 2006; 103: 1494–8.

5. F. Dexter, T. Maxbauer, C. Stout, L. Archbold, R. H. Epstein. Relative influence on total cancelled operating room time from patients who are inpatients or outpatients preoperatively. *Anesth Analg* 2014; 118: 1072–80.

6. R. H. Epstein, F. Dexter. Management implications for the perioperative surgical home related to inpatient case cancellations and add-on case scheduling on the day of surgery. *Anesth Analg* 2015; 121: 206–18.

7. Y. Xiao, P. Hu, H. Hao, et al. Algorithm for processing vital sign monitoring data to remotely identify operating room occupancy in real-time. *Anesth Analg* 2005; 101: 823–9.

8. F. Dexter, A. Macario, F. Qian, et al. Forecasting surgical groups' total hours of elective cases for allocation of block time. Application of time series analysis to operating room management. *Anesthesiology* 1999; 91: 1501–8.

9. R. T. Donham, W. J. Mazzei, R. L. Jones. Procedural times glossary. *Am J Anesthesiol* 1999; 23(5 Suppl): 4–12.

10. D. P. Strum, L. G. Vargas, J. H. May. Surgical subspecialty block utilization and capacity planning. A minimal cost analysis model. *Anesthesiology* 1999; 90: 1176–85.

11. D. P. Strum, L. G. Vargas, J. H. May, et al. Surgical suite utilization and capacity planning: A minimal cost analysis model. *J Med Syst* 1997; 21: 309–22.

12. C. McIntosh, F. Dexter, R. H. Epstein. Impact of service-specific staffing, case scheduling, turnovers, and first-case starts on anesthesia group and operating room productivity: Tutorial using data from an Australian hospital. *Anesth Analg* 2006; 103: 1499–516.

13. F. Dexter, J. Ledolter, R. E. Wachtel. Tactical decision making for selective expansion of operating room resources incorporating financial criteria and uncertainty in sub-specialties' future workloads. *Anesth Analg* 2005; 100: 1425–32.

14. P. Shi, F. Dexter, R. H. Epstein. Comparing policies for case scheduling within one day of surgery by Markov chain models. *Anesth Analg* 2016; 122: 526–38.

15. F. Dexter, R. E. Wachtel, R. H. Epstein. Decreasing the hours that anesthesiologists and nurse anesthetists work late by making decisions to reduce the hours of over-utilized operating room time. *Anesth Analg* 2016; 122: 831–42.

16. R. H. Epstein, F. Dexter. Statistical power analysis to estimate how many months of data are required to identify operating room staffing solutions to reduce labor costs and increase productivity. *Anesth Analg* 2002; 94: 640–3.

17. R. J. Sperry. Of economic analysis. *Anesthesiology* 1997; 86: 1197–205.

18. R. E. Wachtel, F. Dexter, D. A. Lubarsky. Financial implications of a hospital's specialization in rare physiologically complex surgical procedures. *Anesthesiology* 2005; 103: 161–7.

19. F. Dexter, A. E. Abouleish, R. H. Epstein, et al. Use of operating room information system data to predict the impact of reducing turnover times on staffing costs. *Anesth Analg* 2003; 97: 1119–26.

20. A. E. Abouleish, F. Dexter, C. W. Whitten, et al. Quantifying net staffing costs due to

longer-than-average surgical case durations. *Anesthesiology* 2004; 100: 403–12.

21. F. Dexter, R. D. Traub. How to schedule elective surgical cases into specific operating rooms to maximize the efficiency of use of operating room time. *Anesth Analg* 2002; 94: 933–42.

22. I. Ozkarahan. Allocation of surgical procedures to operating rooms. *J Med Syst* 1995; 19: 333–52.

23. J. Wang, F. Dexter, K. Yang. Behavioral study of daily mean turnover times and first case of the day tardiness of starts. *Anesth Analg* 2013; 116: 1333–41.

24. F. Dexter, A. Macario, R. H. Epstein, et al. Validity and usefulness of a method to monitor surgical services' average bias in scheduled case durations. *Can J Anesth* 2005; 52: 935–9.

25. F. Dexter, A. Macario. Changing allocations of operating room time from a system based on historical utilization to one where the aim is to schedule as many surgical cases as possible. *Anesth Analg* 2002; 94: 1272–9.

26. F. Dexter, J. T. Blake, D. H. Penning, et al. Calculating a potential increase in hospital margin for elective surgery by changing operating room time allocations or increasing nursing staffing to permit completion of more cases: a case study. *Anesth Analg* 2002; 94: 138–42.

27. F. Dexter, H. Ledolter. Managing risk and expected financial return from selective expansion of operating room capacity. Mean-variance analysis of a hospital's portfolio of surgeons. *Anesth Analg* 2003; 97: 190–5.

28. L. O'Neill, F. Dexter, R. E. Wachtel. Should anesthesia groups advocate funding of clinics and scheduling systems to increase operating room workload? *Anesthesiology* 2009; 111: 1016–24.

29. A. Macario, F. Dexter, R. D. Traub. Hospital profitability per hour of operating room time can vary among surgeons. *Anesth Analg* 2001; 93: 669–75.

30. L. O'Neill, F. Dexter. Tactical increases in operating room block time based on financial data and market growth estimates from data envelopment analysis. *Anesth Analg* 2007; 104: 355–68.

31. J. T. Blake, F. Dexter, J. Donald. Operating room managers' use of integer programming for assigning allocated block time to surgical groups: A case study. *Anesth Analg* 2002; 94: 143–8.

32. P. T. Vanberkel, R. J. Boucherie, E. W. Hans, et al. Accounting for inpatient wards when developing master surgical schedules. *Anesth Analg* 2011; 112: 1472–9.

33. M. L. McManus, M. C. Long, A. Cooper, et al. Variability in surgical caseload and access to intensive care services. *Anesthesiology* 2003; 98: 1491–6.

34. S. Gallivan, M. Utley, T. Treasure, et al. Booked inpatient admission and hospital capacity: Mathematical modelling study. *BMJ* 2002; 324: 280–2.

35. G. Meyfroidt, F. Guiza, D. Cottem, et al. Computerized prediction of intensive care unit discharge after cardiac surgery: Development and validation of a Gaussian processes model. *BMC Med Inform Decis Mak* 2011; 11: 64.

36. R. E. Wachtel, F. Dexter. Tactical increases in operating room block time for capacity planning should not be based on utilization. *Anesth Analg* 2008; 106: 215–26.

37. F. Dexter, R. H. Epstein, H. M. Marsh. Statistical analysis of weekday operating room anesthesia group staffing at nine independently managed surgical suites. *Anesth Analg* 2001; 92: 1493–8.

38. R. J. Casimir. Strategies for a blind newsboy. *Omega Int J Mgmt Sci* 1999; 27: 129–34.

39. F. Dexter, A. Macario, R. D. Traub, et al. An operating room scheduling strategy to maximize the use of operating room block time. Computer simulation of patient scheduling and survey of patients' preferences for surgical waiting time. *Anesth Analg* 1999; 89: 7–20.

40. F. Dexter, R. D. Traub, A. Macario, et al. Operating room utilization alone is not an accurate metric for the allocation of operating room block time to individual surgeons with low caseloads. *Anesthesiology* 2003; 98: 1243–9.

41. A. E. Abouleish, F. Dexter, R. H. Epstein, et al. Labor costs incurred by anesthesiology groups because of operating rooms not being allocated and cases not being scheduled to maximize operating room efficiency. *Anesth Analg* 2003; 96: 1109–13.

42. S. Freytag, F. Dexter, R. H. Epstein, et al. Allocating and scheduling operating room time based on maximizing operating room efficiency at a German university hospital. *Der Chirurg* 2005; 76: 71–9.

43. J. M. Lehtonen, P. Torkki, A. Peltokorpi, T. Moilanen. Increasing operating room productivity by duration categories and a newsvendor model. *Int J Health Care Qual Assur* 2013; 26: 80–92.

44. R. E. Wachtel, F. Dexter. Review of behavioral operations experimental studies of newsvendor problems for operating room management. *Anesth Analg* 2010; 110: 1698–710.

45. J. J. Pandit, F. Dexter. Lack of sensitivity of staffing for 8 hour sessions to standard deviation in daily actual hours of operating room time used for surgeons with long queues. *Anesth Analg* 2009; 108: 1910–15.

46. A. Prahl, F. Dexter, M. T. Braun, L. Van Swol. Review of experimental studies in social psychology of small groups when an optimal choice exists and application

to operating room management decision-making. *Anesth Analg* 2013; 117: 1221–9.

47. F. Dexter, L. S. Weih, R. K. Gustafson, et al. Observational study of operating room times for knee and hip replacement surgery at nine US community hospitals. *Health Care Manag Sci* 2006; 9: 325–39.

48. F. Dexter, R. P. Dutton, H. Kordylewski, R. H. Epstein. Anesthesia workload nationally during regular workdays and weekends. *Anesth Analg* 2015; 121: 1600–3.

49. F. Dexter, D. Masursky, R. E. Wachtel, N. A. Nussmeier. Application of an online reference for reviewing basic statistical principles of operating room management. *J Stat Educ* 2010; 18(3).

50. R. E. Wachtel, F. Dexter. Curriculum providing cognitive knowledge and problem-solving skills for anesthesia systems-based practice. *J Grad Med Educ* 2010; 2: 624–32.

51. E. Marcon, F. Dexter. Observational study of surgeons' sequencing of cases and its impact on post-anesthesia care unit and holding area staffing requirements at hospitals. *Anesth Analg* 2007; 105: 119–26.

52. A. Junger, M. Benson, L. Quinzio, et al. An anesthesia information management system as a tool for controlling resource management of operating rooms. *Meth Inform Med* 2002; 41: 81–5.

53. R. H. Epstein, F. Dexter. Uncertainty in knowing the operating rooms in which cases were performed has little effect on operating room allocations or efficiency. *Anesth Analg* 2002; 95: 1726–30.

54. A. E. Abouleish, S. L. Hensley, M. H. Zornow, et al. Inclusion of turnover time does not influence identification of surgical services that over- and underutilize allocated block time. *Anesth Analg* 2003; 96: 813–18.

55. F. Dexter, R. D. Traub. Lack of systematic month-to-month variation over one year periods in ambulatory surgery caseload application to anesthesia staffing. *Anesth Analg* 2000; 91: 1426–30.

56. D. Masursky, F. Dexter, C. E. O'Leary, C. Applegeet, N. A. Nussmeier. Long-term forecasting of anesthesia workload in operating rooms from changes in a hospital's local population can be inaccurate. *Anesth Analg* 2008; 106: 1223–31.

57. N. R. Farnum, L. W. Stanton. *Quantitative Forecasting Methods*. Boston: Kent, 1989.

58. F. Dexter, R. H. Epstein. Calculating institutional support that benefits both the anesthesia group and hospital. *Anesth Analg* 2008; 106: 544–53.

59. F. Dexter, R. H. Epstein. Typical savings from each minute reduction in tardy first case of the day starts. *Anesth Analg* 2009; 108: 1262–7.

60. F. Dexter, R. D. Traub, A. Macario. How to release allocated operating room time to increase efficiency. Predicting which surgical service will have the most under-utilized operating room time. *Anesth Analg* 2003; 96: 507–12.

61. F. Dexter, A. Macario, R. D. Traub. Which algorithm for scheduling add-on elective cases maximizes operating room utilization? Use of bin packing algorithms and fuzzy constraints in operating room management. *Anesthesiology* 1999; 91: 1491–500.

62. F. Dexter, A. Macario. When to release allocated operating room time to increase operating room efficiency. *Anesth Analg* 2004; 98: 758–62.

63. F. Dexter, P. Shi, R. H. Epstein. Descriptive study of case scheduling and cancellations within one week of the day of surgery. *Anesth Analg* 2012; 115: 1188–95.

64. F. Dexter, A. Macario, D. A. Lubarsky, et al. Statistical method to evaluate management strategies to decrease variability in operating room utilization. Application of linear statistical modeling and Monte-Carlo simulation to operating room management. *Anesthesiology* 1999; 91: 262–74.

65. F. Dexter, R. E. Wachtel, R. H. Epstein. Event-based knowledge elicitation of operating room management decision-making using scenarios adapted from information systems data. *BMC Med Inform Decis Mak* 2011; 11: 2.

66. F. Dexter, A. Willemsen-Dunlap, J. D. Lee. Operating room managerial decision-making on the day of surgery with and without computer recommendations and status displays. *Anesth Analg* 2007; 105: 419–29.

67. F. Dexter. A strategy to decide whether to move the last case of the day in an operating room to another empty operating room to decrease overtime labor costs. *Anesth Analg* 2000; 91: 925–8.

68. F. Dexter, A. Macario, L. O'Neill. A strategy for deciding operating room assignments for second-shift anesthetists. *Anesth Analg* 1999; 89: 920–4.

69. F. Dexter, R. D. Traub. Statistical method for predicting when patients should be ready on the day of surgery. *Anesthesiology* 2000; 93: 1107–14.

70. F. Dexter, R. D. Traub. Sequencing cases in operating rooms: Predicting whether one surgical case will last longer than another. *Anesth Analg* 2000; 90: 975–9.

71. T. J. Babineau, J. Becker, G. Gibbons, et al. The "cost" of operating training for surgical residents. *Arch Surg* 2004; 139: 366–70.

72. S. Eappen, H. Flanagan, N. Bhattacharyya. Introduction of anesthesia resident trainees to the operating room does not lead to changes in anesthesia-controlled times for efficiency measures. *Anesthesiology* 2004; 101: 1210–14.

73. F. Dexter, R. H. Epstein. Associated roles of perioperative medical directors and anesthesia: Hospital agreements for operating room management. *Anesth Analg* 2015; 121: 1469–78.

74. R. E. Wachtel, F. Dexter. Influence of the operating room schedule on tardiness from scheduled start times. *Anesth Analg* 2009; 108: 1889–901.

75. R. E. Wachtel, F. Dexter. Reducing tardiness from scheduled start times by making adjustments to the operating room schedule. *Anesth Analg* 2009; 108: 1902–9.

76. F. Dexter, R. H. Epstein, E. O. Bayman, J. Ledolter. Estimating surgical case durations and making comparisons among facilities: Identifying facilities with lower anesthesia professional fees. *Anesth Analg* 2013; 116: 1103–15.

77. F. Dexter, R. H. Epstein, J. D. Lee, J. Ledolter. Automatic updating of times remaining in surgical cases using Bayesian analysis of historical case duration data and instant messaging updates from anesthesia providers. *Anesth Analg* 2009; 108: 929–40.

78. V. Tiwari, F. Dexter, B. S. Rothman, J. M. Ehrenfeld, R. H. Epstein. Explanation for the near constant mean time remaining in surgical cases exceeding their estimated duration, necessary for appropriate display on electronic white boards. *Anesth Analg* 2013; 117: 487–93.

79. F. Dexter, J. Ledolter. Bayesian prediction bounds and comparisons of operating room times even for procedures with few or no historical data. *Anesthesiology* 2005; 103: 1259–67.

80. F. Dexter, J. Ledolter, V. Tiwari, R. H. Epstein. Value of a scheduled duration quantified in terms of equivalent numbers of historical cases. *Anesth Analg* 2013; 117: 204–9.

81. F. Dexter, A. Macario. What is the relative frequency of uncommon ambulatory surgery procedures in the United States with an anesthesia provider? *Anesth Analg* 2000; 90: 1343–7.

82. F. Dexter, R. D. Traub, L. A. Fleisher, P. Rock. What sample sizes are required for pooling surgical case durations among facilities to decrease the incidence of procedures with little historical data? *Anesthesiology* 2002; 96: 1230–6.

83. F. Dexter, E. U. Dexter, J. Ledolter. Influence of procedure classification on process variability and parameter uncertainty of surgical case durations. *Anesth Analg* 2010; 110: 1155–63.

84. R. H. Epstein, F. Dexter, E. Piotrowski. Automated correction of room location errors in anesthesia information management systems. *Anesth Analg* 2008; 107: 965–71.

Chapter

9

Operations Management and Financial Performance

Seth Christian

Contents

In its essence, operations management is the process by which one seeks to match supply and demand. This standard economic principle exists in all industries, whether it is an energy company, the big box retailer, or the emergency room of a community hospital. Matching supply and demand can be challenging in the operating room (OR); however, as the supply is relatively constant, demand can fluctuate greatly. For example, the ambulatory surgery center may be fully staffed for ten operating suites every Tuesday. On any given Tuesday, the number of cancellations may spike far above the average, leaving empty operating suites attended by wage-earning employees. Conversely, the surgeon in one room may encounter difficulty during his or her first case of the day, causing the case to run significantly over its allotted time. The schedule of operation for the operating suite is then thrown off.

ORs are, in general, profitable. In fact, ORs generally create seventy percent of a hospital's revenue, while constituting only forty percent of the total expenses of the hospital. In the model of the free-standing ambulatory surgery center, the OR is a profit center. So although the revenue stream is vital, running the OR efficiently with the lowest costs possible becomes increasingly important. The OR manager must, therefore, have a profound understanding of cost structures.

In addition, OR managers should monitor key performance criteria, in order to facilitate management decisions and to improve OR efficiency, safety, and satisfaction. Examples of key performance criteria include contribution margins, case cancellation rates, start-time delays, turnover times, etc. In more recent years, Medicare reimbursement has become partially linked to patient satisfaction and patient outcomes; as a result, many ORs include such criteria when monitoring performance and making management decisions.

Cost Structures

"Profit margin" is defined as the difference between revenues and costs. The profit margin can be increased by improving revenues, or, alternatively, decreasing costs. "Costs" can first be categorized as fixed, variable, or semivariable. "Fixed costs" are costs the OR will incur regardless of volume of surgeries performed and generally account for more than fifty percent of an ORs total expenses. Examples of such costs might include the salary of administrative staff, mortgage, capital equipment, billing costs, and information systems. These costs will be in place whether the OR sees an increase in volume, no change in volume, or even a decrease in volume and are generally long-term costs. "Variable costs" fluctuate based on the volume of cases performed and are generally short-term costs. For example, as more surgeries are performed, more supplies are used, and supply costs increase. If there are no surgeries performed on a given day, no additional supplies will be used. Some costs are "semivariable" or have elements of fixed and variable structures. An example of semivariable cost is a full-time employee (FTE) who is paid on an hourly basis. The first 40 hours of their wages are more or less fixed.

Any overtime pay, however, is a variable cost, which is dependent on OR volume. Labor and materials are the two significant fixed and variable costs in the OR.

As one allocates costs, it is important to differentiate direct and indirect costs. Direct costs are directly associated with the running of the OR. Such costs can be attributed back to a source such as a thyroidectomy or other procedure. All hospitals and ORs must factor in "indirect costs," or "overheads," as well. Overhead costs are allocated costs that are spread among all departments or parts of a business. They often originate from support departments such as laundry, dietary services, and housekeeping. Overhead costs may not be directly attributed to the OR but must be factored into the OR budget.

The OR manager may not be able to influence overhead costs, but does have a hand in establishing direct costs in the categories of supply costs, practice management costs, and personnel costs. "Controllable costs" are costs that can be influenced by a manager's decisions. Staffing and supplies are often costs controllable by OR managers. Several strategies for reducing personnel costs have been utilized in the OR.

Personnel costs include the nurses, surgical technicians, and aides in the OR and postanesthesia care unit (PACU). Anesthesia providers may also be included if they are employed by the hospital or surgery center. Personnel costs can make up to 60 percent of an OR budget. Thus, any variance in these costs can have a great impact on the profitability of the OR. Efficiently allocating full-time, part-time, and salaried OR employees in order to avoid excess overtime or underutilized paid time are key to optimizing labor costs.

Supply costs involve the materials needed by the OR to perform surgeries. This is a major component of the OR budget. Pressure exists to hold costs down as much as possible. Thus, this goal must be kept in mind all the way from purchasing the supplies to the analysis of the supplies' use. The OR must have reliable, vital supplies on hand at all times, while avoiding excess or unused inventory, which raises costs without adding value. Thus, optimizing supply costs can be improved by accountability and engagement of all OR personnel and physicians to reduce waste.

Contribution Margin

In managerial accounting, a key concept to understand is the idea of the "contribution margin." This is a method of looking at the relationship between revenues and costs so that the manager can use them to make decisions regarding planning. The key attribute of this approach is the strict delineation between fixed and variable costs, as fixed costs are more constant and will remain in place regardless of how many surgeries are performed. The contribution margin is defined as the difference between revenues and variable costs.

$$\text{Contribution margin} = \text{revenue} - \text{variable cost}$$

The resulting amount, or contribution margin, is then applied to cover the fixed costs. If the contribution margin is greater than the fixed costs, the firm makes a profit. Conversely, if the contribution margin is less than the fixed costs, the firm suffers a loss. Because contribution margin depends upon revenue, payer mix and reimbursement levels will affect the contribution margin. Payer mix and reimbursement levels can vary greatly between institutions. Thus, when filling OR time, one should focus on procedures with higher contribution margins to improve profits, rather than those with high profit but lower contribution margins. Otherwise, when improving utilization of ORs with low contribution margin procedures, one can decrease margins. This is more easily understood if viewed graphically.

In Figure 9.1, the fixed cost is held fixed at $10,000. Total cost starts at $10,000 then has a positive slope up, based on variable costs. Variable cost is the difference between total cost and fixed cost. The point at which total cost and revenue are equal is the "breakeven point," or the point at which the contribution margin covers the fixed cost exactly.

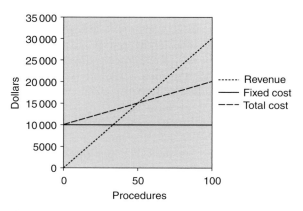

Figure 9.1 Contribution margin.

Any additional contribution margin will be applied to profit. The difference between the revenue and total cost line equals the profit (to the right) or loss (to the left of the breakeven point). For this OR, the break-even point (again, the point at which costs are covered by revenue) is fifty procedures. If this were the data for one week's time, the manager would know that as long as the OR were able to book and perform fifty procedures per week, the unit would not lose money. In addition, any procedures after the fiftieth procedure would be profitable. At any point below fifty procedures, however, the contribution margin would be unable to cover the OR's fixed expenses.

Relationship between Financial and Operational Performance

Although OR managers are not typically responsible for overall financial and operational performance, they must be aware of at least a qualitative relationship between the financial and operational performance of the OR. In order to understand the relationship between operational performance and financial performance, OR managers must have a basic understanding of both financial and managerial accounting. Financial accounting is known as external accounting because the principles of financial accounting aim to create standardized reports with the purpose of comparing organizations within an industry. Managerial cost accounting is known as internal accounting, because it is primarily used as a tool for managers to measure trends in financial performance internally.

Financial accounting statements are composed of four basic documents: (1) the balance sheet, (2) the income statement, (3) the cash flow statement, and (4) the notes to the financial statement.

The balance sheet contains a categorized list of assets and liabilities at the end of an accounting period. It is a picture of the organization's financial position at one point in time, and is often considered the best single indicator of the financial condition of the organization (see Figure 9.2).

The income statement contains a list of all revenues and expenses (Figure 9.3). Revenue for a hospital is generated from both patient care operations and non–patient care operations (parking, cafeteria, research grants, rental space, or equipment sales). Expenses include salaries, benefits, supplies, depreciation, and professional fees.

The cash flow statement contains a list of cash-producing and cash-consuming transactions for the accounting period (Figure 9.4). The cash flow statement shows the financial status in terms of cash flow, rather than according to revenues and expenses in the income statement or accounting entries in the balance sheet.

The notes may include valuable information about the operational status of the organization. Much of the benefit derived from financial statements results from tracking trends in values from one period to the next.

Because healthcare organizations function in different geographic regions and environments while delivering different mixes of services to patient populations, operational indicators make diverse organization more comparable. Many operational indicators are adjusted for case mix and prevailing local wages. Case mix adjustment is a mathematical correction made to account for differences in case type and severity of illness between patient populations. Wage index adjustment is a mathematical correction made to account for differences in employee wages between geographic areas.

Measures of Financial Performance

In addition to the general observation of whether or not an OR is producing enough revenue to meet expenses, financial metrics or indicators can further describe the financial health of the entity. Such measurements describe an institution's ability to meet its responsibilities. For instance, a business can meet its short-term demands by taking on additional debt. This will allow the business to pay its bills at the end of a given month. This, however, is unsustainable in the long term. The business must be able to develop enough equity to meet these obligations. An inability to build such equity will hinder the business from making purchases, developing new technology, or continuing to provide its current standard of service.

Specific financial ratios are also accepted indicators of financial performance (Figure 9.5). "Liquidity ratios" measure the ability to meet short-term obligations. "Capital structure ratios" measure ability to meet long-term obligations. "Profitability ratios" measure ability to generate retained earnings and thus to increase assets. "Activity ratios" measure the efficiency with which assets are used to generate revenues.

Indicators of financial performance expressed as ratios make the information easier to interpret and facilitate benchmarking between similar institutions.

Community Health Care System Balance Sheet

Figure 9.2 Community health care system balance sheet.

Assets (in thousands)		1998		1997
Current assets				
Cash	$	3 364	$	5 990
Cash equivalents	$	6 032	$	4 316
Accounts receivable	$	21 655	$	22 622
Uncollectable allowances	$	766	$	1 046
Charity allowances	$	921	$	1 257
Courtesy allowances	$	98	$	136
Doubtful allowances	$	144	$	201
Contractual allowances	$	4 666	$	1 086
Inventory and supplies	$	1 745	$	2 147
Prepaid expenses	$	1 309	$	1 544
Non-Current assets				
Property, plant, and equipment	$	62 730	$	62 452
Land and improvement	$	4 545	$	3 967
Building and equipment	$	116 997	$	109 648
Construction in progress	$	336	$	1 087
Allowance for depreciation	$	59 148	$	52 250
Restricted assets	$	12 344	$	12 121
Other assets				
Miscellaneous assets	$	1 392	$	830
Total assets	$	110 571	$	112 022

Liabilities and Equities (in thousands)		1998		1997
Current liabilities				
Accounts payable	$	7 406	$	7 895
Accrued liabilities				
Payroll expenses		2 393		3 684
Employee benefits		2 253		2 936
Other liabilities		2 583		2 823
Insurance costs		1 768		1 941
Current portion of long-term debt		1 453		670
Non-current liabilities				
Long-term debt		37 577		37 833
Equity				
Retained earnings		55 138		54 240
Total liabilities and equity		$110 571		$112 022

Operation room managers understand that factors such as reduced OR costs, increased OR operational efficiency, and increased patient volume will improve financial performance.

Liquidity is the measure of an institution's ability to pay its debts or liabilities with its current assets. One can consider this to be "cash on hand." The amount by which assets exceed liabilities is known as "working capital."

$$\text{Working capital} = \text{assets} - \text{liabilities}$$

As an organization's liquidity increases, it has a greater ability to meet its liabilities. If an organization is managed poorly or is struck by unexpected financial hardship, a crisis can ensue when its bills cannot be paid. Such a crisis may be short lived or may be an indication of deeper financial problems. Liquidity is often studied in terms of ratios. The current ratio is the measure of current assets to current liabilities.

$$\text{Acid test} = \left(\text{cash} + \text{cash equivalents}\right) \div \text{current liabilities}$$

Community Health Care System Income Statement

Revenues and Expenses (in thousands)		1998		1997
Revenues				
Patient-care revenues	$	134 101	$	140 684
Other revenues				
Educational programs	$	887	$	886
Research and grants	$	973	$	2 417
Rentals space or equipment	$	2 421	$	971
Sales of medical and pharmacy items to non-patients	$	2 592	$	2 587
Cafeteria sales	$	802	$	801
Auxiliary fund raising and gift shop sales	$	1 143	$	1 141
Parking	$	1 058	$	1 056
Investment income on malpractice trust funds	$	973	$	971
Total revenues	$	144 950	$	151 514
Expenses				
Salaries and wages	$	667 165	$	67 893
Employee benefits	$	13 961	$	16 217
Professional fees	$	8 803	$	12 048
Supplies	$	33 269	$	33 316
Interest	$	4 004	$	3 857
Bad debt expenses	$	5 406	$	6 583
Depreciation and amortization	$	6 898	$	8 022
Restructuring costs	$	5 272	$	628
Taxes	$	252	$	913
Total expenses	$	145 033	$	149 477
Nonoperating gains (losses)				
Revenues from activities unrelated to patient care	$	812	$	833
Gains (losses) from investment of unrestricted funds	$	703	$	621
Gains (losses) from sale of property	$	(534)	$	(360)
Nonoperating gains (losses)	$	981	$	1 094
Excess of revenues and nonoperating gains over expenses	$	898	$	3 131

Figure 9.3 An example of an income statement.

Rarely is this ratio equal to 1. Rather, a very high acid test ratio is approximately 0.3.

Another interesting liquidity ratio useful for making decisions and deciphering financial health of an organization involves the number of "days of cash on hand."

$$\text{Days of cash on hand} = \left(\text{cash} + \text{cash equivalents}\right) \div \text{daily operating expenses} \\ \left(\text{without depreciation}\right)$$

Simply put, this measures the number of days the organization could meet its expenses using solely the cash it has on hand. This indicates an organization's ability to survive a sudden downturn in cash flows. For the manager, or even an investor unfamiliar with operations management, this is a concept that can be missed. This is particularly true in the setting of the freestanding ambulatory surgery center. The capital to make a purchase may be available upfront (the building is financed, the equipment is purchased); however, the cash on hand is insufficient to maintain the operation should volume decrease due to market forces. A rudimentary example may be the ability to purchase the car, but being unable to buy the gasoline to fuel the vehicle.

Capital Structure

Even in healthcare, where the mission is to serve and care for the patient, an OR must generate income. Without doing so, the organization cannot buy equipment or hire additional personnel. As stated earlier, profit margin is the difference between total revenues and total costs. Profitability ratios indicate ability to generate income.

Community Health Care System Cash Flow Statement

Cash flow (in thousands)		1998
Cash flow from operating activities and gains losses		
Revenues and gains greater than (less than) expenses and losses	$	898
Adjustments to reconcile revenues and gains in excess of expenses and loses with net cash provided by operating activities and gains and losses		
Provision for bad debts	$	5 406
Depreciation and amortization	$	6 898
Change in assets and liabilities		
Patients accounts receivable with provision for bad debt	$	4 439.00
Inventory and supplies	$	402.00
Prepaid expenses	$	235.00
Restricted expenses	$	(223.00)
Other assets	$	(562.00)
Account payable	$	(489.00)
Accrued payroll and employee benefits	$	(1 974.00)
Accrued interest	$	(173.00)
Other liabilities	$	(240.00)
Net cash provided by operating activities	$	14 617.00
Cash flows from investing activities		
Purchase of property, plant, and equipment	$	(14 074.00)
Net cash used by investing activities	$	(1 453.00)
Cash flows from financing activities		
Repayments of long-term debt	$	(1 453.00)
Net cash provided by (used by) financing activities	$	(1 453.00)
Net increase (decrease) in cash and cash equivalents	$	(910.00)
Cash and cash equivaents at beginning of year	$	10 306.00
Cash and cash equivaents at end of year	$	9 396.00

Figure 9.4 Community health care system cash flow statement.

$$\text{Total margin ratio} = \left(\text{income} \div \text{total revenues}\right) \times 100\%$$

The total margin ratio simply measures the amount of revenue that contributes to income. This can come from patient care or non–patient care sources.

$$\text{Operating margin ratio} = \left(\text{operating revenues} - \text{operating expenses}\right) \div \text{total revenues}$$

Operating margin excludes non–patient care-related activities and focuses solely on the operational revenues from patient care. This is subsequently usually less than the total margin ratio. Within the OR the main mode of increasing operating margin is by decreasing expenses.

$$\text{Return on equity} = \left(\text{income} \div \text{equity}\right) \times 100\%$$

Finally, return on equity is often considered the primary test of profitability. This measure relates income to equity or net assets of the organization. Equity is determined as the difference between assets and liabilities. The resulting number indicates the rate at which an OR or other organization produces profit relative to its net assets. A higher percentage indicates greater return on equity, and thus greater profitability.

Measures of Operational Performance

Although measures of financial performance are vital to determine the health of an organization's finances, they do not characterize the efficiency by which the organization provides services with the resources at hand. In an ideal model, an organization would utilize resources perfectly. In other words, the OR would consume exactly what is required for its services, no more, no less. Every additional suture required or labor hour needed above this point decreases efficiency. A manager can work to increase operating income by increasing revenues or decreasing expenses. By and large, the overwhelming method for increasing income is by decreasing expenses. These fundamentals are

Community Health Care System Financial Performance Ratios

Ratio	Low	Middle	High
Liquidity			
Current	1.5	2	2.5
Acid test	0.2	0.25	0.3
Days in patient accounts receivable	40	55	70
Days of cash on hand	20	26	32
Capital structure			
Long-term debt-to-equity	0.6	0.7	0.8
Times interest earned	2.4	2.7	3.0
Cash flow-to-debt	0.1	0.2	0.3
Debt service coverage	3.1	3.5	4.0
Profitability			
Total margin	3%	4%	5%
Operating margin	2%	3%	4%
Return on equity	5%	7.5%	10%
Activity			
Asset turnover	0.8	0.9	1.0
Fixed asset turnover	1.5	2.0	2.5
Current asset turnover	3.0	3.5	4.0

Figure 9.5 Community health care system financial performance ratios.

analyzed much like the financial statements through the use of performance ratios (Box 9.1). These ratios are complicated by the fact that case mix is not universal across institutions. A case mix index is therefore applied that weighs a facility's cases and patient illness against an average. A similar index is utilized to adjust for wage differences between regions.

One indicator of interest is the revenue a facility generates per discharge. This can be used for inpatient hospitals as well as ambulatory centers. The net inpatient or outpatient revenues depending on the facility are divided by the number of discharges, adjusted for case mix and wage discrepancy.

$$\text{Net patient revenues} \div (\text{no. of discharges} \times \text{case mix index} \times \text{wage index})$$

A similar indicator can be used to measure the costs incurred per discharge by substituting net costs for revenue. This is again adjusted for case mix and wage.

$$\text{Net patient costs} \div (\text{no. of discharges} \times \text{case mix index} \times \text{wage index})$$

When operating within a large facility, it may be impossible to measure the OR's contribution to costs. Generally speaking, this contribution will be high and may make up the majority of the costs for a typical admission.

As labor costs often make up a large percentage of a facility's total expenditures, it is also important to analyze the efficiency by which labor is used. In an inpatient facility, this is done by taking the number of FTEs and multiplying them by 2080 (the number of hours worked in a year). This product is then divided, once again, by the number of discharges adjusted for case mix and wage.

$$(\text{FTEs} \times 2080) \div (\text{no. of discharges} \times \text{case mix index} \times \text{wage index})$$

The resulting value measures labor productivity. If the number of employees remains constant, a lower value indicates higher labor productivity. That is, labor is being utilized at a greater rate. As the number of discharges (patients) increases, labor productivity will be greater. Although this is generally a positive trend, it does not mean that costs may be lower. A facility may have higher labor productivity as fewer staff are required to see a set number of patients, but if these employees are higher cost, overall labor costs may still be fairly high.

The average unit cost of labor can be measured by measuring the salary per FTE.

$$\text{Total salary} \div (\text{no. FTEs} \times \text{wage index})$$

This indicator can be skewed higher or lower depending on the institution. A facility that utilizes

Box 9.1. Operational Performance Indicators and Suggested Example Values

Occupancy	50%
Length of stay, case mix adjusted	4.5 days
Revenue per discharge, case mix, and wage index adjusted	$5000
Revenue per visit, wage index adjusted	$225
Cost per discharge, case mix, and wage index adjusted	$5,000
Cost per visit, wage index adjusted	$225
Inpatient staff hours per discharge, case mix, and wage index adjusted	135
Outpatient staff hours per visit	6
Salary per full-time equivalent employee, wage index adjusted	$33,000
Capital costs per discharge, case mix, and wage index adjusted	$5400
Outpatient revenue	33%

a smaller number of employees who are also higher-cost employees will have a higher average salary. This does not necessarily indicate greater total labor costs. Likewise, any institution that contracts for services such as dietary or housekeeping will have a greater average salary, as contracted employees are not factored.

Finally, a facility that provides both inpatient and outpatient services can analyze the contribution of outpatient services to overall revenues by calculating the percentage of revenue received from outpatients.

$$\left(\text{Net outpatient revenues} \div \text{total revenues}\right) \times 100\%$$

If a facility is able to maintain a constant level of inpatient revenue stream, an increase in the percentage coming from outpatient services is generally a positive trend. This is secondary to fewer costs associated with such services. If, however, the increase in outpatient revenues is at the expense of inpatient revenues, the result is far less positive.

Process View

Any industry can be seen as more than the products or services it provides. It is important to examine the processes by which the supply is generated. The process is the accumulation of multiple steps or activities. When one analyzes an OR, it is often done from the perspective of the patient. That is, the patient is the

unit of measurement. As patients works their way through the process of outpatient surgery, they will experience many activities, including: registration, preadmit testing, preoperative nursing care, preoperative assessment, transfer to preoperative holding area, procedure in OR, recovery room, outpatient surgery, and finally home. The time the patient spends in each of these activities is called the activity time. If there are gaps in between the activities, the patient is then waiting. This allows one to describe supply–demand mismatches. Waiting times are a consequence of finite supply. In a hospital with unlimited ORs, surgeons, nurses, and anesthesiologists, the patient's waiting time would be zero. Unfortunately, this is rarely the case.

Process performance can be analyzed using three measurements: "volume," "flow time," and "flow rate." Volume is the total number of units within the process at any one time. Flow time is the amount of time required for one unit to flow through the entire process. Flow rate is the rate at which units are passed through the process in flow unit time (units/hour or day). In the OR, the number of patients awaiting surgery, receiving surgery, and recovering from surgery is the volume. The flow time is the average time for a patient to make it through from registration to discharge. The flow rate is usually the number of patients who receive surgery per day. The maximum flow rate is also known as the capacity of the process – that is, the greatest rate at which patients receive surgery and are discharged home. If you are able to increase capacity, supply will be able to meet demand under a greater number of circumstances. These three measurements are related to one another through Little's Law:

$$\text{Average volume} = \text{average flow rate} \\ \times \text{average wait time}$$

Process Capacity and Bottlenecks

Process capacity, or maximum flow rate, is the maximum amount a process can produce during a certain period of time. This is the amount the process can produce even if the process generally produces less than the capacity. One of the foremost goals of operations management is to maximize capacity. One does so by first analyzing the process itself to seek out limits to capacity. These limits may be physical such as having ten ORs, or related to labor, such as lacking an extra nurse for the recovery room. The point at which the process stalls, slows, or is limited by the flow time through an activity is known as the "bottleneck." The bottleneck's capacity is, in turn, the process's capacity. This is the rate-limiting step.

Let's look at a simplified example of process analysis applied to the OR. The process is made up of many steps or activities, starting with patients arriving at registration. First the patients must register to be admitted. This step is staffed by three employees and takes an average of fifteen minutes per patient. Second, patients are admitted to outpatient surgery, where nursing staff check vitals, start IV's, draw any ordered tests, and administer medications, etc. Six nurses, who can see two patients at a time, staff the unit. It takes about thirty minutes to complete this step. Third, once patients are called for, they are moved to preoperative holding area, where a nurse checks all consents, anesthesia providers meet and evaluate patients, and the surgeon checks on the patients. Up to ten patients can be in the preoperative holding area at any one time, and they stay for approximately thirty minutes. Fourth, the patient is brought to the OR for surgery. This facility staffs twenty ORs with an average procedure time of 2 h. Fifth, the patient is moved to the PACU for recovery, where he or she is monitored by nursing staff. The PACU is staffed with four nurses, who can each take two patients. Average time to discharge a patient after arrival is sixty minutes. Sixth, once patients are discharged from the PACU, they returns to outpatient surgery for monitoring and discharge. Owing to the staggered nature of postoperative arrival back in outpatient surgery, the unit is staffed with five nurses who can again take two patients at a time. The average stay is thirty minutes. So, in this example there are six distinct steps that must happen in order.

Table 9.1 lists all the locations/steps in order that the activities are performed. The inventory is the number of patients that can be in the activity at any one time, while the flow time is the average time the activity takes. Using this information, we are able to calculate the capacity for each step. Although the inventory of the registration is lowest among the activities, the flow time is also the shortest. Conversely, flow time is longest in the OR itself, but the high level of inventory allows for higher capacity. The activity with the lowest capacity turns out to be recovery in the PACU, at eight patients per hour. It is the bottleneck, or rate-limiting step. Additional ORs can be opened or registration staff hired, but the maximum capacity will not improve above eight patients per hour.

By analyzing the process, we can seek to determine the bottleneck. In our example, if the manager worked to relieve the bottleneck in the PACU by increasing staffing or decreasing flow time, he or she could work to improve the process capacity.

We can also look at utilization of a process, or how much production is made relative to the maximum production possible.

$$\text{Process utilization} = \text{flow rate} \div \text{process capacity}$$

We can then analyze why a process may not be 100 percent utilized. This may be demand limited if flow rate is decreased due to a lack of demand for the unit produced: for instance, the ORs being underutilized because the number of surgeries booked is low. Going back to our hypothetical OR, if the flow rate is less than eight patients per hour, the PACU is no longer limiting flow through the process. The decreased utilization is due to demand rather than supply. If we then look at each step within the process, we see that the activity with the highest utilization will be the bottleneck of the process. It is also important to keep in mind that the bottleneck can also occur outside of the OR process, such as the ICU or clinic.

Table 9.1 Process Analysis in the OR

Activity	Inventory	Flow time (h)	Capacity (patients/h)
Registration	3	0.25	3/0.25 = 12
Outpatient surgery	12	0.5	12/0.5 = 24
Preop holding	10	0.5	10/0.5 = 20
OR	20	2.0	20/2 = 10
PACU	8	1.0	8/1 = 8
Outpatient surgery	10	0.5	10/0.5 = 20

Table 9.2 Process Capacity of Eight Patients Per Hour

Activity	Inventory	Flow time (h)	Capacity (patients/h)	Utilization (%)
Registration	3	0.25	3/0.25 = 12	6/12 = 50
Outpatient surgery	12	0.5	12/0.5 = 24	6/24 = 25
Preop holding	10	0.5	10/0.5 = 20	6/20 = 30
OR	20	2.0	20/2 = 10	6/10 = 60
PACU	8	1.0	8/1 = 8	6/8 = 75
Outpatient surgery	10	0.5	10/0.5 = 20	6/20 = 30
		Process flow rate = 6 patients/h	Process capacity = 8 patients/h	6/8 = 75

Table 9.3 Process Capacity of 12 Patients Per Hour

Activity	Inventory	Flow time (h)	Capacity (patients/h)	Utilization (%)
Registration	3	0.25	3/0.25 = 12	12/12 = 100
Outpatient surgery	12	0.5	12/0.5 = 24	12/24 = 50
Preop holding	10	0.5	10/0.5 = 20	12/20 = 60
OR	20	2.0	20/2 = 10	12/12 = 100
PACU	10	0.75	10/0.75 = 13.33	12/13.3 = 90
Outpatient surgery	10	0.5	10/0.5 = 20	12/20 = 60
		Process flow rate = 12 patients/h	Process capacity = 12 patients/h	12/12 = 100

If we were to find that the process flow rate was six patients per hour even though our bottleneck capacity was eight patients per hour, our process utilization would stand at 75 percent (Table 9.2). The PACU still stands as our bottleneck, as it has the highest activity utilization of the process, but at this time it is not limiting the OR's production.

If, on the other hand, the process were running at capacity of eight patients per hour with patients waiting to be transferred to the PACU, the process utilization would be at 100 percent. The OR manager now has the opportunity to effect change. An additional PACU nurse is hired and efforts to improve efficiency within the PACU decrease the flow time from 60 to 45 min.

Now more patients are able to complete the process, and capacity has increased to 12 patients per hour (Table 9.3). The PACU is no longer the bottleneck. The ORs and registration are now limiting capacity. An OR manager must also keep in mind that increasing OR utilization can decrease flexibility for surgeons.

One of the main goals of the OR manager is to identify sources of inefficiency that reduce capacity, and then resolve the issues. The manager must seek to identify the bottleneck and work to relieve it; otherwise the OR will be forever limited by that step. Increasing staffing or equipment to every other activity in the process will do nothing but decrease efficiency while increasing cost. However, if one is able to take a process analysis view of the OR, such decisions can be made without missing the true source of the problem. Such a misstep can have the potential to be costly, such as allocating resources towards additional housekeeping staff in hopes of improving turnover times, when the nursing shortage in the PACU has patients recovering in the OR.

Suggested Reading

P. C. Brewer, R. H. Garrison, E. W. Noreen. *Managerial Accounting*, 14th edn. New York: McGraw-Hill, 2012.

G. Cachon, C. Terwiesh. *Matching Supply with Demand: An Introduction to Operations Management*, 3rd edn. Boston: McGraw-Hill, 2011.

R. A. Gabel, ed. *Operating Room Management*. Chicago: Butterworth-Heinemann, 1999.

A. P. Harris, W. G. Zitzmann. *Operating Room Management: Structure, Strategies, & Economics*. St. Louis: Mosby, 1998.

Chapter

10

Reengineering Operating Room Function

Nigel N. Robertson

Contents

Introduction

Operating rooms (ORs) are rightly regarded as important drivers of the productive potential of any healthcare organization. They are often the greatest source of revenue within a hospital system but also have a high cost base that presents an element of risk to the organization if not managed effectively.

Globally, healthcare systems are under ever more pressure to deliver greater efficiency, productivity, and – above all – quality of care within constrained budgets. ORs are increasingly seen as "outliers" by funders and regulators measuring performance improvement through transformational process redesign methodologies such as Lean Six Sigma (LSS).

Modern industrial and commercial complexes are designed and built to seamlessly integrate into the process and functional objectives of the organization. Many examples of such workplaces are available as video clips on the web; readers are particularly directed to one such clip featuring the Volkswagen Phaeton plant in Germany (www.youtube.com – search "VW phaeton factory").

Much of the current hospital stock was built in the 1950s to 1980s. Clinicians were not involved in high-level design until the layout of the building had been determined. By then, it was too late to optimize the OR design and co-locations; many an architect's

plan placed the ICU at a remote location from the OR, much to the chagrin of the putative operators!

The objective of this chapter is to briefly discuss the meaning of efficiency in the context of ORs, outline the concept of LSS, variability, and waste in OR processes and describe ways in which architects and clinicians can work to design facilities that will be fit for purpose. The building process is described and also how to stay in touch with the process to achieve best outcomes. Communication platforms in the OR are also described. Refurbishment of existing buildings is a particular skill, and there is some discussion of this aspect within the chapter. It should be made clear from the outset that there is no single best way to design the OR suite; solutions are contextual; it depends how the organization and clinicians plan to use the unit. Space precludes the creation of an OR design manual; this chapter, however, gives clinicians and managers a toolkit with which to benchmark their facility.

Efficiency, Productivity, and Design

What does the term "efficiency" mean in the OR? Stakeholders in a healthcare system define efficiency in the OR with a range of responses (Figure 10.1) that are discussed in detail in other parts of this book. The objective of delivering efficiency at its simplest level is to produce a realistic schedule that fits the resource available; the schedule for the day has a reasonable

I thank Associate Professor Simon Mitchell and Drs. Charles Bradfield and Chris Chambers for their editorial and proofreading skills; and Ms Diane Newby and Ms Karen Patching for their help in preparing the illustrations.

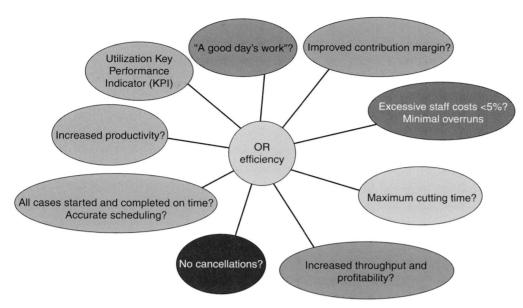

Figure 10.1 OR efficiency, as defined by stakeholder groups in the OR.

probability of filling the OR session without finishing early, finishing late, or cancelling any patients, as described by Pandit et al. [1]. It sounds so simple.

A number of measures of OR activity have been proposed over the past two to three decades, but most of them have significant limitations and can either be manipulated or include major correction factors to enable a merger of quantitative and qualitative datasets. These are discussed in more detail elsewhere in this book.

Recently, Macario produced a scoring system for OR efficiency (Table 10.1) that used existing data and assigned points to eight metrics that he deemed to be important end points of OR efficiency [2]. These included excessive staffing costs, start time tardiness, turnovers, contribution margins, postanesthesia care unit (PACU) admission delays, and cancellations. Efficient units scored more points, and in his editorial Macario succinctly described real-life metrics that all OR clinicians recognize.

Pandit and his colleagues have also developed an elegant model that uses simple data, available in all OR suites, to create a measure of "productive potential" for an OR team [3].

It is important to understand measures of efficiency when designing ORs. Some of the preceding discussion will perhaps have delivered some clues as to the reasons for this; "turnover times" and "PACU admission delays" have an impact on OR efficiency, however it is defined. We therefore need to explore how the design of OR facilities affects these production metrics.

Over the past decade, many healthcare organizations have sought to streamline their operations by adopting methods developed for industry and commerce, such as LSS processing and queueing theory. These have become very attractive to managers, chief executives, and boards as a way to bring some order to the apparently chaotic nature of healthcare.

There is, however, little evidence of systemic success in the literature thus far (although many anecdotal examples are quoted). Skeptics point to the unique variability within healthcare compared with car production lines, for example, as a potent reason to resist adoption of LSS in healthcare. However, as Dr. Litvak at the Institute of Healthcare Improvement and others have pointed out, there are two types of variability: natural and artificial [4]. The former relates to the randomness of patient arrival into the system, the complex and variable nature of their illness, and the length of the treatment episode. This variability may add cost but cannot be eliminated.

Artificial variability, however, is usually the result of a systems limitation or bottleneck, such as a poorly drafted elective surgical schedule or a building

Table 10.1 A Scoring System for OR Efficiency

Metric	Points		
	0	1	2
Excess staffing costs	>10%	5–10%	<5%
Start-time tardiness (mean tardiness of start times for elective cases per OR per day)	>60 min	45–60 min	<45 min
Case cancellation rate	>10%	5–10%	<5%
PACU admission delays (% of workdays with at least one delay in PACU admission)	>20%	10–20%	<10%
Contribution margin (mean) per OR hour	<$1,000/h	$1,000–2000/h	>$2,000/h
Turnover times (mean setup and cleanup turnover times for all cases)	>40 min	25–40 min	<25 min
Prediction bias (bias in case duration estimates per 8 h of OR time)	>15 min	5–15 min	<5 min
Prolonged turnovers (% of turnovers that are more than 60 min)	>25%	10–25%	<10%

Source: A. Macario. Are your operating rooms efficient? A scoring system with eight performance indicators. ***Anesthesiology*** 2006; *105*: 237–40.

capacity and design problem. This form of variability can and should be eliminated.

Waste

Elements of LSS and variability methodology in healthcare constitute a common theme of waste in the system. The following discussion will focus on waste in the OR and how this relates to the design of the OR facilities.

The NHS Institute for Innovation and Improvement in the UK defined seven forms of waste as applied to the healthcare context [5]:

- overproduction – undertaking activity in batches or "just-in-case"
- inventory – refers to materials and also to patients; usually a symptom of poor supply chain or admission/discharge process
- waiting – can apply to patients, staff, material, or equipment
- transportation – excess or inefficient movement of patients or material
- defects – any defect that impacts on a process, including patient cancellation
- staff movement – relates to organization and layout of facility and also to information solutions
- unnecessary processing – using complex facilities or equipment to undertake simple tasks

When these elements are applied to the OR, we start to see the importance of developing an integrated view of design and process.

Waste in the OR Suite – Design Is a Contributor

This concept of waste allows some themes to emerge for both clinicians and managers concerned with OR efficiency. These may now be applied to the OR setting (Figure 10.2):

- overproduction – example: batched patient arrivals for OR sessions
- inventory – example: poor storage layout/ inadequate capacity, leading to uneven supply chain
- waiting – example: poor scheduling, prolonged turnover, tardiness, PACU capacity
- transportation – example: poor layout of OR suite, co-location of related units such as ICU, PACU, sterile supplies; elevators remotely located
- defects – example: cancellations, missing patient information, equipment failure, surgical site infection
- staff movement – example: store rooms remote from OR, lack of surgeon workspace during turnover, use of IT solutions
- unnecessary processing – examples: repeated patient checks in the OR, non–value-added preoperative testing, ambulatory cases in tertiary center OR suites

The first two elements of the design journey are now described: an outline of efficiency and productivity in the OR; and the concept of systematic waste that is influenced by the design of the OR suites.

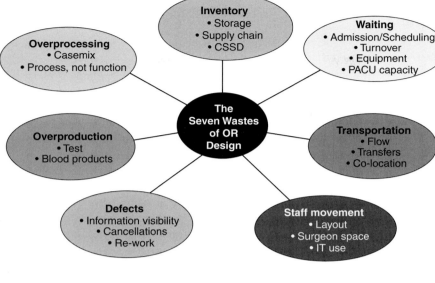

Figure 10.2 Examples of waste in the OR suite. CSSD, Central Sterile Services Department; PACU, Post-Anesthesia Care Unit; OR, Operating Room; IT, Information Technology

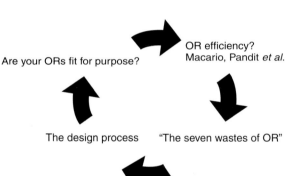

Figure 10.3 The design cycle for OR construction.

Taking these forward, we can then start to formulate a design process that will produce a facility that is fit for purpose (Figure 10.3).

The OR Design Process

Who Is Involved?

Anyone who has built a house will recognize that there are many parties involved: owner, bank, local authority, builder, architect, and others.

Hospitals are enormously complex facilities and require input from a bewildering range of stakeholders (Figure 10.4). Clinicians may have limited experience dealing with many of the representative professions and trades involved, but it is important to be part of the design team from the earliest opportunity to insure

that clinical concerns are met as the process evolves. A tender process will result in selection of a "design and build" team and a project management team that will usually be responsible for delivery of the facility.

Clinicians should be seconded to the latter team from the outset. Crucial decisions that impact on the whole life of the building are often made within the first few weeks and months of the project. Initial footprint and layout plans are often tied to tender documents and budgets. Plan redraws become problematic once the organization and project team has locked them in to target timelines and payment schedules.

Ideally, staff clinicians should be involved and seconded to the project team. The organization must recognize the value of this addition to the team and provide cover for the clinical commitments of their staff.

Clinicians attached to the project team bring authenticity to the design. They can enlist their colleague "champions" to develop a very clear vision of the design features required to support the function of the facility. In our project, I was the design coordinator for the OR suites, and this involved "360" meetings with many stakeholder groups such as:

- clinical user groups
- project executives and board members
- government/funder representatives
- consumer representatives
- construction and project management team members
- architects

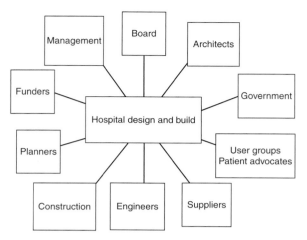

Figure 10.4 The important stakeholders involved in a hospital design and build project.

- engineers/IT consultants/electrical engineers
- building and workforce migration specialists

Many weeks and months of discussion and negotiation are the norm, and it is crucial to gather information, keep an open mind, be nonjudgmental, and, above all, focus on the solution.

Relatively few clinicians have the task of designing an OR facility during their career, and therefore it may seem a daunting prospect.

Site Visits

A useful benchmarking exercise is to visit other recently constructed facilities. The architects engaged on the project will be specialized in the design of hospital facilities and will have previous projects available for scrutiny. These visits are vital for the success of the project for the following reasons.

- A modern hospital facility is substantially different from the current aging hospital stock. A visit demonstrates what is now possible in design and function.
- Architects tend to template the current project from recently completed works. Visiting other hospitals designed and built by the same group will help to develop the vision of the facility and also foster understanding of how they develop a project design.
- Assessment of the environmental aspects of the facility – size and shape of the rooms, corridor widths, storage, color scheme, acoustic

management, etc. – is mandatory. These are all contributors to the "feel" of the building.

- Fixtures such as pendants and booms or minimally invasive surgery (MIS) ORs can be critically appraised from a clinical perspective, with feedback from clinical staff rather than a sales pitch from the company representative.
- A useful if informal cost/utility analysis can be completed on site with the staff and managers.
- Staff working in the facility can be asked to give feedback, both on the design process and an informal "post hoc" audit of the unit. This is especially valuable for benchmarking.
- Meetings with management representatives can be scheduled to gain further feedback on strengths and weaknesses of the design.

Site visits during a project may result in significant variance to the proposed design that may require careful negotiation with architects and funders.

Process Mapping

The success of the project depends on this step. It is crucial to construct a clear picture of the expected caseload, case mix, model of care, and clinical pathways for the planned facility.

If the project is a redevelopment (new hospital building within an existing complex), most processes and pathways will have evolved to fit the old facility. User groups should be given the tools to redesign the capacities and flows to match best practice, and for many this is a potentially stressful exercise requiring good leadership. Professional facilitation and change management will be required. Cultures also become established and may need some transformational change to maximize the benefits of the new facility. This should be tackled early and facilitated.

There are several process issues that have a significant bearing on design.

- Basic demographic statistics
  - Patient numbers
  - Surgical specialties
  - Future population growth/health requirements
- Proposed model(s) of care
  - Hospital inpatient, ambulatory
  - Planned surgery/unplanned/trauma
    - Dedicated unplanned surgery OR required?

- Variable utilization targets, efficiency, urgency
- Clinical pathways
  - Preadmission process
  - Planned/unplanned surgery pathways
  - Postoperative care/discharge

What will emerge is a comprehensive plan describing how the facility is to be used. That plan will then determine the overall size of the unit, the numbers and dimensions of the ORs, the size and configuration of the admission and postoperative facilities, and the requirements for staff amenities. In reality, of course, this cannot be 100 percent accurate given the forecasted nature of future health requirements, but the exercise of compiling a process map is invaluable when discussions commence with architects and planners and this allows staff to revalidate their own practices and benchmark off other similar organizations.

The key is to build as much flexibility into the design as possible. Most buildings have a working life of 40–50 years. Planners are not able to predict all future developments over this time span, and therefore the building will almost certainly be modified. The best designs are simple, flexible, and also fit for purpose.

Getting Started

The project director will map out a process leading to sign-off for the developed design plans that will be converted into building drawings (Figure 10.5). The first step will be high-level floor plans outlining the location of wards and other units within the building. The architects will then meet with the user groups to agree a "schedule of accommodation." This is a set of documents detailing the size, shape, services, fixtures, and fittings of every room in the OR suite, down to the last power and data outlet. It is this information that the architect will use to draft the initial plans, and it goes without saying that a great deal of thought and work is required to get this correct.

The schedule will also detail the width of corridors and size of storage facilities. There are two points to remember here. The first is that storage space is often a victim of "value management," or what is more commonly known as staying on budget; adequate, well-placed storage is essential. The second point is that circulation space (corridors, reception space, etc.) should constitute approximately 35 percent of the total floor area of the unit (Ian Moon, architect, and

McConnel, Smith and Johnson architects, Sydney, Australia, personal communication). The schedule of accommodation will usually be presented in data sheet form, specific to a particular room type such as an OR, an office, or a PACU bed space. Each will have a unique sheet code number.

The architect will want a great deal of detail at this stage; success is facilitated by a clear process map and vision of the functional aspects of the proposed unit. Remember that, as with house building, architects can only design to the brief that they receive. If a detailed brief is not submitted and agreed upon, a stock solution will ensue that may not be fit for purpose.

Architects use computer-aided design (CAD) software to draft plans (Figure 10.6). These software packages allow very complex designs to be clearly displayed and can be redrafted relatively quickly to reflect changes. Object CAD software can now develop three-dimensional computer models of facilities, and more recently building information modeling has been developed as an approach to integrate design, function, budgets, and progress updates to give the project team real-time data on which to base necessary changes more efficiently. Clinicians on the project team should become familiar with these valuable tools.

A set of preliminary design plans will follow, based on the schedule of accommodation. This will be the basis of ongoing discussion and negotiation until sign-off is achieved. Involve all interested stakeholders in this stage, including surgeon representatives (often the most intermittent attendees), infection control, and the radiology service.

Issues to be decided will include:

- size and shape of the ORs and their position in the OR suite
- environmental considerations – windows, natural light, acoustic solutions
- position of fixtures, fittings, and services such as power, gases, and communications within rooms
- advanced features such as MRI and MIS equipment and interventional radiology; special floors and set-downs may be required
- support rooms for the OR (scrub bay, setup room, anesthesia induction room, cleanup room)
- location, as well as size, shape, and visibility, of the reception area and control hub for the OR coordinators and managers
- storage areas – floor area, shape, sterile/nonsterile, co-location to ORs, shelving – fixed/

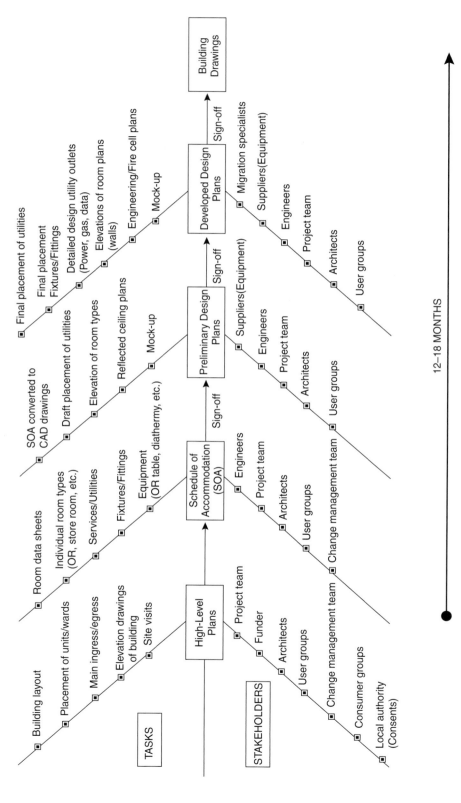

Figure 10.5 High-level building design process map.

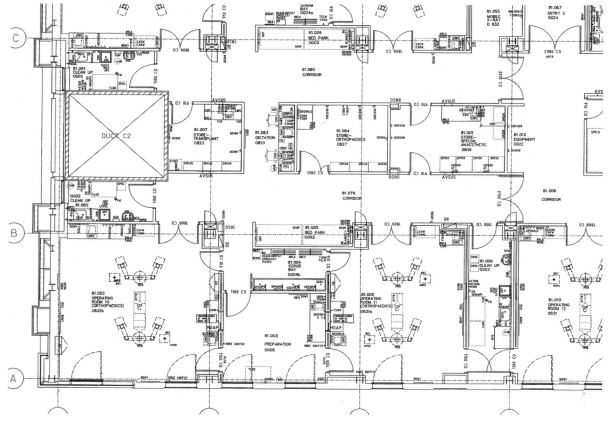

Figure 10.6 A developed design CAD drawing of part of the eighth level of Auckland City Hospital, New Zealand, showing the OR suite. The ORs are situated around the perimeter of the building to maximize natural light use.
Reproduced with the permission of McConnel, Smith and Johnson P/L, Architects, Sydney, Australia.

mobile, required services such as IT, and power outlets for charging equipment

- admission and postanesthesia units – location, floor area, number of patient spaces, staff base positions, fixtures and fittings
- procedure areas for anesthesia blocks, minor procedures
- pharmacy supply – satellite pharmacy, mobile solution, controlled drug management
- ingress and egress routes – how the access ways are designed for patients, staff, supplies, and equipment; emergency egress
- fire and smoke damage prevention measures
- fire and smoke cell design and location of fire alarm control panels

- electrical safety measures and methods – line isolation monitor, residual current devices, equipotential earthing studs
- infection control measures, including ventilation systems and room design
- electrical supply safety, including generator-supplied circuits, uninterruptable power supply (UPS) circuits, location and number of outlets
- sterile supplies and processing unit – within unit or remote? (many will be remote from the OR suite); transport of sterile supplies – dedicated elevators?
- corridors – width, clear, or allow storage of equipment?
- single corridor design or sterile core with outer corridor for nonsterile traffic – this has

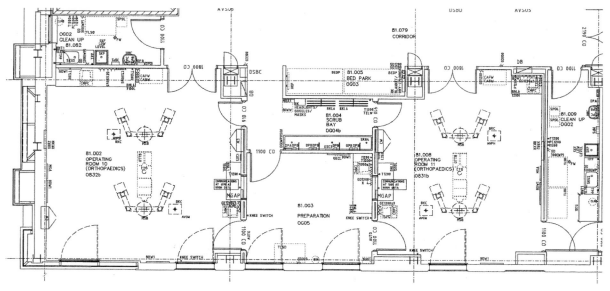

Figure 10.7 Preliminary design CAD drawing of an individual OR "pod."
Reproduced with the permission of McConnel, Smith and Johnson P/L, Architects, Sydney, Australia.

- major implications for many other design considerations
- staff amenities – changing rooms, meal room, offices, internet café, meeting rooms, dictation area, washrooms
- ancillary services – cleaners, trash storage and pick-up, goods inwards area
- links to co-located units such as ICU, high-dependency unit (HDU), etc.
- hospital/OR interface and substerile areas; scrubs-only areas

Clearly, to consider all of the above (and this is not exhaustive) the users will need well-conceived plans of how the unit is to be used. Again, flexibility is the key, coupled with simplicity of design.

Throughout the process, matching of design proposals to the agreed flows and functional mapping will pay dividends. Many iterations of the plans will be circulated before sign-off; keep track of the current version to avoid confusion.

A useful exercise is a mock-up of the OR design. This can be done either in a rented industrial space or at the architect's office and will allow users and other stakeholders to view full-scale facilities and the configurations of rooms; this may avoid costly redraws of final building plans.

OR Dimensions

There is an inexorable trend toward larger ORs as the operating team "footprint" becomes ever larger and more complex. A wide array of designs, sizes, and shapes have been described, including the so-called *barn operating rooms*, where several OR areas are clustered in one physical space, separated only by retractable curtains and each with a discrete ventilation unit (Figure 10.7).

Not all ORs need to be 860 sq ft (80 m^2), an area commonly quoted in some discussion documents. The ideal size of the room depends on the type of surgery that is proposed (and therefore the surgical footprint), the presence of ancillary facilities such as anesthesia induction rooms, and the flow within the OR itself. The configuration of the immediate OR area will also determine the numbers and positions of doors, regarded as dead space by architects when planning the configuration of a room.

At Auckland City Hospital, the largest OR is 700 sq ft (65 m^2), and orthotopic liver transplants are comfortably undertaken in a 650 sq ft (60 m^2) square-sided room. These rooms accommodate the surgical footprint, all of the ancillary equipment (such as C-arms and microscopes), and still have circulation space around the perimeter.

To retain flexibility, a general rule is to keep the OR fixtures such as cupboards and benches to a minimum, unless the OR is going to be used for one type of surgery only (examples would be ophthalmology surgery or endoscopic ambulatory surgery). Relatively "empty" rooms are beneficial for cleaning and infection control purposes.

Special consideration will have to be given for MIS rooms, including those housing robots. These may include such additions as specially strengthened areas on a wall on which to mount plasma screens, an adjacent area for a robotic control console, and added systems cabling behind the walls and in the ceiling space. Such MIS rooms have a software control hub that may need to be located in an adjacent space, and proprietary cabling may be required.

Utilities

Special mention should be made about the provision of power, gases, and communications in the OR.

Utility services become more complex as rooms become larger and more sophisticated. A model of utility supply must be agreed that will service the functions of the room as early as the schedule of accommodation stage. This includes the number and distribution of electrical outlets and their power source. Most, if not all, circuits will be routed through the hospital generator backup supply; a subgroup will also be routed via a battery bank that will provide UPS in the event of generator failure. This supply has a finite capacity, and users will be advised by the engineers how to match the battery bank capacity to the requirements of the unit.

Many ORs now have their power, gas, and data cabling delivered via a boom or pendant, in order to deliver the services to the center of the room and have some ability to locate the services to suit the patient orientation within the OR.

Each boom or pendant needs to be positioned appropriately in the room. There is no "correct" position, and the users need to model the room function and decide on:

- symmetrical versus asymmetrical position within the room
- position relative to the operating table
- articulated or fixed-arm boom/pendant, stalactite pendant
- a solution for the anesthesia machine – freestanding on the floor, docked and lifted on the pendant, or fully pendant-mounted

- numbers and types of power points, gas outlets, vacuum and gas scavenging connection points, and data connection sockets

Space precludes more detailed discussion on this issue here. Most booms and pendants will have a life span of up to 20 years. Some forward thinking and engineering will reduce the chance of a costly upgrade by requesting extra data cabling and draw lines within the housing so that new cabling can be added later without major refit work. Any proprietary cabling for monitoring systems needs to be specified and supplied by the relevant company. Booms or pendants may also be used in ICU, cardiac catheter rooms, and the emergency department; the tender process will require a solution that has the flexibility to suit all locations, and other user groups will be involved in the tender process.

OR Ventilation Systems

It is only 30 years ago that some ORs had no dedicated ventilation system, and more "mature" readers may remember rooms that had opening windows to cool the rooms in summer! Many variations of design have been used since then, ranging from horizontal flow units through laminar, ultra-high-flow systems, to the down-flow hepa-filtered units of today. Engineers and designers have produced well-researched computational flow dynamic or airflow models that appear to deliver the best ventilation and decontamination of the surgical field.

Space precludes detailed discussion on this subject. The main principles are given below.

- The OR is a plenum, relative to the corridors and ancillary rooms – that is the pressure inside is higher than outside.
- Every room should have an individual air handling unit that has independent temperature and humidity control.
- The current best model is a ceiling-mounted down-flow system with a hepa-filtered array above the patient and team with high- and low-level exhausts positioned on the ceiling and opposite walls in the room for even venting.
- The area of the filter array should match the surgical footprint if possible.
- Down-flow rates from the filters above the patient are more important than room air changes per hour (the traditional measure of effectiveness).
- High-flow rooms with large arrays should be used for surgery such as joint arthroplasty, but

traditional "laminar flow" with a curtain around the surgical footprint is not necessary. Indeed, evidence is emerging in the literature of possible inferior outcomes in arthroplasty patients with excess surgical site infection rates from laminar flow rooms.

- The smooth downdraught of air will be disrupted by objects such as lights, booms, and surgical personnel and therefore will not completely wash the surgical site in a laminar fashion.
- Ventilation systems do not, of themselves, prevent infection. They produce an incremental effect in conjunction with other well-documented measures outside the scope of this chapter.

Sterile Supplies and Instrument Processing

Formerly, OR suites had an instrument-processing and instrument-sterilizing unit attached and were designed around a sterile processing core. Many modern facilities, in contrast, have remote surgical sterilizing departments (SSDs), and there are some examples of clusters of regional hospitals being supplied from a single remote, factory-like SSD by truck.

The design of the OR suite determines how the surgical instruments are managed. For example, if a single corridor design is designed to allow natural light into the ORs, this mandates the use of sealed case-carts to achieve separation of clean and used instruments.

A dedicated means of transportation of instruments to and from the SSD is recommended, and a backup route should be formally identified. Users also need to agree on the proportion and type of instruments that can be stored in the OR suite once processed versus those that need to be ordered from the SSD sterile instrument store as required. Flash sterilizers have been extensively used in the past but are not now regarded as best practice and should not be included in the design brief. A software solution linking the procedure booking with the surgeon preference list and the picklist in the SSD is essential, along with a smart storage solution.

The sterile supply chain and process requires a strong systems approach. Clinical staff should sign off the instrument and equipment orders, but it is immensely wasteful of time and energy to have them find missing instruments or correct errors in the picklist.

Admission Unit

Ideally an admission unit should be central and close to the organizational hub of the OR. It should be easily accessed by patients and their families and be of sufficient size to cope with peak traffic. This usually occurs between about 06:00 and 08:00 h depending on the OR start pattern (same start or staggered start), which will determine the required capacity of the unit.

The admission unit can be co-located with the PACU and inpatient preoperative area to facilitate staffing flexibility and cross-functional use of space. Consult rooms or cubicles should be included for interviews, surgery site marking, and last-minute examinations in private. Storage facility for patient records and property is essential. Access to patient records, labs, and a picture archiving and communication system (PACS) is essential for clinicians, especially if the patients have been preassessed outside the facility.

Postanesthesia Care Unit

The floor area and location of the PACU is vitally important. Patient and staff flows through the unit require formal mapping, and the interface to the rest of the building must be determined. Access to ICU and ingress for services including radiology and cardiology for postoperative investigation purposes need to be addressed. The PACU should include a clinical station that is centrally located, capacious, and has good visibility across the unit.

Fixtures such as booms or pendants to deliver utilities into the bed space may be considered.

The PACU may be the best site for a sub-pharmacy, and it should also have its own storage area.

In large units, the recommended ratio for PACU spaces to ORs is 1.5:1, and the bed space area should be approximately 85 sq ft (8–9 m^2), including circulation space. In ambulatory units this ratio can be less, as patients usually progress more rapidly to a step-down unit or may bypass PACU completely. The capacity to provide patient privacy, at least visual privacy, is important. Users may request a subgroup of HDU-type spaces with enhanced monitoring capability for extended PACU stays.

"Waste" Management in the OR

Let us now return to the concept of waste in the OR process and how design may be used to mitigate this.

To recap, the seven wastes cited above are:

- waiting
- transportation
- defects
- staff movement
- inventory
- overproduction
- unnecessary processing

The reader will note the change of order of the individual elements; this reflects their impact on OR suite efficiency.

Waiting

Waiting is probably the biggest source of waste in the OR. In its broadest sense, it can be embedded within all aspects of OR activity, from the admission process to PACU capacity or equipment delivery, and generally can be translated into delay or tardiness in the OR pathway.

Many groups have published papers on start times, turnover, and OR scheduling, over the past decade in particular, and the underlying objective of most has been to improve efficiency, complete more cases in a given time, reduce waiting and delays, and improve profitability by increasing contribution margins.

Areas that have been explored include:

- development of robust preassessment models to reduce admission times and avoid cancellations on the day of surgery
- accurate scheduling of surgery, using historical data, to reduce tardiness and session overruns
- solutions to shorten the turnover time between cases and improve first-case start times
- modeling of flows through the PACU to determine capacity and minimize bed block
- evolution of roles and responsibilities of staff to achieve greater flexibility and productivity in the workforce
- storage, maintenance, and processing solutions for equipment and consumables

Building design can reduce waiting and delays. The list below shows where design features in the OR suite support and facilitate improvements in flow and productivity:

- an admission unit within the suite to process preadmitted patients on the day of surgery
- working in parallel (see below) at the start of the day and also between cases to minimize nonoperative time

- a PACU that is correctly located and sized to deal with the OR workload and has a discharge pathway or step-down unit to smooth flow out of the OR suite
- well-positioned and designed storage areas

Working in Parallel – One Size Fits All?

Many older hospitals (particularly in the UK and Australasia) were designed and built with anesthesia induction rooms. Induction rooms went out of vogue in many places but recent work has been exploring their place in modern practice. Induction rooms are one potential solution in the quest to reduce turnover and nonoperative times, but there are others. Marjamaa et al. compared five scenarios in a computer simulation [6]: the traditional model of sequential induction and surgery in the OR; use of induction rooms; use of a centralized induction area; use of an anesthesia induction team; and finally the more traditional approach to parallel processing, having four OR teams for three surgeons. They found that all of the parallel solutions outperformed the traditional model and that increased costs of personnel were balanced by increased revenue. They commented that cases of less than 2-h duration benefit most from parallel tasking and that the best model for quality of care was the model of one anesthesia team following the patient though the whole process.

Sandberg et al. constructed the "operating room of the future" at Massachusetts General Hospital, with the express intent of running activities in parallel and reducing nonoperative time [7] (Figure 10.8). Patients were transferred from main admission to an induction area within the OR pod, where anesthesia was induced prior to transfer to the OR. Postsurgery, early recovery occurred in a dedicated space within the pod, prior to transfer to the main PACU by perioperative nurses. This model, in conjunction with advances in technology such as mobile operating table tops and a reengineered work process, led to enhanced performance, saving around 38 min per case. Increased staff costs were largely offset by increased revenue.

Two other design models are worthy of comment. The first is the inclusion of a regional block area. This can be utilized well before the scheduled start of the operating list to insert and establish both central neuraxial and major peripheral nerve blocks and can either be staffed by the attending anesthesia team or by a separately rostered "block" team. This area is

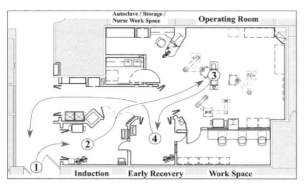

Figure 10.8 The OR of the future; a self-contained pod of perioperative spaces, including a workspace for staff. From Sandberg et al. *Anesthesiology* 2005; *103*: 406–13.

best co-located near the PACU to maximize staffing flexibility and requires adequate space and lighting to perform procedures, as well as equipment such as ultrasound imaging devices and ready access to resuscitation equipment.

The second design is a more radical solution to working in parallel and consists of an instrument preparation room attached to the OR, where the sterile instruments can be decanted and set up by the scrub personnel, either while the previous patient is emerging from anesthesia and the room is being cleaned and set up, or while a prolonged anesthesia induction and setup is undertaken in the OR. The preparation room ventilation is supplied from the same OR air handler and pressures are set such that the prep room is a plenum relative to the OR, thereby eliminating atmospheric contamination from the OR. The advantage of this model is that the patient is induced in the OR by the anesthesia team and is not moved during anesthesia. Once the patient is fully prepared and positioned, the decanted instrument trolleys are wheeled from the ultra-clean prep room into the OR and final patient checks, skin prep, draping, and surgery proceed. This is the design used at Auckland City Hospital (see Figures 10.7 and 10.9). Figure 10.9a and 10.9b show two different process maps of OR procedures with parallel task solutions. Induction rooms are used for short, rapid-turnover cases whereas instrument preparation rooms are used for longer, more complex cases.

Using a combination of these models, Smith et al. set out to reduce nonoperative time and increase throughput for joint arthroplasty cases by utilizing an induction room for block insertion, a sterile setup area for instrument decanting, and a reengineering of roles within the OR team. This group achieved a 50 percent reduction in nonoperative time and higher throughputs that generated a positive margin greater than the incremental cost, making it a cost-effective solution [8].

It appears, then, that a parallel tasking solution is desirable – but which one? This is clearly a crucial question for any design team, as the chosen solution will require a supporting architectural design and real estate with appropriate engineering and utility services to be successful. It should be emphasized that all of the above solutions rely not only on redesign of the facility but also reengineering of processes and reassignment of staff roles. The project group should therefore select a solution that best fits the proposed model of care.

Induction rooms seem to be most effective for relatively short cases, with shortened nonoperative times allowing extra cases to be completed in the allocated session time. For longer and more complex cases, instrument preparation rooms may be more effective, in conjunction with a regional anesthesia block insertion area. The solution is contextual and in theory may produce a mixed design model, with some ORs equipped with induction rooms and others with instrument preparation rooms in the same suite.

Transportation

Unnecessary transportation of patients, equipment, or consumables is extremely wasteful. When applied to OR design, this means ensuring that internal co-locations fit the flow of patients through the OR suite. For example, the admission unit should not be remotely located from the ORs and the PACU should be centrally located within the suite. An important but somewhat counterintuitive concept is that vertical adjacencies may be more convenient than horizontal ones in large facilities. Staff change rooms or patient admission units may be better positioned on an adjacent floor rather than at great distance on the same floor.

OR user groups must also decide how patients are going to be transported to and from the ORs. Routes from the emergency room and radiology need to be mapped and optimized. Bilateral meetings with the emergency room, ward, and radiology user groups are mandatory for success.

Patient transfer solutions should also be considered here. Mobile operating patient trolleys and OR table tops are available to minimize the number of patient

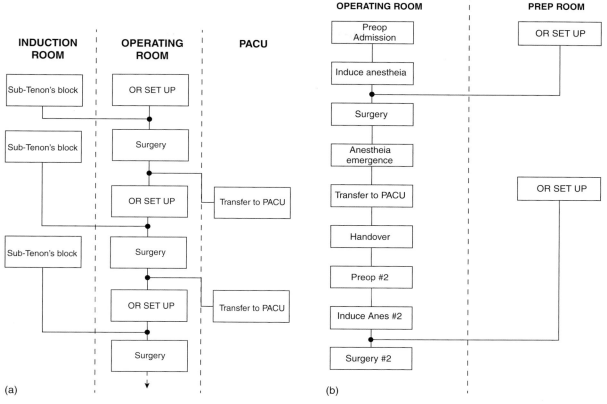

Figure 10.9 (a) and (b) These are two different process maps of OR procedures with parallel task solutions. Induction rooms are used for short rapid-turnover cases whereas instrument-preparation rooms are used for longer, more complex cases.

transfers during the OR stay. These will shorten case times and potentially reduce staff injuries from manual handling of patients.

Transportation of instruments and equipment is a major logistical exercise. Many OR suites do not have the storage capacity to hold all of the instrument inventory; most are held in a clean "warehouse" facility in SSD and transported to the OR either as part of a consignment for a given session or within a case cart for an individual case.

As outlined above, the SSD is often remote from the OR suite in modern facilities, and this necessitates a robust transport solution, such as dedicated elevators or corridors into the OR suite. A secondary or step-down sterile store within the OR suite acts as the receiving area for the sterile instrument pack, and final adjustments can be made prior to transfer to the OR.

Laboratory specimens should either be processed in the OR suite (blood gas analysis or thromboelastography) or transported efficiently to the

lab, for example by compressed air tube network. The route and mode of transport for emergency supplies such as blood products should also be mapped.

Staff Movement

In larger OR suites, staff may spend considerable time transferring patients, sourcing supplies, and travelling to and from staff amenities, change rooms, etc. During the early planning stages, take some time to map out staff flows during the working day. The architect's plans (Figure 10.10) will end up with a myriad of colored lines as different staff members in the user group map their day, but it will yield very valuable information, detailing how the staff will need to move within the unit, and may lead to rearrangement of subunits to minimize unnecessary movement. The solution will be optimized only in conjunction with a review of staff roles and process reengineering.

Surgeons have gaps in their operating day during the nonoperative phase of the OR list. Office space

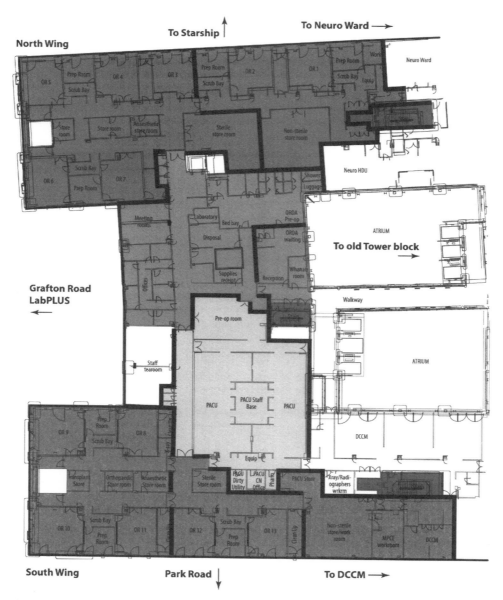

Figure 10.10 This shaded plan is used to map out transport flows and staff movement. The main ingress/egress routes are center right. There is a single-corridor design. The admission and PACU areas are central and the ORs and staff areas are on the perimeter of the building. Reproduced with the permission of McConnel, Smith and Johnson P/L, Architects, Sydney, Australia.

close by the OR (see Figure 10.8) will allow them to complete some office work and also help to keep them in close proximity and available for the next case. This need only be an alcove with a desk and IT hub but will be appreciated and cost-effective. The communication platform in the OR suite will be covered later in the chapter.

Most other innovations to reduce waste in this area are outside the scope of this chapter and will be dealt with elsewhere in the book.

Reducing Defects

Reducing defects is a key feature of LSS processing and in the OR relates to issues such as patient cancellation, wrong site surgery, equipment defects, incorrect information, and scheduling errors. Access to patient information to reduce cancellation and rework has been discussed above.

Most of the measures to reduce defects involve reengineering, and redesigning processes and building design features are mostly related to flow and capacity. Are the admission unit and the PACU large enough cope with peak traffic? How is the ICU capacity calculated to prevent bed block and OR cancellation?

Inventory and Storage

This aspect of design and planning will be mostly about the interface between the ORs, materials management, goods inwards, and SSD; representatives of these services should be involved in planning.

The goals are:

- to establish storage floor area and location in the OR suite
- to map out transport of instruments and consumables to and from the storage areas
- to delineate sterile and nonsterile storage areas
- to negotiate a robust supply chain and minimize inventory held in-house
- to perform a "5S – sort, set, shine, standardize, sustain" exercise to optimize layout, shelving solution, and sustainability of design in the storage areas

This section also includes pharmacy imprest and supply chain mapping. A satellite pharmacy will save time and effort for the OR and anesthesiology staff.

Overprocessing/Overproduction

These two wastes are probably of least relevance to OR design. They refer mainly to process issues but can be of relevance in terms of matching process to design. An example of waste here would be an admission unit that was too small to deal with batched admissions at 06:00 h for the start of the day. The solution is that either the unit has to be designed to fit the process or the process has to be altered to support, for example, staggered OR starts.

Overprocessing refers to developing an over-complicated process when dealing with a simple problem and has little relevance to building design, other than mapping out flows through the unit and as a general principle when signing off plans.

Communication Platforms in the OR

With the advent of health information technology (HIT), the handling of data and information in healthcare has been revolutionized over the past decade. Patient records are rapidly becoming digitized (as are laboratory and radiology data) and stored in vast data warehouses. Clinical records departments are fast becoming IT portals instead of storage facilities.

Within the OR suite, IT platforms are used for:

- logging patient procedures and time stamps for throughput and financial management
- promulgating the OR workload with scheduling software;
- ordering sterile supplies and instruments
- creating electronic health records during procedures (both surgical and anesthesia), including dictation of procedure record;
- computerized provider order entry for medications
- accessing patient information, including labs and radiology
- image generation and management from MIS rooms, including real-time Internet transmission
- generating reports of OR activity for staff/ management/board;
- logging incidents for investigation/audit
- researching patient pathology or drug information via the Internet and online library

It will be apparent from the above list that the physical design of the network within the building and the OR suite is vitally important. It is the OR process that should dictate the IT requirements and design, rather than the converse.

Developments in HIT move with great rapidity, making future-proofing the network problematic. However, if the building is designed with future modification in mind, the network will be relatively easily upgraded.

Currently, most hospitals are constructed with a core network of fiber optic conduit interfacing with copper cabling to individual outlets. Wireless and mobile solutions are also becoming more prevalent, as are "cloud-computing" solutions, in which software platforms and data storage are supplied by a third party. Data warehousing and large servers will often be offsite and should be considered as a continuity issue for ORs.

Timely access to primary care patient information for hospital staff remains a challenge. Here HIT applications will certainly enhance overall care and reduce rework. During the design drawing phase, users will need to specify how the IT solutions will be used (the bullet-point list above includes potential uses), and therefore which network components are required.

Contemporary ORs may have as many as five or six hardware units within them (PCs, PACS, image management systems), all requiring intranet cabled or wireless connections. As wireless and cloud solutions develop, hardware and cable requirements should diminish.

Another mode of communication within the OR is the call system for house staff or orderlies and in the event of a critical incident. The physical design of the call buttons and their location in the OR need some thought, as does the method of communicating with and requesting assistance from outside the OR; this can be auditory, visual, or both.

Visibility of information within the OR will help to reduce both unnecessary staff movement and defects. If, for example, the registered nurse in the OR can see the instrument picklist from SSD online for the next case, he or she will not have to leave the OR to verify availability in person. If the anesthesiologist can see the labs and echocardiography report of the next patient online in the OR, a delay or cancellation may be avoided.

Building Life Span and Renovation

Future-Proofing the Design

Throughout this chapter, the emphasis has been on simplicity and flexibility. Most buildings completed today will have a useful life of 40–50 years and will almost certainly require alteration and refurbishment at some time. The preferred building format at present is to have a structural lattice of concrete or steel beams with concrete or steel beam floors at about 5 meters intervals and suspended false ceilings to give room heights of about 3 meters. The room design and layout within this lattice is usually achieved with a plasterboard or dry-wall solution. This gives the building great flexibility of design and allows alterations to be easily completed. The ceiling space contains much of the infrastructure installations such as air-handler units, plumbing, gas piping, and fixture supports and can be accessed easily for upgrades and repairs.

Future-proofing the capacity of the building is also desirable. Population-based intervention rates almost inevitably lead to expansion of the facility but initial fit-out of all spaces may not be justified in the first few years. Modern building design allows that spaces such as future ORs can be built to a shell stage with services to the space but no fit-out of walls, ceiling, or fixtures, saving initial cost and matching expansion costs to increased revenue at a later stage. The space can be utilized as storage until required. Fit-out can often be achieved with little or no disruption to activity as the external cladding of the building can be removed to facilitate building and installation work.

Many buildings are also designed to support the construction of an additional floor, if required at a future date.

The relatively open design of modern buildings also means that refits of IT hubs and networks are comparatively straightforward.

Renovating an Existing Building

Renovating an existing building presents a fresh set of potential barriers to success, as the building frame is likely to feature:

- solid wall construction, requiring major demolition work
- very limited ceiling space for infrastructure refit, such as air-handler units
- low ceiling height – problematic for modern ceiling-mounted fixtures such as pendants/booms or operating lights
- limited ducting for utility upgrades
- poor flow design and co-locations of rooms
- limited OR and PACU floor area
- remote staff amenities

Careful evaluation early in the project will determine whether the building can be made "fit for purpose." It may be more cost-effective to demolish and build new.

If the decision is to renovate, all of the considerations for a new build pertain, but good problem solving may be required to remediate the building limitations. Often, the full extent of required work is not apparent until the actual demolition and construction has commenced, and therefore the project team needs to build flexibility into the project schedule as well as contingency funding if required for extra works.

Renovation solutions rarely achieve all the design objectives possible in the new building, but with an expert design and build team a satisfactory outcome is possible. Many older buildings will have redundant areas, often vertically adjacent to the proposed renovation that can, when refitted with modern transport solutions, become useful ancillary space for the OR suite. Relocating the SSD off-floor will liberate valuable clinical space within the OR suite, for example. Construction of enlarged air-handler units and cabling for fixtures in the limited ceiling space presents a particular challenge, but again, careful design with the engineers will yield acceptable solutions.

From Plans to Procedures

Staying in Touch

Clinical user groups commonly comment on exclusion from the building process once the design drawings had been signed off. There is usually an 18-month to 2-year construction and fit-out phase for a large installation, and user groups must remain in touch with the process. They will mostly be involved in planning any migration program but should also be taken on site visits on a regular basis.

Clinicians seconded to the building project need to remain involved as integrated members of the team. Engineering schedules will require review, and real-time problem solving is an almost everyday event, as those who have been involved in a domestic building project will attest.

Translation from drawing to framing is never 100 percent, and careful site visits will pick up inaccuracies, such as a missing doorframe or a floor construction anomaly. Horizon-scanning for new technology should continue throughout the project, as last-minute infrastructure may be required before walls or ceilings are finalized. Budget and timeline variances may require clinician input to problem solve and prioritize negotiable and nonnegotiable positions that only clinical experience and contacts can finesse.

Tenders for fixtures such as booms and equipment such as case-carts and anesthesia machines also require attention, with clear, agreed tender processes and objectives.

Handover of the facility from the construction team requires many hours of work to complete facility and utility systems checks prior to migration. Clinical engineering and infection control units must formally sign off the facility as fit for use.

Migration

The organization will hire a specialist migration team to move staff and patients into the new building. This process will take up to a year before the moving date to plan, and clinical scenarios should be modeled to cover any eventuality, including systems failures. Trialing the new ORs prior to moving date is essential, as is a formal sign-off of all the systems and utilities in the OR suite. Successful migration requires meticulous planning and execution and almost merits a dedicated chapter.

Summary

In this chapter, we have explored the concept of design for OR efficiency. We have looked at the potential for good design to reduce or eliminate wasteful process in the OR and we have suggested steps for a successful design process.

The clear message here is that the design of the OR suite should:

- reflect and support the flows and processes, as determined by the organization
- establish simplicity and flexibility as the two main guiding principles
- provide a safe environment that fosters quality health outcomes

The theme throughout has been that design, process, and function cannot and should not be considered as separate entities; they are integral parts of hospital building solutions that, today more than ever, are required to deliver productive, efficient, and effective health outcomes.

References

1. J. J. Pandit, S. Westbury, M. Pandit. The concept of surgical list "efficiency": A formula to describe the term. *Anaesthesia* 2007; 62: 895–903.

2. A. Macario. Are your operating rooms efficient? A scoring system with eight performance indicators. *Anesthesiology* 2006; 105: 237–40.

3. J. J. Pandit, D. Stubbs, M. Pandit. Measuring the quantitative performance of surgical operating lists: Theoretical modelling of "productive potential" and "efficiency." *Anaesthesia* 2009; 64: 473–86.

4. E. Litvak, M. Long. Cost and quality under managed care: Irreconcilable differences? *Am J Manag Care* 2000; 6: 305–12.

5. NHS Institute for Innovation and Improvement. The seven wastes of lean. 2008. www.institute.nhs.uk/quality_and_service_improvement_tools/ (accessed May 2, 2012).

6. R. Marjamaa, P. Torkki, E. Hirvensalo, O. Kirvela. What is the best workflow for an operating room? A simulation study of five scenarios. *Health Care Manag Sci* 2009; 12: 142–6.

7. W. Sandberg, B. Daily, M. Egan, et al. Deliberate perioperative systems design improves operating room throughput. *Anesthesiology* 2005; 103: 406–18.

8. M. Smith, W. Sandberg, J. Foss, et al. High-throughput operating room system for joint arthroplasties durably outperforms routine processes. *Anesthesiology* 2008; 109: 25–35.

Chapter

11

Operating Room Design and Construction
Technical Considerations

Judith S. Dahle and Pat Patterson

Contents

Introduction

For most operating room (OR) leaders, the planning and design of a new surgical suite happen only once or twice in their careers. More than likely, these responsibilities will be added to their normal duties. These complex, multi-year projects are demanding, and there is a great deal to learn and apply within a short time. These projects call for a variety of strengths, including strong organizational skills, the ability to collaborate with other disciplines, and the ability to manage complex projects with deadlines.

Surgery is always a team effort. That's particularly true for an OR design and construction project. The success of the entire project, from the initial meetings to the final approval and move-in, depends on the collaboration among multiple disciplines. That includes not only the clinical disciplines of surgery, anesthesia, nursing, and related disciplines but also the design and construction professions. Working with a multidisciplinary team can be a major benefit because it provides a support system for decision making and an educational opportunity for the OR manager and the entire surgical team. Whether the OR director is a novice or experienced, the key to staying organized is to break the project into phases and to develop a checklist for each phase.

Several essential resources can provide guidance throughout the project. These include the *Guidelines for*

Design and Construction of Health Care Facilities from the Facility Guidelines Institute (FGI) [1], *Planning, Design, and Construction of Health Care Facilities* by the Joint Commission [2], and guidelines and standards of the Association for Professionals in Infection Control and Epidemiology (APIC) [3], among others.

Strategic Program Planning

The building or remodeling of OR suites is a demanding and expensive undertaking. Whether the project is to renovate a current suite or build new ORs, it is important to think about the organization's long-term direction and how that will influence the design and efficiency of the surgical suite. The challenge for management and the design teams is to envision how surgery will be performed in the future. How will new and emerging technology affect the services provided? How will work processes be affected by technology? What will the patient population be like within the next five to ten years? Will the hospital's admissions have a higher percentage of geriatric patients requiring complex surgical care? Are there programs in the community promoting diet and weight loss, which may bring a new bariatric program to the hospital? It is crucial for the organization to define its goals and strategies clearly so the design team may plan for OR processes that will support an efficient, safe, and cost-effective care delivery system for many years.

The first step in the planning process may be to conduct a needs analysis that will help drive decisions throughout the process. In a needs analysis, all of the surgical, anesthesia, and support services identify goals and discuss their anticipated needs for the future. Multiple meetings are needed to gather input from each surgical specialty and anesthesia providers. As part of the analysis, management must identify the reason for the construction: is it to expand space for increasing surgical volume, to redesign the facility for emerging technologies, to better compete with neighboring facilities, to anticipate new services, or to respond to changes in the healthcare delivery model?

The OR leadership team plays a crucial role in strategic planning. They will be asked for data regarding types and volume of procedures. OR directors experienced in this process also recommend gathering detailed financial and market information, including trends, projections for volumes, and case types as well as profitability information [4].

Many more questions need to be addressed during the planning phase such as:

- What are the market demographics?
- What will provide the competitive edge?
- What level of technology will be required?
- What are the pros and cons of the technology costs?
- How much functional space is needed for each OR suite?
- Will there be specialty rooms?
- How much storage will be required?
- Where will storage be located?
- What will the traffic flow be like and how efficient will it be? [4]

Detailed questions for each area, specialty, and technology will be addressed later in the design process when the master planning and design concepts are in place. An effective planning process is essential for the success of the completed project. A successful project will have been designed to be flexible and adaptable for the future. Although trends cannot be predicted with certainty, detailed multidisciplinary planning can help to avoid major design mistakes.

New Construction or Renovation?

As part of the planning process, management may want to evaluate whether to build new OR suites or renovate existing space. Only altered, renovated, or modernized portions of an existing building system – or individual components that have been altered, renovated, or replaced – are required to meet the installation and equipment requirements in the FGI guidelines [1]. A list of exceptions to the guidelines, which apply as long as they do not reduce the existing level of health and safety in a facility, can be found in the 2014 FGI guidelines to help clarify when existing systems or building equipment must be updated.

A variety of conditions affect the feasibility of renovation such as:

- the amount and type of space available for renovation
- mechanical and electrical system limitations
- ability to work within the existing building's boundaries
- location of columns and structural walls
- location of vertical penetrations, such as mechanical shafts, elevators, and fire stairs

In some cases, organizations can renovate and convert existing space for less money than they can build new space. Often, however, renovation costs may exceed new construction costs because of unforeseen conditions, phasing, scheduling, or logistical complexities. There are several issues to consider:

- Converting existing space to new functions frequently requires working with room dimensions, structural grids, and building configurations that force compromises to meet the needs and goals of the project.
- Remodeling often triggers the need to upgrade existing structures to meet current building code requirements. This in turn increases construction costs.
- Renovation can cause disruption of ongoing normal operations and require the relocation of services. Coordination of temporary relocation of services and the sequencing of events on the overall time line may make remodeling more time-consuming than new construction.
- A renovation project may trigger correction of accessibility deficiencies in areas of the facility remote from the proposed renovation.
- A partial renovation can result in the need for dual systems, which may increase operating costs and staff confusion [2].

The Planning and Design Team

The planning and design team should consist of a core group that will remain consistent throughout all phases of the project. The team needs a level of ownership and commitment to the project. The organization's representatives should be a multidisciplinary group from the relevant areas of the facility. The professional consultants on the team include those who will execute the planning, design, and construction. The size of the team varies with the complexity of the project. Additional members function in an advisory role and may attend only certain meetings that require their expertise.

Core members include:

- a representative from administration
- physicians
- nurses
- infection preventionist
- facilities planning/engineering
- architects
- engineers
- finance

Members who provide additional input at times throughout the project include:

- contractor
- equipment/technology planners
- physicists/hybrid rooms
- materials management
- laboratory staff
- support services
- pharmacy staff
- interior designers
- landscape designers for new facilities

An empowered leader from the organization needs to be selected and given the responsibility to keep the process moving forward, on time and within budget. The leader will establish the communication process. This person needs to have facilitation skills and to be flexible, a good manager of people, and responsive to sudden changes.

One person from the consultant role, usually an architect, will take the leadership for coordinating the members representing consulting services. Frequently, this person is helpful in determining when to ask the advisory group or additional members to participate in meetings.

A representative of the architectural firm usually takes the minutes of each meeting, which initially may be weekly, and distributes them to members of the planning and design team. In addition, the architect, in collaboration with the organization's representatives, develops and maintains an organizational tool such as a project evaluation and review technique (PERT) chart. A PERT chart diagrams the project activities and identifies critical tasks, milestones, projected timelines, and primary responsibility for each of the activities. This tool is helpful for the entire team to identify delegated tasks, tasks not assigned, and tasks that may delay the project.

The organization develops a budget as part of the initial preplanning that is revised as the project moves forward and changes are made. The budget is developed in several segments: construction costs, equipment costs, professional fees, escalation fees, and contingency costs. The nurse leader is the clinical expert on the team. All team members look to the nurse leader for recommendations and input about the appropriateness of the design with respect to regulatory requirements from accrediting bodies, state health departments, and others; space allotment; patient safety; and interdepartmental functions, to name a few areas of expertise. It is nursing's opportunity to design an environment that is safe for patients and staff, is efficient, meets the needs of the physicians, and meets the mission and vision of the organization.

The nurse leader has a prominent role as a member of the planning and design team. Initially, this may seem like a daunting task that adds to an already full workload. Although the project may seem overwhelming to a nurse leader who is not familiar with design and construction, it provides a great leadership opportunity. Involving everyone who will be directly affected by the construction and will be working in the new or remodeled area is essential. Collaborating with staff members in the process allows them to feel a sense of ownership in the building effort [5]. Communication about the project with nursing, physician, and support staff helps decrease the staff's stress about the project and brings helpful ideas to the design process. The staff can provide valuable ideas in relation to storage and supply access, types of case carts, OR furniture, and cabinets as well as the location of electrical outlets, data ports, and other design items that affect patient flow. Direct care providers can provide the best input regarding design aspects that will improve safety and efficiency. Nurses who are participating in design and construction for the first time will find that the design team members are willing to share their expertise.

Phases of a Project

Design and construction projects typically follow these six phases:

Planning

The planning phase includes wish list considerations, master planning, setting the vision, and needs analysis. This is the time to gather input from each specialty and to hold meetings with the staff to find out what they envision for the new OR and what the positive and negatives of the current OR may be.

Site visits to other facilities are helpful because they provide OR leaders with an opportunity to see completed ORs and talk to the personnel to learn what works well in their facility and what they would have done differently. It is helpful to take a multidisciplinary group on the site visit.

Schematic

The schematic phase involves drawing a rough outline of the project, including a preliminary room layout, structure, and scope of the project. At this time, the architect begins to prepare diagrams that display the major functions, the structural components, and the approximate size needed for the various functions. The planning and design team members provide important input at this time. There are frequent meetings during this phase, with brainstorming and probing discussions with the architectural firm. A detailed list of ideas is collected, and the architect will develop more in-depth drawings from each of these sessions.

Design Development

In design development, details are added to the design drawings, including electrical outlets; data ports; furniture location; fixtures; and details regarding casework, hardware, and décor. This phase takes several meetings with frequent revision to the plans. The design team should ask many questions and review the plans closely. Every detail of the finished facility needs to be included at this time. The final design is reviewed by the planning team. Then the key decision makers from the organization approve and sign the final plans before they are converted to construction documents. Once this phase is completed, making revisions incurs additional costs.

Construction Documents

During the construction documents phase, all aspects of the design are converted into building plans that a contractor can use to estimate costs, identify issues, and plan construction activities. These documents will be used throughout the construction phase and are used to obtain building permits for the project. At this point, the organization discusses contract conditions with the contractor and the architect. Roles and responsibilities of all participants are defined. During this phase, the design team does not meet as often, and there may be less communication between the architect and other team members. At this time, the architectural firm is detailing the drawings in preparation for the bidding process with the builders.

Construction

During the construction phase, the OR suite is actually built. Before the construction begins, the design team should meet with the contractors to discuss final preparation. These discussions need to include site security, contractor education, storage of materials, barrier placement, infection prevention, and the communication process to be used during the project. Frequent visits to the site, when appropriate, by planning and design team members are advisable. It is important to ask questions. Sometimes what the team saw on the drawings does not look the same during construction. Ask for clarification and explanation of the construction process. Weekly construction meetings provide an opportunity for effective communication and education throughout the project.

Commissioning

Before taking ownership of a building, project, or renovation, the organization must make sure all specifications are met; all requirements are in order for licensure; and all systems, components, equipment are operational [2]. Plumbing; electrical systems; heating, ventilating, and air conditioning (HVAC) systems; fire alarms; and safety systems will be tested at this time.

Considerations for Operational Processes

General Considerations for OR Suites

The size and location of the surgical suite will be determined by the level of care provided. The number

Box 11.1. OR Design: General Principles

- Make each OR at least 600 sq ft (55.74 m²), larger for cardiovascular, orthopedic and other complex procedures. The *Guidelines for Design and Construction of Healthcare Facilities* [1] recommend a minimum of 400 sq ft (37.20 m²) of clear floor space for general ORs, with a minimum of 600 sq ft for ORs performing surgical procedures that require additional personnel and/or large equipment, such as some cardiovascular, orthopedic, and neurosurgical procedures.

- Make the ORs identical to avoid staff having to adjust to new positions and item locations.

- Install adequate wiring, ventilation, and structural reinforcement to accommodate equipment.

- Design ORs for multiple uses because caseloads and surgical techniques may change.

- Include communication tools such as wall monitors and e-mail stations in OR design.

- Make storage space adequate and rapidly accessible; avoid distant storerooms, or expect more onsite hoarding of supplies.

- Design logistics for smooth supply transport and protection of sterile items.

- Design patient transport routes and waiting locations to provide comfort, privacy, and the growing trend toward presence of family members.

of ORs and postanesthesia care unit (PACU) beds and the size of the support areas are governed by the expected workload. Current and future workloads by specialty should have been determined during the preplanning and planning phases (Box 11.1).

The surgical suite will be divided into two designated areas – semirestricted and restricted – defined by the activities performed in each area.

- The semirestricted area includes the peripheral support areas of the surgical suite, including storage areas for clean and sterile supplies; sterile processing rooms; scrub stations; and corridors leading to restricted areas of the surgical suite.

- A central control point may be established to monitor the entrance of patients, personnel, and materials from the unrestricted area into the semirestricted area. Traffic in semirestricted areas is limited to authorized personnel and patients. Personnel in these areas are required to wear surgical attire and cover head and facial hair.

- The semirestricted area may contain entrances to locker rooms, the PACU, and sterile processing areas. Sterile processing is a semirestricted environment but can be entered directly from the unrestricted area or from another semirestricted area.

- The restricted area is a designated space in the semirestricted area of the surgical suite that can be reached only through a semirestricted area. The restricted access is primarily to support a high level of asepsis control, not necessarily for security purposes. Traffic in the restricted area is limited to authorized personnel and patients. Personnel in restricted area are required to wear surgical attire and cover head and facial hair. Masks are required where open sterile supplies or scrubbed persons may be located [1].

Design to Decrease Flow Disruptions

Investigators have used human factors analysis to identify and classify flow disturbances during surgery. The analysis looks at any factor, specifically human factors, impeding work or communication during surgery. Studying cardiac surgery, researchers from the Medical University of South Carolina, Charleston, found that one-third of the disturbances were related to OR physical layout and design [6]. With technological advances in equipment and procedures, the OR has become more complex, potentially disrupting workflow and affecting patient safety. The researchers have also developed a taxonomy to describe the nature of flow disruptions during cardiac surgery.

Six categories of flow disruptions were identified and analyzed in each phase of surgical care (preoperative, operative, and postoperative) with more detailed descriptions within each category.

The main categories were:

- communication (verbal and nonverbal)
- usability (computer, equipment, packaging, etc.)
- layout (equipment, connector positioning, furniture, visibility)
- environmental hazards (slipping, falling, crushing)
- interruptions (phone calls, nonessential personnel, shift changes, etc.)

- equipment failure (surgical, anesthesia, etc.) [5]

Under layout, the researchers described six subcategories of disruptions or areas of interest:

- Connector positioning – wires and tubes entangled or misplaced, which can hinder movement and continuation of a task.
- Equipment positioning – machines and tools may restrict or prevent the movement and actions of the staff.
- Furniture positioning – chairs, OR bed, and desk can cause OR staff to deviate from their original movement.
- Permanent structures positioning – doorways are frequently used in the OR during surgical procedures, preventing continuous movement and possibly causing injury.
- Inadequate use of space – surface and floor space are used inappropriately through clutter, untidiness, congestion, and blockage.
- Impeded visibility – the staff may have objects that obstruct their ability to see at important times in the procedure [6].

Methodology is being developed to help researchers understand the impact of each type of flow disruption.

Evidence-Based Design

Evidence-based design (EBD) is a recent concept fostered by the Center for Health Design (www.healthdesign.org) [7]. In EBD, design and construction are based as much as possible on research evidence, with the goal of producing the best possible outcomes for patients, families, and staff while improving the process of care. The evidence suggests that standardization is one aspect of design that improves patient safety by reducing the risk of errors. For example, when multiple facilities such as ORs are oriented the same way, the staff knows where equipment and supplies are kept. The surgical team knows how the patient will be oriented in the room, reducing the risk of wrong-side surgery. Less time is spent looking for supplies and equipment, which reduces rework, minimizes fatigue, and allows caregivers to focus on direct patient care. Standardization also improves efficiency and productivity and lowers costs [7].

Patient Flow Considerations

The smooth flow of patients from the admitting area to the preoperative holding area, to the individual OR suite, and into the PACU depends partially on an efficient facility design. The planning for patient flow should consider the experience not only of patients but also of family members who accompany the patient on the day of surgery. Patients need to be prepared and wait for surgery in a private environment where the family may stay with them until they are taken into the OR. There also needs to be a quiet area where medical staff can discuss medical issues with the patient and a quiet, comfortable area where families can wait during the procedure. New facilities are often designed with family waiting areas that have features such as natural light, comfortable furniture, data ports and wireless internet access, and play areas for children.

The decision for private rooms or bays in the preoperative area is influenced by the size of the area, the ability to provide patient care efficiently, and the impact of the choice on staffing levels. A common design for patient cubicles is three walls with a curtain across the foot of the bay. This allows patient privacy but provides efficiency and visibility for the nursing staff.

The immediate preoperative area (holding area) needs space to accommodate both patients on stretchers and ambulatory patients who are seated. This area needs to be under the direct visual control of the nursing staff. Provision needs to be made for patients with transmissible infections, developed in collaboration with the infection prevention department. Consideration also needs to be given to the patient mix and the surgical program. Space may be needed for additional equipment, depending on the surgical program planned.

The planning phase for the preoperative space is an opportunity to evaluate spaces that may be used as cross-functional areas during the day. For example, a portion of the PACU may be used as part of the preoperative holding area during the first part of the day. This arrangement can contribute to efficient staffing, particularly if the staff is cross-trained for both preoperative and postanesthesia care, and may decrease the amount of space required for the preoperative holding area.

The planning phase is also the appropriate time to design the communication and documentation systems for the new area, which can have a positive impact on efficiency, safety, and patient and staff satisfaction. The use of information technology can make for a quieter work area, fewer interruptions, and an opportunity for more efficient patient flow. These are examples of how information technology may provide for an improved environment:

- Airport-style tracking systems enable the staff to see the status of individual OR suites, help the staff to anticipate the patient flow, communicate with other departments such as the critical care unit, and keep families informed of patients' progress.
- Wireless communication systems using small phones or badges may be installed to facilitate communication among the nursing staff.
- Audiovisual systems allow surgeons to communicate with the radiology and pathology departments more efficiently and clearly.

Design of Postanesthesia Care Areas

There are specific space requirements for both phase I and phase II postanesthesia recovery areas. A minimum of 1.5 postanesthesia patient care stations per OR is required. When designing the recovery area and determining the number of recovery positions required, the project team should consider the types of surgery and procedures performed, types of anesthesia used, average recovery periods for patients, and the anticipated staffing model. Special consideration is needed if pediatrics is part of the functional program [1].

The phase I level of care applies to patients in immediate postanesthetic recovery in which a 1:1 or 1:2 nurse–patient ratio is maintained, depending on the patient's status. This phase lasts until the patient meets the "critical elements," as recommended by the American Society of Perianesthesia Nurses. During phase II, care focuses on preparation of the patient and family for discharge to home or extended care [8].

The FGI guidelines [1] recommend a separate area for phase I and phase II postanesthesia care, such as a separate step-down area, but this is not always possible because of space. The first concern is to follow the appropriate level of care while maintaining patient privacy.

Maintaining privacy in the preoperative and postoperative areas is a challenge because of limited space. Many facilities have cubicles with three walls and a sliding glass door or a privacy curtain. Others provide separate enclosed patient rooms for preoperative care and discharge preparation, but this design does not provide the flexibility required for efficient patient flow and presents a staffing challenge.

General requirements for postanesthesia care include medication stations, hand-washing stations,

a nurses' station, charting facility, and storage allocations [1]. Involving the PACU staff in planning this area is beneficial because they can provide valuable information about what functions well in the current facility and what does not. The design of the PACU also depends on the functional program. Examples of issues to be considered are whether the PACU will accommodate pediatric patients, intensive care patients, and family visitation and whether the area will care for inpatients as well as outpatients.

Materials Flow

Surgery consumes a large volume of supplies and instrumentation. How these materials are supplied and distributed through the facility has a major bearing on the surgical suite's overall efficiency and on the cost of care.

The flow of materials needs to be planned so the movement of clean and sterile supplies and instruments is separated from contaminated items and waste by space or traffic patterns [9]. The clean storage space needs to be in a moisture- and temperature-controlled area that is free from cross-traffic. The soiled area cannot have direct connection with the ORs. Involving the staff from materials management and sterile processing as well as the OR staff who are most directly involved in supply distribution is important to planning a successful materials flow.

There are several issues to consider for surgical supplies:

- How will supplies be received in the surgical suite? Is there a separate area outside the suite to break down shipping containers so only the clean inner packaging enters the suite?
- What supply chain system will be used for delivery, control, and replenishment of supplies?
- How will supplies be transported to the surgical area and to the individual ORs?
- How much and what type of storage will be needed to accommodate this system, both in the suite and in the individual ORs? Where will sterile supplies be stored so their sterility is not compromised?
- After surgery, how will soiled trash be removed from the suite and stored so patients and clean areas are not exposed to contaminated materials?
- There are several issues to consider for surgical instrumentation:

- Where will instrumentation be processed? In some hospitals, sterile processing is performed within the semirestricted area of the surgical department. In this case, the size and location of the clean and soiled workrooms will be determined in the functional program. In other hospitals, sterile processing is performed outside the suite. In this case, direct but separate paths should be planned between the surgical suite and sterile processing area for both clean and soiled instrumentation. For example, the surgical suite may be on a floor above the sterile processing area, with dedicated clean and soiled elevators connecting the two units.
- Will the surgical suite perform sterilization on an emergency basis? If so, sterilization facilities need to be provided in an area readily accessible to the ORs that complies with guidelines for immediate-use steam sterilization (formerly called flash sterilization). Immediate-use sterilization refers to the processing of items intended to be used immediately and not stored. This process requires the same critical reprocessing steps as any other sterilization cycle, including cleaning, decontamination, and transport of sterilized items [10].

Equipment Storage

Equipment storage is always a challenge. Today's surgical procedures require a variety of large, portable pieces of equipment such as x-ray equipment, stretchers, fracture tables, and warming devices. All of these must be stored in locations that are convenient to the ORs but must be kept out of corridors and traffic [1]. If the surgical suite will be large with specialized ORs, the storage spaces should be readily accessible to the specialized rooms. In new construction, recessed space is frequently planned outside each OR for the storage of a stretcher. Other areas may be designed for large items such as x-ray equipment. In developing the functional program, the planning and design team should list all of the equipment the surgical suite is likely to include and how frequently it is used. That list should be available for reference as the design is developed.

Staff Support Areas

The design of staff support areas can have a major impact on staff satisfaction. These areas include places for changing from street clothes to surgical attire and a lounge for breaks and lunch. The changing areas are required to have lockers, showers, toilets, handwashing stations, and space to change clothing [1].

The lounge area is intended to minimize the need for staff to leave the surgical suite for breaks and meals and to provide convenient access for both the OR and the PACU staffs. The decision about whether to have a combined or separate lounge for physician, nursing, or ancillary staff usually depends on the amount of available space and the philosophy of the organization. There are also regulations for these areas that vary by state and locality.

Though much of the surgical suite design focuses on functionality and efficiency, the design of staff support areas should also consider comfort and aesthetics. The staff's participation is essential in planning an area that will suit their needs. A combination of eating area, lounge, and kitchen is most desirable. If there is an opportunity, the lounge should have windows to allow for natural light and an outside view. Selection of furniture is important for comfort and function. Color selection should consider gender as well as generational, cultural, and geographical preferences.

Ancillary Department Coordination

The physical relationship between the surgical suite and supporting departments is an important consideration. The planning team needs to consider the surgical program and identify all of the services that may be required for each specialty. Generally, the ORs should be located close to the emergency department, radiology department, cardiac catheterization laboratory, and clinical and pathology laboratories. The PACU should be located so patients can be transported easily to the intensive care units. Representatives from pharmacy, interventional radiology, and any department that routinely provides services to the surgical department should be included in discussions about location and information technology that may assist in the coordination of care.

Design of Individual ORs

Space Requirements

A general OR is required to be at least 400 sq ft (37.20 m²) with a minimum clear dimension of 20 ft between fixed cabinets and built-in shelves, according to the FGI guidelines [1]. ORs for surgical procedures requiring additional personnel and/or large equipment, such as cardiovascular, orthopedic, and neurological procedures, require 600 sq ft (55.74 m²). Many hospitals are designing all of the ORs to accommodate the latest technology and equipment, allowing for flexibility in scheduling procedures into any room. The larger rooms, in addition to accommodating the many pieces of equipment today's surgery requires, provide adequate room for the staff to move, allowing for better staff circulation and greater efficiency. Larger rooms also allow clearance for patient transport and the movement of portable equipment. In addition, they provide space for a sitting workstation where clinicians can document care electronically and manage controls for digital imaging and other technology.

Ceiling-Mounted Booms

The use of ceiling-mounted booms in ORs enables equipment and related cords to be kept off the floor, decreasing clutter and allowing for safer movement around the room [11]. In new construction, the space above the ceiling can be designed to include conduit to accommodate utilities and the necessary cabling for equipment mounted on the booms. If the ORs are being remodeled, engineers must assess the ceiling structure to determine the weight-load capabilities before planning to install ceiling-mounted booms. It is a good idea to provide additional capacity to meet future needs.

Retractable utility columns for anesthesia providers provide an efficient, well-organized service area at each end of the room. The columns house medical gases, phone jacks, and data connections. The columns do not eliminate the need for a small anesthesia cart but provide another means to keep the floor free of cords.

Proper placement of ceiling-mounted equipment booms is critical. Booms should be placed on the side of the room away from the OR door where patients enter the room. The articulating arms need to move freely and not interfere with movement of the surgical lights. Physicians and staff who perform minimally invasive video-guided surgery can provide valuable insight on placement of booms and should be involved in site visits to view established facilities. Computer-aided design and simulation are also helpful in visualizing the placement of booms.

Configuration of the OR

During the design process, it is helpful to create a schematic drawing of the individual OR and trace all of the paths personnel may travel during a procedure. The room plan should be evaluated for how it will function during the set-up phase of surgery as well as when the sterile back table has been moved into place during the procedure. Scenarios should also be created for other mobile equipment that comes into the room during surgical procedures. This same process should be used to plan the placement of storage cabinets, workstations, wall-mounted view boxes, white boards, and other stationary devices.

Door placement should be designed to maintain a sterile work zone in relation to the OR bed. There are two doors, one for transporting the patient and personnel and the other for access to the substerile area or central core. The main door should be located to facilitate the transport of the patient by stretcher or by patient bed. The most efficient door placement is to the left of the patient's head. It is also advisable to design all of the OR rooms so the approach to each room is the same. Consistency in design improves safety and efficiency.

Placement of electrical and data outlets is critical for the OR's functionality and efficiency. Even if there are ceiling-mounted booms, additional outlets are required throughout the room. The architect and electrical engineer can provide guidance to the design team about electrical loads per outlet and the types of outlets required. Outlets that will be used in the event of a power failure when the OR is on an auxiliary system are required to be clearly marked. The clinical staff on the design team can provide valuable information about the location of these emergency outlets. It is convenient if electrical outlets can be placed at a higher-than-normal elevation on the wall. Despite wireless technology, hardwiring is still necessary for backup data access. It is a good idea to plan for the future during the construction process by providing for additional electrical and data capacity. It is less expensive to run additional conduit at the time of construction than to add it a few years later when it may require taking an OR out of service for upgrading.

Substerile Space Requirement

In many OR suites, a substerile room is located between each two OR rooms and enhances the rooms' function. Substerile rooms, used for immediate-use sterilization, are typically equipped with a steam sterilizer, a countertop, and built-in storage for supplies [1]. The substerile area may also be in the clean core if the clean core is directly accessible from the ORs. In this case, the substerile area needs to be accessible without traveling through any ORs.

Interior Finishes

Interior elevation drawings will include information about design elements such as cabinets and other casework, wall service details, equipment mounting locations, sinks, plumbing fixtures, and other details [12]. The purpose for cabinets needs to be defined. What will be stored in the cabinets? Do the cabinets all need to be built in, or should some storage be mobile? Cabinet surfaces need to be chosen keeping in mind the surface's durability and ability to withstand frequent cleaning.

Wall finishes must also last through rigorous cleaning and be smooth and seamless. The color needs to be pleasing and relaxing. Floors must be durable, nonskid, capable of handling the movement of heavy equipment, and ergonomically comfortable for staff. Many flooring options are available, including terrazzo, tile, sheet vinyl, and newer products. The design team's interior design representative can provide samples of materials and discuss the pros and cons of each product.

Equipment Planning

Outsourced Equipment Planners

Equipment planning is an essential and time-sensitive element of the planning, design, and construction process. Timing for equipment delivery should be planned so equipment arrives at the correct time for installation and so unnecessary storage is not required because equipment arrives too early. To determine the equipment space, design needs, and budget, an equipment list should be developed as part of the planning phase. The equipment list is necessary not only for the design process but also as a budget guide.

Researching equipment options, cost, and availability can be time-consuming. One option is to hire a company that specializes in planning and purchasing equipment for healthcare facilities. The equipment planner then meets with the project representative to learn about the needs of the project and propose the role the planner can provide. The hospital decides what

level of services to contract for with the equipment planners, weighing the cost of these services against the hospital's own resources for equipment planning.

There are several options when using an equipment planner. The planner can collaborate with the team to identify all of the equipment, from large equipment such as sterilizers, x-ray units, lasers, and OR lights to smaller items such as carts and stools. The planner researches product availability and costs and obtains product information and installation details for the contractors, and then assembles the information in a binder or reference file. In addition, the equipment planning firm can either purchase the equipment itself or coordinate with the hospital's purchasing department. The equipment planner can develop a timeline with the vendors and schedule deliveries according to the construction timeline.

Purchasing Protocol

Whether or not an outside equipment planner is used, the hospital's materials manager needs to be an advisor to the design team, and a decision-making protocol needs to be established for the project. An effective method is needed for evaluating equipment and determining its value related to improvements planned in areas such as patient and staff safety, patient outcomes, best practice, and regulatory requirements. Decisions are needed early in the design process about whether to acquire new or refurbished equipment, purchase equipment through group purchasing contracts, and who will be responsible for each element of equipment planning and acquisition.

A data sheet for each room is used to identify and record types and locations of all necessary room elements and systems. The data sheet may also indicate who will be responsible for purchasing and installation of each element, or this may be completed on a separate document. Data sheets also can function as checklists to confirm all details have been completed prior to the room being used.

Infection Prevention during Construction

Part of the planning for construction includes plans for managing potential risks to patients, staff, and the public during the project [12, 13]. At the beginning of the planning phase for a construction project, the hospital needs to plan for infection control by conducting an Infection Control Risk Assessment (ICRA) [1]. The goal of the ICRA is to mitigate the risk of harm to the patients, staff, and others within or near the construction project. Depending upon the scope of the project, some potential risks are dust and fumes, mold, fungi, water contamination, hazardous material, noise, and vibrations.

The ICRA is a multidisciplinary, documented assessment process to identify and mitigate risks of infection that could occur during construction. This assessment is part of the integrated facility planning, design, construction, and commissioning activities. The ICRA team consists of members with expertise in infection prevention and control; direct patient care; facility design; construction; HVAC; and plumbing systems. The scope of the project dictates whether other members are needed [1].

In addition, patient safety has come to the forefront of hospital design. The 2014 FGI guidelines added a safety risk assessment (SRA), which combines with the ICRA. The purpose of the owner-driven SRA is to foster a proactive approach to patient and caregiver safety by mitigating risks from the physical environment that could directly or indirectly contribute to harm. The project team must identify through the SRA risks involving infection control, patient handling, falls, medication safety, psychiatric injury, immobility, and security [1].

The OR manager on the design team is responsible for participating in both the ICRA and SRA and monitoring adherence with the plans and regulations. A challenge is to make sure the staff understands these risks and that the contractors understand how to work safely in the hospital environment, especially when close to patient care areas [12, 14].

Important resources are the Centers for Disease Control and Prevention's *Guideline for Environmental Infection Control in Health-Care Facilities* [15], the FGI guidelines [1], the Joint Commission's book, *Planning, Design, and Construction of Health Care Facilities* [2], and the APIC standards and guidelines [3].

Interim Life Safety Measures

In addition to infection prevention, the team needs to assess and manage other risks that may arise during construction, such as protecting patients from fire, smoke, and toxic fumes. They must also consider risks that may arise after the structure is occupied. Healthcare must meet the needs of three populations: families/visitors, patients, and staff,

particularly patients who are unable to leave their beds, the OR, or the hospital [16].

During the project, part of the planning team's responsibility is to plan for compliance with Interim Life Safety Measures (ILSM). The National Fire Protection Association 101 (NFPA 101) is part of the interim life safety measures [17]. The NFPA 101: Life Safety Code is used in every US state to address minimum building design, construction, operation, and maintenance requirements necessary to protect building occupants from fire, smoke, and toxic fumes. Life Safety Code is a registered trademark of NFPA. The Life Safety Code can be used in conjunction with other building codes or alone in jurisdictions without a building code. The Centers for Medicare and Medicaid Services and the Joint Commission refer to NFPA 101, as do federal, state, and local fire officials.

Among life safety issues that may need to be considered during construction are the need to redirect occupants because of blocked exits, to alter fire safety systems temporarily, and to construct fire barrier walls altering traffic patterns. Plans to mitigate these and other hazards need to be developed and communicated throughout the affected areas of the hospital. Plans for managing emergencies also must be established before construction begins.

Throughout project planning and construction, the OR manager needs to anticipate potential safety hazards that may surface. An unexpected utility shutdown, for example, is a serious safety concern. As part of the ILSM plan, the manager should be prepared to educate the construction team about the importance of planning for and communicating about any type of event that could potentially affect patients, families/visitors, and staff.

New Technology/Integrated ORs

Advancements in technology have allowed ORs to integrate systems that manage information, audiovisual signals, and radiographic imaging inside and outside of the OR suite. There is some indication that integrated technology can enhance the efficiency of certain aspects of surgical procedures. Small studies have found that compared with a conventional OR, intraoperative efficiency was improved in a dedicated minimally invasive surgery (MIS) OR with permanently fixed equipment [18]. Researchers have also found neck flexion and surgical spine rotation for surgeons and nurses were significantly reduced in a dedicated MIS room [19]. Some of this technology not only enhances efficiency but also improves patient safety through improved and timelier communication among care providers.

Questions that arise during the planning and design of a new suite include how much technology is needed in every room, how much of this technology needs to be integrated, and whether the technology installed today will be compatible with the next phase of technology [20]. To answer these questions, the OR planning team needs to perform extensive research, make site visits, interview other clinicians who have developed integrated ORs, learn from their experience, and develop a list of pros and cons.

General questions for planning for new technology include:

- Will the technology integrate with the hospital's systems?
- How will the technology affect existing processes?
- Will automation actually be more efficient or will it add unnecessary steps to an existing system?
- How many ORs need an imaging system?
- What types of procedures will be performed in these rooms?
- Is an anticipated new service or procedure volume driving the design plan?
- Should the rooms be flexible or specific for certain types of procedures?
- Are all the rooms equipped to handle the new technology?
- If a robotic surgical system is a potential addition, how many surgeons will use it, and will it be cost-effective?
- Will technology be ceiling mounted or floor mounted?
- Will the equipment be wired or wireless?

Hospitals that decide to build integrated ORs should involve stakeholders to identify the goals and desired outcomes of the project to achieve and determine the best return on investment. They also often decide to engage the advice of an unbiased consultant. Organizations that subscribe to services offered by the nonprofit ECRI Institute (www.ecri.org) can seek its advice for objective technical information.

Hybrid ORs

The hybrid OR is a rapidly evolving surgical environment. These technologically advanced rooms, which combine surgical equipment and instrumentation with a fixed and dedicated imaging system, are intended for complex surgical and interventional procedures that require advanced imaging. Examples are hybrid coronary revascularization procedures, percutaneous cardiac valve replacement, and complex brain and spine cases [21]. Industry experts estimate that by 2018, 75 percent of cardiovascular surgeons will be working in a hybrid operating suite, ECRI Institute reports [22].

Evidence on clinical benefits is limited, but some reports indicate that advantages may include shorter patient recovery time due to less physiological stress because multiple procedures can be performed in the same episode, streamlined care delivery, better cross-specialty communication, and potential for revenue growth as conventional ORs and interventional rooms are freed for other procedures [22, 23].

Because hybrid rooms are not only technologically but operationally complex, planning requires the collaboration of multiple disciplines. This includes not only the surgical and interventional disciplines but also administrative and clinical staff, facilities personnel, biomedical engineers, information technology specialists, and equipment vendors. Also important to include are others who are critical to the room's functioning, particularly anesthesia providers, imaging support personnel, and perfusionists [21].

There are several general questions to address in the decision-making process about whether to include a hybrid room(s) in the operating suite:

- Will a hybrid OR be supported by existing interventional and surgical caseloads?
- How will a hybrid OR affect the utilization of other interventional suites and ORs?
- Can a hybrid OR be installed in existing space or will substantial renovation or new construction be needed?
- Is the hybrid OR best located in the interventional or surgical departments? Generally, interventional suites do not have the required ventilation, scrub area, sterilization area, or access to surgical equipment and instrumentation. It may be less expensive and easiest to install the hybrid OR in the surgical suite where those support services are already in place.
- What infrastructure will be needed? Consider in particular the size of the room, ceiling height, and weight-bearing capacity of the ceiling and floor.

- How will the room's space be organized? Consider the positioning of equipment and lights, air flow, and the pattern of movement for patients and personnel. It is helpful to construct a mockup of the room to allow clinicians to test the configuration of space and equipment. Planning teams often also choose to visit existing facilities to learn what works well and doesn't work well for them [21, 24, 25].

Once the decision is made to include hybrid rooms in the facility design, early in the planning the project team should ensure that all members thoroughly understand how the hybrid OR is intended to function. Many manufacturers offer highly specialized, proprietary imaging systems that can be permanently integrated into the OR. Intraoperative CT, MRI, and vascular imaging technologies are common. In many cases, these modalities can be moved into and out of the surgical field via floor or ceiling assemblies, allowing for a clear zone when imaging technology is not needed. Hybrid OR imaging technologies present additional spatial, structural, patient, and staff safety issues that must be addressed by the entire team. Representatives from the imaging equipment manufacturer need to be involved early in the planning phase and throughout the project [1]. In the design of an MRI room, specific requirements must be considered, including obtaining an adequate MRI scan, medical imaging in a high magnetic field, and isolation from radiofrequency artifact. Radiofrequency isolation is one of the more difficult tasks and should receive priority from physicists involved within the project [26].

The minimum clear floor area of 650 sq ft (60.39 m^2) is recommended for a hybrid OR. However, the size of a hybrid OR is highly dependent on the functional requirements of the room as an operating environment as well as the requirements of the imaging equipment. This generally increases the room area requirements. The project team is strongly encouraged to develop a full-scale mockup of the room during design to ensure it will function properly.

Many imaging systems are sensitive to vibration, electromagnetic interference, and other forces. The project team should consult with equipment manufacturers to determine if site readiness testing is required. Also, these imaging systems often use liquid-based cooling, which may cross into the surgical environment, requiring additional protection from dripping.

A hybrid OR with intraoperative magnetic resonance imaging (iMRI) must be designed so the doors swing outward from the room to prevent them from becoming inoperable in the event of a magnet quench [1]. In an MRI magnet quench, all of the electrical energy in the superconducting wire is dissipated as heat, rapidly boiling the liquid helium keeping the magnet cold, turning it into helium gas. The equipment needs to be properly vented to provide for the escape of helium in case of a quench. The consequences of unvented helium are that it can burn. If helium fills the room, displacing the oxygen, unconsciousness can quickly result (www.mriquestions.com/what-is-a-quench.html).

Design Considerations for Ambulatory Surgical Centers

In an ambulatory surgical center (ASC), where patients arrive soon before surgery and are discharged soon after, the admission process and patient flow are prime considerations. The facility needs to be planned so the admission process is convenient for the patient and efficient for physicians and staff. Surgical scheduling and the preoperative assessment program need to be planned so procedures can be scheduled easily, the preoperative assessment is safe as well as convenient, and a limited number of patients are waiting in the admitting area at one time. Preoperative and postoperative areas also need to be planned to balance the need for privacy with smooth, safe, and efficient patient flow.

For an ASC project, it is advisable to have an architect who specializes in the design of outpatient facilities, specifically surgical centers. The design team needs to include members who understand the importance of efficient patient flow.

The detailed size and facility requirements for an ASC can be found in the FGI guidelines [1]. In general in ASCs, the OR size is smaller than in a hospital, and hallway dimensions vary by location. The former class A OR is now termed a "procedure room," which is designated for procedures that are not defined as invasive and that may be performed outside the restricted area of the surgical suite but that may require sterile instruments and supplies. Outpatient ORs, formerly class B and C, are required to have a minimum clear floor area of 250 sq ft (23.25 m^2) and a clear dimension of 15 ft (4.58 m) between fixed cabinets and built-in shelves. Where complex orthopedic and neurosurgical procedures are performed in the outpatient setting, the rooms should have a minimum clear floor area of 600 sq ft (55.74 m²) with a clear dimension of 20 sq ft (6.10 m²). Outpatient surgery also follows the surgical suite guidelines for two areas, semirestricted and restricted [1].

The NFPA Life Safety Code and infection prevention and control requirements apply to the design and construction of an ASC just as they do to a hospital.

The facility's entrance forms the patient's and family's first impression of the ASC's services. The facility needs to be designed so patients can easily enter the building whether they are ambulatory or have assistive devices (such as crutches, a walker, or wheelchair); can find their way easily; and are protected from the elements. A separate exit and patient pick-up area are needed to prevent preoperative and postoperative patients from using the same passageways and/or elevators. The pick-up area needs to be convenient for drivers to access and protected from the elements.

Support services should be planned during the initial phase of the design process. The planning team should conduct a needs assessment for ancillary services such as laboratory (both clinical and pathology), radiology, medical records, central supply, sterile processing, and materials management. Plans for these should be developed as the functional program is designed. The amount and flow of materials are crucial because ASCs often have limited space.

Summary

The information provided in this chapter is intended to guide the OR manager and the surgical team through a design and construction project in the surgical arena, whether the project is small or large. Although the project may appear overwhelming initially, breaking it into phases can make it more manageable. Collaboration among multiple disciplines and input from the end users will greatly assist in a successful outcome.

The essential resources – FGI guidelines [1]; *Planning, Design, and Construction of Health Care Facilities* by the Joint Commission [2]; guidelines and standards of the APIC [3]; and American Society of Anesthesiologists' *Operating Room Design Manual* [26], among others – can provide strong support during all phases of the project. The project team must verify that the most current editions of the essential resources are used. The FGI guidelines are updated every four years, with the next update in 2018. APIC updates its guidelines and standards

regularly. The Joint Commission's *Planning, Design, and Construction of Health Care Facilities* is updated every one to two years.

With these resources as well as a team of qualified professionals and the close involvement of end users, OR leaders can participate in designing and building a project that will meet the quality and safety expectations of patients and clinicians as well as help to fulfill the organization's vision and mission.

References

1. *Guidelines for Design and Construction of Health Care Facilities*. Chicago, IL. Facility Guidelines Institute, 2014.

2. Joint Commission. *Planning, Design, and Construction of Health Care Facilities*, 3rd edn. Oakbrook Terrace, IL: Joint Commission, 2015.

3. Association for Professionals in Infection Control and Epidemiology. Guidelines and standards. www.apic.org.

4. Worley DJ, Hohler S. OR construction project: From planning to execution. *AORN J.* 2008;88:917–41.

5. Saver C. Tips for surviving an OR building project. *OR Manager*. 2008;24(2):18, 21.

6. Palmer G, Abernathy JH, Swinton G, et al. Realizing improved patient care through human-centered operating room design. *Anesthesiology*. 2013;119:1066–77.

7. Center for Health Design. www.healthdesign.org.

8. American Society of PeriAnesthesia Nurses. *Perianesthesia Nursing Standards, Practice Recommendations, and Interpretive Statements: 2015–2017*. Cherry Hill, NJ: ASPAN, 2015. www.aspan.org

9. Association of periOperative Registered Nurses. Guidelines & clinical resources. www.aorn.org/guidelines.

10. Association for the Advancement of Medical Instrumentation et al. *Immediate-Use Steam Sterilization*. Arlington, VA: AAMI, 2011. www.aami.org

11. Brogmus G, Leone W, Butler L, et al. Best practices in OR suite layout and equipment choices to reduce slips, trips, and falls. *AORN J.* 2007;86:384–94.

12. American Society for Healthcare Engineering et al. Joint ASHE, APIC, and SHEA response to electronic faucet technology. June 23, 2011. www.ashe.org/resources/alerts/2011/pdfs/joint_statement_faucets-062311.pdf.

13. Bartley JM. APIC state-of-the-art report: The role of infection control during construction in health care facilities. *Am J Infect Control*. 2000;28:156–69.

14. Bartley JM, Olmsted RN, Haas J. Current views of health care design and construction: Practical implications for safer, cleaner environments. *Am J Infect Control*. 2010;38:S1–S12.

15. Centers for Disease Control and Prevention. *Guideline for Environmental Infection Control in Healthcare Facilities*. Atlanta, GA: CDC, 2003. www.cdc.gov/HAI/prevent/prevent_pubs.html

16. Peck RL, Powers-Jones S. Staying up-to-date on life safety. *Healthcare Building Ideas*. November 1, 2010. www.healthcaredesignmagazine.com/building-ideas/staying-date-life-safety

17. National Fire Protection Association. *NFPA 101: Life Safety Code*. Quincy, MA: NFPA, 2015.

18. Hsiao KC, Machaidze Z, Pattaras JG. Time management in the operating room: An analysis of the dedicated minimally invasive surgery suite. *JSLS*. 2004;8:300–3.

19. Van Det MJ, Meijerink WJ, Hoff C, et al. Ergonomic assessment of neck posture in the minimally invasive surgical suite during laparoscopic cholecystectomy. *Surg Endosc*. 2008;22:2421–7.

20. Eder P, Register JL. Ten management considerations for implementing an endovascular hybrid OR. *AORN J*. 2014;100(3):260–70.

21. Van Pelt J. Hybrid ORs: What's behind the demand? *OR Manager*. 2011;27(5):7–10.

22. ECRI Institute. *What Is a Hybrid OR? Should Your Facility Have One?* Plymouth Meeting, PA: ECRI Institute, 2015. www.ecri.org

23. Bonatti J, Lehr E, Vesely MR, et al. Hybrid coronary revascularization: Which patients? When? How? *Curr Opin Cardiol*. 2010;25:568–74.

24. Mathias J. Planning and staffing a hybrid OR. *OR Manager*. 2011;27(5):10–12.

25. Urbanowicz JA, Taylor G. Hybrid OR: Is it in your future? *Nurse Manage*. 2010;41(5):22–7.

26. American Society of Anesthesiologists. *Operating Room Design Manual*. www.asahq.org/resources/resources-from-asa-committees/operating-room-design-manual

Chapter

12

Operating an Ambulatory Surgery Center as a Successful Business

John J. Wellik

The History of Ambulatory Surgery

In the Early 1800s All Surgery Was "Outpatient Surgery"

Ambulatory surgery can be traced back to the roots of surgery itself. In the 1800s, surgeons would perform surgery in the home of the patient, and with the exception of alcohol and restraints, very little was done to dull the pain. Anesthesia as we know it did not exist for these surgical operations. Drugs such as nitrous oxide and ether had been used recreationally for some time, but physicians did not apply the analgesic and amnestic effects of these agents to the practice of medicine for many years.

Early Anesthesia Was Associated with Significant Morbidity and Mortality

In 1842, a dentist by the name of Horace Wells witnessed a public demonstration of nitrous oxide in Hartford, Connecticut, and later realized that he might be able to use nitrous oxide to extract teeth with very little pain. Wells eventually had one of his own teeth extracted under nitrous oxide anesthesia, but it took several years before nitrous oxide was fully accepted by the medical community [1]. Unfortunately, early anesthetics, including nitrous oxide, had significant morbidity and mortality [2].

Advances in Medicine Necessitated Hospital-based Surgery

For nearly a century, advances in surgery and anesthesia have necessitated that procedures take place in a controlled environment that could only be offered by a large hospital. Even as early as 1927, some physicians,

such as Ralph Waters, argued that their techniques were safe enough to be performed outside the hospital. Waters wrote in his memoirs that his techniques of measuring blood pressure and heart rate frequently made his procedures safe, and that his office-based practice avoided the obstacles of a hospital operating room (OR) as well as patient and surgeon inconveniences [2].

The Evolution of Modern Ambulatory Surgery

The Concept of Ambulatory Surgery Was Revisited in the 1950s

It was not until the 1950s, as a result of a hospital bed shortage, that Canada began revisiting the idea of performing ambulatory surgery. Canadian physicians began performing hernia repairs in the outpatient setting as early as the 1950s. The idea of ambulatory surgery did not become popular in the United States until the 1960s, when John Dillon and David Cohen at the University of California Los Angeles created an outpatient surgery service. Although Canada began performing outpatient surgeries because of a hospital bed shortage, Dillon and Cohen were more interested in the economics of ambulatory surgery and the potential financial implications [2].

Anesthesiologists Pioneer the First Free-Standing Ambulatory Surgery Center

Two anesthesiologists in Phoenix, Arizona – John Ford and Wallace Reed – were also interested in ambulatory surgery because of the potential for improvements in cost containment, reimbursement, efficiency, and convenience. In 1971, John Ford and Wallace Reed created the Phoenix Surgicenter, which is credited with being the first free-standing ambulatory surgery center (ASC) in the United States [2]. The primary goal was to achieve maximum efficiency and patient throughput. To decrease overhead and costs to the patients, they eliminated all unnecessary services that existed in standard hospitals (i.e., cafeteria, transport personnel, excessive laboratory testing).

Several Changes Were Necessary for Ambulatory Surgery to Become Practical

Although physicians were realizing the potential benefits of ambulatory surgery, the practice of medicine was not capable of implementing the concept. Specifically, most surgeries were still very invasive, and anesthetic techniques had complication rates far too high for routine same-day discharge. For this reason, relatively few ASCs were built until the mid-1980s, when several things happened: (1) accreditation programs and standards were established; (2) the US government accepted ASCs and established Medicare reimbursement rates; (3) advances in the field of anesthesiology dramatically reduced the anesthesia-related morbidity and mortality; and (4) development of new surgical instruments such as lasers, enhanced endoscopic techniques, and fiber optics reduced the trauma and recovery time associated with many surgical procedures [3].

In 1980 the United States had approximately 275 ASCs, and approximately 15 percent of all surgeries were done in outpatient facilities [3]. By 1990, the number of ASCs had grown to 1,450 and the flurry of ambulatory surgery organizations continued to expand. The Society for Ambulatory Anesthesia was created, and new drugs were being created to further facilitate ambulatory surgery. Ketorolac, the first parenteral nonsteroidal anti-inflammatory drug approved for severe postoperative pain, was reported to provide the analgesic potency of morphine without associated respiratory depression [4]. By the year 2000, there were approximately 3,000 Medicare-certified ASCs and the number continued to grow throughout the decade, increasing nearly 70 percent to over 5,100 by the close of 2010. The growth has continued in the current decade, albeit at a slower pace with the total approaching 5,500 in 2014 (Figure 12.1).

Although the new regulatory environment and medical advances helped establish an environment

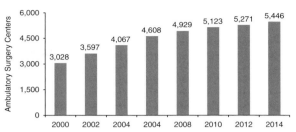

Figure 12.1 Number of outpatient surgery centers, 2000–2014. *Source*: Medicare Payment Advisory Commission, *A Data Book: Healthcare Spending and the Medicare Program, June 2007 and June 2016.*

for ASCs to reap the benefits envisioned over 40 years ago, these were not the only factors for the explosion of ASCs across the country.

Additional Factors Driving the Growth of ASCs

Procedures in ASCs Cost Less

As mentioned earlier, ASCs were designed to maximize efficiency, eliminate unnecessary services, and decrease costs. ASCs are now widely acknowledged to be a cost-effective alternative to the higher-cost inpatient setting. Hospitals have to pay higher overhead, administrative, and facility development costs, which make their per-procedure costs higher than those of ASCs. For this reason, managed care companies, self-insured employers, and government payers prefer to have patients go to lower-cost ASCs [5].

Patients Value the Convenience of ASCs

ASCs are designed to be more convenient for the patient. The architectural layouts are usually designed to maximize throughput. Administrative paperwork is minimized to facilitate faster admission. Family members are allowed to be with the patients during the recovery period, and patients are allowed to leave ASCs relatively quickly after surgery. As a result, patients say they have a 92 percent satisfaction rate with both the care and service they receive from ASCs [6].

Surgeons Value the Efficiency of ASCs

Efficiency is particularly important to surgeons. It takes much less time to prepare an OR in a specialized

ASC for the next patient than in a standard hospital. Improved efficiency allows surgeons to treat more patients in the same amount of time than they would be able to do in a hospital; some surgeons maintain that they can do three times the number of procedures in an ASC as they could in a hospital setting [3]. Many surgeons prefer working in an ASC because they can set the standards for staffing, safety precautions, postoperative care, etc., rather than having these things decided for them by a hospital administrator. Physicians also prefer the greater flexibility in scheduling and more consistent and reliable nurse staffing [5].

Types of ASCs

Practice-Based

Practice-based ASCs are commonly owned and operated by a specific physician group practice. These are equipped and staffed for a single medical specialty and are usually located in or adjacent to offices of a physician group practice. Practice-based or single-specialty centers often require lower capital and operating costs than free-standing ASCs.

Free-standing

Free-standing ASCs are typically owned by a group of local investors, physicians, and/or an investment company. Such ASCs generally serve a broader group of physicians, which compromises the flexibility of scheduling and increases overhead, but adds diversity of revenue levels and patient mix.

Hospital Joint Venture

Surgery centers operated through a hospital joint venture include a hospital or health system in their ownership hierarchy. These ASCs may have been built by the participating hospital as a separate facility dedicated to ambulatory services or, as is becoming increasingly more common, resulted from a merger between previously free-standing and/or practice-based ASCs with large healthcare providers.

Getting Started

Legal Structure and Ownership

ASCs are typically organized as some type of limited liability entity, which affords the individual investors a limitation on personal liability associated with the financial obligations of the center. Limited liability companies (LLCs) are the most common type of legal entity used for an ASC, although limited partnerships may offer some advantages over LLCs in certain states.

As noted previously, there are different types of ASCs and, accordingly, the ownership of the entity will depend upon the type of facility. Practice-based centers may be owned by the group practice or by individual physicians within that practice. Free-standing centers may have ownership split among a number of group practices and/or individual physicians as well as third-party management or development companies. Centers joint ventured with a hospital will include an interest owned by an entity affiliated with the hospital or health system partner.

Anti-Kickback and "Stark Law" Considerations

The ownership and operation of ASCs is subject to comprehensive federal and state regulations. Although the specific provisions of the Social Security Act prohibiting physician referrals to facilities in which they or family members own a financial interest, commonly referred to as Stark Law, generally do not apply to ambulatory surgery services, the overall "anti-kickback" provisions of federal criminal law do apply and must be considered when structuring ownership allocation and investment protocol in a surgery center. These regulations prohibit payment or receipt of any consideration in exchange for referring patients for services that are reimbursed under a federal healthcare program, notably Medicare and Medicaid. The Health and Human Services Office of the Inspector General (OIG) has published regulations outlining certain safe harbors under the anti-kickback statute, including safe harbors applicable to surgery centers. This safe harbor generally protects ownership or investments in surgery centers and payments that are a return on that investment for physicians who refer patients to the center or perform procedures on patients who are referred to the center, if certain conditions are met. These conditions include the following criteria:

1. At least one-third of each physician investor's medical practice annual income must come from performing outpatient procedures that are approved by Medicare for reimbursement in an ASC.
2. At least one-third of the Medicare-eligible outpatient procedures performed annually by

each physician investor must be performed at the surgery center in which the investment is made.

The safe harbor guidelines also allow nonphysician investors who are not employed by, nor in a position to provide any goods or services or refer patients to, the center or the physician investors. Surgery centers that include ownership by a management company, which is typically compensated with a percentage of the center's revenue, or by a hospital, which is likely to be in a position to refer patients to the center or its physician investors, would not satisfy all of the requirements of the safe harbor provisions. However, it should be noted that the safe harbor provisions do not expand the scope of activities that the anti-kickback statute prohibits and the OIG has acknowledged that legitimate surgery center arrangements exist that do not meet all of the safe harbor criteria. Thus, although failure to meet all the safe harbor criteria does not mean that any given surgery center structure is in violation of the law, such structures could be subject to greater scrutiny by regulators.

Governing Board

The organizational documents of the legal entity should outline the specifics of the facility's governance, i.e., number of board members, election protocol, subcommittees, etc. Identifying initial board members with a mix of business, clinical, and interpersonal skills is critical to the successful start-up of the center. Any compensation arrangements for the board members should be mindful of the safe harbor guidelines discussed above. Given that the physician investors, who are the most likely candidates for board positions, may also be the largest utilizers of the facility, any compensation for board service should be clearly tied to time spent on governance issues and be subject to reasonable periodic maximums in order to avoid the appearance of payment for volumes of patient referrals to the center.

Regulatory Approval and Licensing

Certificate of Need Requirement

Healthcare regulations in certain states require that, prior to the construction of new healthcare facilities or the introduction of new services, a designated agency must determine that a need exists for those facilities or services. This process is often referred to as a certificate-of-need (CON) application, which can be time-consuming and expensive. Not all states have CON laws, and for those that do the requirements and process varies, with some providing thresholds for capital expenditures or scope of service that may exempt smaller and/or single specialty surgery centers from the CON review process.

Medicare Provider Application

In order to participate in Medicare, an ASC must satisfy regulations known as conditions for coverage. For a new facility, this is typically accomplished through a direct survey coordinated through the Center for Medicare and Medicaid Services (CMS) after submission of a Medicare provider application. Diligent completion of the application and coordination with CMS on scheduling the survey to coincide with the anticipated facility opening date are critical to avoiding delays in obtaining the Medicare provider number. Although receipt of that provider number directly impacts payment for services performed for Medicare and Medicaid patients, private managed care payers typically will not finalize reimbursement contracts until the facility obtains its Medicare certification.

Business Plan

Specialties, Types of Procedures

Determining the surgical specialties to be accommodated will drive many of the specific assumptions involved in preparing a comprehensive business plan. The number and size of operating and procedure rooms will drive the overall space requirements for the facility. Specific procedures to be performed will dictate the equipment and instrument requirements and budget as well as the staffing plan.

Managed Care Contracting Strategy

A number of surgery centers in recent years adopted "out-of-network" strategies, whereby the facility chooses not to enter into contracts with some or all private managed care payers. In extreme examples, the facility does not apply for Medicare certification. These facilities rely on individual patient payments, or more typically, receipt of out-of-network reimbursement from the patients' insurance carriers. Traditional preferred provider network plans (PPOs) historically have paid a lower percentage of charges to providers of services to their members who do not contract with the carrier. However, with no contracted fee schedule, centers executing these out-of-network strategies were often able to realize higher reimbursement per case at the lower out-of-network percentage of gross charges reimbursement than if they had contracted with the carrier. As the number of facilities pursuing such a strategy grew, so too did efforts by managed care companies to limit their exposure to these facilities. These efforts include: (1) alerting state regulators to practices in which a patient's financial responsibility, which is typically higher due to the higher co-pay percentage and/or deductible for services provided by an out-of-network provider, is waived; (2) providing reimbursement directly to the patient instead of the provider, resulting in the facility needing to collect from the patient well after the date of surgery; and (3) refusing to provide any reimbursement for services provided by specific facilities.

Regardless of an in- or out-of-network approach, estimating reimbursement levels, or net revenue, is one of the most critical steps in developing a pro forma income statement to be included in a business plan. Assumptions regarding the anticipated payer mix within the specific geographic and demographic mix of patients must be made. Understanding the existing payer mix for the practices of the surgeons who will be utilizing the facility is one potential starting point. This is also one area in which working with a management company and/or a hospital partner can be a key differentiator. Not only will those resources be able to assist with a better understanding of the probable payer mix, they may also be able to assist with negotiating higher reimbursement rates through specific provisions of the contracts with the individual payers.

Managed care contracts for ASCs typically will provide for a percentage of Medicare reimbursement as a starting point in setting contracted reimbursement rates for a facility. Achieving as high a multiple or percentage of Medicare rates as possible for those types of procedures that the facility anticipates performing the most should be a key goal in negotiating contracts. In addition, "carving out" specific procedures that are likely to be a focus of the facility and/or are significant with the practices of key physician utilizers should be another goal in contract negotiation. Specifying set reimbursement rates or higher percentages of Medicare for those procedures can have a dramatic impact on the profitability of the facility. Similarly, establishing mark-up percentages on implantable items should be a consideration.

Location

Proximity to the practice offices of identified physician partners is likely to be one of the key drivers in selecting a search area for a new surgery center. Vacant land or a site available for redevelopment is the most viable alternative, as retrofitting an existing building and transforming it into an efficient surgery center is typically not practical. Proximity to the hospital where the physician partners perform surgery currently and where they will probably continue to perform their inpatient cases is also a consideration. There are advantages and disadvantages to surgery centers located on or adjacent to a hospital campus. Although it may offer convenient access for the surgeons, particularly if they also have their practice office on the campus, it also may bring many of the detractions from patient and staff viewpoints, notably traffic congestion, parking difficulty and expense, and suboptimum discharge logistics.

Site Plan

As noted in the introduction to this chapter, efficient patient flow was one of the primary drivers in Dr. Ford and Dr. Reed's design of the first free-standing surgery center in the United States. That goal carries forward to today. The ideal floorplan provides for logical and efficient physical movement of a patient from check-in to discharge with convenient access for staff to cover both preoperative preparation and postoperative recovery. All sterile areas should be confined to contiguous space in the middle of the patient flow. The exterior site plan should allow for staff parking and entrance near the lounge or locker rooms with ample patient parking near the reception and discharge areas, which should be in close proximity to each other but visibly separated for patient privacy and comfort.

Financial Pro Forma

The specific components of the financial pro forma will be discussed in the next section of this chapter. The pro forma provides the basis for determining the amount of external financing required and is also a key requirement in working with lenders to secure the financing.

Key Components of the Financial Pro Forma

Case Volumes

Estimating case volumes and the ramp-up in those volumes during the center's start-up phase is the critical first step in putting together a financial pro forma. Identifying the individual surgeons who are committed to utilizing the center from its inception can be a starting point in arriving at the volume estimates. The routines or practice flows of those surgeons and further, how they, and their scheduling staff, are willing to alter it with the opening of the center must be analyzed. Depending upon where each surgeon is planning on moving cases from, there will probably be pressure to maintain volumes at the facilities they are currently utilizing. These pressures may be unspoken and/or subtle but they should not be underestimated. Preferences in scheduling of OR time as well as the availability of key staff could be altered. Similarly, the influence of the surgeon's scheduler should not be underestimated. Ideally, the surgeon will drive the decision on the volume and types of cases to be scheduled at the new center, but the surgery center staff should work to develop relationships with the key contacts at each surgeon's office.

The number of operating and procedure rooms contained in the facility will ultimately have an impact on the capacity of the case and procedure volumes to be budgeted for the facility. Initially, however, the capacity of the facility is not likely to be a determining factor in estimating case volumes. Rather, the case volume estimates arrived at by analyzing the probable changes in practice patterns for the early surgeon utilizers should drive the decisions on when to "open" how many ORs. Staffing and equipping only those operating and procedures rooms necessary to handle the initial case volumes will be key to controlling the start-up expenses of the center.

Revenue Per Case

The amount of revenue collected per case will be driven by the specific cases performed and the source of payment for each of those cases. The amount of revenue actually collected is often referred to as "net revenue," whereas the amount billed is referred to as "gross revenue" or "gross charges." The gross revenue for a facility will be driven by the "charge master," which will need to be established within the patient accounting system utilized by the facility for tracking patient billings and collections. Most ASCs set their gross charges on a "bundled" basis per procedure, in which there is one all-inclusive charge for a given procedure, rather than the unbundled, detailed line item charge process typically utilized in an inpatient setting. This approach is driven by the reimbursement

schedule utilized by Medicare for ASCs, which in turn is often the basis for managed care contracts, as discussed previously in the Managed care contracting strategy section of this chapter.

The most precise approach to estimating gross and net revenue would be to develop a matrix of anticipated procedures by physician and by reimbursement source. Depending upon the number of anticipated physicians who will utilize the facility and their surgical specialties, this approach may not be practical. A reasonable alternative for a multispecialty ASC would be to arrive at average gross charges by specialty (orthopedic versus gastrointestinal, etc.) and then estimate average reimbursement percentages by payer type (e.g., contracted, out-of-network, workers' compensation, self-pay, Medicare). If implants are anticipated to be a significant component of cases performed at the center (orthopedic, spine, pain stimulators, etc.), the net reimbursement for those items needs to be included in the revenue calculations in order to develop reasonable estimates of anticipated cash flow requirements and sources.

Fixed Versus Variable Costs

Fixed costs

The fixed costs of a facility are those that do not fluctuate based on activity volumes. The most significant of this type of cost is the cost of the facility itself – either rent or a mortgage payment if the facility is owned by the partnership and leveraged. Equipment costs are typically fixed costs as well, most frequently financed through secured leases or bank loans. The third type of fixed cost is associated with the core staffing of the facility – the administrative or management overhead positions as well as the minimum clinical staffing levels required regardless of the number of cases the facility performs. Determining this staffing level and the timing of hiring each position will be one of the keys to controlling start-up losses and cash flow demands.

Variable costs

Variable costs are those that fluctuate (or should fluctuate) based on case volumes. Clinical staffing above the core staffing levels is typically the most significant variable cost, and the cost that needs to be managed most closely in order to control the profitability of the facility as volumes fluctuate. This can be managed in a number of ways, and each has its advantages and disadvantages. Using contract or agency nurses provides the most flexibility in managing hours, as these arrangements allow for staffing as close to an "as needed" basis as possible. However, the per-hour cost of agency nurses will probably be the highest of any of the alternatives. In addition, availability of specific individual nurses is not assured with this approach, leading to "learning curve" inefficiencies, frustration of the surgeons in working with new staff, and worst of all, potential clinical quality issues.

Identifying a sufficient number of dedicated staff willing to "flex" their hours based on case volumes provides the most consistency in the workforce dynamics at the facility. In order to retain these individuals, it may be necessary to guarantee a certain number of hours each pay period and/or confirm that they will continue to qualify for full-time status for benefit purposes. Maintaining benefits, particularly healthcare coverage, is frequently a determining factor for an employee staying in a position. However, the costs to the center for this coverage are significant and can become unreasonable on a cost-per-hour basis if the level of productive hours is consistently below a full-time load.

An alternative to using agency staff to supplement the facility's full-time staff is to develop a group of individuals who are willing to work on an as-needed basis, often referred to as PRNs. These individuals are employees of the facility being paid hourly rather than through an agency, typically resulting in lower hourly rates. Similar to full-time staff, however, the PRN employees may need a commitment of a minimum number of hours per pay period or per month in order to commit to remaining available for work when needed.

After personnel costs, drugs and medical supplies is the other significant cost item that will be driven by case volumes. Standardizing as many items as possible by working with the utilizing surgeons will help with controlling the required investment in supply inventory and also build purchasing leverage with larger quantities. Consistent and complete utilization of preference cards, whereby the surgeons specify supplies to be used for a given type of case, will further assist with controlling supply levels and limiting wasted supplies. Various types of "packs" are available that contain the supplies typically utilized for different types of cases. Although these offer convenience and may simplify the ordering and inventory monitoring processes, they can also increase the amount of wasted supplies and overall supply costs.

Depending upon the types of procedures performed, implantable supplies or devices can be significant drivers of supply costs. Individually expensive items should be stocked on an as-needed basis for specific cases, or on a consignment basis, allowing for payment to the distributor or manufacturer only when the items are used for a case. As previously noted, insurance contracts should allow for reimbursement of many implantable items at a multiple or percentage of costs in addition to the contracted payment rate for many procedures. Maintaining logs detailing receipt and use of these items will insure accurate reimbursement as well as prevent theft or loss due to expiration.

Financing

Facility

Finish-out costs for a surgery center are significant, typically two or three times the cost of constructing the "shell" of a new facility. Real estate developers or landlords will often roll the cost of the finish out into the lease rate for a facility, although the "cap rate" used may not be attractive, given that the owner will factor in payment risks as well as a return above their cost of capital. Another consideration that will impact the monthly and annual cost of rolling finish-out costs into a facility lease rate is the term over which the costs are being amortized. The lease term required in order to achieve a manageable rent level may be for a longer period than the surgery center investors are willing to commit. An approach to arriving at an equitable lease rate for a newly developed surgery center would be to develop an initial rate that is a blend of a shorter amortization period, perhaps 10 or 15 years, for much of the finish out with the core facility construction costs amortized over 20 or 25 years. Lease renewal options should factor in this blended approach, with an appropriate reduction in rate after the finish-out costs have been amortized.

Equipment

Rolling the finish-out costs into a broader financing agreement that also covers the initial equipment is another approach. However, including more than tangible, movable equipment in a financing agreement will increase the interest rate as well as the likelihood of the requirement of personal guarantees from the individual physician investors in the surgery center. Guarantees, while an obvious financial encumbrance for the initial physician investors, can also become a practical and administrative burden for the surgery center business or legal entity as physician owners leave or change ownership interests. The requirement of a debt or lease guarantee will also be an impediment to bringing in new physician investors. Approaches to mitigating these concerns include ensuring that any guarantees are pro rata based on ownership and also "burn off" provisions that provide for elimination of the guarantee over time assuming satisfactory payment experience or other criteria.

Working Capital

In addition to funding the finish out and tangible surgical and business office equipment, funds will also need to be available to cover preopening operating expenses, notably payroll and supplies as well as rent and other fixed costs. Accurately projecting the opening date and tying hire dates and supply receipts to this date will mitigate the preopening expenses and related cash flow requirement.

Monitoring Performance

Once the ASC is operational, monitoring its performance will help insure that it remains viable. As the number of ASCs proliferated, more have failed during their early years of operation with approximately 400 closing or merging with another center since 2010 [7]. Inadequate discipline in monitoring key metrics and not taking appropriate action based upon those metrics was likely a significant contributor to many of these failures.

Operating Metrics

OR Utilization and Scheduling Efficiency

Available OR time is the overriding resource constraint for an ASC. Accordingly, managing utilization of the center's ORs will be a determining factor in its success. Developing and adhering to scheduling protocols is a first step. The computerized patient accounting system used by the facility should have an application to facilitate scheduling of OR time, but regardless of whether the computer system is used or more rudimentary paper schedules are the approach, the protocol for scheduling cases should be clearly documented and thoroughly communicated, both to the center's staff as well as to the schedulers at the physician offices for the center's key surgeons.

The components or considerations of the scheduling protocol should include the following.

- What are the acceptable communication channels for requesting OR time? Having a dedicated scheduling phone line that will not be tied up with other center calls will help insure availability of the line when a surgeon's office wants to schedule a case and that the request gets to the correct person at the center. Although multiple employees could have the ability to add a case to the schedule, it should be clear who at the center "owns" the schedule. If schedule requests are accepted via facsimile, again there should be a dedicated fax line to receive these requests and clear procedures on who is responsible for monitoring these incoming fax transmissions and confirming receipt with the surgeon's office. If email or other electronic means (e.g., the center's website) are allowed for scheduling, considerations for ensuring Health Insurance Portability and Accountability Act compliance are required as well as the follow-up and confirmation procedures noted for scheduling via fax.

- How will block scheduling be handled? Surgeons who intend to be heavy users of the center will probably want to "block out" or reserve certain consistent, recurring periods of time on the center's schedule to insure they have available OR time for their patients. Although this practice can be a huge plus for the center from an OR utilization viewpoint, it can quickly turn into a utilization, and political, nightmare. On the plus side, reserving blocks of OR time indicates an intended practice pattern whereby a surgeon communicates the intent to bring a significant number of cases to the center. Presumably, the surgeon's scheduler knows of the blocked time and will schedule all eligible patients accordingly. The situation turns problematic when multiple surgeons want to block the same prime, early morning time slots as well as when they fail to consistently book cases within their reserved time frames. Mitigating these challenges is another of the many areas in which encouraging the physicians to help manage each other will often yield the best results. The physician governing board should set and help enforce the procedures for prioritizing block schedule requests and releasing uncommitted blocks timely to insure that the benefits of blocked time exceed its disadvantages.

- How much time will be scheduled for each case? One of the primary advantages to a surgeon in using an ASC versus a hospital environment is the predictability of ORs being available when scheduled. Maximizing this advantage requires accuracy in scheduling. Thorough and precise communication with each surgeon and their staff regarding expectations on required OR time for each type of case will contribute to establishing baselines in scheduling. Tracking of actual times against that scheduled will allow for refinement of the scheduling based on experience. Monitoring and recording whether cases start on time, with standard reasons if not, is a key metric to track and report to the center staff and the physician governing board. Elimination of physician controllable delays (e.g., surgeon not arriving as scheduled) is another area in which "self-policing" among the physicians is most effective.

- How much time will be allowed for between cases? Turnaround time between cases is another key metric to be tracked and shared with the center staff. Keeping that time as short and consistent as possible requires clearly documented procedures and duty assignments.

Staffing Management

As previously discussed, staff costs are the largest variable cost within the facility. Accordingly, managing hours is the most critical area in controlling expenses of the center. The best metric for monitoring how effectively the center is managing its staffing is worked hours per case, which should be tracked and charted on a daily basis. In order for the metric to be actionable, the clinical staff hours should be segregated from the business office and management staff. Maintaining consistent worked hours per case as volumes fluctuate is an indicator that staff hours are being managed effectively. This is only possible if the scheduling protocols mentioned earlier are followed and the turnover time between cases is effectively managed.

The ratio of contract or agency hours to total clinical hours is another staffing metric to track on a daily basis. As discussed earlier, use of agency nurses allows for the most flexibility in staffing but typically at the highest incremental cost per hour and also at the risk of reducing physician satisfaction as well as clinical quality. Accordingly, seeing recurring spikes in contract usage other than on days with unusually high case volumes could indicate issues with managing staff absences, whereas seeing consistent use of contract hours would indicate the potential need for adding "permanent" staff.

Supply Management

After staff costs, medical supply costs will be the second highest variable cost. Working with the physician leadership to establish the center's master supply list and minimizing variances from that list due to individual physician preferences is often one of the more challenging tasks in controlling costs. However, reaching a consensus among the physician leaders on basic supplies with reasonable per unit costs can have a significant impact on the profitability of each case while also minimizing the cash required to stock multiple versions of the same item.

Using preference cards for each case can be an effective tool to assist with purchasing supplies and also for monitoring exceptions from the master supply list requested by individual physicians. At the most basic level, a preference card would include all the supplies that a specific physician requires (or requests) for a specific type of procedure. Templates of these cards can be maintained either manually or on an automated basis through the computer system used by the facility. The need for any modifications to the template for a specific patient can be confirmed when scheduling the case with the physician's office.

Although supplies other than implants are typically included in the bundled facility charge for a given procedure, recording actual supply use after completion of a case and pricing out those supplies will facilitate benchmarking of supply costs between physicians performing the same procedures. This allows the physicians to work together on identifying supply cost saving opportunities to enhance the center's profitability.

Financial Metrics

The center's monthly financial reports should facilitate monitoring of key financial metrics in comparison to the budget and historical performance. The sample income statement in Figure 12.2 outlines some

Center Name
Income Statement Variance Analysis
Month ended MM/DD/YYYY

	Actual	Budget	Prior Year	Variance Budget	%	Variance Prior Year	%
Cases	346	295	249	51	17.3%	97	39.0%
REVENUE							
Gross patient revenue	$510,551	$438,075	$266,609	$72,476	16.5%	$243,942	91.5%
Contractual adjustments	237,502	232,180	146,690	5,322	2.3%	90,812	61.9%
Net revenue	273,049	205,895	119,919	67,154	32.0%	153,130	126.7%
EXPENSES							
Personnel costs	69,123	63,425	47,225	5,698	9.0%	21,898	46.4%
Drugs and medical	43,104	35,400	25,181	7,704	21.8%	17,923	71.2%
Repair and maintenance	5,044	5,500	3,937	(456)	(8.3%)	1,107	28.1%
Purchased services	8,762	6,000	2,836	2,762	46.0%	5,926	209.0%
Minor equipment and instruments	598	500	290	98	19.6%	308	106.2%
Utilities	3,720	3,700	3,483	20	0.5%	237	6.8%
Non-medical supplies and expenses	4,247	4,000	3,939	247	6.2%	308	7.8%
Professional fees	250	300	420	(50)	(16.7%)	(170)	(40.5%)
Sales expense	796	1,000	702	(204)	(20.4%)	94	13.4%
Insurance	1,772	1,950	1,772	(178)	(9.1%)	0	0.0%
Provision for bad debts	6,783	8,220	5,332	(1,437)	(17.5%)	1,451	27.2%
Lease and rent expense	17,906	17,741	16,368	165	0.9%	1,538	9.4%
Non-income taxes	2,889	3,000	2,797	(111)	(3.7%)	92	3.3%
Total operating expenses	164,994	150,736	114,282	14,258	9.5%	50,712	44.4%
EBITDA	108,055	55,159	5,637	52,896	95.9%	102,418	193.6%
EBITDA %	39.6%	26.8%	4.7%	78.8%	(294.0%)	66.9%	438.2%
Depreciation expense	14,512	18,008	13,644	(3,496)	(19.4%)	868	6.4%
Interest expense	5,263	7,468	6,124	(2,205)	(29.5%)	(861)	(14.1%)
Total non-operating expenses	19,775	25,476	19,768	(5,701)	(22.4%)	7	0.0%
Pretax income (loss)	$88,280	$29,683	($14,131)	$58,597	197.4%	$99,835	706.5%
Ratio analysis:							
Gross patient revenue / case	$1,476	$1,485	$1,071	($9)	(0.6%)	$405	37.8%
Net revenue / case	$789	$698	$482	$91	13.1%	$308	63.9%
Salaries and benefits / case	$200	$215	$190	($15)	(7.1%)	$10	5.3%
D&M / case	$125	$120	$101	$5	3.8%	$23	23.2%
Other operating expense / case	$153	$176	$168	($23)	(13.3%)	($16)	(9.3%)
Total operating expense / case	$477	$511	$459	($34)	(6.7%)	$18	3.9%
EBITDA / case	$312	$187	$23	$125	67.0%	$290	1279.5%
Bad debt % of net revenue	2.5%	4.0%	4.4%	(1.5%)	(37.8%)	(2.0%)	(44.1%)

> EBITDA Earnings before interest, taxes, depreciation and amortization is a key measure of profitability and cash flow

Observations:

Volumes are ramping up nicely with current year cases 17% ahead of budget and 39% above prior year.

Gross revenue per case is right on budget and 38% ahead of prior year, which is primarily attributable to changes in specialty mix and/or complexity of cases performed consistent with what was planned.

Net revenue per case is 13% ahead of budget and 64% above prior year indicating an improved payor mix as well as more favorable contracts.

Personnel costs are above budget and prior year in total dollars due to the higher case volumes and complexity of cases, but are below budget on a per case basis indicating success in managing staffing levels and mix to actual case volumes. The per case increase of 5% over prior year is generally consistent with wage increases.

Drugs and medical expense per case are in line with budgeted levels but up significantly from prior year as a result of the increased complexity of cases.

Other operating expenses are generally consistent with budgeted amounts in total dollars but below budget and prior year on a per case basis reflecting the leverage potential of spreading these more fixed expenses over the higher case volumes that were achieved.

Bad debt expense as a % of net revenue is running lower than budget and prior year, which indicates good collection results.

Figure 12.2 A sample income statement.

of the more critical metrics and provides some typical observations based on the month's results.

In addition to monitoring and taking appropriate action based on the center's income statement metrics, the balance sheet also deserves some attention. Cash is likely to be the most important line item on the facility's balance sheet to the physician investors; however, managing it requires focus on several other line items, notably: accounts receivable, inventory, accounts payable, and cash distributions.

Accounts Receivable

Utilizing tools within the center's patient accounting computer system will be key to managing the center's accounts receivable. With respect to monitoring the center's summary balance sheet, ensuring that accounts receivable per the balance sheet equals the total reported by the detail of patient balances maintained within the patient accounting system at each month end is a key control. Discrepancies could reflect receipts that are deposited but not posted to the appropriate patient balance in the patient accounting system or, more concerning, receipts that have been posted to a patient's account but were not subsequently deposited to the center's bank account.

The accounts receivable aging report provided by the patient accounting system will categorize patient balances into "buckets" by the number of days that have elapsed (e.g., less than 30, 30–60, 60–90, etc.) since the date of service. The system should also facilitate categorization of the balances between amounts due directly from the patient (deductible, co-pay, etc.) and the amounts due from the insurance carrier. Proper presurgery screening procedures should facilitate collection of a majority of the amounts due directly from the patient on or before the date of surgery. Procedures for timely and consistent follow-up for any remaining patient balances should be clearly documented and adhered to in order to minimize any write-offs incurred by the facility. These procedures should also outline when, or if, a patient account should be turned over to a collection agency and written off as a bad debt. Decisions also need to be made as to whether the facility will offer payment terms to the patient for their responsibility. This has become a more common request with the higher deductible and co-pay levels that employers and insurers are transferring to individuals. Third-party financing companies have developed programs specifically for healthcare providers and may provide an attractive alternative to requiring center employees to deal with this aspect of the patient relationship.

For insurers with whom the center is "in network," the majority of amounts due should be collected within 30 days of the date of service. Significant delays beyond that time frame would indicate issues with the accuracy of filing claims and/or following the process required by the insurer. Monitoring the day's sales outstanding (DSO) in accounts receivable is a good metric to track on a monthly basis to insure collections are being received on a timely basis. The metric is calculated by determining the average daily net revenue and then dividing the month end accounts receivable by that amount. Using the most recent 2 months of revenue will level out daily fluctuations and also provide for the normal collection lag. For example, if net revenue for January and February totaled $450,000 and February's accounts receivable balance was $270,000, the DSO would be 35 (i.e., $450,000 divided by 59 days equals average daily revenue of $7,627, which when divided into the $270,000 accounts receivable balance yields the DSO metric of 35 days).

Inventory

There are different approaches to accounting for inventory within a center's financial statements. Technical accounting rules would require that all supplies be recorded to inventory on the balance sheet when purchased and then recorded as expense when used for a surgical case. While most patient accounting systems do provide for tracking depletion of inventory by case in conjunction with the preference card utility discussed previously, using this for all supplies is typically not practical given the low dollar cost of routine supplies used in essentially all surgeries. The most simplistic approach to addressing this challenge is to record initial supply purchases to inventory and then expense any subsequent replenishment. However, this approach does not correctly reflect increases in inventory as volumes increase, nor properly account for more expensive supplies used in certain cases.

A hybrid approach is to expense routine supplies as purchased and track certain items such as implants or unique physician-requested items through inventory. Another, slightly more sophisticated, approach is to record all supply purchases to inventory and then record depletion of routine supplies on an average cost per case with implants or other specialty items expensed only as used. Regardless of the approach used to record inventory and expense supply costs, performing a physical count of supply items in inventory periodically is necessary in order to adjust the amount on the facility's balance sheet to reflect supplies actually on hand and to insure that any expired or damaged items are disposed of and recorded as expense. A complete count should be conducted at least annually with more frequent (quarterly if not monthly) counts of items more prone to waste as well as individually expensive items.

Significant monthly fluctuations in the amount of inventory reflected on the facility's balance sheet would indicate that the approach used for expensing supplies is not properly matching the expense with the revenue being generated by cases performed each month, which could yield misleading income statement results.

Accounts Payable

Managing which bills are paid when can be a stressful aspect of managing the surgery center's business operations, particularly during the start-up phase. Entering invoices into the center's accounting system on a timely basis will insure that there is an accurate record of amounts payable and will facilitate use of the tools and reports provided by the system to manage payments effectively. Similar to the accounts receivable aging reports provided by the patient accounting system, the accounts payable module should provide an aging report of invoices and other items that are payable. Efficient use of the center's available cash will require balancing payment of invoices promptly enough so as not to jeopardize the center's credit history with the desire to maintain, and ultimately distribute, the center's cash.

Cash Distributions

At the most basic level, the financial goal of the center will be to distribute sufficient cash to provide an attractive rate of return to the investors. Once the center begins collecting revenue from cases performed, there will probably be pressure from some of the investors to begin distributions quickly and, on an ongoing basis, pressure to keep those distributions as high as possible. However, commencing distributions too quickly or being overly aggressive with the amounts being distributed can lead to significant issues, including jeopardizing the facility's credit rating if it is unable to pay bills timely. Accordingly, the approach to determining reasonable distribution levels should be one that is fully vetted with the center's governing board, preferably with input from a financially disinterested business expert, probably either the center's outside accountant or a representative of the third-party management company. As a rule of thumb, once a facility has achieved somewhat stable volume levels, a minimum of 2 weeks' routine operating expenses should be maintained when making a cash distribution. Other considerations should include upcoming debt payments or other nonrecurring obligations as well as any potential cash reserves for new equipment purchases.

Satisfaction Surveys

Monitoring and measuring the satisfaction levels of the center's "customers" will provide the management team and governing board with an assessment of how the center is perceived. The key groups to be surveyed include physicians, patients, and employees. Including a mix of questions or statements requiring objective responses or rankings with opportunities to provide narrative commentary provides the most actionable survey results. Maintaining some level of consistency in the survey items will facilitate tracking of results over time and evaluation of progress toward meeting and exceeding the expectations of all the constituent groups who will ultimately determine the long-term success of the surgery center.

References

1. R. D. Miller, L. I. Eriksson, L. A. Fleisher, J. P. Wiener-Kronish, W. L. Young. *Miller's Anesthesia*, 7th edn. New York: McGraw-Hill, 2008.

2. S. Springman. *Ambulatory Anesthesia: The Requisites in Anesthesiology*. New York: Mosby, 2006.

3. R. Frey. Ambulatory surgery centers. *Gale Encyclopedia of Surgery: A Guide for Patients and Caregivers*. 2004. www.encyclopedia.com/doc/1G2–3406200021.html (accessed May 10, 2012).

4. P. G. Barash, B. F. Cullen, R. K. Stoelting, M. Cahalan, M. C. Stock. *Clinical Anesthesia*, 6th edn. Baltimore, MD: Lippincott Williams & Wilkins, 2009.

5. C. Jahnle, K. A. Rebane. Ambulatory surgery centers – Fragmented industry poised for consolidation. *Ambulatory Surgery Center Business Review*. Winter 2003.

6.   Ambulatory Surgery Center Association. Ambulatory surgery centers: A positive trend in health care. www .ascassociation.org/advancingsurgicalcare/aboutascs/ industryoverview/apositivetrendinhealthcare/ (accessed November 30, 2016).

7.   Medicare Payment Advisory Commission. A data book: Healthcare spending and the Medicare program. June 2016. www.medpac.gov/docs/default-source/data-book/june-2016-data-book-health-care-spending-and-the-medicare-program.pdf (accessed December 1, 2016).

Chapter

13

Influence of Patient- and Procedure-Specific Factors on Operating Room Efficiency and Decision Making

Markus M. Luedi, Thomas J. Sieber, and Dietrich Doll

Contents

Beyond providing patient safety and surgeon access to scheduled operating room (OR) time, a goal of efficient OR management must be the reduction of overutilized OR time, that is to say, reducing the positive difference between total hours of cases performed (including turnover times) and the allocated OR time per surgical list [1]. The glossary of the Association of Anesthesia Clinical Directors defines turnover time as the "time from prior patient out of room to succeeding patient in room time for sequentially scheduled cases" or "any time when they [the surgeons] are unable to operate . . . thus . . . the time between the end of surgery on one case and the beginning of surgery on the next case" (Figure 13.1) [2]. We will use the term turnover time to mean the interval from when a procedure is completed until the next procedure begins – the procedure/surgery finish (PF) to procedure/surgery start time (PST) interval in Figure 13.1, as this term is more commonly applied in Europe.

Whereas anesthesiologists have focused on technical improvements and patient safety for almost a century, analysis of the influence of patient- and procedure-specific factors on OR efficiency and decision making is relatively recent. We discuss these OR leadership aspects in this chapter.

Patient-Specific Issues for OR Efficiency and Decision Making

Anesthesiologists often can reasonably predict the time that will be needed to prepare a patient, and

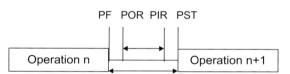

Figure 13.1 Definitions of turnover time according to the Association of Anesthesia Clinical Directors. Procedure/surgery finish (PF): "Time when . . . the physician/surgeons have completed all procedure-related activities on the patient." Patient out of room (POR): "Time at which patient leaves OR." Patient in room (PIR): "Time when patient enters the OR." Procedure/surgery start time (PST): "Time the procedure is begun." Here, we use the broader interval, PF to PST, to refer to turnover time. Adapted from [3].

thus, optimize turnover time [4]. However, it can be difficult to accurately predict induction times in elderly, high-risk patients. Given ongoing demographic changes with an ever increasing share of elderly, high-risk patients, age and ASA physical status have become important considerations for OR leadership and management.

Evidence derived from linear and generalized linear multivariate techniques suggests that patient age and ASA physical status are useful parameters for predicting key figures such as the 50th and 95th percentiles of median turnover times. The 95th percentile is used, e.g., if OR leadership wants to minimize turnover times at any costs, whereas the 50th percentile is used when considering median data. The use of age- and ASA physical status–based turnover time tables (Tables 13.1 and 13.2) for OR scheduling

Table 13.1 50th Percentiles of Age- and ASA Physical Status–Dependent Median Turnover Times (min) of Trauma Surgery Cases in a German Hospital

Age	ASA 1, median [95% CI]	ASA 2, median [95% CI]	ASA 3, median [95% CI]	ASA 4, median [95% CI]
0–20	45.8 [43.8, 47.6]	50.1 [47.9, 58.6]	35.7 [not available]	52.7 [not available]
20–40	51.5 [47.1, 54.9]	49.1 [46.8, 53.5]	61.0 [not available]	not available
40–60	44.5 [41.4, 48.6]	48.2 [46.9, 49.6]	56.2 [49.6, 61.8]	61.9 [not available]
60–80	43.3 [31.8, 45.4]	50.1 [48.1, 52.1]	55.3 [53, 57.2]	69.2 [42.8, 75.9]
>80	82.35 [not available]	51.8 [48.3, 63.4]	59.3 [58, 62.3]	66.9 [57.5, 74.5]

The Association of Anesthesia Clinical Directors' second definition of turnover time is used (procedure finish to procedure start time (PF-PST): "any time when they [the surgeons] are unable to operate ... thus ... the time between the end of surgery on one case and the beginning of surgery on the next case." Adapted from [3].

Table 13.2 95th Percentiles of Age- and ASA Physical Status–Dependent Median Turnover Times (min) of Trauma Surgery Cases in a German Hospital

Age	ASA 1, median [95% CI]	ASA 2, median [95% CI]	ASA 3, median [95% CI]	ASA 4, median [95% CI]
0–20	79.6 [67.5, 84.6]	87.8 [69.2, 94.3]	37.1 [not available]	52.7 [not available]
20–40	87.8 [77.0, 91.4]	83.0 [73.9, 89.1]	82.6 [not available]	Not available
40–60	68.6 [58.1, 83.2]	77.7 [75, 81.4]	81.5 [69.6, 88.4]	66.4 [not available]
60–80	67.3 [44.2, 85.2]	82.8 [78.1, 86.2]	88.3 [82, 91.8]	83.3 [74.8, 88.9]
> 80	95.1 [not available]	80.5 [75.3, 87.5]	89.8 [84.6, 93.6]	90.0 [75.2, 92.6]

The Association of Anesthesia Clinical Directors' second definition of turnover time is used (PF-PST: "any time when they [the surgeons] are unable to operate ... thus ... the time between the end of surgery on one case and the beginning of surgery on the next case." Adapted from [3].

decisions was shown to enable improvements in the predictive accuracy, e.g., by 21 percent for trauma surgery cases in a German hospital. Such instruments allow OR leadership to schedule more accurately and, thus, to reduce overutilized OR time by optimizing allocation of patients to several ORs, to schedule overlapping induction rooms, and to improve logistics of prioritizing transportation of advanced age/high ASA physical status patients to the OR [3].

Such institution-specific OR management decision tables do not require advance estimation of any uncertain patient characteristics; both, age and ASA physical status are usually known well in advance of a scheduled case. However, OR turnover times are complex phenomena that depend on numerous other factors such as timely availability of staff, room cleaning, supervision ratio of anesthesia residents, time of day preparation of surgical instruments, etc. Age- and ASA physical status–related reduction of overutilized OR times also correlate with the number of add-on cases, the duration of the workday [5], and the specific surgical team because of heterogeneity

among specialties. A comprehensive inclusion of all contributing factors into a turnover time table is not realistic. However, it is appropriate and necessary to apply multivariate analytic techniques to develop strategies strategies for predicting turnover times. To operate efficiently, OR staff needs appropriate knowledge.

Given the evident demographic changes, hospital-specific age and ASA physical status tables for turnover times are useful for lists that include many short operations in geriatric cohorts in settings with overlapping induction rooms, or where ORs with differences in predicted over- and underutilization are available, or when transporters are scarce, e.g., in early mornings when all ORs are to be started [3].

List-Specific Considerations for OR Efficiency and Decision Making

Traditionally, the type of anesthesia and procedure, as well as the specific surgeon, are used to predict case durations. In a small case series, Dexter showed that systematically requesting an update for case duration from a surgeon did not improve OR management decision making in thoracic or spinal surgery [6]. However, more sophisticated approaches based on current evidence in different surgical arenas have proved useful.

In outpatient or day-care surgery, for example, it was shown that causes of unplanned hospital admission and prolonged stay were mainly related to surgical issues such as blood loss, longer than anticipated duration of the surgery, or intraoperative haemoglobin concentrations. However, unplanned hospital admission and prolonged stay were also caused by patient-dependent factors such as advanced age, female gender, postoperative nausea and vomiting, and postoperative pain scores, by anesthesiological factors such as the type of anesthesia (e.g., regional versus general), and by OR factors such as prolonged preoperative wait time [7].

In a study aimed at uncovering patient- and procedure-dependent factors influencing case time variability in pediatric surgery, Bravo et al. showed that pediatric surgeries, in contrast to adult surgeries, were characterized by a 'long-tailed' distribution, and often exhibited unpredictably long case duration [8]. Thus, unlike scheduling for adult lists, a scheduling approach personalized for individual surgeons or a "pooled" approach across surgeons was not helpful. They found that a regression tree improved predictions for very few procedures after excluding extreme cases, and turnover time for most procedure types remained unpredictable and independent of the surgeon. The authors recommended not using surgeon-specific scheduling. They concluded that "daily management of pediatric operating rooms will require compensatory overtime, capacity buffers, schedule flexibility" [8].

Anesthesia Technique-Specific Implications for OR Efficiency and Decision Making

In a meta-analysis of 26 clinical trials (1,874 patients) to determine whether regional anesthesia compared to general anesthesia decreased surgical time (a major determinant of variable OR costs) it was found that regional anesthesia did not significantly decrease surgical time [9].

However, in a comparison between settings with general anesthesia without induction rooms and settings with regional anesthesia and induction rooms, it was found that anesthesia-controlled times for outpatient anterior cruciate ligament reconstruction surgeries were significantly shorter in the latter setting [10]. A similar study in outpatients undergoing upper limb surgery found that the use of a "block room" to perform brachial plexus anesthesia reduced anesthesia-related OR time. In addition, brachial plexus anesthesia was shown to shorten recovery times [11].

In a prospective cost-effectiveness comparison between Desflurane and Isoflurane, Beaussier et al. found that, although Desflurane was significantly more expensive than isoflurane, postanesthesia care unit occupancy was significantly reduced, allowing admission of at least one additional patient. The gain was independent of duration of the surgery or of the time of day a patient was admitted to the postanesthesia care unit. The authors pointed out that "using new halogenated anesthetic agents with faster rates of elimination may outweigh the incremental cost" [12].

Organizational Issues on OR Efficiency and Decision Making

In an analysis of short-term optimization of first-case starts, service-specific staffing, case scheduling, and turnover, McIntosh et al. showed that productivity can be increased only moderately because existing workload and staffing are fixed properties. More important considerations were appropriate managerial decisions, such as appropriate OR allocations 2–3 months ahead of the day(s) of surgery [13]. Hospitals that treat emergency patients daily face the challenge of providing immediate resources for anesthesia and subsequent surgery. Almost by definition, an emergency case creates conflict potential in a daily OR routine. Thus, a procedural setting based on fair and rational priorities and processes is essential.

Case sequencing rules have a considerable impact on the peak of activity in post anesthesia care units. Intuitively, scheduling longest cases first might be a promising sequencing rule to minimize overutilized OR time and concomitant delays in admission to the post anesthesia care unit. However, using a discrete event simulation experiment that included a wide range of scenarios, Marcon et al. showed that scheduling longest cases first required more post anesthesia care unit staffing during, increased overutilized OR time, and resulted in more days – with at least one delay in post anesthesia care unit admission – thus, perhaps counterintuitively, scheduling longest cases first does not smooth the flow of patients entering the post anesthesia care unit [14].

In their milestone study on the numbers of emergency surgeries completed in a 7-h workday, Torkki et al. showed that anesthesia induction rooms can increase the number of operations per room. They found that, although mean surgery times did not change, nonoperative time decreased by >40 percent when anesthesia was induced in an induction room outside the OR [15].

Whereas the advantages of dedicated ORs for surgeons are well studied and understood, evidence regarding anesthesiology is only just emerging. In a retrospective case–control study, Roberts et al. assessed the impact of dedicated ORs for patients with femoral neck fractures. They found that overutilized OR time ("after-hour surgery") decreased significantly in a setting where dedicated orthopedic ORs were implemented. In addition, significantly fewer patients were admitted to intensive care postoperatively, and exhibited less postoperative mortality, stroke, infection, myocardial infarction, and heart failure [16].

Contrary to older studies, using a "quasi-experimental controlled time-series design" Van Veen-Berkx and colleagues showed that use of dedicated ORs in emergency surgery reduced overutilized OR time ("overtime"), and was superior to use for emergency surgery of ORs where time was allocated within scheduled lists [17]. Heng et al. described similar results ("decreasing overruns in elective rooms"). Also, patients were discharged more than one day earlier (16.0 vs. 14.7 days; $p = 0.12$) following implementation of dedicated emergency ORs [18].

The duration of cardiac surgeries is highly variable, which poses a major challenge for OR leadership and management. In an effort to increase accuracy of forecasting operation times and to identify factors that impact operating theatre productivity in cardiac surgery, Lehtonen et al. simulated an operating theater with a linear regression model of operation times from 2,603 patients. They identified the type of operation and the head surgeon as factors that most influenced operation length. The strongest impact on OR efficiency was the availability of an induction room outside the operating theatre to reduce nonoperative time; whereas, improved forecasts of surgery time did not impact productivity [19]. These results, in conjunction with the German study on impact of age and ASA physical status on OR turnover time, suggest that efforts to reduce turnover times make the most sense for lists with many short operations in geriatric cohorts.

Summary

Provided that accurate patient-, procedure-, and hospital-specific data are available, any institution can use specific multivariate technique modeling with patient- and procedure-specific factors to minimize turnover times. The gain is a reduction in overutilized OR times of surgical lists. Using these approaches, OR leadership specifically has an opportunity to reduce turnover times in lists with many short operations in geriatric cohorts. However, tactical decisions such as selectively expanding OR resources for specific surgeons are likely to have more impact.

Sophisticated tools are emerging that promise to allow optimization of OR efficiency and decision making based on list-specific considerations. Current evidence indicates that specific, separate consideration must be given to inpatient and outpatient lists and to adult and pediatric lists. Putatively more expensive measures such as the establishment of anesthesia induction rooms, list-specific ORs, shorter acting volatile anesthetics, or regional anesthetic approaches might turn out to increase efficiency, and thus, be cost-effective.

Specific managerial efforts always have to be addressed within the entire context of OR leadership and management, and should include factors such as improving personal accountability, streamlining procedures, and fostering interdisciplinary teamwork.

References

1. Dexter F, Epstein RH, Traub RD, et al. Making management decisions on the day of surgery based on operating room efficiency and patient waiting times. *Anesthesiology* 2004; 101: 1444–53.

2. Glossary of times used for scheduling and monitoring of diagnostic and therapeutic procedures. *AORN J* 1997; 66: 601–6.

3. Luedi MM, Kauf P, Mulks L, et al. Implications of patient age and ASA physical status for operating room management decisions. *Anesth Analg* 2016; 122: 1169–77.

4. Escobar A, Davis EA, Ehrenwerth J, et al. Task analysis of the preincision surgical period: An independent observer-based study of 1558 cases. *Anesth Analg* 2006; 103: 922–7.

5. Doll D, Wieferich K, Erhart T, et al. Waiting for Godot: An analysis of 2622 operating room turnover times. *Eur J Anaesthesiol* 2014; 31: 388–9.

6. Dexter EU, Dexter F, Masursky D, et al. Prospective trial of thoracic and spine surgeons' updating of their estimated case durations at the start of cases. *Anesth Analg* 2010; 110: 1164–8.

7. Junger A, Klasen J, Benson M, et al. Factors determining length of stay of surgical day-case patients. *Eur J Anaesthesiol* 2001; 18: 314–21.

8. Bravo F, Levi R, Ferrari LR, et al. The nature and sources of variability in pediatric surgical case duration. *Paediatr Anaesth* 2015; 25: 999–1006.

9. Dexter F. Regional anesthesia does not significantly change surgical time versus general anesthesia – A meta-analysis of randomized studies. *Reg Anesth Pain Med* 1998; 23: 439–43.

10. Williams BA, Kentor ML, Williams JP, et al. Process analysis in outpatient knee surgery: Effects of regional and general anesthesia on anesthesia-controlled time. *Anesthesiology* 2000; 93: 529–38.

11. Armstrong KP, Cherry RA. Brachial plexus anesthesia compared to general anesthesia when a block room is available. *Can J Anaesth* 2004; 51: 41–4.

12. Beaussier M, Decorps A, Tilleul P, et al. Desflurane improves the throughput of patients in the PACU. A cost-effectiveness comparison with isoflurane. *Can J Anaesth* 2002; 49: 339–46.

13. McIntosh C, Dexter F, Epstein RH. The impact of service-specific staffing, case scheduling, turnovers, and first-case starts on anesthesia group and operating room productivity: A tutorial using data from an Australian hospital. *Anesth Analg* 2006; 103: 1499–516.

14. Marcon E, Dexter F. Impact of surgical sequencing on post anesthesia care unit staffing. *Health Care Manag Sci* 2006; 9: 87–98.

15. Torkki PM, Marjamaa RA, Torkki MI, et al. Use of anesthesia induction rooms can increase the number of urgent orthopedic cases completed within 7 hours. *Anesthesiology* 2005; 103: 401–5.

16. Roberts TT, Vanushkina M, Khasnavis S, et al. Dedicated orthopaedic operating rooms: Beneficial to patients and providers alike. *J Orthop Trauma* 2015; 29: e18–23.

17. van Veen-Berkx E, Elkhuizen SG, Kuijper B, et al. Dedicated operating room for emergency surgery generates more utilization, less overtime, and less cancellations. *Am J Surg* 2016; 211: 122–8.

18. Heng M, Wright JG. Dedicated operating room for emergency surgery improves access and efficiency. *Can J Surg* 2013; 56: 167–74.

19. Lehtonen JM, Kujala J, Kouri J, et al. Cardiac surgery productivity and throughput improvements. *Int J Health Care Qual Assur* 2007; 20: 40–52.

Chapter

14

Operating Room Management in the Perioperative Surgical Home and Other Future Care Models

Juhan Paiste, John Schlitt, and Thomas R. Vetter

Introduction

The Perioperative Surgical Home (PSH) seeks to remedy present widely fragmented and overly costly perioperative care in the United States [1–4]. The PSH relies upon rigorous process standardization, evidence-based best practices, as well as robust coordination and integration of care. Shared decision making among the patient and all providers is emphasized. Its highly patient-centered approach guides the patient and their family members through the complexities of the perioperative "journey" – especially during transitions of care – along the entire continuum from the decision for surgery to the postdischarge phase (Figure 14.1) [4–6].

As this new patient care model continues to be defined and implemented, there will be many successful variants of the PSH, predicated on the local infrastructure, resources, internal/external forces, and the degree of collaboration among its many institutional stakeholders [1, 7]. Furthermore, a successful PSH model is not be a static entity but undergoes continuous evolution, with an attendant incremental expansion of specific services and scope [8].

An integrated care pathway is a structured multidisciplinary care plan that details the essential steps in the care of all patients with a particular clinical problem or undergoing a specific procedure [9]. "The aim of [an integrated] care pathway is to enhance the quality of care across the continuum by improving risk-adjusted patient outcomes, promoting patient safety, increasing patient satisfaction, and optimizing the use of resources" [10].

The growing number of Enhanced Recovery After Surgery protocols [11], the Bundled Payments for Care

Improvement [12], and Comprehensive Care for Joint Replacement [13] programs promulgated by the US Centers for Medicare and Medicaid Services' (CMS) Innovation Center, and other surgical procedure-specific integrated care pathways are the fundamental building blocks and operational components of a PSH model (Figure 14.2).

After first defining value in perioperative care and summarizing the nascent but seismic value-based changes in healthcare reimbursement, this chapter will describe representative, practical performance improvement tools for operating room (OR) management and tangible examples of optimizing value in OR management. Lastly, attention will be specifically focused on the increasing use and even further expanded role of the ambulatory surgery center (ASC) within the PSH model.

Definition of Value in Perioperative Care

Leading health economist Michael Porter has posed the central question, "What is value in healthcare?" and defined it as the ratio of health outcomes achieved per dollar spent [14]. This simple quotient can be expanded to include several specific outcome domains in its numerator [15]:

- Value = [quality + safety + (patient and provider satisfaction)] ÷ [cost]

The combination of expanded health insurance coverage under the 2010 Patient Protection and Affordable Care Act, more robust economic and job growth, the increased prevalence of chronic medical

THE PATIENT'S PERIOPERATIVE JOURNEY

← INTEGRATED TRANSITIONS OF CARE ACROSS PERIOPERATIVE CONTINUUM →

PHASE OF CARE	PRE-OPERATIVE	INTRA-OPERATIVE	POST-OPERATIVE	POST-DISCHARGE	
POINT OF CARE	SURGICAL CLINIC PREOPERATIVE ASSESSMENT, CONSULTATION & TREATMENT CLINIC	SAME DAY SURGERY OPERATING ROOM POST-ANESTHESIA CARE UNIT	INTENSIVE CARE UNIT AND/OR ROUTINE INPATIENT UNIT	INPATIENT REHABILITATION AND/OR SKILLED NURSING FACILITY	OUTPATIENT REHABILITATION AND/OR HOME HEALTH CARE
PATIENT'S PERSPECTIVE	DECIDING ON SURGERY ANTICIPATING SURGERY PREPARING FOR SURGERY	UNDERGOING MY PLANNED SURGERY	RECOVERING FROM MY PLANNED SURGERY		RETURNING TO MY NORMAL FUNCTION
LOCATION	HOME	HOSPITAL OR AMBULATORY SURGERY CENTER	NON-HOME		HOME
KEY COMPONENTS	MEDICAL OPTIMIZATION PREHABILITATION POST-DISCHARGE CARE PLANNING	← OPIOID-SPARING, MULTIMODAL ANALGESIA → ← THERAPEUTIC AND FUNCTIONAL ACTIVITY GOALS → ← FORMAL TRANSITIONAL CARE MANAGEMENT →			

Figure 14.1 The patient's journey across the entire perioperative continuum.

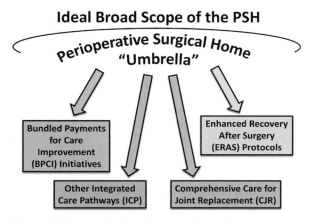

Figure 14.2 The optimal broad scope of the PSH.

conditions, and an aging population are expected to result in a continued greater demand for healthcare goods and services in the United States [16]. It is anticipated that by 2023, a projected 19.3 percent of the US gross domestic product will be spent on healthcare [17]. Between 2010 and 2014, the number of surgical admissions in the United States decreased from 18 to 13 admissions per 1,000 individuals [18]. Nevertheless, surgical procedural care currently accounts for nearly half of all inpatient hospitalization expenses in the United States [19]. Fragmentation and inefficiency in surgical care delivery, defensive medicine, discordant incentives between stakeholders who deliver versus who pay for this care, and a lack of emphasis on delivering *value* are contributing to excessive surgical expenditures [20, 21].

Rather than continuing to reward volume regardless of quality of delivered care, the US Department of Health and Human Services intends to increase the proportion of Medicare value-based purchasing from 30 percent at the end of 2016 to 50 percent by the end of 2018 [22]. The Medicare Access and CHIP Reauthorization Act (MACRA) of 2015 [23] was yet another major shift in payment toward value that has direct perioperative implications [3]. MACRA has established policies to transform physician payments from a system that rewards volume to one that recognizes value. The Merit-Based Incentive Payment System allows clinicians to continue to be reimbursed under traditional fee-for-service, but with their payments annually adjusted – upward or downward – based on their performance on several domains, including clinical quality, use of health information technology, resource utilization, and clinical practice improvement activities [3]. The Advanced Alternative Payment Model is intended for clinicians who elect to participate in alternative practice models and are willing to accept significant shared financial risk for the quality and effectiveness of their patient care [23].

Created in 2015, the Health Care Transformation Task Force (http://hcttf.org/) is an industry consortium that has brought together patients, providers, payers, and purchasers, from both the private and public sectors in the United States, to transform provider and hospital reimbursement from the traditional, volume-based, fee-for-service contracts instead to predominately linked to value-based care [24]. This task force is committed to shifting 75 percent of nongovernmental healthcare payments to value-based arrangements (i.e., contracts) by 2020 [24].

Such fundamental changes in payment models collectively represent a "burning platform" that will necessitate an equally fundamental change in perioperative care delivery models in the United States [15].

Achieving Optimal Value in OR Management

Surgical care generates substantial revenue for hospitals, but it is also one of the largest drivers of cost within the hospital [25]. The healthcare reform mandate to cut costs, while simultaneously providing care to millions of previously uninsured Americans, will significantly affect hospital ORs and surgical services.

As hospitals face a range of mounting financial pressures and their operating margins (profits) are decreasing, it is vitally important to understand the profitability of surgical cases, which is measured by the contribution margin. The contribution margin is revenue minus variable costs and is typically between $1,000 and $2,000 per OR hour [26]. Naturally, this

contribution margin materializes only during actual surgical procedure time. The OR profit (surplus) is defined as revenue minus fixed cost (maintenance of facilities, information systems, OR apparatus, etc.) and variable cost (salaries, implants, disposable supplies, medications, etc.). Variable cost usually is less than half of fixed cost [25].

Despite the OR being such a mainstay for hospitals' profitability, there are little published, formal data on true OR costs, as there are far too many variables to accurately determine how much one minute of OR time costs [27]. Hospital administrators tend to use a ballpark estimate of $15–20 per OR minute cost for a basic surgical procedure and potentially more for higher complexity cases. This cost estimate is calculated by dividing all OR expenses (salary and benefits, supplies, drugs, services, depreciation) by the total number of OR hours available for surgical cases [28]. Although OR costs and potential profits are subject to many variables, one thing is certain: time is the most valuable OR resource.

Requisite effective organization and successful operation of perioperative services in turn require clearly defined governance structure, accountable leadership and representation by all stakeholders: namely, surgeons, anesthesiologists, nursing, and administration. Tactical and strategic decisions made by the diverse OR leadership should be guided by earlier stated value proposition – to deliver the highest quality surgical care safely and efficiently with the lowest cost possible, and in an environment, that is satisfying for the patients and healthcare providers.

Numerous factors can constrain OR productivity and efficiency, including infrastructure, human resource management, case scheduling variation, process and work flow, as well as technology and information management limitations [29]. The manufacturing industry has developed and implemented several techniques to manage their processes and to maximize efficiency. LEAN and Six Sigma are two such methodologies that can be used at both the work unit and organizational level. LEAN is a process that continually reduces waste and improves workflow to efficiently produce a product or service that is perceived to be of high value to those who use it [30]. Six Sigma is an alternate method to reduce process variation through the rigorous application of process metrics collection and statistical analysis. Increased efficiency results in enhanced productivity, decreased personnel costs, reduced waste, and increased financial performance [31].

The first step in any perioperative process improvement effort is to develop a value stream map of patient flow that details the event location, personnel needs, and information technology requirements, alternative pathways, key performance elements at each step, and potential bottlenecks. Once a detailed value steam map is developed, multidisciplinary teams are tasked to redesign workflow based on LEAN and/or Six Sigma methodologies.

Addressing the following areas in the perioperative patient care continuum may yield significant improvement opportunities: (1) streamlining and standardizing the preoperative case scheduling and patient clinical evaluation and testing processes; (2) designing surgical case scheduling processes that support improved OR utilization through decreased underuse and overuse of OR resources (decreased surgical volume variation); (3) reducing OR nonoperative time by improving efficiency of nonoperative processes (e.g., patient transport time, OR turnover/cleaning time); (4) standardizing processes to capture, enter and report required patient information; and (5) improving employee engagement and teamwork among and across all surgical service constituents [32].

Increasing Use and Expanded Role of the ASC in the PSH Model

Over the last 30 years, advances in surgery, anesthesia, and analgesia have made it possible to discharge patients home the same day as a surgical procedure. As a result of these clinical advances, as well as the introduction of the Medicare inpatient prospective payment system, there has been a tremendous increase in the number of outpatient surgeries performed nationwide [33]Between 1981 and 2005, the number of outpatient surgeries performed has grown almost tenfold, from 3.7 million to almost 32 million annually. In 2014, outpatient procedures represent over 60 percent of all surgeries performed [34].

In light of these significant procedural volumes and based upon the 2010 (and still current) Affordable Care Act, it is important to understand the role that the ASC can play in the PSH model and the value-based healthcare equation.

In order to fully appreciate the current and potential role of the ASC, one must first understand the definition of an ASC. An ASC is a freestanding facility, not associated with a hospital. This differs significantly from a hospital outpatient department (HOPD), which is 100 percent owned by the hospital and is reimbursed at a different rate by the CMS. There are significant differences between an ASC and an HOPD (Table 14.1).

It would seem apparent that an ASC would be a significantly less expensive alternative to the HOPD for outpatient surgery. This is supported by existing literature that shows that common outpatient procedures like cataracts and endoscopy procedures can be performed at up to 50 percent less cost in an ASC versus an HOPD. Furthermore, patient expenses, represented by the copayment to the facility, can be more than 50 percent lower at an ASC when compared to an HOPD [35].

However, in today's medical environment there has been a recent trend towards conversion of ASCs to HOPDs [36]. This is due to the widening gap between reimbursements for surgical cases at these two different types of facilities. The Medicare Prescription Drug, Improvement, and Modernization Act of 2003 froze ASC payment updates. Furthermore, between 2008 and 2012 Medicare phased in a new system for ASC payments based on the outpatient prospective payment system. The rates were set so that for any outpatient procedure, payment to an ASC would be no more than 59 percent of payment made to a hospital, phased in fully by 2012 [37]. This potentially limits the ability of an ASC to put the resources in place to develop a sustainable PSH model.

When one examines the value-based equation – basically the ratio of quality divided by cost – this above reimbursement trend seems to decrease the intrinsic value of outpatient care. The question then becomes: How can we utilize the ASC to increase the value provided for outpatient surgery?

A simple answer to this key question would be to move a significant number of procedures being done in an HOPD to an ASC setting. However, this answer is not as simple as it seems. Opponents of this strategy will claim that an ASC is only equipped to handle the noncomplex medical patient. Furthermore, they will claim that an HOPD provides a superior level of care to the complex medical patient. Interestingly, some studies indicate that the highest-risk Medicare patients were less likely to visit an emergency department or to be admitted to a hospital following outpatient

Table 14.1 Characteristics of an ASC versus a HOPD

	ASC	HOPD
Reimbursement	On average receives 56% of amount paid to an HOPD and cannot be more than 59% of that paid to an HOPD	Higher reimbursement for comparable services
Surgical procedures	No CMS-defined "inpatient procedures" are permitted to be performed	100% of all procedures can be performed
Planned overnight stays	Not allowed	Allowed
Ownership and control	Can be owned by physicians	Must be wholly owned by the hospital. Hospital has all operational responsibility
Licensure and operations	Can be independently licensed and operated	Must be operated under same license as hospital
Clinical and financial integration	May work with physicians who do not have hospital privileges.	All staff must have hospital privileges. Must share income and expenses with hospital
Location	Able to be freestanding in any location	Must be within 250 yards of hospital main campus, or within 35 mile radius with satisfaction of additional requirements
Public awareness	No specific requirements	Patients must be made aware that they are in a hospital setting and will be billed accordingly

surgery if they were treated in an ASC, regardless of medical complexity [37]. There is also evidence that procedures take on average 31.8 fewer minutes at an ASC [37]. These data speak to the ability of an ASC to be convenient and efficient for both patients and providers.

The current CMS regulation on extended recovery in an ASC setting is another major limitation of the strategy to shift procedures to an ASC. CMS clearly states that in order to maintain CMS certification, an ASC should have no planned overnight stays [38]. Furthermore, CMS has a defined list of "inpatient procedures" and "outpatient procedures." Medicare patients currently cannot undergo any inpatient procedures at an ASC, regardless of their overall medical condition [38]. With the development of the PSH, especially its protocols and pathways for patient optimization, there is an enormous opportunity to perform more complex surgical procedures in an ASC setting [39]. However, some of these surgeries will require an outpatient designation and at least one overnight stay.

In order to expand the role of the ASC in the PSH model, a new approach must be considered. First, CMS must consider increasing ASC reimbursement. There should be a requirement that this will occur only if the same quality thresholds are met in the ASC setting versus the hospital setting. This increase in reimbursement will allow the ASC to put resources in place to adopt and to execute the PSH model, which is a keystone in maximizing the value equation. Furthermore, as CMS continues to be at the forefront of value-based innovation, as evidenced by its bundled payment initiatives, it will be necessary to afford an ASC the opportunity to provide extended recovery to include at least one overnight stay.

ASCs play a critical role in the healthcare system. They are efficient, quality, low cost alternatives to hospital-based care. In order to increase their use and expand their role in the PSH model, pivotal changes to the current CMS environment need to be considered.

Conclusion

The PSH concept has generated ample, thoughtful, yet at times spirited dialogue in the US anesthesiology community and literature [1–6, 16, 40–42]. It remains to be seen if the PSH is a prescient and sustainable redesign – or a quixotic notion that will ultimately crumble under the weight of its overly ambitious scope and attendant major "ask" and "lift" (in management speak). Nevertheless, advocates and skeptics of the PSH presumably agree upon the continued vital role of anesthesiologists in successful OR management. Furthermore, anesthesiologists have demonstrated expertise in risk assessment and quality improvement. They are thus well positioned to serve as leaders in any perioperative care environment and model of the future [43].

References

1. Kain ZN, Vakharia S, Garson L, et al. The perioperative surgical home as a future perioperative practice model. *Anesth Analg.* 2014;118(5):1126–30.

2. Vetter TR, Boudreaux AM, Jones KA, Hunter JM, Jr., Pittet JF. The perioperative surgical home: How anesthesiology can collaboratively achieve and leverage the triple aim in health care. *Anesth Analg.* 2014;118(5):1131–6.

3. Schweitzer M, Vetter TR. The perioperative surgical home: More than smoke and mirrors? *Anesth Analg.* 2016;123(3):524–8.

4. Cannesson M, Kain Z. The perioperative surgical home: An innovative clinical care delivery model. *J Clin Anesth.* 2015;27(3):185–7.

5. Vetter TR, Goeddel LA, Boudreaux AM, Hunt TR, Jones KA, Pittet JF. The perioperative surgical home: How can it make the case so everyone wins? *BMC Anesthesiology.* 2013;13:6.

6. Goeddel LA, Porterfield JR, Jr., Hall JD, Vetter TR. Ethical opportunities with the perioperative surgical home: Disruptive innovation, patient-centered care, shared decision making, health literacy, and futility of care. *Anesth Analg.* 2015;120(5):1158–62.

7. Vetter TR, Ivankova NV, Goeddel LA, McGwin G, Jr., Pittet JF. An analysis of methodologies that can be used to validate if a perioperative surgical home improves the patient-centeredness, evidence-based practice, quality, safety, and value of patient care. *Anesthesiology.* 2013;119(6):1261–74.

8. Vetter TR, Barman J, Hunter JM, Jr., Jones KA, Pittet JF. The effect of implementation of preoperative and postoperative care elements of a perioperative surgical home model on outcomes in patients undergoing hip arthroplasty or knee arthroplasty. *Anesth Analg.* 2016.

9. Kinsman L, Rotter T, James E, Snow P, Willis J. What is a clinical pathway? Development of a definition to inform the debate. *BMC Med.* 2010;8:31.

10. Schrijvers G, van Hoorn A, Huiskes N. The care pathway: Concepts and theories: An introduction. *Int J Integr Care.* 2012;12:e192.

11. Ljungqvist O. Sustainability after structured implementation of ERAS protocols. *World J Surg.* 2015;39(2):534–5.

12. Press MJ, Rajkumar R, Conway PH. Medicare's new bundled payments: Design, strategy, and evolution. *JAMA.* 2016;315(2):131–2.

13. Center for Medicare & Medicaid Services. Medicare program: Comprehensive care for joint replacement payment model for acute care hospitals furnishing lower extremity joint replacement services. Final rule. *Fed Regist.* 2015;80(226):73273–554.

14. Porter ME. What is value in health care? *N Engl J Med.* 2010;363(26):2477–81.

15. Vetter TR, Jones KA. Perioperative surgical home: Perspective II. *Anesthesiol Clin.* 2015;33(4):771–84.

16. Vetter TR, Pittet JF. The perioperative surgical home: A panacea or Pandora's box for the specialty of anesthesiology? *Anesth Analg.* 2015;120(5):968–73.

17. Sisko AM, Keehan SP, Cuckler GA, et al. National health expenditure projections, 2013–23: Faster growth expected with expanded coverage and improving economy. *Health Aff (Millwood).* 2014;33(10):1841–50.

18. Health Care Cost Institute. Health care cost and utlization report 2015. December 12, 2016. www .healthcostinstitute.org/wp-content/uploads/2015/10/ 2014-HCCUR-10.29.15.pdf.

19. Weiss AJ, Elixhauser A, Andrews RM. Characteristics of operating room procedures in U.S. hospitals, 2011. Statistical Brief #170. 2014.

20. Cormier JN, Cromwell KD, Pollock RE. Value-based health care: A surgical oncologist's perspective. *Surg Oncol Clin N Am.* 2012;21(3):497–506.

21. Fry DE, Pine M, Jones BL, Meimban RJ. The impact of ineffective and inefficient care on the excess costs of elective surgical procedures. *JACS.* 2011;212(5):779–86.

22. Burwell SM. Setting value-based payment goals – HHS efforts to improve U.S. health care. *N Engl J Med.* 2015;372(10):897–9.

23. Clough JD, McClellan M. Implementing MACRA: Implications for physicians and for physician leadership. *JAMA.* 2016;315(22):2397–8.

24. Health Care Transformation Task Force. *Major health care players unite to accelerate transformation of the U.S. health care system.* Washington, DC: Qorvis MSLGROUP, 2015. http://hcttf.org/releases/2015/ 1/28/major-health-care-players-unite-to-accelerate-transformation-of-us-health-care-system.

25. Macario A, Vitez TS, Dunn B, McDonald T. Where are the costs in perioperative care? Analysis of hospital costs and charges for inpatient surgical care. *Anesthesiology.* 1995;83(6):1138–44.

26. Macario A. Are your hospital operating rooms "efficient"? A scoring system with eight performance indicators. *Anesthesiology.* 2006;105(2):237–40.

27. Macario A. What does one minute of operating room time cost? *J Clin Anesth.* 2010;22(4):233–6.

28. Park KW, Dickerson C. Can efficient supply management in the operating room save millions? *Curr Opin Anaesthesiol.* 2009;22(2):242–8.

29. Harders M, Malangoni MA, Weight S, Sidhu T. Improving operating room efficiency through

process redesign. *Surgery*. 2006;140(4):509–14; discussion 14–6.

30. Schweikhart SA, Dembe AE. The applicability of Lean and Six Sigma techniques to clinical and translational research. *J Investig Med*. 2009;57(7):748–55.

31. McDaniel RR, Jr., Lanham HJ. Evidence as a tool for managerial action: A complex adaptive systems view. *Health Care Manage Rev*. 2009;34(3):216–8.

32. Cima RR, Brown MJ, Hebl JR, et al. Use of Lean and Six Sigma methodology to improve operating room efficiency in a high-volume tertiary-care academic medical center. *J Am Coll Surg*. 2011;213(1):83–92; discussion 3–4.

33. Leader S, Moon M. Medicare trends in ambulatory surgery. *Health Aff (Millwood)*. 1989;8(1):158–70.

34. *Chartbook 2016: Trends affecting hospitals and health systems*. Washington, DC: American Hospital Association. www.aha.org/research/reports/tw/chartbook/2016/tableofcontents.pdf (accessed January 31, 2107).

35. Ambulatory Surgery Center Association. Ambulatory surgery centers: A positive trend in health care 2012. www.ascassociation.org/communities/community-home/librarydocuments/viewdocument?DocumentKey=7d8441a1-82dd-47b9-b626-8563dc31930c.

36. Szabad M, Freerks M, Bushee MM. Reverse migration? A trend of ASC conversion to HOPD2013. www.mcguirewoods.com/news-resources/publications/health_care/reverse-migration-whitepaper.pdf.

37. Munnich EL, Parente ST. Procedures take less time at ambulatory surgery centers, keeping costs down and ability to meet demand up. *Health Aff (Millwood)*. 2014;33(5):764–9.

38. Centers for Medicare and Medicaid Services. 42 CFR Part 416: Medicare Program; Update of Ambulatory Surgical Center List of Covered Procedures; Interim Final Rule. www.cms.gov/Medicare/Medicare-Fee-for-Service-Payment/ASCPayment/downloads/1478-ifc.pdf.

39. Erhun F, Malcolm E, Kalani M, et al. Opportunities to improve the value of outpatient surgical care. *Am J Manag Care*. 2016;22(9):e329–35.

40. Prielipp RC, Morell RC, Coursin DB, et al. The future of anesthesiology: Should the perioperative surgical home redefine us? *Anesth Analg*. 2015;120(5):1142–8.

41. Warner MA, Apfelbaum JL. The perioperative surgical home: A response to a presumed burning platform or a thoughtful expansion of anesthesiology? *Anesth Analg*. 2015;120(5):1149–51.

42. Kain ZN, Hwang J, Warner MA. Disruptive innovation and the specialty of anesthesiology: The case for the perioperative surgical home. *Anesth Analg*. 2015;120(5):1155–7.

43. Holt NF. Trends in healthcare and the role of the anesthesiologist in the perioperative surgical home – The US perspective. *Curr Opin Anaesthesiol*. 2014;27(3):371–6.

Chapter

15

Non-Operating Room Locations

John M. Trummel, Brenda A. Gentz, and William R. Furman

Contents

Introduction

The term NORA is an acronym for non–operating room anesthesia. It refers to the practice of anesthetic care in any location other than an operating room (OR) or obstetrical suite and is sometimes called "offsite anesthesia." Providing anesthetic care in a NORA setting poses unique clinical and management challenges. Many of these are well known to anesthesia providers. A unique operational aspect of the NORA environment can be a relatively high volume of brief procedures and the rapid turnover time, especially in endoscopy suites and pediatric procedure areas. The location may be at a considerable distance from skilled assistance and the anesthesia personnel may be relatively unfamiliar with the facility and the location of critical equipment. In addition, nonsurgical proceduralists and their staff may be unaccustomed to, or even dismissive of, important anesthesia and safety processes. This may lead to conflicts over clinical care priorities in the pre-, intra-, and postprocedural periods. Nonsurgical proceduralists and their staff may also be unacquainted with basic elements of perioperative business management. These include efficient scheduling, standard preprocedural and preanesthetic evaluation, postprocedural recovery and discharge processes, communication with administrative staff from other departments, different and possibly competing staffing models, requirements

for billing of anesthesia services, and the principles of procedural quality and safety. Mismanagement of offsite anesthesia can adversely impact efficiency and the ability of a department to offer these services.

The goal of this chapter is to address management problems common to anesthesia care outside the OR. The areas that tend to have the greatest clinical activity for most practices are endoscopy, radiology and cardiac care, and these will be highlighted. Other areas where NORA services may be provided include the emergency department, intensive care units and pediatric units. The general principles and issues apply across all NORA sites.

Common Challenges

To effectively provide anesthesia in any NORA site, as indicated in Box 15.1, it is necessary to meet external regulatory requirements, develop a scheduling and administrative structure and approach, make decisions about preprocedural evaluation requirements, determine staffing models, define appropriate postanesthetic recovery care, bill and collect for services, and provide safety and quality oversight. In short, all the elements relevant to OR anesthesia pertain to each NORA location, but they usually must be developed separately from the OR as NORA tends to take place outside the structures and functions of conventional OR services.

The Regulatory Environment

Regulatory and professional standards that affect NORA practice are promulgated by both governmental and nongovernmental organizations (Box 15.2). Governmental regulatory bodies consist of national and local entities, such as the Centers for Medicare and Medicaid Services (CMS) and state departments of health, insurance, and justice. Nongovernmental agencies that exert jurisdiction over NORA care include The Joint Commission (TJC) and various professional medical specialty organizations, including the American Society of Anesthesiologists (ASA).

TJC plays a prominent role in defining care standards for anesthetic care provided both in and out of the OR. CMS often adopts TJC's standards when it writes conditions of participation relative to Medicare and Medicaid. TJC's International Accreditation Standards for Hospitals is a publication that defines standards for anesthesia and surgical care in hospitals worldwide.[1] It specifically states that its standards "are applicable in any setting in which anesthesia and/or procedural sedation are used, and surgical and other invasive procedures that require consent are performed." This includes "hospital operating theatres, day surgery and day hospital units, dental and other outpatient clinics, emergency services and intensive care areas" (in other words, all OR or NORA locations). Sedation and anesthesia services must "meet professional standards and applicable local and national standards, laws, and regulations." TJC puts emphasis on providing similar care, adhering to the same standard, to all patients throughout the entirety of a healthcare organization. When developing and approving specific institutional policies, it therefore is necessary to avoid significant care variation across anesthetizing settings.

Other organizations also have positions with respect to NORA care. The ASA has an important role in promulgating standards, guidelines and practice parameters and has published many of interest in the areas of qualifications to administer anesthesia, safety, pre- and postprocedural care and definitions of sedation. Several relevant statements and advisories are listed in Table 15.1. Other specialty organizations, including the four gastroenterology-related organizations listed in Box 15.2, publish opinions and guidelines on the topic of anesthesia, sedations, and periprocedural NORA care. The American Society for Gastrointestinal Endoscopy Standards of Practice Committee publishes its guidelines and standards of practice for proceduralists on the internet.[2]

Scheduling and Administration

The number of personnel needed by an anesthesiology department to manage the scheduling and administration of NORA services depends on the case volume. If this task is not integrated into the daily work of OR scheduling personnel, it will require one or more staff tasked with multiple administrative roles. If it is integrated into the daily work of the OR scheduling personnel, it will have the potential to consume a considerable amount of their time. For busy anesthesiology practices, a medical director for NORA services is often necessary. This is

---

[1] https://jointcommissioninternational.org/assets/3/7/Hospital-5E-Standards-Only-Mar2014.pdf (accessed 2 January, 2017).

[2] http://asge.org/publications/publications.aspx?id=352 (accessed January 2, 2017).

Table 15.1 ASA Statements and Advisories Relevant to NORA

Care	Pub Date
Statement on Nonoperating Room Anesthetizing Locations	Oct 2013
Advisory on Granting Privileges for Deep Sedation to Non-Anesthesiologist Sedation Practitioners	Oct 2010
Statement on Granting Privileges for Administration of Moderate Sedation to Practitioners Who Are Not Anesthesia Professionals	Oct 2011

an individual on the anesthesiology staff with a specific interest in NORA who acts as a liaison to multiple other departments, addressing both clinical care questions and administrative issues as they arise. Key personality characteristics for this role are a high level of patience and courtesy because of the need to interact with other physicians and staff who may not intuitively understand some of the basic vocabulary and expectations commonly shared by the people who work in the OR environment. Some conversations and explanations may need to be repeated frequently.

The primary duties of administrative staff are to ensure accurate scheduling and to deal with billing and staffing issues. Personnel in this role need to work closely with scheduling staff from other departments. It is helpful to have someone who can analyze data as well. These roles can be shared among several people or tasked to one person, depending on the level of workload on the NORA service and the skillset of staff members.

Efficient scheduling is one of the more difficult day-to-day administrative tasks in NORA because the anesthesia cases in a NORA site tend to be a subset of the total clinical work in that area. It may be helpful to have a specific person who routinely deals with NORA scheduling (both in the anesthesia department and in the requesting service) because there are significant nuances to the job that make it difficult to be done by someone unfamiliar with the role or by a different person each day. Relationship building across departments can make scheduling challenges easier to resolve.

There are several models for case scheduling. One traditional model has a central anesthesia scheduler make appointments and try to fill time in the daily schedule. In this model, the anesthesia assignment might be viewed as a virtual OR block with open scheduling for any service that requests it. The anesthesia scheduler is tasked with balancing and

organizing these requests. Unlike an actual OR, where the patients come to the anesthesia teams, in this model the anesthesia teams travel to the patients at the various procedural sites. Services requiring anesthesia must call to book cases and receive time assignments according to an open booking system. This model favors greater efficiency for the utilization of the anesthesia personnel's time but may be less efficient with respect to the utilization of the procedural site and its equipment. It typically is better suited to low volume settings and can become highly inefficient when individual specialties each have a large volume of cases.

As an example, suppose that the radiology department schedules one MRI with anesthesia in the middle of the day. If the anesthesia team is delayed arriving from a prior procedure at a different NORA site, this will lead to the magnet being unused during that delay. It may also result in further delays in the MRI schedule for the remainder the day. In addition, the anesthesia team will subsequently be late for any other NORA cases scheduled at other sites. This will cause underutilization of the anesthesia team and underutilization of resources at these other sites as well. If the total NORA demand for anesthesia is low, extra time can be built into the schedule to account for these delays, but as the volume increases, this model tends to become tightly coupled so that even a small delay will have an increasingly magnified effect on the schedule as the day progresses. Whether this model is preferable for a facility should be evaluated in terms of the overall impact on all service lines affected.

Economically, the example above may have limited effect on the anesthesia providers and may even be beneficial. In this model, the anesthesia team is mostly fully engaged when needed and there should be fewer days where a team is on duty but utilized only part of the day. While this is advantageous for the anesthesiology department, for other departments it is less efficient. In an aligned healthcare environment where the institution and the anesthesiology practice try not to suboptimize each other in order to achieve individual success, the additional anesthesia collections would have to be compared to the cost to the institution in terms of lost facility fee revenue from the decreased number of total MRIs performed each day. The financial impact of facility fees tends to be greater than that of anesthesia professional fees, so a decision that reduces the number MRIs performed might not be economically sound, even if it reduces anesthesia team underutilization. But if this type of delay merely forestalls the time of completion of the MRI schedule without diminishing the amount of revenue generated by the facility, the savings in anesthesia team labor cost (if any) should be compared to any savings in MRI suite labor and overtime (if any). As a result, when the facility is relatively underutilized, this traditional model may be most cost-effective. It also tends to have a more favorable impact on the anesthesia team members, who typically do not like to wait and may become irritated if they are delayed in an induction area with an anesthetized patient until a scanner room has been vacated by the previous patient.

A different scheduling option is to assign specific block times to individual services and require that they schedule their nonemergent cases in those blocks of time only. Offering individual services block time frequently allows easier scheduling for other clinical departments and can be very efficient if the time is highly utilized. For the anesthesia teams it reduces complexity because it means they are assigned to one area and work there all day, rather than traveling from one location to another. This allows the anesthesia team to spend most of their time providing clinical care and less of their time traveling for place to place and setting up in a new location. It can also reduce the amount of time spent by anesthesiology department staff on scheduling administration, however some control over case booking, specifically the control of time allocation, may be lost. In either model a specific administrative liaison in the anesthesiology department is usually necessary unless NORA volume is very low.

Block time scheduling is typically advantageous for high volume services, as is common in busy endoscopy suites and pediatric oncology clinics. The potential disadvantage is that the anesthesia team is at risk of significant underutilization on a day when the specific NORA service does not use all its block time or does not schedule cases appropriately. This can be partially solved by releasing unbooked time to other services in advance if the time on the schedule is not filled by a specified date. Often, it makes the most sense for an anesthesiology department to adopt a hybrid approach to NORA scheduling. This perspective is similar to the operational approach to efficiency and scheduling in ORs (see Chapter 16). In such a model, block time is offered to busy services and ad hoc

scheduling through the anesthesia department is used for lower volume services. No matter what scheduling paradigm is used, it is important to continually assess predicted versus actual times and use this data to optimize utilization.

Preprocedural Evaluation

Some amount of preprocedural evaluation is required prior to any anesthetic or procedural sedation. There are several issues that need to be considered when conducting and documenting this evaluation in the context of NORA. First, there are specific minimum standards and regulations to meet. Second, the lines of authority (who controls and is responsible for completing the preprocedural evaluation process) needs to be clearly defined. This determines accountability for assuring that required medical information is obtained, documented and available to all members of the care team in a timely fashion, for all patients. Third, policies for updating this information must be in place. Finally, cost and patient convenience must be considered.

Both TJC and the CMS have requirements for preanesthesia evaluations. TJC hospital standard PC 03.01.03 which requires that a preoperative assessment be documented before anesthesia or surgical treatment and requires that this assessment include the patient's medical, physical, psychological, and spiritual/cultural needs. In addition, TJC standards require reevaluation of the patient immediately before initiating moderate or deep sedation and before anesthesia induction. In addition, CMS requires that the evaluation of any patient who has received deep sedation, general anesthesia, or regional anesthesia (but not moderate sedation) be performed by a provider qualified in anesthesia during the first 48 h after the procedure. Neither organization has any other recommendation on adequate preoperative evaluation or timing.

The ASA practice advisory for the preanesthesia evaluation addresses preanesthetic concerns for both operating and non-OR anesthetics [1]. The preanesthesia evaluation involves the gathering of available data as well as obtaining additional missing information and ordering specific testing or specialty consultation, all at the discretion of the anesthesiologist, for the purpose of educating the patient, organizing resources for perioperative care, or formulating plans for intraoperative care, postoperative recovery, and perioperative pain management. While the advisory does not definitively address timing of the evaluation, it does suggest that patients having procedures of low invasiveness could probably be evaluated as late as the day of the procedure.

The requirement for a preprocedural history and physical exam, apart from the preanesthesia evaluation, is based on external regulatory mandates. The requirement for the timing of a complete or limited history and physical exam prior to NORA care is at the discretion of the institution. Most institutions require a complete history and physical within 30 days of general anesthesia and major surgery. While there is no scientific support for this requirement in terms of timing, it does provide a means for the anesthesia team to gain access to pertinent medical information for the assessment of the severity of patient's medical condition. A simple solution is to require the same standard for all episodes of anesthetic care both in and outside of the OR. However, the requirement for a complete history and physical exam may be burdensome and of little or no added value for many patients who are having a relatively minor procedure (such as a screening colonoscopy). It may be reasonable to have a less rigorous policy for minor or less invasive procedures that are performed outside of the OR. In any case, all service lines should be made aware of the requirement to avoid conflict and unnecessary delay on the day of service.

Preanesthetic laboratory testing of asymptomatic patients, a prominent feature of anesthesia care in decades past, is no longer recommended in the anesthesiology community, as it does not make an important contribution to the process of perioperative assessment and management of the patient. The American Society of Gastrointestinal Endoscopy concurs that routine laboratory testing for patients undergoing endoscopy is not warranted and should be ordered only for specific diagnostic indications [2].

No matter how the medical information on the patient is gathered, the anesthesia team must have access to it prior to the procedure in order to plan and conduct a safe anesthetic. This can be especially challenging in a tertiary medical center that configures its process for acceptance of subspecialty referrals in an "open access" mode. The meaning of "open access" is that patients can be scheduled by a referring provider on a first-come, first-served basis and with no requirement for approval or a preprocedural consultative visit. Such patients are unknown to the anesthesia team until they present, often after being transferred by ambulance, in the procedural suite as an urgent add-on case just before the time of the procedure.

The policy for preoperative evaluation should be consistent across the institution. One option to ensure this would be to have all electively scheduled NORA patients seen in the preanesthesia testing (PAT) clinic. This might be feasible for small NORA volume institutions, but as mentioned above would be very inconvenient and logistically difficult in a busy endoscopy referral practice. At high NORA volumes, the burden of seeing these patients would have a significant manpower impact on the PAT clinic. It is generally considered more practical to reserve PAT access to patients with specific indications, such as significant medical comorbidities, or to those scheduled to undergo more invasive NORA procedures (such as transvascular aortic valve replacement [TAVR] or cerebral angiography). For most NORA patients, telephone screening by a nurse might suffice to gather and document the information that will be desired on the day of the procedure. Whatever approach is chosen, the various proceduralists who utilize the anesthesia service must understand the algorithm. This helps reduce last-minute conflicts and the need to make decisions with incomplete and possibly inadequate medical information.

Staffing Models, with Emphasis on Gastrointestinal Endoscopy

Staffing models vary widely across the country. This variation is driven by cost and efficiency considerations, reimbursement models, staff availability and local regulations. Various organizations have published standards that may impact anesthesia staffing decisions. Four main anesthetic care models have been utilized in the United States in NORA settings: nurse-administered propofol deep sedation with proceduralist medical direction; anesthesia care team practice with medical direction of a Certified Registered Nurse Anesthetist (CRNA) or anesthesiology assistant by a physician anesthesiologist; physician anesthesiologist personally provided care (with or without a trainee); and CRNA-independent practice (in states where CRNA-independent practice is an option).

Registered Nurse–administered propofol-based deep procedural sedation (sometimes signified by the acronym NAPS) has been extensively described for gastrointestinal endoscopy and to a lesser degree for some cardiology procedures. This delivery model is controversial and there has been significant debate regarding the training and qualifications necessary to safely administer propofol. While the safety of this practice is beyond the scope of this chapter, available literature has not revealed significant safety issues in the populations where it has been used. The use of NAPS has been advocated by four major gastroenterology societies (American Gastroenterological Association, American Society for Gastrointestinal Endoscopy, American College of Gastroenterology, and American Association for the Study of Liver Diseases) as a cost-effective way to deliver the advantages of propofol. This was initially based on relatively small clinical trials (75–80 patients) that compared nurse-administered propofol to midazolam plus meperidine in the hands of gastroenterologists and found the propofol protocol to be effective, well tolerated, and characterized by rapid recovery [3, 4]. One of these studies included 75 patients for whom exhaled gas capnography was part of the protocol, a feature not widely utilized in clinical gastroenterology endoscopy practice. In both studies, the nurses administering propofol were all Advanced Cardiac Life Support–certified, in keeping with the ASA recommendation that any provider utilizing propofol for sedation should have the education and training to rescue a patient from the effects of general anesthesia. The controversy regarding NAPS is focused on the question of whether the nurse and the gastroenterologist are sufficiently capable of rescue, which implies airway management, circulatory support, and resuscitation skills.

The extent of utilization of NAPS is unknown. The practice is precluded in locations where the safety question has led to restrictions and prohibitions by licensing agencies and state regulatory bodies. Where the option is available, local financial and social incentives may come into play. Some anesthesiology practices see NAPS as unwelcome competition; others may lack the manpower to provide propofol for all endoscopic procedures. As a result, anesthesiologist opposition is variable. On the other hand, many proceduralists are unenthusiastic about accepting the burden and liability risk that comes with sedation and prefer to leave this to anesthesia providers. Finally,

reimbursement differs by payer. Some insurance companies provide separate compensation for anesthesia services while others bundle it with the procedural payment. CMS has recently unbundled payment for moderate sedation from payment for the screening colonoscopies. As a result, endoscopists may bill separately for this service if it is provided by them. If they don't provide it, their Medicare allowable payment is reduced. This economic decision may increase the proceduralists' desire to supervise the sedation process. Some payers have also denied payment for anesthesia services for screening colonoscopies unless the patient meets specific requirements, such as a history of prior intolerance to sedation, ASA III or higher physical status, a difficult airway, morbid obesity, or procedural complexity.

For most gastrointestinal endoscopic procedures, especially screening colonoscopies and straightforward upper endoscopies, the availability of an anesthesia team and propofol enhances the efficiency and productivity of the endoscopy suite. Time from arrival in the procedural room to readiness for the procedure to commence tends to be shorter than when intravenous midazolam and a narcotic are administered by nurses under the direction of the endoscopist. Similarly, time from completion of the procedure to recovery and discharge are typically much shorter when propofol is used. As a result, the anesthesia team's impact on the endoscopy suite is to increase the number of procedures that can be done in a day. Since gastrointestinal endoscopy suites typically have a positive contribution margin to their facility, institution leadership may be willing to bear the expense of anesthesia staffing in the endoscopy suite.

For the anesthesia staff working in the endoscopy suite, the rapid turnover and short duration of cases means there will be a heavy workload. Anesthesiologist personally providing care and CRNAs practicing independently in this setting learn to be very efficient and operate using a very standardized approach to all but the most complicated cases. Anesthesiologists who provide medical direction to CRNAs in this setting typically take on the duty of preparing the patients before anesthesia and completing required documentation, which the CRNAs manage the procedural care, typically with propofol infusions. The team approach can be more efficient in terms of turnover time, making the added cost worthwhile. For the physician anesthesiologist, the pace of work is such that medically directing three endoscopy rooms requires stamina and organization; medically directing four, and keeping pace with endoscopists who work quickly, can prove impractical or impossible.

For the anesthesia staff working in other NORA sites, the higher the level of complexity of the procedures or the greater the medical complexity of the patients, and the greater the distance from support and supplies the more likely the care team model is favored. Therefore, for cardiac electrophysiology studies, and for many interventional cardiologic, neurologic, and other radiologic procedures, the team model tends to be preferred. For noninvasive imaging procedures (CT, MRI, PET), it is more common to use a single provider.

Recovery

The location and staffing needs for NORA recovery depends upon the volume of cases, the nature of these cases, and the comorbidities of the patient. Recovery from a short endoscopic procedure utilizing propofol is quite different from a general anesthetic for a TAVR. Short-acting anesthetics are the norm for short outpatient procedures such as upper and lower gastrointestinal endoscopies, and recovery area is often located in or adjacent to the preprocedural preparation area and patients who received anesthesia care may be comingled with patients recovering from nurse-administered moderate sedation. One study estimated that a total of six pre- and postprocedure beds could adequately serve a four-procedure endoscopy suite [5]. Patients who have received only propofol, and patients who have received mild or moderate sedation, are typically sufficiently recovered at the completion of their procedure for what is referred to as phase II recovery. This phase of care is able to be staffed at a lower nurse to patient ratio (one nurse to four patients, maximum) than those who have received general anesthesia (one nurse to two patients, maximum).

Phase I recovery is usually required after more complex cases, usually in the postanesthesia care unit or even the critical care setting, depending on the complexity of the case and institutional practice. When the TAVR was first introduced, it was common to perform an intubated general anesthetic with pulmonary arterial pressure monitoring, and to ventilate the patient in the ICU after the procedure. With time and refinements in operative technique, the level of anesthetic invasiveness has been able to be modified in many institutions.

Billing

Anesthesia services for NORA cases are compensated using the same systems as for OR anesthesia. Therefore, billing and collection practices for NORA should be nested in the anesthesiology department's OR revenue cycle process. Under the fee for service model, anesthesia care is reimbursed based on anesthesia base units specific to the type of procedure and time units based on the duration of the procedure. The anesthesia base units are procedure specific and not dependent on location. CMS takes the lead in defining the number of anesthesia base units for each type of procedure. When CMS reduces payments for a procedure, commercial payers typically strive to amend their payment rules accordingly. CMS is currently exerting downward financial pressure on the healthcare community in an effort to diminish the practice of offering anesthesia services and propofol to healthy patients undergoing screening colonoscopies.

Safety and Quality Oversight

Nonsurgical proceduralists often do not share the normative understandings of anesthesia-related safety concerns that most surgeons understand. As a result, many basic things anesthesiologists take for granted, such as the importance of reliable suction and continuous oxygen saturation or exhaled carbon dioxide monitoring, may not be intuitive to gastroenterologists, cardiologists, and radiologists. For this reason, it is incumbent on the anesthesiology department to formulate the safety and quality requirements for anesthetic care in a non-OR site and monitor it. Typical points of conflict, where negotiation and collaboration are required, include access to the patient during the procedure, room configuration (if a new location is being planned), level of monitoring, access to resuscitative equipment, and processes for medication availability and handling.

Operational Issues Unique to NORA in Radiology

Anesthesiologists tend to view the practice of anesthesia care in the radiology department as a single location, much like another OR. Administratively, however, the various radiologic subspecialties typically function somewhat independently. Therefore, NORA in radiology often features several distinct services: MRI, CT, interventional radiology, interventional neuroradiology, and body scanning with interventions, to name a few.

If none of these radiological subspecialty services has a full day's caseload, the anesthesiology department might allocate a team to provide care to "patients in radiology" on that day. Challenges arise, and dissatisfaction results, when one service's patients are delayed, causing a delay for the next service. The key to addressing these challenges lies in overcoming the "silo mentality" where the personnel in each subspecialty service profess no accountability or connection to one another and manage their own internal schedules for their own benefit. This is a role for the medical director of NORA services.

One reason why personnel might be motivated to work in this manner is financial. From the facility's point of view, it might actually be optimal to keep the MRI scanners maximally utilized, with as little downtime as possible between cases. From that perspective, it might seem acceptable to delay an anesthesia case a few minutes by fitting another scan into the schedule ahead of the anesthesia case. The decision to impose such a delay might seem sensible to the MRI personnel, especially if they are unaware of the medical condition of the case to follow in interventional radiology or insensitive to the needs of the anxious MRI patient whose induction of anesthesia is being delayed.

Additional roles for the medical director of NORA services in the radiology context include standardizing anesthesia practices in accordance with MRI magnet safety, keeping the institution's monitoring current in terms of technology, and supporting safety and pediatric-friendly practices for the care of children undergoing MRIs and other radiologic procedures. The first role is one where the personnel in the radiology department are expert and can provide guidance; the others are areas where the medical director may need to educate radiology personnel and promote their engagement and cooperation. Anesthetic practice has become very safe and adverse events have become infrequent. As a result, nonanesthesiologists sometimes find it hard to understand the need for rigorous safety practices.

Neuro-interventional radiology is an area that has seen rapid growth over the past several years.

These procedures are generally performed in an angiography procedural room or a hybrid OR. The proceduralists may be neurosurgeons, neurologists, or neuroradiologists, who perform cerebral angiograms, and treat aneurysms, arteriovenous malformations, and vascular occlusions. Common procedures include aneurysm coiling, arteriovenous malformation occlusion, carotid angioplasty and stenting, intracranial clot removal or dissolution in patients with acute stroke, and therapy for intracranial vasospasm. Considerations in terms of planning for these procedures include anesthetic type, recovery location, impact on neurosurgical coverage and need for urgent OR access.

Most of these procedures are done under general anesthesia because controlled ventilation and immobility are requested by the proceduralist. However, simple angiograms and carotid procedures may be amenable to moderate sedation. Many neuro-interventional procedures require overnight observation or inpatient care, so recovery takes place in the postanesthesia care unit or ICU. Frequently, these procedures are urgent or emergent. Hospitals that serve as stroke centers have specific requirements in terms of minimum time from arrival to procedure room access, which requires specific call coverage for these cases. Finally, there remains a small risk of intracerebral hemorrhage requiring an emergent open operative procedure. This requires transport to the OR for surgical intervention if a hybrid room is not used, and a neurosurgical nursing team must be available for such a contingency.

Summary

The appearance and growth of procedural practices outside the OR have tested the flexibility and inventiveness of the anesthesiology community. Some NORA contexts feature high turnover of short, mainly low complexity procedures performed on generally healthy patients, while others feature complex interventions on complex and compromised patients with serious comorbidities. The venues often feature less ergonomically optimal conditions than those to which anesthetists are accustomed in the OR, posing potential safety risks to the patient, and the procedural area personnel often do not seem to be attuned to these risks. Despite these challenges, NORA environments provide medical services that patients need. The procedures are usually less invasive than an alternative surgical operation, but they can only be accomplished with the involvement of an anesthesia team. For these reasons, despite the challenges and inconveniences these procedure entail, it appears that the future of medical care will continue to include a growing component of NORA. The anesthesiology community is uniquely positioned to lead and guide this growth in an efficient and safe manner.

References

1. American Society of Anesthesiologists Committee on Standards and Practice Parameters. Practice advisory for preanesthesia evaluation: An updated report by the American Society of Anesthesiologists Task Force on Preanesthesia Evaluation. *Anesthesiology* 2012; 116(3): 522–38.

2. American Society for Gastrointestinal Endoscopy Committee on Standards of Practice. Routine laboratory testing before endoscopic procedures. *Gastrointest Endosc* 2014; 80(1): 28–33.

3. Vargo JJ, Zuccaro G, Dumot JA, et al. Gastroenterologist-administered propofol versus meperidine and midazolam for advanced upper endoscopy: A prospective, randomized trial. *Gastroenterology* 2002; 123(1): 8–16.

4. Sipe BW, Rex DK, Latinovich D, et al. Propofol versus midazolam/meperidine for outpatient colonoscopy: Administration by nurses supervised by endoscopists. *Gastrointest Endosc* 2002; 55(7): 815–25.

5. Day LW, Belson D, Dessouky M, Hawkins C, Hogan M. Optimizing efficiency and operations at a California safety-net endoscopy center: A modeling and simulation approach. *Gastrointest Endosc* 2014; 80(5): 762–73.

6. Cravero JP, Blike GT, Beach M, et al. Incidence and nature of adverse events during pediatric sedation/anesthesia for procedures outside the operating room: Report from the Pediatric Sedation Research Consortium. *Pediatrics* 2006; 118(3): 1087–96.

Chapter

16

Efficiency and Scheduling

Brian C. Spence and William R. Furman

A working definition of efficiency is the ability to produce desired results without wasting materials, time, or energy. In the context of operating room (OR) scheduling, the chief desired result is the ability to accommodate the operative needs of the patients of the healthcare facility without wasting resources. The relevant resources in this situation are time and space. The fundamental decisions to be made in the pursuit of efficiency involve allocation of space (rooms) to patients (and their surgeons) at particular times.

Decision making related to OR scheduling has been categorized as strategic, tactical, or operational, depending on the time frame [1]. Strategic decisions, such as the choice of how many ORs to build or whether to construct or expand an ambulatory surgery center, are made and carried out over the course of one to three years. Tactical decisions, such as whether to allocate additional OR time to specific subspecialties, are made approximately one year in advance. That topic, covered in more detail in Chapter 8, relates to the time frame required to recruit personnel, acquire specialty equipment, and if necessary obtain financing, and then construct or renovate ORs for specific purposes.

Operational decision making is the term for the day-to-day, weekly, and monthly allocation decisions that promote optimally efficient utilization of the ORs that have been planned, built, fitted out, and staffed. A key goal of operational decision making is to achieve high efficiency by minimizing underutilization and overutilization of OR resources [2]. In this context, underutilization represents time when an OR is not in use but is staffed, and overutilization represents time when an OR is in use beyond the time period for which staffing was planned and scheduled. Underutilization

typically represents time during which employees are being paid at their regular rates but may not be productive. Overutilization typically results in additional costs, often at an overtime pay premium.

The task of simultaneously minimizing both underutilization and overutilization on a daily basis is usually the responsibility of the anesthesiologist-in-charge for the day (synonyms include "coordinator," "floor runner," "board runner"), who collaborates with the OR charge nurse for the day. These daily operational leaders function within a framework of rules for OR case scheduling and pursue a general goal that intuitively translates as, "try to fit all the cases into the available rooms in a way that makes them all end as close to 5 p.m. (or some other specific end time) as possible, with the fewest minutes of rooms and number of rooms running later." Many OR coordinators perform their role instinctively. This chapter will focus on operational decision making in the OR.

Prior to Day of Surgery: Building the Schedule

The daily schedule of OR cases tends to be very fluid. As a result, the task of assigning anesthesia staff (and OR nursing staff as well) to rooms and patients is almost always deferred until mid-day one business day prior. Depending on local culture and habit, the coordinator may accept the schedule that is produced by the nursing and scheduling staff, or may take an active role engaging with the OR nursing and surgical leadership in an effort to address scheduling choices that appear inefficient. This activity is invariably based on an unscripted cognitive process where there is little published wisdom to provide guidance.

Most experienced coordinators attempt to address the common scheduling issues: gaps between cases, instances where a surgeon has multiple cases that do not follow one another in the same room, and apparent underrepresentations of the amount of time needed for cases. The latter issue receives particular attention when it causes the room to appear falsely scheduled to end on time, especially when a late finish is not in the staffing plan and the late finish will result in unplanned overtime stays for staff who are not expecting to be detained. Very granular knowledge of operative procedures and the relative abilities and tendencies of individual surgeons is necessary in order to know when to intervene and attempt to alter the schedule. Sometimes the effort only leads to conflict, administrative time consumed, and an insignificant gain in efficiency, if any. Deft application of interpersonal skills and emotional intelligence [3] are sometimes more valuable than chronological precision.

The framework of the OR system on which the day is built is the surgical schedule. There are two basic models for OR booking. One, usually referred to as block allocation, is where time is reserved for individual surgeons or groups of surgeons (typically groups within a surgical specialty) who have the ability to book into predesignated blocks of OR time. These blocks of time are protected from being booked by other surgeons or services. In its purest form, the block allocation is inviolable and protection is preserved until the start of the day of surgery. The other model is open booking, in which all cases are added to the schedule on a "first come is first served" basis. Both have relative merits and drawbacks, and as a result features of open scheduling are used within most block allocation systems.

Open scheduling might appear to be more flexible and accommodating in terms of time allocation for surgeons, as they can book into any available time that aligns with their availability and needs. This approach would seem to offer an opportunity to schedule optimally, with minimal underutilization or overutilization, because the scheduling office can control the times that are offered to the surgeons. However, if the exact time the surgeon prefers is not available, underutilization may result, a consequence of fragmentation of available time. For example, if surgeon A requests but cannot be given a first case start at 7:30 a.m. because there is already a case in every room at 7:30, surgeon A might opt to utilize the entire morning for some other activity or procedure. Surgeon A's next preferred time might be 12:30 p.m. If the OR schedule does not have any room where cases are scheduled so that they will be completed and the room turned over at exactly 12:30 p.m., there will be a period of underutilized time between the completion of the last scheduled case and the 12:30 p.m. start of surgeon A's case. In practice, open scheduling is more suitable for OR suites with a small number of rooms, or for selected single-specialty rooms within a larger OR suite. Typical examples are four- to six-room ambulatory surgery centers, or the two to four cardiac surgical rooms in a larger OR suite.

Block scheduling is better suited to larger, more complex OR environments where the full spectrum of specialty services are provided. It is predicated on the expectation that each service has the case volume needed to reliably fill the number of days or half-days per week allocated to it. In return for prohibiting other services from scheduling into Surgeon B's time, Surgeon B is expected to fill the time with his or her cases. In practice, most institutions set a time point prior to which Surgeon B must fill the block. This "release time" might be any number of business or calendar days prior to the date of surgery. Beyond that point, unfilled time in the block becomes available to all surgeons and this part of the schedule changes to the open model. Many institutions vary the release time by service, in recognition that some services and surgeons provide care to a more elective population (such as prostatectomies, total joint replacements, cataract surgery), while others treat a population that should have access to an OR on a few days' notice (such as orthopedic trauma, brain tumors, detached retinas). In addition, some time is typically reserved for emergency cases on the day of surgery.

Block scheduling encourages more efficient use of the OR. It communicates an expectation to surgeons and services that they will use their allocated time. It facilitates monitoring of utilization and identification of chronically underutilized blocks, which can be reallocated to surgical services that show a need for additional time. The implicit threat that a surgeon or service will lose a block, and therefore lose some flexibility and convenience in scheduling, serves as a motivator for surgeons to try not to lose allocations. In theory, this should be a means for improving efficiency, since one way for a surgeon to retain a block is to fill it and minimize underutilization. Unfortunately, two other ways to retain a block are (1) to overutilize (operate slowly, doing in five hours what another surgeon does in three), and (2) exert political influence. In practice, many institutions find it costly in terms of working relationships to take OR block time away from anyone.

Another advantage of block scheduling is that it allows specialized and service specific equipment (such as a robot or an operating microscope) to remain in a specific room every day. This makes it immediately available, decreasing room turnover times, and reduces the risk of damage during relocation.

Block scheduling is inherently less flexible than open scheduling. A pure block schedule does not have an intrinsic ability to easily accommodate combined service cases such as mastectomies followed by breast reconstruction. It also provides obstacles to short-term changes in surgical schedules, such as might occur if surgeon asks to operate on a different day of the week than usual for a short period either because of a case backlog or a personal scheduling need.

In response to these challenges, most large OR suites find it preferable to maintain a block schedule or a hybrid version that combines service-specific blocks with some open block time. The open blocks are not assigned to any specific surgeon or service, but are instead available to anyone and may be booked well in advance of the day of surgery. In addition, if the OR suite has a policy for releasing unbooked block time some number of days prior to surgery, this time becomes available as part of the open time pool as well, and can be used to accommodate additional elective cases, or more urgent unplanned cases.

In theory, the short-term allocation and forfeiture of block time, which is a tactical decision (see Chapter 8), should not be based on utilization [4], but on the reality of the current caseload. In the longer term, strategic decisions about increasing OR capacity should be based on the institution's financial goals and capacity to sustain the costs of meeting its nonremunerative missions. In practice, however, in most institutions the availability heuristic frequently wins out; utilization data are at hand and the social pressure to apply them can be irresistible.

In a perfect world, every surgeon would take the same amount of time to do each procedure, with neither intersurgeon variability nor intrasurgeon variability. The procedure scheduled by the surgeon would always be congruent with the procedure performed, historical times would always be accurate, surgeons would never prompt their staff to understate the time required for a procedure and would never schedule more cases than they could complete by 5:00 p.m. without notifying the OR desk in advance. Every surgeon would have the same number of hours of surgery to do each week, and they would always tell the OR scheduling office well in advance about their anticipated time away for meetings and vacations so that their time could be released for others to use. Under those circumstances, it would be easy to know exactly how much time to allocate to each surgeon or service. Underutilization would be minimized and overutilization would be due to unplanned emergency cases where life and limb were imperiled.

In the real world, none of the above obtains and much of it is beyond human control. The application of historical and utilization data are imperfect, but commonly used. Where that is done, the rules for booking and forfeiting OR time in the block schedule need to be clear, robust, and not subject to excessive manipulation by one constituency to its own advantage.

On the Day of Surgery: Managing the Schedule

The tactical decision to allocate block time to a particular surgeon or surgical service in order to maximize efficiency occurs several weeks to months in advance. However, on the day of surgery it is the operational decision making that will be used to minimize under and overutilization and get the existing caseload accomplished within the given workday. The published schedule is a starting point, but each day some cases will take longer than scheduled, others will take less time, some cases will be cancelled, and some will be added (electively, urgently, or emergently).

For the anesthesiologist in the role of coordinator, the task may be explained as follows: decide how to change the schedule in response to all of the above unpredicted events. What cases should be reassigned earlier or later, and in what room? How should the added cases be assigned? Can every case on the schedule be completed, or will some have to be deferred to a future date? How much inefficiency will result? Can you minimize underutilization and overutilization and still optimize patient care (not defer cases unnecessarily)? How much underutilization can you tolerate? How much overutilization can you tolerate? How much risk of overutilization will you accept?

Although it is clear that the coordinator is expected to strive to accommodate as many cases as possible, there may be subtle incentives to tolerate underutilization. Staff do not complain much about being able to take a break or finish early. They might reinforce the behavior of a coordinator who dismisses them early by smiling and showing appreciation. They would be less likely to do so in return for being assigned another case. The additional labor costs of underutilization are small. In some work environments, when staff are dismissed early the employer might save some hourly wages, but in others, the assigned staff are paid whether there is a case for them to do or not, especially near the end of the day.

There may be explicit incentives to avoid overutilization. In small amounts, additional overtime work may be desired by staff as an earning opportunity, but beyond that point, morale may be adversely impacted, and staff do complain about missing time with their families or missing commitments because of unanticipated late workdays. The additional labor costs of overutilization are generally greater than those of underutilization. Overtime hours are usually paid at a premium, well above the standard hourly rate.

The monetary cost of overtime hours, while considerable, is generally understood to be less than the operational cost of losing cases to competitors. The performance of the coordinator is judged to have not been efficient, in retrospect, if there has been potentially avoidable underutilization on a day when there is also substantial overutilization (late-running cases that should have been accommodated earlier during the day). However, at the moment when an opportunity presents itself to accommodate an added case in an underutilized room, the coordinator does not know with certainty whether the decision to accept that added case will result in an overrun. In short, the coordinator sees an opportunity to reduce underutilization but is taking a risk that doing so will lead to increased overutilization.

Some OR coordinators are decidedly risk-averse, and avoid placing an added case in an open slot if they perceive any risk that the case will take longer than advertised. Others are less risk-averse. One study examined the impact of an operational OR manager's risk appreciation and demonstrated that bolder (non–risk-averse) managers made decisions that resulted in significantly less underutilized OR time compared to risk-averse OR managers, while not having a significant increase in overutilization [5]. In other words, the OR managers who were not risk-averse accommodated more patients, avoided underutilization, and incurred only minimal increases in overutilization. They were, therefore, more efficient.

Summary

The strategic and tactical decision making that provides the framework for the surgical schedule and OR are vital for any healthcare institution because the OR is a major revenue generating resource. However, it is the operational decision making that influences the day-to-day productivity of the OR and ultimately produces the surgical schedule that generates that revenue. In this regard, the role and performance of the anesthesiologist-in-charge is pivotal. It is essential that strategic, tactical, and operational decisions be aligned. Even more importantly, it is critical that the operational decisions be made in a manner that maximizes OR efficiency by minimizing under- and overutilization while simultaneously supporting the institutional mission of providing safe and effective healthcare to patients.

References

1. Dexter, F., J. Ledolter, and R. E. Wachtel, Tactical decision making for selective expansion of operating room resources incorporating financial criteria and uncertainty in subspecialties' future workloads. *Anesth Analg*, 2005; 100(5): 1425–32, table of contents.

2. Strum, D. P., L. G. Vargas, and J. H. May, Surgical subspecialty block utilization and capacity planning: A minimal cost analysis model. *Anesthesiology*, 1999; 90(4): 1176–85.

3. Goleman, D., What makes a leader? *Harv Bus Rev*, 1998; 76(6): 93–102.

4. Wachtel, R. E., and F. Dexter, Tactical increases in operating room block time for capacity planning should not be based on utilization. *Anesth Analg*, 2008; 106(1): 215–26, table of contents.

5. Stepaniak, P.S., et al., The effect of the operating room coordinator's risk appreciation on operating room efficiency. *Anesth Analg*, 2009; 108(4): 1249–56.

Chapter

17

Operating Room Budgets
An Overview

Steven Boggs and Sanjana Vig

What Is a Budget?

According to *Webster's Dictionary*, a budget is "a plan used to decide the amount of money that can be spent and how it will be spent." From this simple definition many different types of budgets can be derived:

- Academic departmental budgets
- Large nonacademic departmental budgets
- Multispecialty group
- Single specialty private practice groups
- Sole proprietorship.

This chapter is intended to familiarize readers with the basic terminology common to all budgets. It is also intended to highlight the advantages and risks associated with the budgeting process and to illustrate how the reader can utilize budgets in managing an anesthesia department, a perioperative service and procedural and operating room (OR) services.

As forward-looking documents, budgets help an enterprise or department evaluate its financial performance over time and plan for various fiscal contingencies in the future. Budgeting and planning are related but not identical [1]. Planning can be for 1 year, 3 years, 5 years or longer, while budgets have historically been made for 1-year periods. Viewed in this way, budgets contribute to strategic planning but in themselves are not sufficient for that purpose. Many changes may occur over the course of multiple 1-year periods, so merely adding five 1-year budgets together is not the same as developing a comprehensive 5-year strategic plan. An organization's long-term strategic plan will drive financial objectives and will, therefore, ultimately drive the budgetary process.

Volatility in revenue streams for healthcare, the necessity to evaluate service lines against external and internal factors and increasing competition in the healthcare market has forced many organizations to abandon slower, more resource-intensive budgeting processes for more nimble forecasting. This has led some healthcare organizations to move from an annual budget to nonbudgetary planning. We will discuss this option after we discuss some of the basics of traditional or classic budget formation.

Traditional Budget Formation

Both for-profit and not-for-profit enterprises have to create budgets. While the tax implications may differ between the two entities, each must remain financially solvent to continue to provide services. In certain circumstances, oversight requirements are such that a budget must be provided to regulators or other officials in order to comply with their fiduciary responsibilities.

The typical budgeting cycle is that the organization's finance function sends out a request for information. This request will specify categories that each department (anesthesia being one of these) needs to fill out for the next year. Categories include salaries, benefits, requirements for capital improvements, administrative costs and all other items that have previously been included in the budget.

This method of annual budgeting has both advantages and disadvantages. It allows the entry of new data so that financial planning for the next year may occur. Alternative outcomes can be considered and management can weigh the possibilities of various scenarios (see Table 17.1). The enterprise can use the budget so assembled – when each department contributes its requirements – so that the enterprise can choose where to allocate resources. By reviewing historical data and weighing strategic decisions, the organization can allocate resources to areas that are profitable and, perhaps more importantly, identify areas that constitute financial drag.

However, budgeting contains risks that must be managed appropriately. The business must remain flexible in implementing tactical and strategic decisions when budget variances do occur. The organization must always be ready to adapt to changing circumstances and be ready to act on current information, rather than being constrained by budget categories.

Budgeting is not a science and despite the fact that it is quantitative in nature, a budget is only as good as the assumptions that are made. Managers in large departments may cushion their projected budget requirements so that their allowances for travel, R & D and other categories are never reduced when annually reviewed, even if such a reduction would be better overall for the organization. If the budget is only created once a year there is a strong tendency for departments to seek as much funding as they can get at that time, regardless of need, so that they do not have to reapply later in the year when funds may be limited.

Boxes 17.1 and 17.2 further break down and illustrate the advantages and disadvantages of budgets.

Accounting Statements

Before considering types of budgets, it is important to briefly review the fundamental accounting statements [2]. There are three basic statements, the Balance Sheet, the Income Statement and the Statement of Cash Flows. Unlike a budget, these documents are historic in nature and review the performance of the entity over the course of the past year.

1. The *Balance Sheet* presents a *quantitative* view of a company's financial condition at a given moment and is comprised of three parts, assets, liabilities and the difference between the two, net assets (also known as equity). This statement is analogous to an x-ray, giving a captured view of the entity at a point in time. This fundamental equation of accounting is highlighted below:

$$\text{Net assets} = \text{assets} - \text{liabilities}$$

As can be seen in the Statement of Financial Position from Mount Sinai (Figure 17.1), important categories in this document are both current assets and liabilities and total assets and liabilities. It is important to keep an eye on current assets (C/A), which are resources that are readily available to an organization at that time, including cash, investments and receivables. Current liabilities (C/L) are what an entity has to pay within that year (debts, accounts payable, compensations/benefits, third-party settlements). Calculating the ratio of C/A to C/L is important sign of a hospitals ability to meet all of its financial requirements. This ratio is called the Current Ratio and is preferred to remain above 2:1.

For not-for-profit entities, e.g., hospitals and healthcare organizations, net equity is typically listed as net assets. This is the difference between total assets and total liabilities and again is a financial indicator of the organization's financial health.

2. The *Income Statement* or *Statement of Activities* reports an entity's financial performance over a specific accounting period. Also known as the profit and loss statement, it reports how an entity incurs its revenues and expenses through both operating and nonoperating activities. In this way, the Statement of Activities shows performance over a given period of time, similar to the information derived from an anesthetic record.

The statement of activities (Figure 17.2) includes operating revenue, operating expenses and then a category of other items that do not fit neatly into these categories:

- Revenue – from patients, other (research/academic, investments)
- Expenses – salaries/benefits, supplies/outside services
- Operating gain and loss – aka income earned after expenses are paid, or the bottom line
- Excess of revenues over expenses – the money actually earned from all parts of the business, or OR
- Revenues less expenses result in operating gains/loss
- Operating gain/loss = operating revenues – operating expenses.

3. The *Statement of Cash Flows* (Figure 17.3) illustrates how changes in balance sheet accounts and income affect cash and cash equivalents, and breaks

Table 17.1 Sample Anesthesia Department Scenario Report

	2016 projected	2017 base	2017 optimistic	2017 pessimistic
Revenue				
Cardiac anesthesia	23,145	25,235	27,345	22,164
Neuroanesthesia	11,765	12,985	15,399	11,970
Pediatric anesthesia	8,598	9,658	11,237	9,010
General anesthesia	35,908	37,956	41,453	35,211
Orthopedic anesthesia	24,445	26,123	28,223	25,800
Interventional pain	18,202	20,100	22,984	18,900
Net revenue	122,063	132,057	146,641	123,055
Expenses				
Cardiac anesthesia	19,450	21,568	20,945	19,945
Neuroanesthesia	9,143	10,200	11,123	9,900
Pediatric anesthesia	7,374	8,956	9,856	8,145
General anesthesia	31,231	32,876	38,276	31,201
Orthopedic anesthesia	21,890	23,528	25,342	22,398
Interventional pain	15,301	16,869	19,487	16,101
Administration	14,956	15,786	16,123	15,213
Net expenses	119,345	129,783	141,152	122,903
Operating margin	2,718	2,274	5,489	152
Operating margin percent	2.23%	1.72%	3.74%	0.12%

Box 17.1. Advantages of Creating a Budget

Planning orientation	Forces administrators to think about long term consequences/ effects of their decision making
Model scenarios	Allows prediction of results of different management decisions; can estimate financial impact of each result
Profitability review	Helps companies remain focused on profitable business areas and those needing improvement
Assumptions review	Reevaluation of business assumptions helps to continuously align business goals with changing environments.
Performance evaluations	For example, ties bonuses/incentives to employee performance; helps drive budget changes
Predict cash flows	Good for short term budgeting; unpredictable for future/long term
Cash allocation	Drives administrative decisions regarding which assets to invest in
Cost reduction analysis	Helps decide which cost reduction targets to pursue
Shareholder communication	Helps convey information to investors

the analysis down to operating, investing and financing activities. A fluid input/output graph for a patient would indicate that a very healthy, highly trained athlete could risk death if running through the Mohave Desert without water. Likewise, an otherwise viable enterprise can face bankruptcy if insufficient cash reserves are available for ongoing requirements.

Budget Categories

Revenue Budget

Of the types of budgets, the revenue budget is most central to a business' ongoing viability. This budget reflects the revenue expectations of management for the coming year.

Box 17.2. Disadvantages of Budgets

Inaccuracy	If any part of budget creation assumptions change, then actual results can vary from predictions
Rigid decision making	Decisions occur once a year; as yet no system exists to review previous assumptions in the event that the environment changes
Time required	Making budgets is time consuming
Gaming the system	There may be dishonesty during budget creation; falsify cation of information so results are better than predictions
Blame for outcomes	Nonadherence to a budget can create cause for blame
Expense allocations	Administrators may disagree about how funds are allocated
Use it or lose it	In order to maintain expense allocations for their department, managers may authorize unneeded spending
Tunnel vision	Budgets may lead managers to only consider financial outcomes; there is no qualitative perspective

I. The Statement of Financial Position

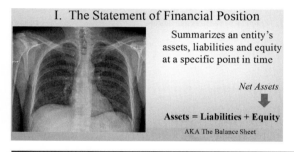

Summarizes an entity's assets, liabilities and equity at a specific point in time

Net Assets

Assets = Liabilities + Equity

AKA The Balance Sheet

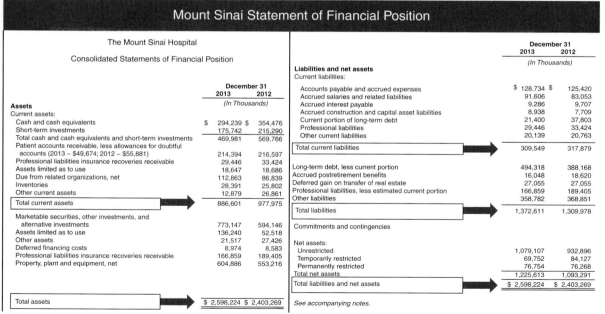

Figure 17.1 (a) Statement of financial position. (b) Example of a balance sheet.

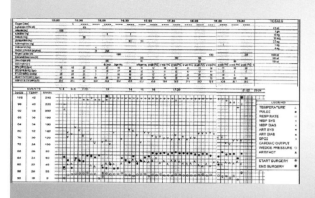

II. Statement of Activities

Reports the financial performance of an entity over specific period of time

Revenues (*incoming* monies)

Expenses (*outgoing* monies)

Also known as:

- Profit and Loss Statement

- Statement of Revenue and Expense

- Operating Statement

- Income Statement

Interesting because it is a direct result of business operations

Statement Of Activities

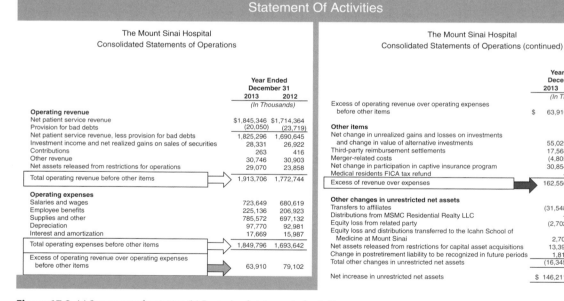

The Mount Sinai Hospital
Consolidated Statements of Operations

	Year Ended December 31	
	2013	2012
	(In Thousands)	
Operating revenue		
Net patient service revenue	$1,845,346	$1,714,364
Provision for bad debts	(20,050)	(23,719)
Net patient service revenue, less provision for bad debts	1,825,296	1,690,645
Investment income and net realized gains on sales of securities	28,331	26,922
Contributions	263	416
Other revenue	30,746	30,903
Net assets released from restrictions for operations	29,070	23,858
Total operating revenue before other items	1,913,706	1,772,744
Operating expenses		
Salaries and wages	723,649	680,619
Employee benefits	225,136	206,923
Supplies and other	785,572	697,132
Depreciation	97,770	92,981
Interest and amortization	17,669	15,987
Total operating expenses before other items	1,849,796	1,693,642
Excess of operating revenue over operating expenses before other items	63,910	79,102

The Mount Sinai Hospital
Consolidated Statements of Operations (continued)

	Year Ended December 31	
	2013	2012
	(In Thousands)	
Excess of operating revenue over operating expenses before other items	$ 63,910	$ 79,102
Other items		
Net change in unrealized gains and losses on investments and change in value of alternative investments	55,029	27,249
Third-party reimbursement settlements	17,568	41,623
Merger-related costs	(4,805)	–
Net change in participation in captive insurance program	30,854	8,470
Medical residents FICA tax refund	–	21,916
Excess of revenue over expenses	162,556	178,360
Other changes in unrestricted net assets		
Transfers to affiliates	(31,548)	(16,098)
Distributions from MSMC Residential Realty LLC	–	60
Equity loss from related party	(2,702)	–
Equity loss and distributions transferred to the Icahn School of Medicine at Mount Sinai	2,702	(60)
Net assets released from restrictions for capital asset acquisitions	13,392	8,014
Change in postretirement liability to be recognized in future periods	1,811	(1,240)
Total other changes in unrestricted net assets	(16,345)	(9,324)
Net increase in unrestricted net assets	$ 146,211	$ 169,036

Figure 17.2 (a) Statement of activities. (b) Example of statement of activities.

The revenue budget has two portions. First is the income budget, which includes earnings from provision of services, auxiliary services, financial activities (e.g., rent), investment revenue, donations and grants. Due to an increasingly volatile healthcare environment, there is increased uncertainty about payment rates and reimbursement. Therefore, it is important that all assumptions made when creating this type of budget be appended to and fully understood when constructing this part of the budget.

Second is the expenditure budget, which includes costs of employees (a major portion of the budget for any anesthesia department), materials and supplies, office, interest, and depreciation expense. Expenses

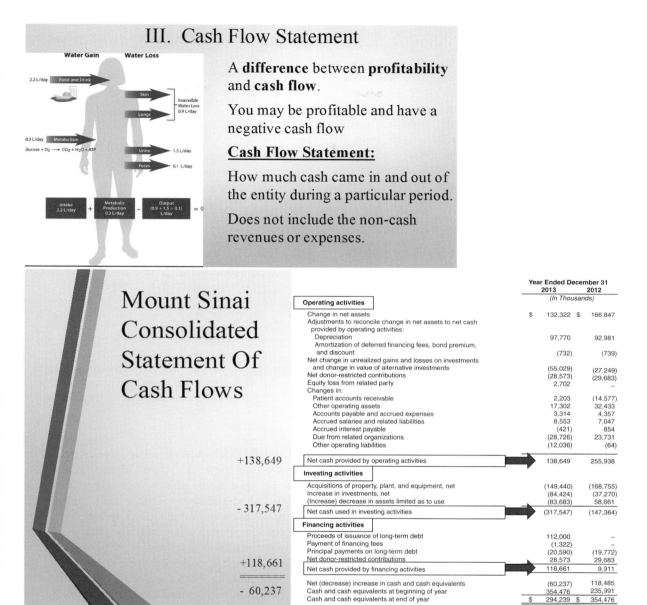

Figure 17.3 (a)Statement of cash flows. (b) Example of statement of cash flows.

are more predictable in nature but allowances for unexpected expenses must also be made.

Depending on the size of the entity, revenue budgets can be broken down into sections. For example, for an anesthesia department the revenue budget could be broken down by location should the department provide services outside of the OR; or, it could be broken down by division: cardiac, neurosurgical, obstetrical, pediatrics, trauma, etc. Evaluating the revenue budget by service line can help allocate resources appropriately. If a service line is not profitable it is useful to identify that fact, even if reduction of service is not an option.

Compensation Budget

For anesthesia departments or groups, salary and related expenses constitute a large portion of the budget. The compensation budget, therefore, is one of the largest budgets that must be formulated. Budget items in this category include actual salaries and social security taxes, Medicare taxes and federal unemployment taxes.

Benefits are also incorporated and include health insurance, dental and pension benefits (401(k)) and pension matching. In addition, there must be budgetary consideration for the difference between employees on salary and those paid on an hourly basis. For hourly workers, overtime must be accounted for. Monthly or annual bonuses must also be taken into account.

Capital Budget

If an enterprise, department, or group plans to purchase or lease a major asset, it is imperative that an analysis of the costs, benefits and advantages of purchasing the asset be made. A capital asset will provide benefits for years to come and will likewise, take a period of time to pay for. The value of the asset will be depreciated over the useful life of the asset. Building and additions to facilities and equipment are typical capital budget items.

The goal of a capital budget analysis is to make a decision, "yes or no," whether to lease or buy an asset. There are various tools available for this analysis, which are beyond the scope of this chapter. They would include Net Present Value analysis, Payback Method, Internal Rate of Return and Bottleneck Analysis. However, a capital acquisition should either increase revenue or reduce costs for the organization.

Research and Development Budget

To develop a robust academic department, it is essential that a department support its faculty in application for funding for research. Administration must understand the nature of research awards and where to apply for funding. Some typical sources of funding for anesthesia research include [3, 4] (see Box 17.3):

- National Institutes of Health (NIH)
- Patient-Centered Outcomes Research Institute
- Agency for Healthcare Research and Quality (AHRQ)
- Foundation for Anesthesia Education and Research
- International Anesthesia Research Society
- Anesthesia Patient Safety Foundation
- American Heart Association.

Box 17.3. Types of NIH Awards

F	For predoctoral and postdoctoral fellowships, as well as training for experienced scientists who wish to change career directions.
K	For career development. Most mechanisms are for junior investigators, but a few are for mid-career and senior investigators.
P	For program projects or centers. For large, multi-project efforts that typically include a diverse array of research activities.
R	Research projects. There are also resource grants, such as the R24 and R25 mechanisms.
T	For training predoctoral and postdoctoral researchers and for conferences.
U	Cooperative agreements used when there is a substantial programmatic involvement between the awarding institute and center at NIH and the investigator's institution.
Trans-NIH	A variety of broad-reaching, cross-institute programs, such as the "NIH Roadmap Initiatives" and the DP1 and DP2 mechanisms.

For the NIH (and other awarding agencies frequently follow NIH), there are several considerations. The applicant must differentiate between direct costs and facility and administration (F&A) costs. Direct costs are those which can be identified specifically with a particular sponsored project, instructional activity, or any other institutional activity, or that can be directly assigned to such activities relatively easily with a high degree of accuracy. F&A costs benefit more than one cost objective, and are not readily assignable to the cost objectives specifically benefitted, without effort disproportionate to the results achieved.

The NIH also allows two types of budgets. A modular budget is permitted if the direct costs are less than $250,000 per year, the grant type is of a certain type (R01, R03, R15, R21, R34) and the applying organization is based in the United States. Otherwise, a detailed budget is required and involves completion of various sections:

Section A and B: Personnel
Section C, D and E: Equipment, Travel, and Trainee Costs

Program Director/Principal Investigator (Last, First, Middle):

BUDGET FOR ENTIRE PROPOSED PROJECT PERIOD
DIRECT COSTS ONLY

BUDGET CATEGORY TOTALS	INITIAL BUDGET PERIOD (from Form Page 4)	2nd ADDITIONAL YEAR OF SUPPORT REQUESTED	3rd ADDITIONAL YEAR OF SUPPORT REQUESTED	4th ADDITIONAL YEAR OF SUPPORT REQUESTED	5th ADDITIONAL YEAR OF SUPPORT REQUESTED
PERSONNEL: *Salary and fringe benefits. Applicant organization only.*					
CONSULTANT COSTS					
EQUIPMENT					
SUPPLIES					
TRAVEL					
INPATIENT CARE COSTS					
OUTPATIENT CARE COSTS					
ALTERATIONS AND RENOVATIONS					
OTHER EXPENSES					
DIRECT CONSORTIUM/ CONTRACTUAL COSTS					
SUBTOTAL DIRECT COSTS (Sum = Item 8a, Face Page)					
F&A CONSORTIUM/ CONTRACTUAL COSTS					
TOTAL DIRECT COSTS					

TOTAL DIRECT COSTS FOR ENTIRE PROPOSED PROJECT PERIOD $

JUSTIFICATION. Follow the budget justification instructions exactly. Use continuation pages as needed.

Figure 17.4 Example of budget categories.

Section F: Other Direct Costs

Looking at a sample budget from the AHRQ, one can see the various categories included in the required budget (Figure 17.4).

Administration Budget

Support functions, which cannot be accounted for elsewhere, are generally listed in the administration budget. This would include budgeting for executive, accounting, HR, treasury, IT, and legal departments.

Creating this budget requires consideration of multiple factors, including: employee compensation, the largest portion of this budget; historical basis, or using numbers from a previous year (these must be verified as changes may have occurred); step costs, for instance additional OR staffing during a period of expansion; zero-base analysis, which recreates the budget from the ground up and justifies the need for each expense.

Although administrative expenses are usually fixed within a certain range, they must be continuously reexamined as changes in other budgets can affect administrative costs.

Types of Budgets

Budgets can be prepared either from a top-down or a bottom-up approach. There are advantages to each. A top-down approach is generally quicker to implement and reflects exactly the goals of senior management. However, this type of budgeting is not as granular and may not capture all of the important information that would be added in a bottom-up budget. The bottom-up budget is more detailed but takes much more time and work to develop. The end-users are the individuals who contribute the information so this type of budget is much more specific. Consequently, it is also more expensive to create.

Traditional Line-Item Budget and Incremental Budgeting

With a traditional line-item budget, allowable spending inputs are placed on salaries, benefits, supplies and other categories. Similar to this is the incremental budgeting process where each category of funds in the budget is assumed to be approximately that of the prior budgetary period.

Incremental budgets are not as labor and time intensive as other budgeting techniques. The primary advantage of this budgeting technique is its ease of creation and the basic understanding needed to interpret the data. However, there are several disadvantages to this approach. In using adjusted historical numbers, future budgets are created automatically with little review. As a result, inefficiencies and budgetary slack are carried forward. Departments and managers intentionally overestimate expenses and underestimate revenues so that their budget will not be reduced in the next budgetary cycle.

Large changes in budget requirements are often overlooked and resource allocations to certain areas are perpetuated, regardless of whether or not it is required. Risk taking is not accounted for with this technique, as there is little room for new activities or ventures to take place. Consequently, this type of budget may misallocate funds to underperforming units and not allow the organization the capital it needs to invest in new, novel initiatives [5, 6].

Zero-Based Budgeting

Zero-based budgeting [7] is a process that calls for a top-to-bottom analysis of budgeted expenditures and requires the justification of each item in the budget. The budget is then created, based *not* upon historical allocations but on what is actually needed regardless of prior funding. This is the opposite of the more traditional incremental budgeting, which involves minor adjustments to historical values.

Peter Pyhrr of Texas Instruments (TI) is considered the "father of zero-based budgeting," using it at TI in 1962 and then writing about it in *Harvard Business Review* in 1970. Subsequently, Jimmy Carter used this process while governor of Georgia and then implemented it throughout government agencies when he became president.

A zero-based budget can eliminate excess spending and help an enterprise focus on key business objectives for the given budgetary period. However, direct costs of goods or services are one area that falls outside of this analysis. Direct costs are only incurred once a sale (or, in healthcare, a revenue generating event) has taken place.

Developing a zero-base budget involves several key elements:

1. *Develop* decision packages, which give management the information needed to rank one business activity against another. Information to consider includes:
   i. Purpose of the activity
   ii. Business consequence of not performing it
   iii. Alternatives to performing that activity
   iv. Costs and benefits of the activity
   v. Performance metrics related to it

Guidelines for package development involve taking into account product, or service, changes, geographical areas to target (or out of OR locations to serve), facility size, and number of staff.

2. *Rank* decision packages in order from most to least important. Preliminary rankings are most often done by lower level managers, as they are most intimately knowledgeable about the on goings of their division. Senior level management takes these opinions into account when deciding where to allocate funds or make changes.

Zero-based budgeting helps managers focus on, and identify, key business activities and maintain the mission of the business. By ensuring that each expense is justified in its use, budgets are also controlled for inflation and wasteful spending. While doing these things requires a lot of time and effort, it is prudent to continuously review a business' dealings so as to ensure critical areas of the business receive the funds that they need and waste is reduced

Performance-Based Budgeting

Performance-based budgeting (PBB) attempts to link inputs to outcomes [8, 9]. This budgetary methodology has typically been utilized in the public sector. However, with the advent of corporate performance management the goals and objectives of an organization are detailed and measurements and tools are developed to measure performance (key performance indicators [KPIs]). For healthcare, with its obvious emphasis on outcomes, this

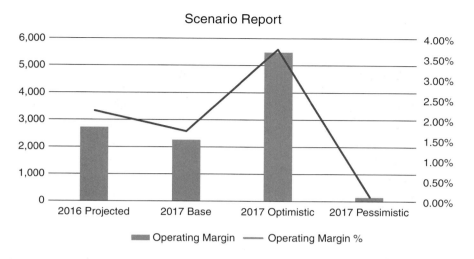

Figure 17.5 Scenario projections.

budgetary technique has obvious implications, linking strategy and planning as it does.

Advantages of PBB are considered to be increased accountability, better performance management and improved resource allocation [10]. It is suggested that managers use the KPIs from PBB to improve operational efficiency instead of using it as a punitive technique. For a competitive non–public sector marketplace, however, the utility of this budget technique remains to be demonstrated.

Operating Without a Budget

A growing number of organizations – initially outside of healthcare and now within healthcare – have recognized that the traditional budgeting process has grown too time and cost intensive for the return that it yields for the organization. Furthermore, the information that an annual budget produces is often not useful to management by the time it is actually finalized. Planning cycles now stretch out beyond 5 years (20+ quarters) and while the level of detail required by management to make certain actions may not be that which is seen in a traditional annual budget, the pairing of strategic planning and budgeting has become more important. Finally, computer systems have significantly increased their capacity to perform "what-if" scenario evaluation so that the consequences of various decisions can be weighted.

All of these factors have led a growing number of organizations to rethink the utility of the annual budget [11–14]. Some healthcare organizations have made the decision to operate without a budget [15]. They have reallocated some of the time and funds that previously were used to create annual budgets into creating rolling forecasts that allow the organization to ensure that financial performance is in line with the strategic plan. This technique also allows continuous feedback between operations and finance [16–19].

Advantages of rolling forecasting include:

- Improve efficiency by pushing organizational change
- Reduce funds and time expended to create the annual budget
- Emphasize continuous performance improvement
- Agility to changes in the healthcare marketplace increased
- Ensure that forecasting is always current
- Extends the planning horizon.

To create a rolling forecast, an organization:

1. Creates its strategic plan
   - Determines capital allocations
   - Creates targets for operating margins, volume, cost, profitability
   - Consider alternative outcomes (what-if scenarios)
     - Reimbursement decreases
     - Increases or decreases in patient volume (competition)
     - Loss of specialty group
     - FTEs
     - Payer mix changes

2. Determines how to organize high-level units for monitoring (i.e., service lines versus clinical specialty)
   - Identify KPIs for each service line
   - Information delivered to appropriate party at the right time.
     - Executives receive higher level KPIs and Dashboards
     - Directors receive consolidated results, outliers, explanations
     - Managers received detailed reports

Budgeting Procedures

To create an annual budget it is important that every party contributing to the budget package receive strict timelines for submission of information. While the budget can be created with certain items outstanding, it cannot go forward with most items missing, e.g.,

- Revenue
- Compensation
- Capital
- Research and development

Each department must contribute its forecasts for all budget elements. This includes revenue projections, compensation categories including bonus and benefits, capital requirements and funds to be devoted to R & D. The rationale of the budgetary model must be reviewed for both ongoing applicability and errors in assumptions.

Once the budget has assimilated all new data and checked for validity it is then submitted to senior management for approval. Once approved, a traditional year-long budget is the operating blueprint for the organization and variances are measured against this budget for the next year.

Budget Reporting

Whether an annual or a rolling budget is prepared, regardless of the amount of detail involved, management requires an ongoing estimation of performance of the organization, department or unit against projections. Consequently, some data collection system is absolutely essential to compare budget or projected results against actual results.

Variances are reported as both absolute numbers and also as percentages of the total category. Variances can be displayed either in tabular form (variance from monthly projection) or graphically, allowing

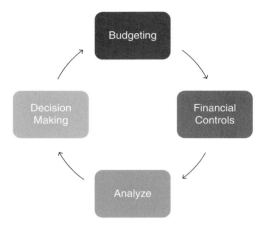

Figure 17.6 Scenario projections.

assimilation of large amounts of data, to illustrate the cumulative divergence from budget targets.

Budgeting Controls

Before a budget is finalized, it undergoes numerous changes. As a result, within any company, there may be more than one version of the budget. Ensuring that everyone is on the same page requires some budgeting controls. Some simple controls include labeling the final version as "FINAL" and creating document protections so that it cannot be tampered with.

Integration controls can help mitigate any problems with the budget not being used; for instance, including budgeted forecasts when reporting actual results and mentioning it during performance appraisals.

The process of budgeting controls may be represented as in Figure 17.6.

Summary

Budgeting is a critical element in conserving and deploying resources for departmental and hospital management. With the reduction in operating margins for hospitals it has become more imperative to make realistic assumptions about anticipated revenues and expenses for all healthcare entities. While budgets used to be static documents, frequently created once a year with great time and expense, now more nimble, strategically important assumptions are made with time projections much further into the future. Familiarity with these changes in budgetary techniques will be a useful tool for individuals involved in departmental and hospital management.

References

1. *Five approaches to effective budgeting and forecasting in healthcare.* axiomEPM, 2016. www.hfma.org/brg/pdf/ Ebook%205%20approaches%20to%20effective%20 budgeting%20in%20healthcare-final.pdf

2. *A primer on hospital accounting and finance for trustees and other healthcare professionals* (4th ed.). Kaufman Hall, 2009. http://dhss.alaska.gov/ahcc/Documents/ meetings/201306/PrimerHospAcctFinance4thEd.pdf.

3. NIH grant application. https://grants.nih.gov/grants/ forms/all-forms-and-formats.htm

4. http://med.stanford.edu/anesthesia/research/funding .html

5. *Does your budgeting process lack accountability? How effectively you monitor variances will tell you.* Kaufman Hall, 2016. www.kaufmanhall.com/resources/ does-your-budgeting-process-lack-accountability-0

6. Newbert A, Sutton J. Has the annual budget outlived its usefulness? February 23, 2016. Healthcare Connection, Crowe Horwath.

7. Pyhrr PH, Zero-base budgeting. *Harvard Business Review* 1970; 48(6): 111–21.

8. Yaisawarng S, Burgess JF. Performance-based budgeting in the public sector: An illustration from the VA health care system. *Health Economics* 2006; 15(3): 295–310.

9. Robinson M, Duncan L. A basic model of performance-based budgeting. International Monetary Fund, Fiscal Affairs Department. Technical Notes and Manuals 2009, 09/01: 1–16.

10. Birshan M, Engel M, Sibony O. Avoiding the quicksand: Ten techniques for more agile corporate resource allocation. *McKinsey Quarterly* 2013. www.mckinsey .com/business-functions/strategy-and-corporate- finance/our-insights/avoiding-the-quicksand

11. The World Bank, Poverty Reduction and Economic Management Network (PREM) notes. February 2003, 78: 1–4.

12. Akten MGM, Scheiffele MA. Just-in-time budgeting for a volatile economy. *Mckinsey Quarterly* 2009. www.mckinsey.com/business-functions/ strategy-and-corporate-finance/our-insights/ just-in-time-budgeting-for-a-volatile-economy

13. Meyers R. Budgets on a roll. *Journal of Accountancy* 2001. www.journalofaccountancy.com/issues/2001/ dec/budgetsonaroll.html

14. Miller D, Fau AM, Fau SS, Hackman T. How rolling forecasting facilitates dynamic, agile planning. *Healthcare Financial Management* 2013; 67(11): 80–2, 84.

15. Ellison A. This health system threw out its annual budget – Here's why. *Becker's Hospital Review*. www .beckershospitalreview.com/finance/this-health- system-threw-out-its-annual-budget-here-s-why .html

16. Berger S. Knowing the limitations: Rolling forecasts and hospital financial planning. *Healthcare Insights*. http://blog.hcillc.com/blog/knowing-the-limitations- rolling-forecasts-and-hospital-financial-planning

17. Teach E. No time for budgets: Yesterday's budgets are too slow for today's volatile world. Here's how to pick up the planning pace. May 27, 2014. ww2.cfo.com/ budgeting/2014/05/time-budgets/

18. Zeller TL, Metzger LM. Good bye traditional budgeting, hello rolling forecast: Has the time come? *American Journal of Business Education* 2013; 6(3): 299.

19. Johnson H. Rolling budgets catching on: More efficient and flexible forecasting tools. *Crain's New York Business* 2011. www.crainsnewyork.com/article/20110731/SUB/ 307319999/rolling-budgets-catching-on

Chapter

18

Preoperative Evaluation and Management

Alicia G. Kalamas

Contents

Physician-directed preoperative clinics underpin the success of a patient's journey through the surgical continuum of care. These clinics not only allow for early identification and mitigation of perioperative risk [1–3], but also have been shown to improve hospital resource utilization [4, 5]; enhance patient satisfaction [6]; reduce duration of hospital stay [7, 8]; mitigate operating room (OR) delays and cancellations [9, 10]; facilitate medication reconciliation [11]; and potentially reduce in-hospital mortality [12].

In this chapter we discuss six topics: (1) components of comprehensive preoperative risk assessment; (2) various models for the delivery of preoperative care; (3) value of early remote triage; (4) nuts and bolts for starting a preoperative clinic; (5) economics of preoperative evaluation and management; and (6) embracing the preoperative clinic.

Components of Comprehensive Preoperative Risk Assessment

There is growing recognition that proper preoperative preparation goes well beyond the anesthesiologist's assessment of anesthetic risk. With the advent of new anesthesia techniques, innovative drugs, enhanced training, pulse oximetry, and capnography, anesthesia-related mortality risk has declined sharply over the past 40 years. Contemporary estimates of mortality solely attributable to anesthesia are quite low (1 in 100,000) [13]. Conversely, all-cause 30-day surgical mortality for elective non–day surgery approaches 1 in 50 [14]. Understanding and identifying the factors that contribute to patient perioperative risks is the first step towards proper preoperative preparation.

Risks associated with surgical hospitalization can be divided into four categories: (1) patient factors; (2) surgical factors; (3) anesthetic management; and (4) care coordination. The overarching goal of preoperative evaluation and management, therefore, is to identify risk factors from within these categories; implement risk mitigation strategies; and communicate information broadly to all members of the healthcare team in a systematized fashion.

Patient Factors

For several comorbid conditions, a robust literature exists to define the effect of a given patient risk factor on outcomes. For example, multiple risk indices have been developed to predict major adverse cardiac events (e.g., myocardial infarct; sudden cardiac death). One of the most widely used indices is the Revised Cardiac Risk Index (RCRI). The RCRI includes five patient risk factors with approximately equal prognostic importance: coronary artery disease; congestive heart failure; history of cerebral vascular accident (stroke or TIA); diabetes; and renal insufficiency. The presence of ≥2 of these factors has been shown to identify patients at moderate (7%) and high (11%) risk for postoperative cardiac complications. Furthermore, patients with at least three of these factors have an increased risk for cardiovascular complications during the ensuing 6 months, even if they do not experience major cardiac complications during their surgical hospitalization [15].

Tools such as the RCRI, therefore, not only allow for identification of candidates for whom further testing (e.g., stress tests) or other management strategies (e.g., perioperative beta blockade) may be beneficial, but also allow for identification of low-risk patients for whom additional evaluation or management is unlikely to be helpful (and may in fact be harmful).

Similarly, several patient-related factors such as chronic obstructive pulmonary disease, age older than 60 years, American Society of Anesthesiologists (ASA) class of II or higher, functional dependence, obstructive sleep apnea, and congestive heart failure have been shown to increase the risk for postoperative pulmonary complications. Postoperative pulmonary complications play a significant role in overall morbidity and mortality in patients undergoing non-day surgery. Consequently, early identification of at-risk patients allows for targeted and timely implementation of evidence-based risk-reduction strategies, including preoperative inspiratory muscle training, incentive spirometry, deep breathing exercises, and neuroaxial blockade [16, 17].

Identification and optimization of diabetes is one of the most important goals of a preoperative clinic, as several large-scale clinical trials have established a link between poor glycemic control, postoperative complications, hospital length of stay and mortality [18–23]. Preoperative clinics, when properly utilized, can be leveraged to coordinate all stakeholders (primary care provider, endocrinologist, anesthesiologist, surgeon, and hospitalist) to ensure adequate pre-, intra-, and postoperative glycemic control. Importantly, referral to a preoperative clinic for comprehensive management of an elevated HbA1c was shown to reduce the incidence of prolonged hospitalization and complication rates during the first year after surgery in patients undergoing elective total joint arthroplasty [24].

Many of the commonly used tools for predicting perioperative risk have substantial limitations as they are based on single organ systems and do not take a patient's physiologic reserve into consideration. Yet an aging population has led to increased numbers of older patients presenting for surgical evaluation with tremendous heterogeneity in terms of overall health status and ability to withstand stress. While there is no standardized method for assessing physiologic

reserves, the concept of frailty has been introduced as a phenotype characterized by age-associated declines in lean body mass, strength, and endurance [25]. Several studies have shown that frailty independently predicts postoperative complications, length of stay, discharge to a skilled or assisted living facility, and mortality [26–28]. Newer assessment tools have been developed and validated including the Hopkins Frailty Score and Fried frailty criteria and may prove beneficial when weighing the risks and benefits of surgery and engaging patients and their families in shared decision making [29].

While documentation and optimization of existing medical conditions is paramount, equally important is identification of those previously unrecognized conditions that may impact a patient's perioperative course (e.g., obstructive sleep apnea [OSA]). This is not to suggest, however, that "routine" testing of all presurgical patients is justifiable, either medically or financially. Rather, a proper health history coupled with screening questionnaires such as those used for detecting OSA (e.g., STOP-Bang questionnaire) are valuable tools to help guide the appropriate ordering of diagnostic, rather than screening tests [30]. Screening tests in presurgical patients are time consuming, costly, and false-positive results expose patients to risky and unwarranted additional assessments [31, 32].

Surgical Factors

While patient factors play a significant role in predicting postoperative complications, predictions of postoperative outcome must also take into account the invasiveness of the proposed surgical procedure. Every surgical procedure elicits a stress response, initiated by direct tissue injury, pain, and anxiety. This response sets off a predictable cascade of physiologic and metabolic events (tachycardia, hypertension, fever, immunosuppression, protein catabolism, and water retention) through direct activation of the sympathetic nervous system and hypothalamic-pituitary-adrenal axis. The severity of this stress response, which begins with induction of anesthesia and peaks postoperatively, is directly related to the extent and duration of the surgical procedure.

The vast majority of surgical procedures can be considered safe (mortality risk of <1%). However, there is a >200-fold difference in the incidence of all-cause death between the highest- and lowest-risk surgeries, with the most invasive and lengthy procedures associated with the greatest risk of adverse outcome (e.g., vascular surgery adjusted adverse outcome incidence of 5.97% compared to only 0.07% for breast surgery). Hence for purposes of risk stratification, the traditional classification of surgical procedures as high or low risk appears inappropriate. Fortunately, a recently published observational population-based study of 3.7 million surgical procedures in the Netherlands provides a detailed and contemporary overview of postoperative mortality for the entire surgical spectrum [33] The results of this study may eventually serve as a reference standard for surgical outcome in Western populations.

Anesthetic Management

Morbidity and mortality are rarely attributable directly to anesthesia. However, there are several anesthesia-related factors beyond the choice of anesthetic agents that must be taken into consideration when safely preparing a patient for surgery. Both the safety of the anesthetizing location and selection of anesthetic provider are critical components of any perioperative risk mitigation strategy.

The demand for anesthesia care in support of procedures performed outside the OR (out-of-OR) has dramatically increased in recent years. While these procedures are relatively straightforward and often minimally invasive, the delivery of safe out-of-OR anesthesia is complicated by a variety of factors – cramped dark rooms, unfamiliar surroundings, and fewer supporting staff and resources relative to OR suites. All of these factors can lead to delays in recognition and treatment of respiratory depression, offer poor access to the patient, and place patients at increased risk for catastrophic consequences. Data from the ASA Closed Claims Project demonstrates that monitored anesthesia care in remote locations poses a seven-fold risk of oversedation and inadequate oxygenation/ventilation compared to the OR. Similarly, the severity of patient injury is greater in remote locations, with the proportion of death directly attributable to anesthesia almost double that seen in the OR [34].

Awareness and vigilance can minimize the risk of patient injury in these challenging settings. However, this requires careful identification of patients at highest risk for adverse events (e.g., OSA, morbidly obese, elderly, debilitated patients). Unfortunately

there is a frequent misperception that out-of-OR procedures are "benign" in nature. In addition, there is often a failure to recognize that patients treated in remote locations tend to be older, sicker, and more likely in need of emergent care than patients receiving care in OR settings.

A specific out-of-OR location that warrants special consideration is the freestanding surgical center. Freestanding surgical centers are not connected to a hospital and therefore access to both specialized medical resources and emergency care is limited. For these reasons certain patient populations are not suitable candidates for these surgical suites, as immediate access to *all* available health resources must be assured for even the most minor of procedures. Based on data collected through the National Survey of Ambulatory Surgery by the Centers for Disease Control, almost half of ambulatory surgery visits in the United States occur in freestanding centers each year [35].

As the obesity epidemic and aging US population expand, so too will the demand for surgical services in freestanding surgical centers and other remote locations. For both obese and aged patients, the presence of multiple chronic diseases demands heightened awareness of the location of, staffing models for, and resources available to out-of-OR care settings as part of any comprehensive perioperative risk mitigation strategy.

Care Coordination

The surgical episode of care is unfortunately highly fragmented. This is due in large part to care provision via disparate services and providers. Consequently, information that originates with the patient subsequently flows along many pathways to physicians, nurses, pharmacists, and other care providers. Despite large investments in information technology, providing the correct information, when needed, to the appropriate care providers continues to be problematic. As a result, failures of information transfer and communication errors among care providers can lead to mistakes in care provision and patient harm [36]. To compound this issue, communication deficits are not discrete events; namely, information loss in one phase of care can potentially compromise safety in a downstream phase of patient care.

While effective and standardized communication among healthcare professionals during the perioperative period has been shown to facilitate surgical safety

[37], few organizations have developed a systematized approach to ensure essential information is preserved. Integrated care pathways (ICPs) – also known as multidisciplinary pathways of care, care maps, and collaborative care pathways – offer one such approach for standardized communication. First introduced in the early 1990s in the UK, ICPs are structured, multidisciplinary plans of care for patients with similar diagnoses or symptoms [38]. The ICP specifies the interventions required for the patient to progress along the continuum of care. In addition, the ICP delineates these interventions against a timeframe (measured in hours, days, or weeks) and/or patient care milestones designed to support clinical management. ICPs are inherently "patient-focused," as they view the delivery of care in terms of the patient's journey through the system and place emphasis on the coordination of care across different disciplines and sectors.

In practical terms, the ICP can act as the single record of care, with all members of the multidisciplinary team required to record their input into the ICP document. This documentation also provides each healthcare professional with information about the patient's condition over the course of therapy and beyond (e.g., referral back to primary care physician). ICPs are designed explicitly to ensure that no step in a care continuum (e.g., management of anticoagulation therapy) is missed. To accomplish this, ICPs codify the foreseeable clinical actions that represent best practice for most patients most of the time. They also include prompts for care providers to confirm critical steps have been completed at each appropriate point in the care continuum. A few large integrated health systems such as Intermountain HealthCare [39] and Geisinger [40] have successfully implemented care pathways with substantial clinical and financial benefit.

Development of comprehensive care pathways can be a daunting task, involving buy-in from several stakeholders (e.g., surgery, anesthesia, nursing, hospital administration) and until recently few organizations have developed and implemented ICPs. However, changing reimbursement structures are challenging physicians and hospitals to embrace patient-centered care models designed to improve quality and to reduce the cost of care. One such care model, the perioperative surgical home (PSH), is an innovative practice model that has been proposed by the ASA [41].

The PSH is a continuum of patient-centered care coordinated by a multidisciplinary team focused on standardization and coordination throughout the perioperative period, including postdischarge. ICPs, developed and shared by all stakeholders, will be central to the success of this effort.

With regard to the surgical episode of care, the preoperative assessment is the natural point of entry into an ICP. Consider, for example, a patient on Coumadin who requires perioperative use of bridging anticoagulation (e.g., Lovenox) to prevent thromboembolism. Proper management of this patient requires (1) discontinuation of Coumadin preop; (2) initiation of Lovenox preop; (3) discontinuation of Lovenox 24 h prior to surgery; (4) lab draw day-of-surgery to verify International Normalized Ratio (INR) is normalized; (5) reinitiation of therapeutic Lovenox and Coumadin postop; (6) daily INR measurements; (7) discontinuation of Lovenox when the patient is therapeutic on Coumadin; and (8) follow-up with the patient's primary care provider to ensure the patient's INR is stable on the reinitiated Coumadin dose. Failure to initiate any one of the above mentioned steps at the appropriate point in time could have grave consequences.

In order to initiate cross-disciplinary and longitudinal planning for surgical patients (as outlined above), Dr. Angela Bader and her colleagues at the preoperative clinic at Brigham and Woman's Hospital have effectively used email communication with patients' healthcare providers to facilitate critical discussions, workup new clinical findings, and initiate conversations on goals of care. They found that communication via email was a highly effective means for alerting all stakeholders to the patient's current health status and creating a forum to allow for asynchronous discussion among busy providers [42]. As such, preoperative clinics are perfectly positioned to facilitate information exchange among providers, integrate recommendations into a comprehensive perioperative plan, and serve as the cornerstone of a successful PSH model.

Various Models for the Delivery of Preoperative Care

Surgical patients, even those with significant comorbidities, are seldom admitted to the hospital in advance of their procedure for preoperative care. Instead, preoperative assessment and risk management occur in the outpatient setting for the vast majority of patients. Four models for preoperative assessments exist: (1) the patient visits a preoperative clinic days in advance of their procedure; (2) a telephone interview is the sole basis for the evaluation; (3) the patient is seen by the primary care provider; or (4) an evaluation is performed at bedside, day-of-surgery, in the preoperative holding area. Each of these approaches has merit for subsets of patients, but none is appropriate for all patients all of the time given patient heterogeneity.

Preoperative Clinics

Physician-directed preoperative clinics devoted exclusively to the preoperative evaluation of patients allow for comprehensive patient assessment. The focus of these clinics is to evaluate risk by taking into account the patient, the procedure, and anesthesia-related factors. In addition, these clinics typically have system-based processes in place to facilitate coordination of care across the entire surgical care continuum. That is, physician-directed preoperative clinics focus not only on identifying perioperative risk but also on implementing risk mitigation strategies and communicating this information to the entire healthcare team.

Not surprisingly, these clinics allow for early identification and mitigation of perioperative risk. In addition, they have been shown to improve hospital resource utilization by reducing unnecessary preoperative consults and laboratory tests; enhancing patient satisfaction; reducing duration of hospital stay; mitigating OR delays and cancellations due to inadequate assessment or patient preparation; facilitating medication reconciliation, and potentially reducing in-hospital mortality. However, performing an exhaustive in-person evaluation for every patient prior to the day of surgery is cost prohibitive and unnecessary.

Telephone Interviews

The majority of hospitals and surgical centers do not have dedicated preoperative clinics due to the substantial costs associated with sizable staff and physical space requirements. Instead they rely upon telephone interviews typically conducted by Registered Nurses (RNs). This approach is less costly, but has several shortcomings: (1) overreliance on formulaic questionnaires that are not specific to the particular patient's situation; (2) failure to capture the breadth and depth of information required to properly assess risk; and (3) consumption of an unnecessary amount

of time and clinical resources. In addition, phone interviews typically occur the day before surgery, leaving little time to properly address perioperative risk. This model relies heavily on mid-level providers to merely *collect* information without adequate processes in place to order the appropriate diagnostic tests, follow through on risk management, optimize patient outcomes, and reduce adverse events.

Primary Care Providers

Primary care providers are often asked by surgeons to evaluate and "clear" a patient for surgery. The goal of this evaluation is to determine the risk of the proposed procedure to the patient and to optimize management of preexisting medical conditions. Primary care providers, however, are often ill-prepared to comment on several of the non–patient-related risks that one may encounter during a surgical admission. A patient's primary medical provider may be well suited to assess and optimize that patient's medical conditions, but may be less familiar with the specifics of the procedure itself. These include anesthetic considerations and the systems-related issues that may pose risk to patients (e.g., monitoring on the wards for patients with obstructive sleep apnea). Consequently, a dangerous misconception exists; namely, the belief that when a primary care provider has "cleared" a patient for surgery, the patient can automatically be assumed to be a good candidate for anesthesia, the surgical procedure, and all risks associated with the surgical episode of care.

To complicate matters, providers who are unsure of what is expected from them during this preoperative assessment often order myriad tests such as blood work, EKGs, chest x-rays, and cardiac stress tests out of concern for "missing something." However, it is now appreciated that extensive routine testing is not justifiable, either medically or financially, and an excessively aggressive approach to preoperative testing may lead to specious, risky, and unwarranted assessments. This likely explains why medical consultation by physicians not specifically trained in perioperative evaluation and management has been shown to be associated with increased mortality and hospital stay [43].

Day-of-Surgery

Delaying the preoperative evaluation until the day-of-surgery creates a potentially dangerous situation; namely, an inherent bias to downplay perioperative risk factors such that surgery can proceed as planned. There are several reasons for this: a medical team that is intent on proceeding with their case; an OR suite and staff that have been mobilized; and a nervous patient who has mentally prepared for and made work and home-life arrangements to accommodate the surgery. Fortunately most healthcare delivery systems within the United States recognize the inherent dangers and financial consequences of delaying preoperative assessment to the day-of-surgery. Consequently, this model is not commonly employed.

There is widespread disagreement regarding the best model for delivering preoperative care because none of the approaches described above optimizes for the individual needs of each patient. Collectively these approaches result in a subset of patients who are not appropriately evaluated for perioperative risk and another subset of patients who are unnecessarily subjected to exhaustive evaluations and diagnostic tests that are not indicated. The answer to optimal preoperative assessment for all patients lies in careful triage based on each patient's medical history. Such triage can identify those patients in need of aggressive preoperative management and those who can safely proceed to surgery with minimal management.

Value of Early Remote Triage

While there is no consensus on the optimal approach to preoperative assessments, there is widespread acceptance that certain patient populations are more likely than others to benefit from an in-person clinic visit and/or diagnostic testing. Healthy patients with no/low perioperative risk can be safely "fast-tracked" to the day-of-surgery with little hospital staff intervention. Patients with modifiable risk factors should ideally be identified far enough in advance (e.g., proximate to the time of surgical scheduling) to allow ample opportunity to intervene in a meaningful way. The challenge to date has been finding a system that allows for accurate triage of those presurgical patients who require intense preoperative clinical resources – lengthy phone calls, in-person visits, diagnostic testing – and those who do not.

To facilitate presurgical patient triage, many hospitals rely on RN-initiated phone-based interviews. These interviews use static preformulated questionnaires to elicit the patient's preoperative medical history. Unfortunately, the static nature of these questionnaires makes it difficult for the nurses administering them to capture the breadth and depth of information required for proper triage. Consequently, it is common that important elements of the patient's medical history are missed by RN phone triage and only identified upon further questioning on the day-of-surgery. Two studies have shown that nurses are better at 'ruling out' patients who did not need additional assessment rather than 'ruling in' patients who need to be seen [44, 45]. Such omissions leave patients vulnerable to adverse events; result in day-of-surgery delays and cancellations; and do not effectively tailor the intensity of preoperative assessment to each patient's needs. In turn this leads to suboptimal care, low patient satisfaction, and excess cost.

To overcome some of the shortcomings inherent in the manual capture of patient medical histories by clinicians, Dr. Michael Roizen developed one of the first computer software programs for preoperative assessment, Health Quiz, in the early 1990s [46]. However, the slower-than-anticipated adoption of the electronic health record (EMR) markedly inhibited the success of Health Quiz. Since that time many authors have validated the use of automated techniques to gather health histories and have found a low discrepancy when comparing the outputs generated by an automated questionnaire with those gathered via person-to-person interviews.

Building upon the Health Quiz concept, the Cleveland Clinic created HealthQuest in the late 1990s as a "home grown" solution. HealthQuest is an outpatient preoperative evaluation computer program designed to triage presurgical patients. Patients are administered a computer based questionnaire. Responses to questions are coded to create a HealthQuest Score, using a scale of 1 (healthy) to 4 (multiple complex medical issues). The HealthQuest Score is used to guide the timing and level of required preoperative evaluation. This triage system was tested over a 3-year period in 63,941 outpatient surgical patients. Of these, 22,744 (35.6%) did not require a visit with a healthcare provider prior to the day-of-surgery, as guided by the computer assigned HealthQuest Score and surgical classification scheme. In addition, patient interview time, patient dissatisfaction with the preoperative process, and the average monthly surgical delay rate all decreased during the study period [47]. While The Cleveland Clinic continues to reap enormous benefits from triaging their patients using HealthQuest, most institutions do not have the manpower nor surgical volume to support

A stepwise approach to determining the timing and nature of the preoperative assessment for elective non-cardiac surgery

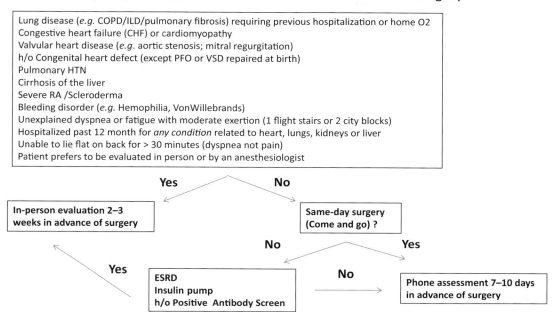

Lung disease (*e.g.* COPD/ILD/pulmonary fibrosis) requiring previous hospitalization or home O2
Congestive heart failure (CHF) or cardiomyopathy
Valvular heart disease (*e.g.* aortic stenosis; mitral regurgitation)
h/o Congenital heart defect (except PFO or VSD repaired at birth)
Pulmonary HTN
Cirrhosis of the liver
Severe RA /Scleroderma
Bleeding disorder (*e.g.* Hemophilia, VonWillebrands)
Unexplained dyspnea or fatigue with moderate exertion (1 flight stairs or 2 city blocks)
Hospitalized past 12 month for *any condition* related to heart, lungs, kidneys or liver
Unable to lie flat on back for > 30 minutes (dyspnea not pain)
Patient prefers to be evaluated in person or by an anesthesiologist

Yes — No

In-person evaluation 2–3 weeks in advance of surgery

Same-day surgery (Come and go) ?

No — Yes

Yes

ESRD
Insulin pump
h/o Positive Antibody Screen

No

Phone assessment 7–10 days in advance of surgery

Figure 18.1 A stepwise approach to determining the timing and nature of the preoperative assessment for elective noncardiac surgery.

development and maintenance of such a sophisticated "home grown" software solution.

Perhaps the two most important elements of a preoperative health history are a *current* medication list and a *current* review of systems. Data within EMRs, however, are highly perishable and therefore cannot be relied upon for making perioperative management decisions. Eliciting up-to-date information directly from the patient can be quite time consuming. While it is widely recognized that using mid-level providers as scribes is not an effective use of healthcare resources, little emphasis has been placed on finding ways to directly engage patients in the process of clerical data entry. In fact, none of the commercially available hospital-wide EMRs has developed a patient portal capable of eliciting a *comprehensive* health history directly from the patient.

Unlike many other industries that have been revolutionized by the wave of self-service the Internet provides, medicine has lagged behind in its acceptance of the Web as a means for communication and, therefore, has been reluctant to enter the arena of web-based applications. However, the internet can be utilized as a telemedicine portal and there are a handful of commercially available web-based preoperative assessment tools. Many of these products are offered either on a per-click basis or for a nominal annual licensing fee, thus eliminating the large upfront and ongoing maintenance costs typical of traditional hardware and software based information technology products [48–50]. That notwithstanding, web-based assessment tools have yet to be widely accepted and adopted.

In the meantime, organizations can use paper-based questionnaires that can be self-administered at the time of the surgical visit to determine the nature and timing of the preoperative assessment (in-person versus phone consultation). See Figure 18.1.

Nuts and Bolts for Starting a Physician-Directed Preoperative Clinic

The first step in planning a preoperative clinic is to define the clinic's mission. In its most robust form, a preoperative clinic should be designed to identify and mitigate *all* risk factors that impact a patient's surgical hospitalization. In essence, a well-functioning preoperative clinic serves as the epicenter for the surgical episode

Box 18.1. Operational Goals of Physician-Directed Preoperative Clinic

1. Triage ALL surgical patients proximate to their initial surgical consultation to determine need for in-person evaluation versus phone consultation (Figure 18.1)

2. Retrieve all relevant health records (e.g., cardiac) prior to formal preoperative evaluation

3. Make contact with all surgical patients no less than 7 days prior to scheduled surgical date (to ensure adequate time for medication management, etc.)

4. Perform a comprehensive risk assessment taking into account the 4 broad sources of risk

5. Determine need for further testing/subspecialty consultation

6. Develop a strategy aimed at optimizing patient's preexisting medical conditions/mitigating perioperative risk

7. Communicate findings with surgeon and primary care provider/agree upon plan that will carry patient through entire surgical hospitalization

8. Codify plan in the form of a document (e.g., care plan) that will follow patient throughout and beyond surgical hospitalization

9. Educate patient

of care. For this to occur, however, representatives from hospital administration, surgery, anesthesia, and nursing must explicitly define and agree to the operational goals (Box 18.1) of the clinic and implement a standardized system for communicating information between any and all providers who will interact with patients during the surgical continuum of care.

Once the goals of the clinic have been defined, the clinic structure can be developed and individual roles delineated. A medical director should be appointed. Ideally this person will have a background in both anesthesia and internal medicine. Hospitalists are well suited for this position as well. In situations where hospitalists are used to staff a preoperative clinic, however, there should be a plan in place for immediate access to an anesthesia consultant should questions arise regarding anesthetic options, appropriateness of anesthetizing location, and/or airway management.

The clinic medical director is responsible for developing protocols, guidelines, and care pathways in conjunction with their surgical, medicine, and anesthesia colleagues. The medical director should also educate the residents and mid-level providers who staff the clinic day-to-day. In addition, a clinic manager (typically a RN) should be appointed to ensure there is adequate infrastructure and support for the administrative and nursing staff. Preregistration, laboratory work, and EKGs can either be performed within the clinic (one-stop shop) or patients can be directed to other parts of the hospital for these services.

Appointments should be scheduled only after the patient has been triaged. This triage should occur proximate to the patient's initial visit in the surgeon's office, thereby allowing ample time for medical optimization, required testing, and/or subspecialty consultation. Triage should be performed by a highly experienced nurse practitioner or physician assistant who can determine if additional information is required prior to formal perioperative risk assessment. Failure to make the correct triage decision or to secure relevant health records prior to formal evaluation has potentially negative consequences downstream – adverse outcomes, low clinic throughput, high cost, low patient satisfaction. Thus it is imperative that a robust triage system be in place and that triage is conducted by a highly experienced member of the preoperative assessment team. Once triaged, patients can be scheduled for either a phone consultation or in-person visit (where appointment duration is consistent with the complexity of the patient's care). When possible, patients should be evaluated a minimum of 7 days prior to their surgical date to ensure ample time for medication management.

At the time of formal evaluation, the health history and all pertinent medical records are reviewed. Additional tests or subspecialty consultation can be arranged and a formal risk assessment takes places. Patients suitable for care pathways or protocols are identified (e.g., obstructive sleep apnea, perioperative beta blockade) and special arrangements are made (e.g., move a diabetic to first case of the day; order STAT potassium day-of-surgery for a dialysis patient). Personal communication between the clinic Medical Director, surgeons, primary care providers, and the anesthesia consultant ensures that any questions or concerns regarding the patient's condition and appropriateness for surgery are discussed. This avoids day-of-surgery delays and potential cancellations secondary to questionable patient suitability for surgery.

Once risk has been assessed and a plan devised, this information must be communicated to all members of the healthcare team. This communication is often conducted via an EMR. Unfortunately, both progress notes and best practice alerts within EMRs are frequently overlooked. The alerts can result in a type of "fatigue" whereby the provider, after receiving too many alerts, begins to ignore and/or override the alerts. Prolonged alert fatigue can negatively impact patient care as important alerts may be ignored [51]. Introduction of checklists, on the other hand, has been associated with a significant decline in the rate of complications and death from surgery. While the exact mechanism of improvement is not known when a checklist-based program is in place, the evidence of improvement in surgical outcomes is substantial [52]. Therefore, the development and consistent use of patient checklists should serve as the foundation for and communication of a patient's perioperative management plan.

Once established, the perioperative plan must be effectively communicated to the patient. Patients should receive explicit information on medication management and pertinent information concerning the surgical process, including anticipated length of stay and probable outcomes. For communication of preoperative information to be effective, the information should be available in many forms, such as visual, auditory, or face-to-face education. Preoperative teaching has several well documented advantages, including decreased length of stay, less demand for analgesia postoperatively, and increased patient satisfaction [53, 54]. Despite the known benefits of patient education, this component of preoperative preparation is unfortunately often overlooked.

Economics of Preoperative Evaluation and Management

Given today's cost conscious environment, there are concerns about appropriate resource use in nonrevenue generating areas. Preoperative evaluation falls within this category for most hospital administrators. They view preoperative evaluation as a cost-intensive operation for which they receive no incremental reimbursement. That is, sending a patient through a preoperative clinic or phone-based preoperative evaluation is considered part of the surgical service provided by the hospital and therefore is bundled within the global reimbursement for the surgical fee. Consequently, the adoption of physician-directed preoperative clinics has been slow.

Physician-directed preoperative clinics, however, have consistently demonstrated value in excess of the cost of the evaluation itself via their impact on patients' health status; improved resource utilization; and reduced day-of-surgery delays and cancellations. In fact, use of physicians to evaluate patients and order indicated tests was shown to have the potential for reducing preoperative testing costs by several billion dollars without negatively affecting patient care.

Furthermore, inadequate preoperative evaluation is a contributory factor in adverse operative outcomes. Of the first 6,271 incidents reported to the Australian Incident Monitoring Study, 11 percent of the reports listed inadequate preoperative evaluation as a contributing factor. Well over half of the incidents were considered preventable. The investigators did not make an estimate of the economic impact of these adverse cases, but many of the adverse outcomes noted – case cancellation (5%), unexpected death (4%), prolonged hospitalization (7%), and use of intensive care facilities (9%) – are understood to rapidly consume resources [55].

In addition to realizing cost savings, proper preoperative preparation has the potential to generate incremental revenue for a hospital by justifying (1) increased disgonsis-related group reimbursements for co morbidities that would otherwise have been overlooked and (2) reimbursement for professional fees. "Usual preoperative care" as performed immediately prior to a procedure is not a billable service. However, physicians and physician extenders are entitled to separate reimbursement for professional fees if the service does not fall within the Medicare surgical global period. In addition, the following requirements must be met: (1) the consultation is being performed at the request of another practitioner seeking advice regarding evaluation and/or management of a specific problem; (2) the request for the consultation and the reason for the request are recorded in the patient's medical record; and (3) after the consultation is provided the practitioner prepares a written report of their findings.

Finally, as patients take on more responsibility for their healthcare decisions with the rise of consumerism, well executed preoperative evaluation can serve as a competitive differentiator for surgical providers. Given a patient's first encounter with a healthcare facility is often during a preoperative evaluation, it is imperative that hospitals and surgical centers critically assess patient experience and satisfaction during the preoperative evaluation process. Length of time waiting and overall time spent in a preoperative clinic correlate inversely with patient satisfaction. Long patient waiting times due to late start/finish of appointments are the result of poor triage, incomplete health information, suboptimal operational workflow, and poorly defined staff goals and incentives. Consequently, hospital administrators and preoperative clinic Medical Directors would be well served to mitigate these issues to ensure a positive patient experience.

Embracing the Preoperative Clinic

In today's competitive surgical environment, efficiency, quality, and patient satisfaction are important criteria by which consumers and their insurers select healthcare providers. Increasingly only those hospitals and surgical providers that deliver high quality care and high patient satisfaction at an affordable price will maintain their financial viability. Consequently, there is growing appreciation for the health and economic benefits of proper perioperative evaluation and management; yet hospitals and surgical providers continue to struggle with optimizing the flow of patients through the surgical episode of care. The solution to this dilemma lies in proper perioperative evaluation and management via physician-directed preoperative clinics.

Perioperative evaluation and management is complex and requires close coordination and cooperation between several members of a multidisciplinary team. Physician-directed preoperative clinics, when properly designed and managed, can achieve this coordination by serving as the epicenter for patients' surgical care, both inpatient and outpatient. The benefits these comprehensive clinics can offer are well documented, yet there adoption has been inhibited by the substantial investment of capital and ongoing operating expense they require. Fortunately, the costs of starting and managing these clinics can be substantially reduced through the use of best practice workflow techniques; timely, remote triage of patients to the right level of care; evidence-based perioperative management; and well-managed reimbursement. As such they should be embraced by clinicians, administrators, and patients alike for the important benefits they can deliver to surgical care.

References

1. Parker BM, Tetzlaff JE, Litaker DL, Maurer WG. Redefining the preoperative evaluation process and the role of the anesthesiologist. *J Clin Anesth* 2000; 12: 350–6.

2. Parsa P, Sweitzer B, Small SD. The contribution of a preoperative evaluation to patient safety in high-risk surgical patients: A pilot study (abstract). *Anesth Analg* 2004; 100: S147.

3. Correll DJ, Bader AM, Hull MW, Hsu C, Tsen LC, Hepner, DL. Value of preoperative clinic visits in identifying issues with potential impact on operating room efficiency *Anesthesiology* 2006; 105(6): 1254–9.

4. Fischer SP. Development and effectiveness of an anesthesia preoperative evaluation clinic in a teaching hospital. *Anesthesiology* 1996; 85: 190–206.

5. Tsen LC, Segal S, Pothier M, Hartley LH, Bader AM. The effect of alterations in a preoperative assessment clinic on reducing the number and improving the yield of cardiology consultations. *Anesth Analg* 2002; 95: 1563–8.

6. Hepner DL, Bader AM, Hurwitz S, Gustafson M, Tsen LC. Patient satisfaction with preoperative assessment in a preoperative assessment testing clinic. *Anesth Analg* 2004; 98: 1099–105.

7. Halaszynski TM, Juda R, Silverman DG. Optimizing postoperative outcomes with efficient preoperative assessment and management. *Crit Care Med* 2004; 32(suppl): S76–86.

8. Vazirani S, Lankarani-Fard A, Liang LJ, Stelzner M, Asch SM. Perioperative processes and outcomes after implementation of a hospitalist-run preoperative clinic. *J Hosp Med* 2012; 7(9): 697–701.

9. Ferschl TA, Sweitzer B, Huo D, Glick DB. Preoperative clinic visits reduce operating room cancellations and delays. *Anesthesiology* 2005; 103: 855–9.

10. Emanuel A, MacPherson R. The anaesthetic pre-admission clinic is effective in minimising surgical cancellation rates. *Anaesth Intensive Care* 2013; 41: 90–4.

11. van den Bemt PM, van den Broek S, van Nunen AK, Harbers JB, Lenderink AW. Medication reconciliation performed by pharmacy technicians at the time of preoperative screening. *Ann Pharmacotherapy* 2009; 43(5): 868–74.

12. Blitz JD, Kendale SM, Jain SK, Cuff GE, Kim JT, Rosenberg AD. Preoperative evaluation clinic visit is associated with decreased risk of in-hospital postoperative mortality. *Anesthesiology* 2016; 125(2): 280–94.

13. Guohua L. Epidemiology of anesthesia-related mortality in the United States, 1999–2005. *Anesthesiology* 2009; 110(4): 759–65.

14. Noordzij PG. Postoperative mortality in the Netherlands: A population-based analysis of

surgery-specific risk in adults. *Anesthesiology* 2010; 112: 1105–15.

15. Lee TH, Marcantonio ER, Mangione CM, et al. Derivation and prospective validation of a simple index for prediction of cardiac risk of major noncardiac surgery. *Circulation* 1999; 100: 1043–9.

16. Qaseem A, Snow V, Fitterman N, et al. Risk assessment for and strategies to reduce perioperative pulmonary complications for patients undergoing noncardiothoracic surgery: A guideline from the American College of Physicians. *Ann Intern Med.* 2006; 144: 575–80.

17. Katsura M, Kuriyama A, Takeshima T, Fukuhara S, Furukawa TA. Preoperative inspiratory muscle training for postoperative pulmonary complications in adults undergoing cardiac and major abdominal surgery. *Cochrane Database Syst Rev* 2015; 5(10).

18. Marchant MH Jr, Viens NA, Cook C, Vail TP, Bolognesi MP. The impact of glycemic control and diabetes mellitus on perioperative outcomes after total joint arthroplasty. *J Bone Joint Surg Am* 2009; 91(7): 1621–9.

19. Han HS, Kang SB. Relations between long-term glycemic control and postoperative wound and infectious complications after total knee arthroplasty in type 2 diabetics. *Clin Orthop Surg* 2013; 5(2): 118–23.

20. Miller JA, Webb MR, Benzel EC, Mroz T, Mayer E. Association between hemoglobin A1c and reoperation following spine surgery. *Neurosurgery* 2016; 63 Suppl 1: 193.

21. Guzman JZ, Iatridis JC, Skovrlj B, et al. Outcomes and complications of diabetes mellitus on patients undergoing degenerative lumbar spine surgery. *Spine* 2014; 39(19): 1596–604.

22. Walid MS, Newman BF, Yelverton JC, Nutter JP, Ajjan M, Robinson JS Jr. Prevalence of previously unknown elevation of glycosylated hemoglobin in spine surgery patients and impact on length of stay and total cost. *J Hosp Med* 2010; 5(1): E10–4.

23. Underwood P, Seiden J, Carbone K, et al. Early identification of individuals with poorly controlled diabetes undergoing elective surgery: Improving A1C testing in the preoperative period. *Endocr Pract* 2015; 21(3): 231–6.

24. Kallio PJ, Nolan J, Olsen AC, Breakwell S, Topp R, Pagel PS. Anesthesia preoperative clinic referral for elevated Hba1c reduces complication rate in diabetic patients undergoing total joint arthroplasty. *Anesth Pain Med* 2015; 5(3): e24376.

25. Fried LP, Tangen CM, Walston J, et al. Cardiovascular Health Study Collaborative Research Group. Frailty in older adults: Evidence for a phenotype. *J Gerontol A Biol Sci Med Sci* 2001; 56(3): M146–56.

26. Makary MA, Segev DL, Pronovost PJ, et al. Frailty as a predictor of surgical outcomes in older patients. *J Am Coll Surg* 2010; 210(6): 901–8.

27. Robinson TN, Wallace JI, Wu DS, et al. Accumulated frailty characteristics predict postoperative discharge institutionalization in the geriatric patient. *J Am Coll Surg* 2011; 213(1): 37–42.

28. McIsaac DI, Bryson GL, van Walraven C. Association of frailty and One-year postoperative mortality following major elective noncardiac surgery: A population-based cohort study. *JAMA Surg* 2016; 151(6): 538–45.

29. Revenig LM, Canter DJ, Taylor MD, et al. Too frail for surgery? Initial results of a large multidisciplinary prospective study examining preoperative variables predictive of poor surgical outcomes. *J Am Coll Surg* 2013; 217(4): 665–670.

30. Nagappa M, Wong J, Singh M, Wong DT, Chung F. An update on the various practical applications of the STOP-Bang questionnaire in anesthesia, surgery, and perioperative medicine. *Curr Opin Anaesthesiol* 2017; 30(1): 118–25.

31. Bryson GL, Wyand A, Bragg PR. Preoperative testing is inconsistent with published guidelines and rarely changes management. *Can J Anaesth* 2006; 53: 236–41.

32. Chung F, Yuan H, Yin L, Vairavanathan S, Wong DT. Elimination of preoperative testing in ambulatory surgery. *Anesth Analg* 2009; 108: 467–75.

33. Noordzij PG. Postoperative mortality in the Netherlands: A population-based analysis of surgery-specific risk in adults. *Anesthesiology* 2010; 112: 1105–15.

34. Metzner JI. Risks of anesthesia at remote locations. *ASA Newsletter* 2010; 74(2): 17–18.

35. National Survey of Ambulatory Surgery. www.cdc.gov/nchs/nsas/about_nsas.htm

36. Nagpal K. MRCS information transfer and communication in surgery. *Ann Surg* 2010; 252(2): 225–39.

37. Haynes AB, Weiser TG, Berry WR, et al. A surgical safety checklist to reduce morbidity and mortality in a global population. *N Engl J Med* 2009; 360: 491–9.

38. Middleton S. *Integrated care pathways: A practical approach to implementation.* Oxford: Butterworth-Heinemann, 2000.

39. Jimmerson C, Weber D, Sobek DK. Reducing waste and errors: Piloting lean principles at Intermountain

Healthcare. *Joint Commission Journal on Quality and Patient Safety* 2005; 31(5): 249–57.

40. Paulus RA, Davis K, Steele GD. Continuous innovation in health care: Implications of the Geisinger experience for health system reform. *Health Affairs* 2008; 27(5): 1235–45.

41. Kain ZN, Vakharia S, Garson L, et al. The perioperative surgical home as a future perioperative practice model. *Anesthesia & Analgesia* 2014; 118(5): 1126–30.

42. Chow VW, Hepner DL, Bader AM. Electronic care coordination from the preoperative clinic. *Anesth Analg* 2016; 123(6): 1458–62.

43. Wijeysundera DN. Outcomes and processes of care related to preoperative medical consultation. *Arch Intern Med* 2010; 170(15): 1365–74.

44. Vaghadia H, Fowler C. Can nurses screen all outpatients? Performance of a nurse based model. *Can J Anaesth* 1999; 46: 1117–21.

45. Barnes PK, Emerson PA, Hajnal S, et al. Influence of an anaesthetist on nurse-led, computer-based, pre-operative assessment. *Anaesthesia* 2000; 55: 576–80.

46. Lutner RE. The automated interview versus the personal interview. Do patient responses to preoperative health questions differ? *Anesthesiology* 1991; 75(3): 394–400.

47. Parker BM, Tetzlaff JE, Litaker DL, et al. Redefining the preoperative evaluation process and the role of the anesthesiologist. *J Clin Anesth* 2000; 12(5): 350–6.

48. Ehrenfeld JM, Reynolds P, Hersey S, Campbell BA, Sandberg WS. *Pilot Implementation & Assessment of a Computerized Preanesthetic Assessment Tool.* Abstract A 851, Annual American Society of Anesthesiologists Meeting 2011, Chicago, USA.

49. Walia A, Sierra-Anderson R, Robertson A. *Feasibility of Using a Web-based Patient Portal to Directly Elicit a Comprehensive Medical History from Veterans.* Abstract S-104, International Anesthesia Research Society, Annual Meeting 2011, Vancouver, Canada.

50. Lobo E, Feiner J, Cahlikova R. *Web-based Mobile Health: Novel Ways to Engage Patients in Their Care and Reduce Healthcare Costs for Hospitals and Patients.* Abstract TO-P437 , International Health Economics Association, Annual Meeting 2011, Toronto, Canada.

51. Kreimer S. Quality & safety. Alarming: Joint Commission, FDA set to tackle alert fatigue. *Hosp Health Netw* 2011; 85(6): 18–9.

52. Haynes AB, Weiser TG, Berry WR, et al. A surgical safety checklist to reduce morbidity and mortality in a global population. *N Engl J Med* 2009; 360: 491–9.

53. Kruzik N. Benefits of preoperative education for adult elective surgery patients. *AORN J* 2009; 90: 381–7.

54. Coulter A. Effectiveness of strategies for informing, educating, and involving patients. *BMJ* 2007: 335.

55. Kluger MT, Tham EJ, Coleman NA, et al. Inadequate pre-operative evaluation and preparation: A review of 197 reports from the Australian incident monitoring study. *Anaesthesia* 2000; 55: 1173–8.

Chapter

19 Identifying Bottleneck Constraints to Improve the Preoperative Evaluation Process

Mitchell H. Tsai, Elie Sarraf, Kyle R. Kirkham, and Terrence L. Trentman

Contents

The real trouble with this world of ours is not that it is an unreasonable world, or even that it is a reasonable one. The commonest kind of trouble is that it is nearly reasonable, but not quite. Life is not an illogicality; yet it is a trap for logicians. It looks just a little more mathematical and regular than it is; its exactitude is obvious, but its inexactitude is hidden, it's wildness lies in wait.

– Chesterton [1]

Introduction

The perioperative surgical home represents a framework to transform the healthcare delivery process. From total joint pathways to enhanced recovery after surgery protocols, anesthesiologists and perioperative leaders are finding themselves increasingly involved in discussions extending beyond the intraoperative period [2]. For anesthesiologists, this platform should sound familiar. Since 1994 with the inception of the preoperative evaluation clinic by Fisher at Stanford University [3], anesthesiologists have recognized that preoperative evaluation, and now optimization, may be critical for a subset of the surgical patient population. These discussions are essentially breaking down the barriers between different periods of time in the perioperative process and bringing forward the implications of coordinated anesthesia and surgical care across the life cycle of a patient.

However, these developments have not been without obstacles or difficulties. Kain et al. have commented on the operational, administrative, and financial barriers [4]. For instance, they identified the difficulty in scaling the coordination necessary to make sure that all patients adhere to protocols. For anesthesiologists, they recognized the lack of professional training when it comes to implementing LEAN management techniques and team-building skills. In the current fee-for-service model, proponents of the perioperative surgical home have yet to lay down a definitive fiscal plan that reimburses anesthesiologists for the additional services provided as the architect. Overriding these concerns, Kain et al. pointed out that our specialty has two core values: an underlying commitment to individuals in pain and a "compelling commitment to improve the care and safety of our patients." How we achieve these in the future will most likely change.

Although the preoperative process represents a module of the perioperative period, we believe that the lessons, thus far, from the perioperative surgical home scale down and provide an effective framework to identify bottleneck constraints. In this chapter, we will identify and discuss potential obstacles to the redesign of a preoperative system at an institution. For instance, some readers may encounter administrative and financial obstacles. Other readers may find themselves with a lack of local expertise or collaboration with their surgical and nursing colleagues. For now, we will concentrate on the following issues:

1. Organizational management and leadership
2. Systems optimization
3. Financial and healthcare resource constraints
4. Information technology
5. Anesthesiology as big business
6. Social and cultural factors

Then, we will explore a framework to transform the preoperative process and view the necessary changes from the perspective of a different healthcare system. Underlying this entire chapter is the understanding that improving the preoperative process will create a bottleneck somewhere else in the system. Constant vigilance, unwavering dedication, and an unflappable belief in building a sustainable system are necessary.

Organizational Management and Leadership

Before approaching any change process, anesthesiologists should have a basic understanding of the difference between management and leadership. In a *Sense of Urgency*, Kotter clearly delineates the responsibilities and tasks for managers and leaders [5]. For managers, the tasks of planning, budgeting, organizing, staffing, and problem solving are all directed at creating predictable, stable processes. By contrast, leaders are responsible for establishing direction, aligning employee's values, motivating individuals and ultimately, inspiring change. For many physicians, the distinction between these two skill sets is important because undergraduate and graduate medical education focuses solely on the fine-tuning of management skills. Should anesthesiologists approach a systems-based change with management skills, they might find themselves alone, inciting conflict, and worst, negatively affecting patient care.

So how do anesthesiologists create and lead change in perioperative processes? Mintzberg viewed management and leadership as right-sided and left-sided neurocognitive skills [6]. Traditionally, the leftside is equated with analytic, data-driven skills, not dissimilar to the responsibilities of any manager. The rightside is usually associated with artistic and emotional processes; this is where the art of leadership comes into play. Anesthesiologists involved in creating change should appreciate that both sides of the brain are necessary. There will be times when inspiring individuals and laying out a vision is critical. Other times, there will be a need to make sure that budgets are met and staffing is available. The key to being an effective manager/leader is the ability to decide which skill set to use. Most times, human beings resort to their strengths and physicians may rely on management skills (i.e., telling someone what to do) when leadership, or listening skills would be more appropriate.

Anesthesiologists leading any change effort should understand that the dynamic set up between management and leadership should create tension, specifically, creative tension. In *Leading in a Culture of Change*, Fullan points out the fallacy of management and the myth of leadership [7]. Pure management systems are essentially at equilibrium; they are static. Think of a finely tuned manufacturing process where the management teams understand the necessary inputs and can quantify the outputs. By contrast, leadership, through adoption of the latest management technique or blind, sweeping culture changes, usually creates an exhausted, aimless organization. It is rare that change leadership follows a checklist or a recipe. Fullan believes that leadership, true leadership, is the practice of creating a learning organization. In these organizations, leaders may arise from any level of an organization. On an individual level, they understand that leadership requires a moral purpose; the opportunity to invest for the long term; a network of relationships and accountability; a platform to disseminate knowledge; and the time for sense-making. The opportunities for adopting this recursive practice in the preoperative setting will be echoed in the remaining sections.

Systems Optimization

While in depth review of optimization can be explored elsewhere [8], the method can be summarized as finding an ideal condition, given the constraints at hand, that will result in the lowest "cost" to the system. The cost of establishing a new preoperative process will consist of a variety of other metrics that will influence decision making. A simple example of a cost function would be setting the thermostat in the middle of winter in Vermont; in this case:

$$J = F_{comfort}\left(temperature\right) + F_{cost}\left(temperatures\right)$$

With $F_{comfort}$ demonstrating the effect the temperature has on a person's comfort, F_{cost} the effect of temperature on monetary cost and J being the "cost function" that we seek to minimize. It is important to note several points in this example:

1. Each individual function is constructed in such a way that "lower is better."
2. $F_{comfort}$ in this situation is dependent on the person living in the house: two individuals may perceive comfort with different ideal temperature. This will influence the "weight" applied to the individual function, which determines how strongly it impacts J. A heavily weighted function will ensure a stronger cost/penalty if it, individually, is not minimized.
3. Comfort has other dependencies that are influenced by individual preferences: one person may wish to wear t-shirt and shorts while at home, while another may be equally comfortable in woolen pajamas.

One immediately notes the tradeoffs between cost and comfort although they are not always reciprocal. Increased temperature will result in increased cost but beyond a certain temperature as an individual becomes uncomfortably hot. Reciprocally, below a certain temperature the cost may become catastrophic (e.g., after a water pipe freezes and then bursts).

Cost functions should be generated for any change in a preoperative period and can be used to guide decision making during the implementation period, and as a component of the continuous improvement process. The concept of bottleneck constraints fits within the paradigm of optimization and needs to be properly understood when seeking to minimize the cost function. Again, these bottlenecks may appear upstream or downstream.

Finally, in the preoperative evaluation setting, it is important to identify the variables that can impact the "cost function" in order to identify the areas that may be optimized. The opportunities – this list is not inclusive – may include the following:

1. Cost of the system which also includes infrastructure cost

2. Operating room (OR) time lost for cancelled cases
3. Cost to society including time lost due to travel or clinic visit; this includes lost wages, lost job productivity for not only patients but also supporters who would assist the patient (e.g., parents or children of the young/elderly patient)
4. Patient satisfaction
5. Physician satisfaction
6. "Quality metrics" that influence reimbursement
7. Procedure reimbursement, which can only be modified as a function of the operating surgeons' skills

The above variables may be modified at both "macro" and "micro" levels. A macro change may be represented by a decision to centrally locate a preoperative clinic, establish a telephone call center, or simply relying on a note from the primary physician with a full assessment performed at the day of surgery. The micro level change would be more focused and specific (i.e., where to locate clinic/call center or minimizing preoperative laboratory tests for specific surgeries). We return to the idea that "macro" and "micro" decision are made in parallel when we examine a platform to streamline preoperative testing patterns.

Healthcare Resource and Financial Constraints

Over the past two decades, there has been a proliferation of preoperative evaluation processes. While the preoperative evaluation clinic remains the gold standard, many anesthesiology groups and academic departments have adopted telephone-based preoperative centers and web-based technologies [9, 10]. The system which develops at each institution is the end result of a myriad of administrative decisions, the preference of the anesthesiology and procedural groups, the information technology infrastructure, and the flexibility of the primary care network. Under the current fee-for-service reimbursement system, preoperative evaluation processes represent a fixed cost for most institutions [11]. For many, anesthesiologists may find themselves at the heart of this constraint. The world of accounting, business plans, and return on investment has usually taken a backseat to clinical outcomes, surgeon satisfaction, and quality measures. However, anesthesiologists need to develop the business acumen and language in order to build the value proposition for a preoperative process. For some anesthesiologists and perioperative managers, additional professional training may be a suitable route [12, 13]. For others, mentorship and administrative experience may suffice, which remains as a standard practice in many corporate environments.

One of the bottleneck constraints an anesthesiologist may encounter is the inability to find the appropriate clinical care provider for a specific task. For physical preoperative evaluation clinics, there are the medical directorship, clinical personnel, and administrative roles. For example, our institution created a telephone-based preoperative assessment center in the 1990s. Today, every patient undergoing surgery at our hospital receives a telephone-based evaluation. The University of Vermont Medical Center does not have a physical preoperative evaluation clinic, although surgeons have the option to call and schedule a clinic visit should the patient's condition or comorbidities warrant further evaluation by an anesthesiologist. During the workweek, nurses call patients at home or at work, and conduct a review of systems, educate the patient on the perioperative process, and answer any questions about the perioperative process. Lozada et al. showed that patients largely prefer a telephone-based preoperative assessment and one would be tempted to presume that this is due to the minimal disruption in their lives compared to an office visit [14]. Yet, have we fully optimized the resources and staffing of the telephone-based preoperative center? Is there a way to increase the efficiency of information transfer using the institutional electronic medical record? Can we better prepare patients for surgery? Are we duplicating services already covered by the surgeon's office?

Govindarajan has argued that the study of healthcare systems outside of the United States affords the opportunity to understand the waste, redundancy, and inefficiencies of the current American system [15]. From this perspective, he describes the resource optimization framework for a rural healthcare system in India. For the United States and the rest of the world, cataract surgery is the most common procedure performed. For the United States, there is already a shortage of ophthalmologists and this labor shortfall is even greater worldwide. In India at the Aravind Eye Care Center, where "necessity spans innovation," healthcare policy maker and hospital administrators recognized the traditional work schedule for an American surgeon made it difficult, if not impossible, to hire the number of surgeons to fully staff

an operational, functional ophthalmology surgical center. The hospital administrators prioritized the surgeon's expertise and clinical skillset in the OR and developed a system whereby the clinic and preoperative processes were handled by mid-level healthcare providers and technicians. In turn, the new framework lowered the fixed costs of delivering care.

This framework can be applied in the preoperative processes which have proliferated across the United States [9, 10]. Under the current anesthesia reimbursement system, the preoperative evaluation is included in the Base Unit for each surgery or procedure. Again, we know that preoperative clinics reduce cancellation rates and on an operational level, the decision to fund preoperative clinics represented a financial hedge against the impact of a cancelled case on the day of surgery. Yet, there is little discussion on how best to staff a preoperative process. Fischer's model and many other models rely on a physician, anesthesiologist or primary care physician, as the captain at the helm [3]. But is it really necessary for a physician to evaluate each patient before surgery? Does the anesthesiology group have the labor force to staff a preoperative clinic? Consider that Philips et al. showed that for the patient evaluated at an ophthalmology clinic before surgery, providers identified a new, chronic condition in less than 1 percent of patients and none of the new diagnoses delayed surgery [16].

Again, the authors believe that neither an anesthesiologist nor financial support should be a bottleneck constraint to a better preoperative process. Historically, anesthesiologists evaluated all surgical patients at the bedside, decided what laboratory or diagnostic tests were necessary to optimize the patient, and educated the patient about the type of anesthesia they would receive. Today, we know that preoperative evaluation clinics and telephone call centers can be staffed by nurses or mid-level providers [14]. For healthy, low-risk patients undergoing low-risk surgical procedures, we could also argue that the clinical attention from a mid-level provider might be a poor match of clinical skillset and patient demands. Perhaps a nurse or medical assistant could guide this patient through surgery. In fact, web-based technologies and clinical decision support systems (sans healthcare provider) have already demonstrated similar efficacies with a lower cost [17, 18]. Using the value-based proposition where value equals outcomes divided by the cost of delivering the care, better optimized preoperative processes inherently provides more value [19].

We started this section with a discussion on the optimization of resources and staffing for preoperative evaluation processes and we end with a note on the opportunities of eliminating this bottleneck constraint. At the Mayo Clinic, Trentman et al. demonstrated that a simplified algorithm and optional screening tool enabled surgeons to appropriately target patients for a preoperative evaluation [20]. To restate, they were able to generate cost savings by optimizing the appropriate level of care for each patient and using the available, remaining resources to target patients with diabetes. Similarly, Davenport et al. demonstrated that preoperative risk factors account for 33 percent of the cost variation, 23 percent of the work relative value units, and 20 percent of the complications downstream [21]. In other words, a patient's preoperative risk factors account for a large proportion of the cost variation. The discussion of financial constraints should ultimately recognize that the healthcare system is currently unsustainable. Anesthesiologists should lead effort towards financial stewardship by optimizing the preoperative resources the necessary to provide safe and effective care [22].

Information Technology

In *Nonzero*, Wright argued that the increasing efficiency of information transfer underlies the basis of human civilization [23]. Over the past two decades, anesthesiology groups have driven the transition from a paper-based record to an electronic database [24]. The predominant literature supporting the importance of IT for anesthesia-driven processes is during the intraoperative period, where documentation and billing compliance errors are reduced [25–27]. However, a recent retrospective review by Chow et al. showed that electronic communication could advance patient-centered care by transmitting clinical information in a timely manner [18]. We also note that there are well-developed papers laying out the infrastructure necessary to develop an effective, efficient anesthesia information management system [28]. As the capabilities of the electronic medical record continue to expand, anesthesiologists need to continue to lead not only the adoption of the platform, but building of the infrastructure to support an array of nonclinical, administrative functions. Depending on the environment, the adoption of an electronic medical record or database may or may not be a constraint.

Porter believes the underpinning transformation to a value-based healthcare delivery system is the recognition that information technology is pivotal [19]. The decision to use information technology should be driven by the opportunity to improve preoperative processes. However, Archer et al. clearly laid out the four potential obstacles:

1. Physicians' autonomy
2. Lack of "buy-in" and support
3. Skewed incentive structures
4. A short-term view for returns on investment [29]

The skills required to build these capabilities are closer to industrial engineering and scientific programming than to medical informatics. At our institution, we have a clinical informatics lead with previous experience as a registered nurse in the OR. She leads a team that bridges the gap between technical and clinical stakeholders. This team has helped our organization drive the change from a paper-based system to a fully accepted perioperative clinical system that currently encompasses the preoperative and intraoperative period. With this team and the automation of documentation, we have been able to drive to clinical improvements based on clinical documentation, build a preoperative evaluation interface, and fully operationalized an anesthesia scheduling system replete with preoperative patient information.

While our institution has found a fair amount of success in using IT to streamline the preoperative process, it should also be recognized that this solution can be challenging to implement for smaller hospitals and small, private anesthesia practices. Even if these locations or groups were able to invest in the startup cost of building the IT infrastructure necessary for this process, they would also require ongoing maintenance of the system with its own cost structure. This would include the hiring and staffing of several positions, including that of a "clinical informatics lead" as described previously. One option to minimize the system overhead of the preoperative process would be either to outsource or consolidate with multiple other institutions, thereby distributing the overhead cost amongst multiple parties as described below.

Anesthesiology Meets Wall Street

In 2012, Galinanes commented on the increasing popularity of mergers amongst anesthesiology groups [30]. Two years later, there were over 80,000 anesthesiologists and nurse anesthetists in the United

States performing an estimated 40,000,000 anesthetics annually and driving the $19 billion American anesthesia industry [31]. The financial reach of anesthesia-driven healthcare services is even noted on the American stock exchanges. For instance, MEDNAX/American Anesthesiology (NYSE:MD) and Team Health Holdings (NYSE:TMH) are listed on the New York Stock Exchange [32]. In 2014, further consolidation of the anesthesia industry occurred when AmSurg Corporation, a publicly traded operator of ambulatory surgery centers, acquired Sheridan Healthcare for $2.4 billion. Again, this $2.4 billion represents almost 10 percent of the anesthesia services provided on an annual basis. Today, 13 percent of the anesthesiology groups in this control employ nearly 75 percent of the anesthesia healthcare providers. Readers may find that the local and regional anesthesia markets are dominated by five major players – MEDNAX, NAPA, Sheridan Healthcare, USAP, and TeamHealth.

From an operational and strategic perspective, these mergers and acquisitions make financial sense [33]. With the passage of the Accountable Care Act, larger groups can create capital pools under risk-sharing arrangement models and access capital for infrastructure investments (e.g., anesthesia information management systems, electronic quality metrics, web-based preoperative evaluation processes). Matching the recent mergers of the healthcare insurance industry, the consolidation of anesthesia groups should provide negotiating leverage, the opportunity to transfer high reliability processes and scale operational efficiencies such as a telephone- or web-based preoperative assessment system or electronic reporting systems.

However, what are the true day-to-day implications for anesthesiologists? It has been noted that hospital administrators are expecting more and more of their anesthesia providers with a concomitant demand to increase efficiency and demonstrate quality. For instance, anesthesia teams are asked to increase coverage throughout the hospital for ICU/critical care, obstetrics, acute pain management, non-OR anesthesia cases, and other services. Traditionally, the financial model for anesthesia groups included labor subsidies payments for staffing these underserved, inefficient areas [34, 35]. With the consolidation of the anesthesia industry, anesthesia providers may find that their negotiating capabilities are relegated to the administrators of large consolidated anesthesia groups.

We have included this brief discussion on the trends in the anesthesiology industry because we believe that anesthesiologists should appreciate the opportunities afforded by and the constraints imposed from the aggregation of anesthesia services. Anesthesiologists examining the preoperative process may find that another practice uses a telephone-based preoperative center and its expansion may be limited by the number of nurses. On the other hand, some may discover that the variability of clinical practice as it pertains to the preoperative testing patterns may increase as group with historically different practice patterns become a single entity. Again, before embarking on a journey to change the preoperative process, anesthesiologists should understand the local, departmental, and institutional context within which they work. No organization or department is too big to fail.

Social and Cultural Factors

Until recently, the development of preoperative processes has focused primarily on the infrastructure resources and financial implications of well-honed systems. There has been little research into the social and cultural factors directly or indirectly affecting the patients and their families [36]. Further, Ankuda et al. showed that 13 percent of patients undergoing elective surgery showed informed consent deficits, usually related to sociodemographic and language factors [37]. However, the impact of the preoperative process may be significant, especially for patients with chronic conditions. For example, Montori et al. showed that diabetes management improved when patients were directly involved with the decision-making process [38]. In a similar vein, Wilson et al. showed similar outcomes for patients with asthma [39]. The fact that both chronic conditions, diabetes and asthma, have implications for the anesthetic care and perioperative pathways should encourage anesthesiologists to develop a better understanding of the processes, especially when shared decision making can reduce the cost of delivery care.

Shared decision making in the preoperative process can also help reduce bottlenecks which occur on an operational level [40]. Chandrakantan and Saunders argued that the shared decision making process can be used in the preoperative evaluation of higher-risk patients. Charles et al. suggested that shared decision-making processes have the following characteristics:

1. There are two participants, physician and patient
2. Information is shared
3. Consensus is built in a step-wise fashion
4. An agreement is reached on the treatment plan [41]

From a system-based perspective, anesthesiologists may discover that a shared decision-making framework may assist patients and help them develop not only an appreciation of the risks and benefits of a surgical procedure, but also a deeper understanding of the implications of anesthesia. In the long run, anesthesiologists may be able to reduce the costs of care by reducing rates of unnecessary surgery or delaying such procedures. For example, in 2012, Group Health in Washington State demonstrated that a shared decision-making educational platform reduced both surgery rates and costs for total joint replacements [42]. Although this study was observational, the authors brought forward a broader discussion of the anesthesiologist's role. Despite these findings, readers should be wary of the argument that delaying a surgery can be cost-saving because it only takes into account the insurance and immediate health cost. In order to move shared decision making forward, anesthesiologists need to facilitate conversations with surgeons, hospital administrators and insurance companies.

A Preoperative Platform

The opportunities to decrease variability in preoperative testing patterns remain. Wijeysundera et al. demonstrated a lack of consistency and a large degree of variability amongst different hospitals in a Canadian province [43, 44]. The same holds true for American systems. In the Pacific Northwest, Thilen et al. demonstrated that in an integrated healthcare system, different surgical subspecialties order preoperative tests without any prudent guidance or clinically driven processes [45]. Mackey argued that any effort designed to decrease variation in medical practices has been "hampered by (1) a lack of understanding of the fundamental link between outcomes variation and medical quality improvement, (2) physicians practicing with an individualist, artisan-like approach in a fragmented medical

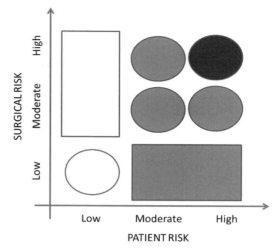

Figure 19.1 ASA/ACA guidelines redrawn in a 3×3 matrix.
White circle: Low-risk patient, low-risk surgery. Any tests ordered for patients in this category are an unnecessary expense.
Gray rectangle: Moderate/high-risk patients, low-risk surgery. The current ASA/ACA guidelines do not delineate the type of anesthetic for the case. For certain cases (e.g., carpal tunnel releases, cataracts), the risk of the regional anesthetic is minimal.
White rectangle: Low-risk patients, low- to high-risk surgery. The ASA has recommended that healthcare providers should not order baseline diagnostic cardiac testing in asymptomatic patients with stable cardiac disease undergoing low- or moderate-risk noncardiac surgery [49, 50].
Black circle: High-risk patients, high-risk surgery.
Gray circles: Moderate-risk patients, moderate-risk surgery; moderate-risk patients, high-risk surgery; and high-risk patients, moderate-risk surgery.

practice environment, and (3) individual physicians and individual institutions relying on their own practice outcomes data for quality improvement" [46].

Again, the variability in the system cannot be emphasized enough despite associated additional healthcare costs and patient morbidity. These findings lie in stark contrast to the financial, operational, and clinical opportunities framed by the Perioperative Surgical Home. Here, Dexter and Wachtel have pointed out that there are ultimately two strategies that will result in net cost reductions with the perioperative surgical home [47]. The first strategy suggests that anesthesiologists should aim to reduce unnecessary interventions in the preoperative period that provide little or no benefit to the patient. To advance the discussion on reducing variability in preoperative testing patterns, we have redrawn the guidelines set forth by the ACC/AHA as a three by three matrix (Figure 19.1).

Using this matrix, the anesthesiologist should be able to design a road map to better understand the opportunities available when assessing which preoperative tests are necessary before surgery. In addition, we are able to elucidate how variability affects the healthcare system when we use this matrix as a starting point to discuss medical quality improvement in a fragmented healthcare delivery system. Again, any reduction in unnecessary perioperative testing can reduce healthcare costs in two ways: not testing or reducing false-positives [48].

By framing the discussion of the preoperative evaluation for surgical patients with this matrix, we show that there are several opportunities to fundamentally change the way we deliver perioperative services. For instance, patients in the *blue circle* (low-risk patient, low-risk surgery) and *yellow rectangle* (moderate/high-risk patient, low-risk surgery) do not need any further cardiac risk stratification or a history and physical by a primary care physician, regardless of the risk of the patient, provided the patient is a reliable historian and the team can undertake a proper medical history. Working in concert, anesthesiologists, surgeons, and administrators can now develop processes to minimize preoperative tests patterns.

By example, anesthesiologists could work collaboratively with ophthalmologists to redesign the perioperative process for patients undergoing cataract surgery. Ideally, the anesthesiologist (or preassessment nurse) reviews the history and the surgeon performs a brief physical exam. This fulfills the compliance requirements for a preoperative history and physical. Although patients with cardiac disease deserve a more thorough review, most times, patients have stable cardiac conditions. A web-based or telephone preoperative evaluation with the appropriate anesthesiologist oversight should suffice and most educational points can be performed over the phone (e.g., patients taking antiplatelet medications can be instructed to discontinue their medications in an appropriate time interval before surgery). By using this platform as a basis to build a different healthcare delivery system, the knowledge and framework should be expanded to other specialties. More importantly, the reduction of variability for this subset of patients has financial ramifications for a large, tertiary academic healthcare system [51, 52]. These opportunities currently exist, can be implemented immediately, and are based on research and national consensus statements.

Continuous Process Improvements

Presciently, Shafer recognized that the current process improvements are limited in scope [53]. He concluded:

> Missing . . . are data showing improved outcomes, costs reduction, or successful implementation of the "triple aims" of the Perioperative Surgical Home. Opinion, reflection, and dialogue are important . . . However, opinion is not a substitute for data.

For anesthesiologists interested in the preoperative process, the preeminent study dates back to Fisher's in 1994 [3]. Six years later, Wu and Fleischer commented that the development of the perioperative surgical home necessitated an individual responsible for outcomes measurements [54]. Anesthesiologists need to drive these changes with transparent, data-driven processes utilizing electronic medical records and clinically relevant outcomes data.

For most physicians, the decision to build a process is not dissimilar to a hospital CEO's strategic initiative to build a new patient unit. However, the process should not stop once the bricks and mortar are up. The impetus behind the perioperative surgical home lies in the fact that anesthesiologists work at the nexus of all the healthcare providers for the care of the surgical patient [55]. With the changing healthcare environment, current anesthesiologists may find their nonclinical, systems-based skills lacking, while program directors are looking for direction and strategies to ensure that future anesthesiologists are trained to build multidisciplinary teams and to create effective processes change. Rathmell and Sandburg argued that anesthesiologists should approach process improvement with scientific rigor and minimal confirmation biases [56].

In the past two decades, we have seen the proliferation of various preoperative healthcare delivery models and a growth of literature supporting the establishment of standardized preoperative processes. We have been inundated with a plethora of studies demonstrating how we should design our preoperative processes. Hartnett et al. demonstrated that improving the clinical and organizational aspects of the preoperative process increases patient satisfaction [17]. However, it is rare that patient satisfaction is seen as a bottleneck constraint. More often than not, patient satisfaction scores serve as the ends, and not the means, for changes in clinical processes. Ultimately, we are missing the literature that describes the obstacles, barriers, and mountains which the authors overcame to implement their strategies and operationalize their healthcare delivery process.

While other authors have reviewed the economic and operational advantages of a preoperative testing clinic [57–60], the time is ripe for a technological and cultural shift for the preoperative evaluation. We believe that improving this process requires the systems-based engineering perspective Sandberg adopted for operationalizing an anesthesia information management system. In its basic form, it follows:

1. Process modeling to create a reference process against which actual process progress can be compared, seeking noteworthy exceptions
2. Data integration of multiple electronic sources and different data types
3. Continuous process monitoring by recursive queries of the AIMS and other database to identify process exceptions
4. Pushing data to key stakeholders, seeking to provide the right information to the persons who need it, at the time when it most useful [26]

In addition to the above, it is important for the relevant stakeholders to delineate the organizational priorities with clear goals as benchmarks that can be used for improvement. These stakeholders will help delineate the different weights that each metric/cost function variable will have in order to properly allocate effort and resources.

Embedded in the model above is Deming's continuous process improvement: study, plan, do and act [61]. We have used this recursive framework throughout this chapter to address not only the bottleneck constraints one may encounter when they journey down a strategic decision to build a different preoperative evaluation process, but also to identify the numerous opportunities to continuously refine a system. Anesthesiologists should be acclimated to working in an environment with constraints. We do this each day with every patient when we design and implement an anesthetic plan based upon the comorbidities of the patient and the needs of the surgeon.

An Outside Perspective: The Canadian Single-Payer Experience

The provision of core health services in Canada is governed by the Canada Health Act [62]. This national legislation establishes core principles, from which the country's provinces are responsible for all aspects of providing care. The Canada Health Act is founded on five core principles:

1. Public administration – health insurance must be administered by a public authority on an nonprofit basis
2. Comprehensiveness – all necessary health services must be insured
3. Universality – all insured residents are entitled to the same level of care
4. Portability – residents can move between jurisdictions in the country without a change in their coverage
5. Accessibility – all insured persons should have reasonable access to healthcare and, in addition, all physicians and hospitals must be reasonably compensated for the services they provide

Within this framework there is considerable latitude for the structure of care delivery models and, notably for physicians, compensation structures. As such, the adoption of structures that parallel the Perioperative Surgical Home model varies between jurisdictions along similar stress points as US models. Where most successful, the system has addressed the key points raised in this chapter and accounted for some of the bottleneck constraints.

Canadian physicians, by and large, function as independent contract providers to the single provincial payer in each jurisdiction. Hospital privileges enable anesthesiologists to provide care in publicly funded institutions but physician compensation is derived from fee structures, which are uniform across jurisdictions. The relationship internal to institutions therefore depends heavily on a leadership model that promotes collaboration with the managerial structure of the hospital. This relationship extends through all levels of the perioperative period resulting in a greater focus on leadership skills development than managerial ability. The Royal College of Physician and Surgeons educational CanMEDS competency framework, which has gained international traction, was revised in 2015 to replace "Manager" with "Leader" in recognition of the importance of this shift when navigating the complex system of healthcare [63].

Cost constraints in single payer system, and the trade-offs within decisions, follow similar patterns to other systems when the question revolves around optimization. In the single-payer environment system level macro costs are frequently at the forefront however, with micro level decisions perceived to impact macro program or institutional opportunities or opportunity costs in a zero sum finding scheme. Anesthesiologists must make value arguments very clear in this environment, with a business case that emphasizes a savings impact in order to argue for infrastructure support associated with programs like the Perioperative Home.

Similar to the examples presented above, Canadian models of preoperative evaluation and testing are not static in their design. The incorporation of video and telephone capabilities was an early modification to accommodate the geographical constraints of small remote communities. Large suppliers for these services, like the Ontario Telemedicine Network, provide private sector innovation despite the single-payer funding source [64]. The emphasis on appropriateness of care and grassroots campaigns like Choosing Wisely have considerable traction in this environment [65]. In a move of support, the Canadian Anesthesiologists' Society Choosing Wisely recommendations all address preoperative care and the choice of testing used during preoperative assessment and optimization [66].

Where successful, integration of Canadian anesthesiologists into preoperative patient optimization as part of overall care pathways has largely depended on a compensation structure that directly supports this model. Most anesthesia practices in the single-payer Canadian systems function predominantly on a fee for service model with compensation set at a provincial level between the government payer and physician representation organizations negotiating for all physicians simultaneously. When participation in perioperative care is recognized in the reimbursement structures, pre- and postoperative continuity of anesthesiologists is promoted. The relationship within hospitals is freed to focus on clinical care, with the physician compensation removed from the equation. However, institutional resource constraints remain significant with nursing, allied health and infrastructure costs borne by the hospital. In a similar vein, many jurisdictions in Canada continue to struggle with equivalent challenges to American perioperative surgical home proponents who seek appropriate compensation models to support this additional workload.

In short, the success of structured preoperative evaluation processes and their full integration into the Canadian single-payer model has occurred to a variable degree across jurisdictions, as in the United States. Where compensation models support this structure, the system efficiency benefits of this model align with the physician resources and full integration has occurred. In these models, the opportunity and effectiveness of efforts like Choosing Wisely can flourish, representing a significant value addition toward system sustainability and quality of perioperative care.

Conclusion

At the American Society of Anesthesiologists annual meeting in 2016, keynote speaker Michael Porter laid out a framework to transform the healthcare system in America [67]. For far too long, physicians and hospital administrators had created a broken system devoid of value. From the physicians' perspective, the goal of evidence-based medicine was to demonstrate that certain treatments provided better outcomes. However, physicians failed to recognize the cost of providing these treatments. On the other hand, hospital administrators implemented cost-cutting strategies in order to bend the cost curve in healthcare. These management techniques mostly ignored the outcomes of the treatments, alternatives, or research and development necessary to improve healthcare at the patient or population health level. By defining value as outcomes divided by the cost of healthcare delivery, Porter's framework brings together both components [68].

Porter believes that the measurement of outcomes and the associated healthcare costs need to be measured beyond the patient–physician encounter. For instance, for patients with osteoarthritis of a hip joint, the value-based framework extends beyond the actual surgical replacement of a patient's hip and whether or not the anesthesiologist administered an antibiotic at the appropriate time interval. In fact, he argues that value of any healthcare delivery system should include the time interval between when the patient is asymptomatic to the actual diagnosis. In short, the longer the period of time the patient is asymptomatic, the better the value proposition. For anesthesiologists, this is nothing new. Anesthesiologists have long understood that the preoperative process plays an important role in the perioperative care of surgical patients on several levels. In terms of patient safety and cardiac outcomes, anesthesiologists and cardiologists have fine-tuned a risk stratification system that lowers the risk of cardiac morbidity and mortality. On an operational and financial level, the benefits of a well-honed preoperative process are well defined.

So where do we go from here? Porter laid out the following structural framework for any physician or healthcare administrator:

1. Create integrated practice units
2. Measure outcomes and costs
3. Move into a bundle payment care cycles
4. Integrate delivery across facilities
5. Expand valued services across a geographical region
6. Build an information technology platform [68]

We have touched upon many of the agenda items in this chapter, but ultimately, by identifying the bottleneck (or constraints) in the preoperative process, anesthesiologists and perioperative leaders are essentially creating value. For instance, if an academic anesthesiologist is deciding whether to pursue a physical preoperative clinic or to build a web-based information technology platform, then they should understand the limitations (or opportunities) present in each process. A physical preoperative clinic limits the ability to integrate delivery across several facilities, but may make it easier to deliver care an integrate practice unit. By contrast, the president of a large, private practice anesthesiology group may view the constraint of the preoperative process as the number of anesthesiologists that may be available. Again, the six agenda items and the bottlenecks discussed in this chapter create a recursive and self-reinforcing matrix. In closing, we hope that the reader will be able to create a continuously improving, sustainable preoperative process that acknowledges the guidelines available from our national societies and challenges the status quo at the local, institutional level. At a minimum, we hope that the reader ventures forth and puts forward a plan of action.

References

1. Bernstein PL. *Against the gods: The remarkable story of risk*. Wiley, 1996 (p. 331).

2. Kain ZN, Vakharia S, Garson L, et al. The perioperative surgical home as a future perioperative practice model. *Anesth Analg* 2014; 118(5): 1126–30.

3. Fischer SP. Development and effectiveness of an anesthesia preoperative evaluation clinic in a teaching hospital. *Anesthesiology* 1996; 85: 196–206.

4. Kain ZN, Hwang J, Warner MA. Disruptive innovation and the specialty of anesthesiology: The case for the perioperative surgical home. *Anesth Analg* 2015; 120(5): 1155–7.

5. Kotter JP. *A sense of urgency*. Harvard Business Press, 2008.

6. Mintzberg H. To fix health care, ask the right questions. *Harv Bus Rev* 2011.

7. Fullan M. *Leading in a culture of change personal action guide and workbook*. John Wiley, 2014.

8. www.dcsc.tudelft.nl/~bdeschutter/pub/rep/06_001.pdf

9. Foss JF, Apfelbaum J. Economics of preoperative evaluation clinics. *Curr Opin Anaesthesiol* 2001; 14(5): 559–62.

10. Pollard JG. Economic aspects of an anesthesia preoperative evaluation clinic. *Curr Opin Anaesthesiol* 2002; 15(2): 257–61.

11. Sibert KS, Schweitzer MP. Alignment of perioperative care with future models of payment. *ASA Newsletter* 2014; 78(10): 26–8.

12. Larson DB, Chanlder M, Forman HP. MD/MBA programs in the United States: Evidence of a change in health care leadership. *Acad Med* 2003; 78(3): 335–41.

13. Desai AM, Trillo RA Jr, Macario A. Should I get a master of business administration? The anesthesiologist with education training: Training options and professional opportunities. *Curr Opin Anaesthesiol* 2009; 22(2): 191–8.

14. Lozada MJ, Nguyen JT, Abouleish A, Prough D, Przkora R. Patient preference for the pre-anesthesia evaluation: Telephone versus in-office assessment. *J Clin Anesth* 2016; 31: 145–8.

15. Govindarajan V, Ramamurti R. Delivering world-class health care, affordably. *Harvard Business Review* 2013; 91(11): 117–22.

16. Phillips MB, Bendel RE, Crook JE, Diehl NN. Global health implications of preanesthesia medical examination of ophthalmic surgery. *Anesthesiology* 2013; 118(5): 1038–45.

17. Harnett MJ, Correll DJ, Hurwitz S, Bader AM, Hepner DL. Improving efficiency and patient satisfaction in a tertiary teaching hospital preoperative clinic. *Anesthesiology* 2010; 112: 66–72.

18. Chow VW, Hepner DL, Bader AM. Electronic care coordination from the preoperative clinic. *Anesth Analg* 2016; 123(6): 1458–62.

19. Porter ME. What is value in health care? *N Engl J Med* 2010; 363(26): 2477–81.

20. Trentman T, Graber RC, Goss DG, Didehban R, Hagstrom SG, Fowl RJ. Identification of appropriate patients for preoperative evaluation: A quality improvement project. *J Hospital Administration* 2016; 5(2): 73–9.

21. Davenport DL, Henderson WG, Kauri SF, Mentzer RM, Jr. Preoperative risk factors and surgical complexity are more predictive of costs than postoperative complications: A case study using the National Surgical Quality Improvement Program (NSQIP) database. *Ann Surg* 2005; 242: 463–8.

22. Butterworth JF, Green JF. The anesthesiologist-directed perioperative surgical home: A great idea that will succeed only if it is embraced by hospital administrators and surgeons. *Anesth Analg* 2014; 119(5): 896–7.

23. Nonzero WR. *The logic of human destiny.* Vintage, 2001.

24. Halbeis CBE, Epstein RH, Macario A, Pearl RG, Grunwald Z. Adoption of anesthesia information management systems by academic departments in the United States. *Anesth Analg* 2008: 1323–9.

25. Spring SF, Sandberg WS, Anupama S, Walsh JL, Driscoll WD, Raines DE. Automated documentation error detection and notification improves anesthesia billing performance. *Anesthesiology* 2007; 106: 157–63.

26. Sandberg WS, Sandberg EH, Seim AR, et al. Real-time checking of electronic anesthesia records for documentation errors and automatically text messaging clinicians improves quality of documentation. *Anesth Analg* 2008; 106(1): 192–200.

27. Kheterpal S, Gupta R, Blum JM, et al. Electronic reminds improve procedure documentation complicance and professional fee reimbursement. *Anesth Analg* 2007; 104(3): 592–7.

28. Shah NJ, Tremper KK, Kheterpal S. Anatomy of an anesthesia information management system. *Anesthesiology Clin* 2011; 29: 355–65.

29. Archer T, Schmiesing C, Macario A. What is quality improvement in the preoperative period? *Anesthesiology* 2002; 40(2): 1–16.

30. Galinanes F. The increasing consolidation of our industry. *ASA Newsletter* 2012; 76(2): 52–3.

31. www.beckershospitalreview.com/hospital-management-administration/waking-up-to-the-consolidating-anesthesia-marketplace.html

32. www.beckersasc.com/anesthesia/frenetic-consolidation-the-anesthesia-market-today-where-ascs-fit-in.html

33. Halzack NM, Rock-Klotz J. Medicare physician compare – Not just for doctor shopping! *American Society of Anesthesiologists Monitor* 2016; 80(11): 12–4.

34. Abouleish AR, Zornow MH, Levy RS, Abate J, Prough DS. Measurement of individual clinical productivity in an academic anesthesiology department. *Anesthesiology* 2000; 93: 1509–16.

35. Abouleish AE, Prough DS, Barker Sj, Whitten CW, Uchida T, Apfelbaum JL. Organizational factors affect comparison of the clinical productivity of academic anesthesiology departments. *Anesth Analg* 2003; 96: 802–12.

36. Gravel K, Legare F, Graham ID. Barriers and facilitatators to implementing shared decision-making in clinical practice: A systematic review of health professionals' perceptions. *Implementation Sci* 2006; 1: 16.

37. Ankuda CK, Block SD, Cooper Z, et al. Measuring critical deficits in shared decision making before elective surgery. *Patient Educ Couns* 2014; 94: 328–33.

38. Montori VM, Gafni A, Charles C. Shared treatment decision-making approach between patients with chronic conditions and their clinicians: The case of diabetes. *Health Expect* 2006; 9(1): 25–36.

39. Wilson SR, Strub P, Buist AS, et al. Shared treatment decision-making improves adherence and outcomes in poorly controlled asthma. *Am J Respir Crit Care Med* 2010; 181(6): 566–77.

40. Nelson O, Quin ED, Arriaga AF, et al. A model for better leveraging the point of preoperative assessment: Patients and providers look beyond operative indications when making decisions. *Anesth Analg Case Reports* 2016; 6: 241–8.

41. Chandrakatan A, Saunders T. Perioperative ethics issues. *Anesthesiology Clinics* 2016; 34: 35–42.

42. Arterburn D, Wellman R, Westbrook E, et al. Introducing decision making aids at Group Health was linked to sharply lower hip and knee surgery rates and costs. *Health Aff* 2012; 31: 2094–104.

43. Wijeysundera DN, Austin PC, Beattie WS, Hux JE, Laupacis A. Variation in the practice of preoperative medical consultation for major elective noncardiac surgery. *Anesthesiology* 2011; 116(1): 25–34.

44. Wijeysundera DN, Austin PC, Beattie WS, Hux JE, Laupacis A. A population-based study of anesthesia consultation before major noncardiac surgery. *Arch Intern Med* 2009; 169(6): 595–602.

45. Thilen SR, Bryson CL, Reid RJ, Wijeysundera DN, Weaver EM, Treggiari MM. Patterns of preoperative consultation and surgical specialty in an integrated healthcare system. *Anesthesiology* 2013; 118(5): 1028–37.

46. Mackey DC. Can we finally conquer the problem of medical quality? The systems-based opportunities of data registries and medical teamwork. *Anesthesiology* 2012; 117(2): 225–6.

47. Dexter F, Wachtel RE. Strategies for net cost reductions with the expanded role of expertise of anesthesiologists

in the perioperative surgical home. *Anesth Analg* 2014; 118(5): 1062–71.

48. Balk EM, Earley A, Hadar N, Shah N, Trikalinos TA. Benefits and harms of routine preoperative testing: Comparative effectiveness. *Comparative effectiveness reviews*. Agency for Healthcare Research and Quality, 2014.

49. Chung F, Yuan H, Yin L, Vairavanathan S, Wong DT. Elimination of preoperative testing in ambulatory surgery. *Anesth Analg* 2009; 108(2): 467–75.

50. Correll DJ, Hepner DL, Chang C, Tsen L, Hevenlone ND, Bader AM. Preoperative electrocardiograms: Patient factors predictive of abnormalities. *Anesthesiology* 2009; 110: 1217–22.

51. Tsai MH, Polk JD. The hidden cost of variability. *Anesth Analg* 2011; 113(2): 431.

52. Tsai MH, Black IH. The devil in the details. *Anesthesiology* 2012; 117(2): 425–6.

53. Shafer SL. Anesthesia & Analgesia's 2015 collection on the perioperative surgical home. *Anesth Analg* 2015; 120: 866–7.

54. Wu CL, Fleisher LA. Outcomes in perioperative medicine and anesthesiology: Into the next millennium. *Anesthesiol Clin North Am* 2000; 18: 633–45.

55. Butterworth JF, Green JF. The anesthesiologist-directed perioperative surgical home: A great idea that will succeed only if it is embraced by hospital administrators and surgeons. *Anesth Analg* 2014; 119(5): 896–7.

56. Rathmell JP, Sandberg WS. Anesthesiologists and healthcare redesign. *Anesthesiology* 2016; 125(4): 618–21.

57. Foss JF, Apfelbaum J. Economics of preoperative evaluation clinics. *Curr Opin Anaesthesiol* 2001; 14(5): 559–62.

58. Pollard JG. Economic aspects of an anesthesia preoperative evaluation clinic. *Curr Opin Anaesthesiol* 2002; 15(2): 257–61.

59. Yen C, Tsai M, Macario A. Preoperative evaluation clinics. *Curr Opin Anaesthesiol* 2010; 23: 167–72.

60. Edwards AF, Slawski B. Preoperative clinics. *Anesthesiology Clinics* 2016; 34: 1–14.

61. www.deming.org/theman/theories/pdsacycle

62. http://laws-lois.justice.gc.ca/eng/acts/C-6/

63. Frank JR, Snell L, Sherbino J, editors. *CanMEDS 2015 physician competency framework*. Royal College of Physicians and Surgeons of Canada, 2015.

64. https://otn.ca/

65. www.choosingwisely.org/

66. http://choosingwiselycanada.org/recommendations/anesthesiology/

67. www.asahq.org/annual%20meetingold/go%20 anesthesiology%202016/keynote%20speaker

68. Porter ME, Lee TH. The strategy that will fix health care. *Harv Bus Rev* 2013; 91(12): 24.

Anesthesia Practice Management

Sonya Pease

Contents

Introduction

Anesthesia practice management today requires a unique set of survival strategies as payment cuts brought by the shift from fee-for-service to value-based reimbursement payment methodologies change the traditional approach to revenue cycle management. Surviving and thriving in this new healthcare environment requires functional knowledge of the fundamentals of how anesthesia is uniquely paid as a specialty as well as effective anesthesia practice management tactics around staffing, operational performance, contracting, regulatory compliance, technology, and revenue opportunities in value-based care models.

The success of the anesthesia practice is critical not just to the members of the practice that it employees but also to the healthcare organization with which it contracts because:

- Nearly 30 percent of all US hospitalizations require a surgical procedure that typically represents a cost 2.5 times more than hospital stays for medical treatment alone [1].
- Typically 50 percent of a healthcare organization's total overhead is driven by surgery and perioperative costs but represents 50–70 percent

of the Healthcare organizations total net revenue [2].

- The anesthesiology service routinely takes care of the top 5 percent of high-risk patients that consume 50 percent of the annual healthcare expenditures nationwide [3].
- Nearly 80 percent of hospitals are paying the anesthesia group a subsidy due to poor payer mix, fair market value compensation demands, anesthetizing location demands, and revenue cycle performance challenges [4].

Put succinctly, surgery and perioperative services are the major driver in hospital profit margins today so it is imperative that the anesthesia practice show value by optimizing operational and financial performance for the anesthesia practice itself, as well as the hospital or healthcare organization to which they provide services [5].

This chapter has three main sections; the first section will focus on the fundamentals of the fee-for-service billing methodology and quality measures unique to anesthesiology, the second section will focus on value-based payment methodologies as define by current legislation, and the third section will focus on key competencies and concepts necessary to run a successful anesthesia practice.

Section 1. Fundamentals

The Healthcare Financial Management Association defines revenue cycle as "all administrative and clinical functions that contribute to the capture, management, and collection of patient service revenue." In other words, this process represents the full cycle of administrative functions required to create and generate a patient account to the eventual collection (or write-off) of payment for those services provided. Managing the revenue cycle components of the anesthesia practice requires understanding the basics of fee-for-service billing as applicable to the different types of staffing models. Fee-for-service billing represents the classic payment method for services based on the anesthesia services provided independent of the quality of the care provided.

Practice Staffing Models

There are numerous ways to provide anesthesia services ranging from independent contractor open medical staff type models to small group practices, large single or multispecialty group practices or employment directly with a healthcare facility or organization. Within each structure also exists various care delivery models, including all-physician, all–Certified Registered Nurse Anesthetist (CRNA) and blended care team models. Each structure and model offers distinct advantages and disadvantages. Just as providers make patient care decisions based on risks and benefits, anesthesia business owners must make business decisions based on the needs of its patient population, the healthcare organization's needs, the financial risks and liabilities of each structure in a particular practice setting, as well as the preferences of the key stakeholders involved.

Independent contractor practice. Individual physicians or CRNAs act as sole proprietors or as single-member corporations; often contracting services directly to specific facilities or surgeons. While independent practice offers the physician or CRNA the highest level of professional independence and entrepreneurial advantages, the economic challenge of covering practice overhead coupled with the increasing difficulty of meeting hospital administrative demands make the long-term sustainability of single-provider practices, or even a coalition of multiple single providers difficult to sustain. This is demonstrated by the proportion of physicians in solo and two-physician practices having trending down from 40.7 percent to 32.5 percent between 1998 and 2006 [6].

Group practice. Group practice remains the prevalent anesthesia practice structure in the United States with small practices of 10 physicians or less and medium practice groups of 11–50 physicians representing the largest population in the 2011 Medical Group Management Association survey. The private practice group model offers a high level of independence and autonomy while also facilitating options for structured work hours, standardized call rotation, and group collaboration to share knowledge, experience and expenses to an extent that is not possible in individual provider practices. While the potential to realize these group practice benefits certainly exists, the absence of strong practice leadership and the variance in individual work ethics, personalities, and practice preferences can divide the practice and threaten its viability.

Larger groups consisting of more than 50 physicians continue to gain market share, both as anesthesia-only and multispecialty practices. These larger entities offer less autonomy and professional independence than their smaller counterparts, but can provide greater opportunity for sharing administrative workload, thus positively impacting quality of life for practice members. Large groups may also offer benefits such as internal continuing medical education (CME) activities, research, online resources, and career advancement opportunities within the organization. In addition, large group practices typically maintain a lower operating cost per physician due to greater economies of scale, and can negotiate additional revenue streams outside of fee-for-service revenue by doing work that cannot be billed for but results in better patient care and has monetary value for hospital partners which may in turn improve margins and related physician compensation. Large groups may also be better positioned to employ or contract professional management services to improve financial outcomes through improved leadership structure and robust resources around recruiting, quality reporting, and billing.

Direct healthcare provider employment. An increasingly common choice for many anesthesia clinicians is entering into an employment agreement with a healthcare facility or large facility-based medical practice, either privately owned or managed by a professional management company. These employers offer numerous advantages over the self-dependence of private practice where the practice must depend upon revenue generated or subsidies provided to offset market deficiencies such as disproportionate percentage of underinsured or government payers. Large facilities or facility-based medical groups typically offer compensation packages that include some level of financial security in the form of a guaranteed base salary somewhat immune to fluctuations in practice volumes or payer mix. They also offer economies of scale similar to large multispecialty group practices that leverage more favorable payer contracts and can offset losses across services reducing overall costs. Most also offer expanded benefit packages with structured retirement plans, choice of insurance packages, paid CME, and broader access to state and federal employee benefits like Family Medical Leave.

The Anesthesia Care Team Model

Once group structure is determined, the choice of care delivery model remains. Both all-physician (and all-CRNA) and care team model practices offer unique benefits and disadvantages. Almost all anesthesia care is provided either personally by an anesthesiologist or by a nonphysician anesthesia provider such as a Certified Anesthesiologist Assistant (CAA) or CRNA. Nonphysician providers function most often under the direction or supervision of a licensed physician – typically an anesthesiologist although, in some circumstances, a nonanesthesiologist physician such as a surgeon or cardiologist may supervise the delivery of anesthesia care.

The anesthesia care team model typically consists of an anesthesiologist directing nonphysician providers at an MD-to-CRNA/CAA ratio ranging from 1:1 to 1:4. Higher supervision ratios can be utilized compliantly depending on the practice environment and patient needs but understanding the intricacies of billing is critical. There are very specific guidelines for billing under the "medical direction" model as there

are well-defined steps that must be taken to be compliant. When billing a case as medically directed the maximum allowable cases an anesthesiologist may bill concurrently is four and the seven steps of medical direction must be followed. These seven steps are:

- perform a preanesthetic examination and evaluation
- prescribe the anesthesia plan
- personally participate in the most demanding procedures of the anesthesia plan including, if applicable, induction and emergence
- ensure that any procedure in the anesthesia plan that the anesthesiologist does not perform are performed by a qualified anesthetist
- monitor the course of anesthesia administration at frequent intervals
- remain physically present and available for immediate diagnosis and treatment of emergencies
- provide the indicated post anesthesia care

If one or more of the above services are not performed by the anesthesiologist, the service is not considered medical direction and usually requires billing the case as "supervision" or as an independent service provided by the CRNA where applicable.

The care team staffing model has been shown to improve access to anesthesia services by expanding the number of anesthetizing locations, increasing opportunities for parallel processing so work that was once done in a linear fashion can occur concurrently, and freeing physician providers for rapid access to areas of greatest clinical need and other perioperative coordinating activities.

State regulatory bodies license nonphysician anesthesia providers and set the conditions under which they can work. These parameters may vary profoundly by state. Some states, for example, require physician supervision of CRNAs while others allow CRNAs to work independent of physician supervision. CAAs always function within an anesthesia care team model and are always directed by an anesthesiologist. In addition to the consideration given to the level of physician supervision desired by the facility and its medical staff in the delivery of anesthesia services, developing an intimate familiarity with the state requirements for supervision of nonphysician anesthesia providers for the state and Medicare region is imperative in determining the practice model.

Billing Fee-for-Service

Reimbursement for anesthesia services is unique from all other medical specialties. At one time, hospitals paid anesthesiologists directly for their services. This practice was replaced by a fee-for-service structure based on a percentage of the surgeon's fee. Today, anesthesia transaction code sets determine how electronic claims are submitted to payers. Increasingly, these new standards require anesthesiologists to provide the surgical code in addition to the anesthesia code on claims. Several key resources are therefore vital for the billing function of the anesthesia practice.

For the past 40 years, the Relative Value Guide (RVG) published by the American Society of Anesthesiologists (ASA) has linked the relative value of anesthesia services to the American Medical Association catalog of Current Procedure Terminology (CPT). The CPT catalog provides widely accepted medical nomenclature and the associated numeric codes used to report medical procedures and services under public and private health insurance plans. The RVG contains the most up-to-date CPT codes with full descriptors for anesthesia services and provides a valuation of the work performed, called a base unit value. A third tool, the ASA Crosswalk, provides the CPT anesthesia code that most specifically describes the anesthesia service for a particular diagnostic or therapeutic CPT procedure code. Typically, anesthesia codes are site specific while a single surgical or procedural code could apply to multiple anatomical sites. Accurate identification of site, therefore, becomes critical to selection of the correct anesthesia code.

Once a code is assigned, a base unit value is calculated that includes all associated anesthesia services associated with that particular procedure in that specific anatomical location, including pre- and post-operative assessments, fluid administration, and interpretation of basic anesthesia monitoring data. Units of time, measured in minute increments, are then added to base units. Base units plus time units comprises the basic fee-for-service charge for anesthesia care provided.

Modifiers such as physical status of the patient, unusual anesthesia circumstances, anesthesia services beyond those associated with the base code, complex positioning or multiple procedures are then submitted in addition to the basic base and time units to arrive at the final valuation for the services provided. The anesthesia practice may also bill some services as flat fee codes which are negotiated for particular procedures

Box 20.1. Examples of Modifier Codes for Billing for Professional Anesthesia Services

AA Services provided personally by the anesthesiologist

AD Services delivered by nonphysicians under the medical supervision of a physician who has more than four concurrent anesthesia procedures under supervision at the same time

QK Services provided by a nonphysician, but medically directed by a physician who has two to four procedures under medical direction at the same time

QX Service provided by a CRNA with medical direction by a physician

QY Indicates an anesthesiologist medically directing only one CRNA

QZ Service provided by a CRNA without medical direction by a physician

with individual payers. These flat fee codes are all inclusive of base units, time units, and any applicable modifier codes. An example of a flat fee service may include the placement of an intravascular line or placement of a regional block for post op pain control. Total charges for the care of any particular patient may include base units, time units, appropriate modifier codes as well as charges for flat fee procedures [7].

Billing for professional anesthesia services takes on additional complexity in the care team model. In addition to the coding process described, additional modifier codes are added to indicate the type of provider involved in delivery of care and the level of supervision if any provided.

Examples of these codes are in Box 20.1.

The Centers for Medicare and Medicaid Services (CMS) has outlined specific anesthesia guidelines for the delivery of anesthesia services that delineate rules and regulation for healthcare facilities to maintain their Conditions of Participation. These rules outline how anesthesia services are furnished within a facility and the survey procedures used to evaluate delivery of services. Failure to function and code within these guidelines can result in both financial and regulatory risk to the practice.

It is vital that anesthesia leadership become intimately familiar with the requirements for compliant coding and billing as well as the requirements for compliance with CMS regulations. Anesthesia billing operations or any outsourced service need to ensure compliance requirements are met and that proper documentation exist to support all billing operations.

Regulatory Reporting Compliance

Medical quality assurance is every clinician's job, but there are specific areas in which an engaged anesthesia service partnering with effective hospital leadership can have a profound impact on reportable regulatory measures for both the healthcare organization and anesthesia group. The Surgical Care Improvement Program (SCIP) was a national campaign launched in 2005 to substantially reduce surgical mortality and morbidity through collaborative efforts of the perioperative team and clinicians involved but have now been retired due to the fact that performance on these measures was so successful they were no longer differentiating for quality improvement purposes. The specialty of anesthesia now has a defined measure set of anesthesia specific measures defined by the Physician Quality Reporting System (PQRS) that will be transitioning to the Merit-Based Incentive Performance (MIPS) quality performance category starting in 2017 [8].

The eight PQRS measures, now called MIPS quality measures, defined within the anesthesia subspecialty set that can be reported to meet the quality measure component of the regulatory reporting requirement may require changes in clinical practice and workflow within the perioperative environment. Unlike the previous SCIP measures that were more process oriented, these measure move more in the direction of improving care by improving performance around specific clinical areas where evidence-based medicine supports improved patient outcomes and fewer perioperative complications.

Failure to report MIPS quality measures, at the time of the writing of this text can result in a potential loss of revenue for specific patient populations.

The current anesthesia MIPS subset of quality measures includes:

- Measure #44 – Percentage of isolated coronary artery bypass graft surgeries for patients aged 18 years and older who received a beta-blocker within 24 h prior to surgical incision for improved morbidity and mortality.
- Measure #76 – Percentage of patients, regardless of age, who undergo central venous catheter (CVC) insertion for whom CVC was inserted with all elements of maximal sterile barrier technique, hand hygiene, skin preparation, and, if

ultrasound is used, sterile ultrasound techniques followed for prevention of catheter-related bloodstream infections.

- Measure #404 – The percentage of current smokers who abstain from cigarettes prior to anesthesia on the day of elective surgery or procedure for prevention of postoperative complications.
- Measure #424 – Percentage of patients, regardless of age, who undergo surgical or therapeutic procedures under general or neuraxial anesthesia of 60 min duration or longer for whom at least one body temperature greater than or equal to 35.5°C (or 95.9°F) was recorded within the 30 min immediately before or the 15 min immediately after anesthesia end time for prevention of postoperative complications.
- Measure #426 – Percentage of patients, regardless of age, who are under the care of an anesthesia practitioner and are admitted to a PACU in which a postanesthetic formal transfer of care protocol or checklist that includes the key transfer of care elements is utilized.
- Measure #427 – Percentage of patients, regardless of age, who undergo a procedure under anesthesia and are admitted to an ICU directly from the anesthetizing location, who have a documented use of a checklist or protocol for the transfer of care from the responsible anesthesia practitioner to the responsible ICU team or team member.
- Measure #430 – Percentage of patients, aged 18 years and older, who undergo a procedure under an inhalational general anesthetic, AND who have three or more risk factors for postoperative nausea and vomiting, who receive combination therapy consisting of at least two prophylactic pharmacologic antiemetic agents of different classes preoperatively or intraoperatively.
- Measure #463 – Percentage of patients, 3–17 years of age, who undergo a procedure under an inhalational general anesthetic, AND who have two or more risk factors for postoperative nausea and vomiting, who receive combination therapy consisting of at least two prophylactic pharmacologic antiemetic agents of different classes preoperatively or intraoperatively.

In addition to these MIPS quality measures listed above, other components described in the new legislation include reporting practice improvement activities, resource use, and advanced care information further elaborated in another chapter. Many healthcare facilities do not understand the complexities of anesthesia services and the lost revenue opportunities that result when anesthesia services fail to report these measures. It is the responsibility of anesthesia leadership, therefore, to ensure optimal performance for these reporting requirements especially in anesthesia service contracts where the hospital is paying the anesthesia group a subsidy.

Section 2. Value-Based Care

CMS Part A has not paid hospitals for patient care costs related to preventable problems like surgical site infections and retained objects since 2008, a financial reality healthcare organizations have had to strategize and make tough business decisions around for many years forcing more emphasis on quality improvement as well as more cost-effective care for patients. Physicians and clinicians paid through Medicare Part B have previously had the luxury to voluntarily report quality measures for additional incentive pay in years past but effective January of 2017 penalties now apply for failing to report quality measures in conjunction with services provided. Value-based care essentially changes the classic fee-for-service payment methodology by reducing the payment or potentially paying a bonus in addition to the base payment dependent on the quality of the care delivered as determined by the defined set of regulatory quality measures applicable to a specific specialty.

MIPS and Alternative Payment Model

In April of 2015 the Medicare Access and CHIP Reauthorization Act (MACRA) was passed by a supermajority vote of the US House and Senate. This replaced the previous payment system for providers called the sustainable growth rate formula. MACRA establishes two paths for Part B reimbursement going forward. One path is the MIPS that consolidates existing quality measures as described above and adds clinical practice improvement activities; this path does not require the anesthesia group to take on any additional risk to collect payment beyond successful reporting of the quality components. The other path in the new legislation is the Alternative Payment Model (APM) in which the physicians providing care accept some level of risk for the total costs of the services and expenses incurred over which they have some control.

Figure 20.1 Illustrates the projection of Part B payments under the MIPS path of the legislation.

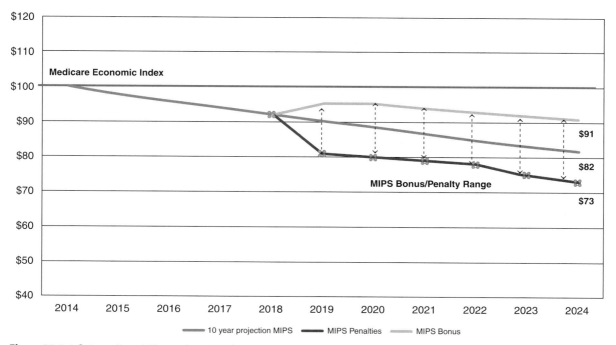

Figure 20.1 Inflation-adjusted 10-year change in physician payment under MIPS.
Data abstracted from the Congressional Budget Office Report [9].

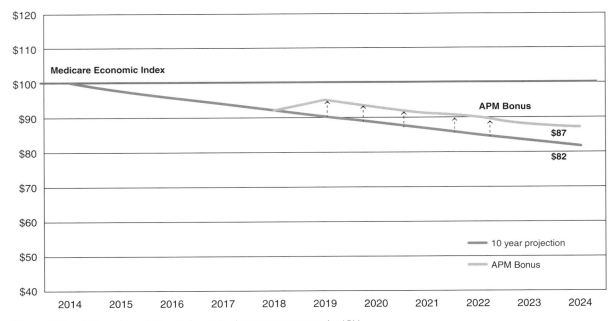

Figure 20.2 Inflation-adjusted 10-year change in physician payment under APM.
Data abstracted from the Congressional Budget Office Report [9].

Penalties and potential for some upside bonus payment will apply but overall the payment for services provided will deteriorate by approximately 18 percent over the 10-year projection. Figure 20.2 Illustrates the projection of Part B payments under the APM path of the new legislation. Penalties are avoided on this path since this road requires taking on risk which allows for some upside bonus payment but overall the payment for services provided will deteriorate by approximately 18 percent as well over the 10-year projection [9]. Figure 20.3 points out the potential for gain sharing in these new APMs of care; this would be accomplished by either contracting with the healthcare facility for bonus payments achieved through performance of specified quality measures or through defined shared savings achieved within a bundled payment type arrangement. A good example of this would be the Coordinated Care of Joint Replacements initiative, a mandatory bundled payment around total lower extremity joint replacement surgeries that creates a single spending target for all healthcare services provided during a 90-day clinical episode of care. This bundled payment is inclusive of the hospital stay, all physician services provided, outpatient care, home health, postacute facility services, as well as cost and penalties associated

readmissions. If the total costs spent are less than the target spend and the quality measures meet threshold on the entire episode of care, then a positive reconciliation payment is made to the healthcare facility mandated to the bundle. Funds generated through the successful performance of these bundled episodes of care can then be shared with the providers who helped drive the financial and quality success of the episode of care.

APMs are payment models such as accountable care organizations or the Medicare Shared Savings Program that meet three major requirements:

- Participants must use certified electronic health record (EHR) technology.
- Clinician pay is based on performance and successful reporting of quality measures.
- The participants bear more than a nominal risk for monetary losses.

APMs create financial incentives to inspire coordination of care across treatment settings within the acute care facility as well as the postacute care facility (skilled nursing facilities) to reduce unnecessary services, and provide guaranteed cost savings to the payer. CMS has set a goal of having 50 percent of all Medicare fee-for-service payments made by APMs

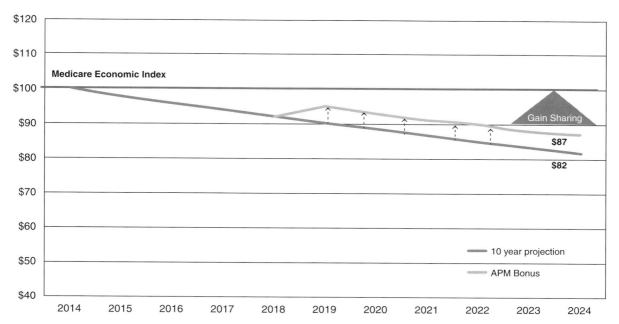

Figure 20.3 Inflation-adjusted 10-year change in physician payment under APM with gain sharing opportunity noted by triangle. Data abstracted from the Congressional Budget Office Report [9].

and 90 percent of all payments linked to quality or value by 2018 [8]. The vast majority of private health plans have similar timelines to transition to value-based care. Anesthesia practices need to be well informed and active participants in these new models of care and payment methodologies by seeking opportunities to engage in perioperative leadership and performance improvement activities for financial upside.

Population Health Management

Population health management is an extension of value-based care at its best, this term refers to the process of managing a population of patients through clinically innovative cost avoiding strategies focused on preventative medicine rather than treating illness and complications to establish improved overall health outcomes for the population such that less expensive healthy patients exist. How the specialty of anesthesiology can impact an entire geographic population where the goal is to avoid costly acute hospital-based care may seem daunting but less so when you take into account population health starts with patient engagement, education, and optimization of chronic disease which is the foundation of the perioperative surgical home model of care.

Just as the emergency room is the front door of the hospital for patients coming into an acute care stay in an unscheduled fashion; surgery is the front door for patients coming into the hospital for the most part in a scheduled fashion. Anesthesia groups have the opportunity to be leaders and collaborators with their healthcare systems by optimizing this "front door" as only the anesthesiologist can truly bridge the huge disconnect between what the primary care physicians can do and the operating room (OR). Through improved communication and integration across service lines throughout the different phases of care and coordination of care, targeting prevention of complications and less costly postoperative care options, anesthesiology is best situated to manage the entire perioperative book of business.

Leadership and work involved in standing up new patient care delivery models are efforts not traditional paid by current payment methodologies making it mission critical to ensure the anesthesia group leadership is well aligned with the healthcare organization they serve. Funding of nonclinical time can be recognized by shared savings when financially successful episodes of care are reconciled or through many other mechanisms such as leadership stipends, comanagement agreements or incentive performance payments.

Section 3. Key Competencies

Beyond the fundamentals of staffing and billing come the intricacies of actually managing the anesthesia group successfully on multiple fronts. This section provides a fairly high level discussion of some of these key areas.

Contracting Anesthesia Services

When negotiating a contract for delivery of anesthesia services, both the anesthesia practice and the healthcare facility must establish and clearly define mutual goals and desired outcomes to ensure success for all parties. Healthcare organizations generally seek to partner with anesthesia groups that are willing to build and structure a team that supports the culture and needs of the healthcare organization. Likewise, the organization and its key stakeholders must be willing to consider and adapt to recommendations for a practice model and structure that allows the anesthesia group to optimize clinical outcomes while maintaining the highest degree of financial independence.

Hospitals and healthcare facilities seeking an anesthesia partner typically issue a request for proposal (RFP) in which the facility issues a formal invitation to multiple anesthesia groups to submit a proposal.

The RFP process for both the anesthesia group and the healthcare facility starts with a very detailed and thoughtful analysis of the anesthesia needs of the organization. This analysis helps ensure facility leadership has developed an understanding of the exact services required and the optimal manner in which they may be provided. A well-structured RFP provides sufficient information for anesthesia practices to not only determine the services being sought but also to obtain critical insight into the environment in which those services will be provided. If not present in the RFP, anesthesia practice leaders should request the following information before submitting their response.

1. Facility demographics including location, size, classifications (community, trauma, for-profit, not-for-profit, etc.), governance structure, and leadership.
2. Status of current anesthesia services, including group structure (independent providers, group, etc.), model (all MD, Care Team, etc.), number of each type of provider, and contract expiration date.

3. Detailed listing of all anesthetizing locations, including number of locations staffed by client personnel at different times of the day for each day of the week. This should include expectations for workflow support that may require additional providers, such as extra rooms used to flip cases in procedural areas, expectations for staffing variation by shift, and depth and intensity of call coverage.
4. Information about caseloads, including service lines; frequently performed procedures; case/patient volumes, including surgery, deliveries, and C-section rate; and ancillary services like endoscopy, cardiac catheterization lab, and interventional radiology. The percentage of ancillary volumes supported by anesthesia should be indicated, including the same type of day-of-week and hour-of-day detail provided for surgery volumes and any available information about volume trends by procedure area and service line.
5. Expectations and requirements for anesthesia provider specialty training and skills, such as pain, cardiothoracic and pediatric fellowship training or transesophageal echocardiography anesthesia, and regional pain management skills.
6. Patient demographics (age, gender) for procedure areas and the facility as a whole.
7. Payer mix information for the procedure areas and for the facility as a whole, including trends in payer mix and reimbursement by payer.
8. Information about organizational governance of the medical staff and where anesthesia fits into the model, including specific bylaws or relationships with other facilities or parent organizations that may impact the anesthesia management structure.
9. Clearly defined service expectations details; for example, in-house 24 × 7 coverage of the Labor and Delivery unit, participation in hospital quality or service initiatives like HealthGrades, reduction in ER to OR times for trauma patients, or presurgical phone calls to patients.
10. Details about any strategies in the 5-year business plan of the facility that will impact provision of anesthesia services through increased or decreased volumes, major changes in payer mix, loss or acquisition of major service

lines or medical staff providers, and facility expansion plans.

The RFP process should provide the opportunity for serious candidates to tour the anesthetizing locations to observe existing patient flow, physical plant, and anesthesia equipment. It should also require all parties to keep confidential any information disclosed by either the healthcare organization or practices submitting proposals. Otherwise, the parties may be reluctant to release detailed information about their internal business plans and performance, making it difficult to accurately align proposed goals and services with those of the facility.

Once a facility has identified a potentially suitable anesthesia practice to be its business partner, it is critical that all the appropriate stakeholders engage in discussions, including the facility's C-suite members with administrative oversight of the procedural areas; chief financial officer; key medical staff members (including chiefs of surgery, obstetrics, and cardiology); and departmental leaders in perioperative services, obstetrics, and other anesthetizing locations.

Recruiting

Recruiting and retaining talented anesthesia providers is a critical function of anesthesia leadership, secondary only to maintenance of clinical excellence. The costs associated with recruitment of a single anesthesiologist may range from $25,000 to $50,000 and even reach $100,000 for high-demand subspecialists with advanced training and skills. Successful recruiting requires detailed knowledge of the hospital or healthcare facility work environment, including case mix and surgeon or proceduralist expectations.

Once candidates are identified, the practice should gather information that includes credentials related to education, certifications, and licensure; work history; personal goals and attributes; and references. As the interview process necessarily exposes the candidate to the facility, it is critical that practice leadership perform full due diligence before any on-site visits. Today's hiring process also may include personality and leadership style assessments for key hires to identify gaps and performance potentials that may impact the group with the goal to prevent hires that may not be successful within a specific culture and reduce staff turnover.

The information-gathering phase should include requests to candidates to explain employment gaps, past and current malpractice, litigation, and/or disciplinary actions, and other details about education and employment history. Sufficient time should be allowed to follow up on any questionable items prior to the interview. Ideally, at least two members of the practice should conduct a preliminary interview with the candidate by phone, exploring any areas that have been at the root of past issues for the practice with former group members as well as areas recognized as highly desirable in the work environments of the practice.

Only candidates who pass the initial background review and are found to be probable matches in the initial phase of the selection process should advance to an on-site interview. On site, candidates should have the opportunity to interact with numerous members of the practice, facility leadership, and key members of the medical staff. Interview questions should focus on areas not covered by the curriculum vitae and be designed to gain insight into the candidate's opinions and ideas, knowledge and experience, as well as work style, interpersonal skills and leadership capabilities. For instance, the interviewer may ask the candidate to provide extemporaneous examples of work experiences that expose his or her strengths and weaknesses, team skills, and interpersonal relationship style.

Special care is advised when vetting PRN (as needed) or locum tenens (temporary) staff. While they may step in to fill the position of a permanent staff member for an extended period of time, their goals and work habits may not be fully aligned with those of the practice and the facility. Many practices make the critical mistake of assuming exemplary clinical skills are sufficient to be a successful member of the practice when, in fact, clinical skills are a minimal qualification for success. Consult with a human resource specialist to gain information about material that cannot be discussed in the hiring process to avoid risk of equal employment violations.

Scheduling

Scheduling coverage for the practice is a complex task that goes well beyond the simple task of assigning staff to shifts and rooms. Effective scheduling begins with determining the true needs of each anesthetizing location. Rarely are anesthesia coverage needs static throughout the day or throughout the week. In high volume, complex departments like surgery, work with department leadership to use data from the surgery information system to determine actual capacity demands by hour of day and day of week. Smaller department's use manual scheduling logs or review patient records assessed over several weeks or months. This extra effort will help avoid gaps in coverage during busy periods and wasted resources during downtimes.

Any scheduling methodology must take into consideration not only staff preferences but also shift equity, fair distribution of responsibilities, limits on consecutive work hours, numbers of day and night shifts, on-call needs, weekend-off requests, and absences for personal time off. Also of vital importance is the employment status of staff members. In practices where nonphysician providers and support personnel (CRNAs, AAs, and anesthesia techs) are salaried, the added expense of overtime can be avoided if the typical workload remains reasonable over the 40-h week. However, if the workweek consistently runs past 40 h or the personnel works on an hourly basis, use historical caseload data to staff the practice with adequate staff to work late hours.

Consider creating a long-range schedule with vacations, weekend call, and weeknight call occurring in a consistently repeating rotation. This type of schedule offers the greatest predictability for planning one's personal life in advance, since call commitments are predictable and occur with consistent repetition. The rotating schedule also offers the easiest option for covering postcall days off and/or days with spikes in volume. Staff members who need a particular day or series of days off can then swap with assigned teammates as needed. Conversely, staff members can make scheduling requests in advance, and the schedule can be built around those personal preferences.

Information Technology

EHRs have become ubiquitous within healthcare in part due to incentive programs mandated by Medicare and Medicaid but also due to business needs around clinical care, billing operations, regulatory, and quality compliance items. Eligible providers, including many anesthesiologists, have benefited from these financial incentives with more than 479,000 healthcare providers receiving payment for participation as of October of 2015 [10]. Current EHR incentive programs published by CMS will focus on advanced use of certified EHR technologies that support health information exchange and interoperability, allow for advanced quality measurement, and maximize clinical effectiveness and efficiencies [10].

Despite the fact that nearly 97 percent of hospitals nationwide have implemented a certified EHR technology nearly 50 percent do not have advanced solutions that include an Anesthesia Information Management System (AIMS) for electronic data capture within the OR and perioperative environments [11]. The perioperative environment has challenges that make implementation of an AIMS very costly and potentially disruptive to clinical workflow efficiencies, the main reason there has been a lag in adoption in this area. But as technology has advanced AIMS have become a catalyst for the transformation of anesthesia care delivery through the use of innovative smart logic and patient centered care pathways enabling clinicians to work smarter not just harder.

The anesthesia practice must recognize the financial investment an AIMS solution is, whether it is the healthcare organization or the group itself bringing in the technology there needs to be a designated trusted anesthesia leader engaged in the implementation to ensure a cost-effective solution maximizes the IT investment by meeting the needs of a particular environment. As technologies continue to advance, incorporating cognitive computing and even artificial intelligence solutions into the perioperative environment, there will be system wide organizational change as traditional workflows that once occurred in parallel become more seamlessly integrated around spending time and resources only on value added care.

Evaluating the Practice

It was traditionally quite simple for a facility to assess the performance of its anesthesia provider relative to their expectations for service. Expectations were so consistent, they were easily defined as "The Four A's," ability, availability, affordability, and affability. Which meant: provide quality care, be on time, remain financially independent from the organization, and act in a professional manner. Today, the expectations of healthcare organizations have grown to also encompass financial accountability and better patient outcomes.

A great anesthesia department operates almost seamlessly with no disruptions in daily patient flow where the results of satisfaction surveys from patients and surgeons speak for themselves and all regulatory departmental functions operate smoothly. Beyond the appearance of a well-functioning anesthesia department proper evaluation of the anesthesia department requires some objective criteria.

Look at the data. The delivery of anesthesia services can either facilitate throughput and performance in procedural care areas or hinder it. Review key performance indicators, including patient throughput, day-of-procedure cancellations, and case turnover times. Once identified, these performance indicators can be tied to performance benchmarks. Throughput indicators such as on time starts, turnover times, and case delays cause and frequency are a measure of the group's responsiveness to daily operational needs of the client. Day-of-procedure cancellations and timeliness of pre- and postanesthesia assessment are indicative of the quality of the preanesthesia clearance process and attention to patient outcomes. Great practices will have access to and proactively deploy proven tools for improving performance in these areas, including access to perioperative management specialists, Lean Manufacturing techniques, and ongoing quality improvement cycles.

Review quality outcomes. Quality management is a regulatory requirement for anesthesia departments. This includes ensuring case reviews are completed, effective peer review is in place and effective remediation for quality issues is deployed. Great anesthesia groups develop strong relationships with the healthcare facility's quality assurance/quality management, risk, and regulatory compliance departments. They also have their own internal audit process and routinely have their quality outcomes, documentation compliance, and regulatory performance reviewed by an objective, knowledgeable outside source with programs in place to ensure benchmark performance on all measures. In addition, they actively support and provide required Focused Provider Performance Reviews on new providers and Ongoing Provider Performance Reviews on active members of the practice. Great practices maintain their anesthesia policies and procedures in current compliance with ASA standards as well as those of the healthcare facility's specific accreditation partner – typically The Joint Commission or Healthcare Facilities Accreditation Program.

Evaluate the leadership. Effective anesthesia physician leadership and organizational governance are key to running a great practice. Lack of effective leadership triggers problems both internally and externally as the cohesiveness of the group decays, commitment to standards declines and support of the healthcare facility's interests take second chair. Effectiveness as a group leader depends less on tenure or years of experience and more upon possession of key leadership skills. The anesthesia leader must either possess or have immediate access to current evidence-based knowledge on effective perioperative management and clearly understand how the department of anesthesia impacts the day-to-day effectiveness of the procedural care area. The leader must possess the interpersonal skills to build relationships with and engender trust from even the most recalcitrant member of the medical staff. It is not necessary that the leader have active clinical experience in all specialty areas served, but superior knowledge in anesthesia fundamentals is imperative. The leader must also commit to devoting adequate time to maintaining up-to-date expertise in anesthesia quality and compliance standards, and to monitoring and assessing the performance of the anesthesia staff relative to those standards.

Examine the credentials of the providers. While there are numerous highly qualified providers who practice anesthesia absent board certification and specialty certifications, the presence of these credentials is an outward measure of the group's overall clinical qualifications. At a minimum, physician members should be board-eligible and actively pursuing certification. Mid-level nonphysician providers should be actively licensed with no restrictions. The great anesthesia practice will ensure all its members meet these requirements. If specialty services are offered, such as cardiothoracic anesthesia, pain management, and neonatal, all providers who participate in the service should be experienced and qualified and at least one member should hold active fellowship-level training in the discipline. Policies and protocols for specialty services should be clearly delineated and all providers serving the specialty should have mentored introduction to the service.

Assess the group's financial strength and stability. Financial sustainability has a profound effect on both the members of the practice and its healthcare facility partner. In assessing financial strength and stability, determine if the practice has internal or external resources to provide expertise in managing payer relations and billing. A great anesthesia practice will be a good steward of its financial potential, contracting favorable terms with payers, carefully documenting patient care to support optimal billing, and coding in full compliance with regulatory guidelines. Failure in any of these pursuits could lead to inadequate cash flow, which could cause the practice to become dependent upon financial support from the healthcare facility, even in markets with a favorable payer mix. Obviously, not all healthcare markets can sustain an independent anesthesia practice, but even in those difficult markets, a great anesthesia practice will accurately forecast any shortfalls and actively work to reduce any financial support. Financial performance should be assessed regularly through structured meetings where transparency is assured and mutual goals are aligned.

Evaluate the ability of the group to respond and adapt. The optimal anesthesia partner is well versed in the challenges that face its partner healthcare facility in the areas of healthcare reform. These challenges include new provisions for pay-for-performance and transformation funding in which more integrated systems of care linked with improved outcomes ensure optimal global payments that encompass the entire patient episode of care. In addition, procedural services – particularly in the perioperative environment – are typically the largest single source of revenue for healthcare organizations. Inefficient OR scheduling and patient throughput or poor staffing utilization, therefore, can have significant financial impact on the organization. As the major stakeholder throughout perioperative services, the great anesthesia practice should have well-developed programs to help ensure the healthcare facilities financial success as well as its own.

Reforming an Underperforming Practice

When evaluation of the anesthesia practice identifies gaps in performance, creating an action plan for improvement is imperative. This may require practice leadership to share results with the healthcare facilities leadership to develop a plan to improve performance. Just the act of voluntarily sharing performance data with the healthcare facility partner can increase its confidence in the anesthesia practice as the healthcare facility has most likely already been assessing the data themselves.

Reengineering an existing practice is a daunting task for even the most experienced leader. The ongoing demands of providing anesthesia services to an active caseload demand time and attention, and the practice may simply lack the skill set required to accomplish the required transformation. In these instances, practice leaders may want to consider seeking outside management support.

To turn around an existing practice, consider the following guidance to address some of the most fundamental practice issues.

Poor performance. When benchmarks and goals are not being met, performance improvement plans must be put in place. As suggested earlier, a meeting between practice and healthcare facility leaders may help prioritize efforts. Then begin by attacking one metric at a time. While initiating an analysis of the entire preoperative process may be the initial inclination, the department is likely to be overwhelmed by the scope of this exercise. In place or in conjunction with a full assessment, choose a component easily controlled to start, such as ensuring charts on all elective cases are reviewed, anesthesia admission orders are written, and a tentative anesthesia plan developed.

Many issues are not problems of process but rather problems of communication or interpersonal conflict. The anesthesia provider interacts with professionals at all levels of the healthcare organization and is therefore in a unique position to improve communication and change paradigms. Bring the anesthesia team together to utilize the goodwill and political capital they hold as perioperative leaders to affect behavioral changes in healthcare peers.

Quality deficiencies. Meeting quality metrics begins with a shared commitment to improvement. A thorough assessment of each provider in the practice may reveal some do not understand the metric, do not understand the importance of meeting the requirements, are not committed to fulfilling their responsibility to meet the goal, or a combination of all these factors. Anesthesia leaders must clearly communicate the importance of meeting quality metrics and follow through to ensure all providers are compliant with established standards. Establish a system of effective peer review to identify individual providers who perform below benchmarks or whose clinical practice does not represent the highest level of patient care. Use any variance from expected performance as a learning opportunity for the whole team.

Ineffective leadership. Ineffective leadership in the anesthesia practice presents a difficult challenge for both members of the group and healthcare facility leaders. The failure of a group to internally discipline itself or to create a culture of citizenship built on professionalism, effective communication, and accountability can create an environment of conflict. The measure of a leader in the clinical environment, particularly a close-knit environment like anesthesia, is the ability to foster this culture and to apply effective professional discipline when the culture is breached. Underperforming providers decrease the productivity of the entire group, and an effective leader will quickly progress these individuals through a performance improvement plan, culminating with removal from the group, if required. Both members of the anesthesia group and facility leadership should not confuse being well-liked or clinical expertise with being an effective leader. Unfortunately, the leader may be the underperformer. In this case, facility medical staff leadership may be called upon to help effect a change. This may best be accomplished by bringing in a management consultant or by encouraging the members of the group to move the practice under the management of a larger anesthesia management group.

Underperforming or underqualified providers. The anesthesia group is no better than the sum of its parts. Since anesthesia practice, even in groups, involves periodic solo practice – while on call, for example – even one poor performer can impact the entire group. Poor clinical practice is actually the easiest issue to address. Providers with deficiencies should be offered immediate remedial training. Clinical performance is a base expectation for overall performance, so if performance does not improve to benchmark or above, the provider should be removed.

The situation becomes more complex when providers are clinically competent – perhaps even exceptional – yet lack the certifications required by medical staff, such as Anesthesia Boards or Cardiac Fellowship. Some deficiencies can be overcome with structured study assignments, workshops, and CME offerings, but if medical staff bylaws or the contract with the facility requires all providers to be board-eligible or -certified, group leadership has no option but to require this of its providers.

Even more challenging is dealing with the problem provider who meets all clinical, credentialing, and regulatory standards, yet fails to blend with practice or client personnel as a team. Others may meet all expectations, including those required for effective teamwork, but commit some transgression, such as drug diversion or inappropriate behavior with a member of the staff. The optimal way to deal with these situations is to have in place a zero-tolerance policy for any behavior detrimental or counter to the best interests of the facility partner. Tolerance by members of the practice, which may stem from a desire to buy forbearance for their own behaviors, will likely be viewed as lack of commitment to the facility and its patients and will, over time, decrease the stability of the contract and the practice.

The solution to each of these issues is straightforward: set a standard, measure performance, execute a performance improvement plan – and if appropriate, remove those who do not comply.

Financial instability. Anesthesia has a fiduciary responsibility to the members of the group and the healthcare facility partner to maintain the highest possible level of financial integrity and independence. Payer contracting and billing is complex and time consuming, and it may be tempting for anesthesia leadership to seek support from the healthcare organization rather than to apply the necessary resources needed to optimize the group's own reimbursement. A sufficient proportion of anesthesia proceeds must be allocated to high-quality financial management of the group's business concerns. To facilitate financial independence, the healthcare organization must work in partnership with the anesthesia group to create efficiencies in the procedural care areas to conserve resources. Financial success and independence can also be fostered by allowing the anesthesia provider latitude in negotiating favorable payment terms with payers rather than expecting it to fall in lock-step with facility contracts.

Anesthesia practices often sabotage their own success by cutting corners to reduce costs associated with contract management, coding, and billing. A high quality practice management firm, or even an anesthesia-specific billing firm, may dramatically improve receipts, reducing dependence on the healthcare organization and increasing the stability of the contract. Processes should be in place to automate patient eligibility verification, track and pattern denials, provide automated concurrency tracking and billing, and speed payment postings. The healthcare organization should require annual evidence of these and other advanced financial practices to ensure contracted providers optimize their own financial support. If the practice is performing all possible due diligence for financial management and is still unable to meet contracted expectations, then the parties should perform additional more extensive analysis to determine possible causes for anesthesia financial shortfalls and explore costly inefficiencies in resource utilization that may need to be better allocated.

Summary

Effective practice management positions the anesthesia practice to optimize opportunities for partnership with the healthcare organization that maximize practice efficiencies, improves reportable measures, ensures quality patient care, and increases patient satisfaction. Even a practice successfully meeting all of these goals should seek further opportunities to leverage the relationship between the practice and the healthcare facility through clinical innovation and leadership.

Value-based care links payment for services to quality outcomes. This creates an opportunity for anesthesia to support optimal outcomes on clinical measures in the procedural environment; and with the frequent interaction between anesthesia provider and patient in the continuum of care, anesthesia is also perfectly positioned to drive patient satisfaction. The "great" anesthesia practice will not have to be forced into this role but, rather, will embrace it as a way to ensure the mutual success of the practice and its healthcare facility partner. By aligning goals with the healthcare partner and attending to the success of the surgeon, the nurse leader, the administrator and the patient the anesthesia practice ensures their anesthesia services contract remains secure.

References

1. AS Resnick, D Corrigan, JL Mullen, LR Kaiser. Surgeon contribution to hospital bottom line – Not all are created equal. *Annals of Surgery* 2005; 242 (4): 530–9.

2. C Clark. Surgical admissions bring 48 of hospital revenue. March 4, 2014. www.healthleadersmedia.com/quality/ahrq-surgical-admissions-bring-48-hospital-revenue#

3. SB Cohen. The concentration of health care expenditures and related expenses for costly medical conditions. October 2014. http://meps.ahrq.gov/mepsweb/data_files/publications/st455/stat455.pdf

4. H Greenfield. Anesthesia 101: Anesthesia subsidy drivers. http://enhancehc.com/anesthesia-101-anesthesia-subsidy-drivers/

5. W Panza, R Dahl. What hospital CEOs need to know about surgical services: 4 strategies for protecting OR revenue. *Surgical Directions* 2013.

6. A Liebhaber, JM Grossman. Physicians moving to mid-sized, single-specialty practices. *Tracking Report* 2007; 18: 1–5.

7. *Medicare Claims Processing Manual.* Chapter 12: Physicians/Nonphysician Practitioners. www.cms.gov/Regulations-and-Guidance/Guidance/Manuals/downloads/clm104c12.pdf

8. The merit-based incentive payment system: MIPS scoring methodology overview. www.cms.gov/Medicare/Quality-Initiatives-Patient-Assessment-Instruments/Value-Based-Programs/MACRA-MIPS-and-APMs/MIPS-Scoring-Methodology-slide-deck.pdf

9. T Hayford, L Nelson. CBO's analysis of financial pressures facing hospitals identifies need for additional research on hospitals' productivity and responses. September 8, 2016. www.cbo.gov/publication/51920

10. Center for Medicare and Mediciad Services. HER incentive program basics. www.cms.gov/regulations-and-guidance/legislation/ehrincentiveprograms/basics.html

11. The Office of the National Coordinator for Health Information Technology. Adoption of HER record systems among US non-federal acute care hospitals. ONC Data Brief No. 23, April 2015. www.healthit.gov/sites/default/files/data-brief/2014HospitalAdoptionDataBrief.pdf

Defining the Anesthesia Value Proposition

Jody Locke

Contents

Anesthesia can be a particularly paradoxical specialty. On the one hand, its practitioners claim to enjoy the shortest decision cycle of any medical specialty. It is said there is no clinical challenge they cannot address and resolve in a matter of 10 or 15 s. And yet, when faced with the sweeping changes taking place in healthcare, they often become paralyzed like deer in a headlight. Timely and reliable data about a patient's every physiological response to the anesthetic and surgery makes for confident decision making in the operating room (OR), but most have no such tools to guide them outside the OR. The skills that have been so carefully honed for patient management still have yet to be consistently applied to effective practice management. Like kids playing in heavy surf, most are still recovering from the last wave when the next one comes crashing down. What used to be hours of boredom punctuated by moments of sheer terror seems to have evolved into a state of chronic anguish and frustration, at least for those who are paying attention to the state of the specialty.

When we survey the current anesthesia landscape it is littered with the vestiges of so many once proud and productive practices. So many good providers with all the best intentions have had to find new places to work. While anesthesia is focused on managing patients safely and securely through the trauma of surgery, no one seems to be managing the specialty safely and securely through the trauma of healthcare reform. The disruption has been pervasive and unpredictable. The specialty that prides itself on being able to prepare for the unexpected has been caught totally off guard.

The values and aspirations that anesthesiologists and their managers bring to the relationship with hospital administrators reflect a long history of balancing a need for personal independence with a professional reality of interdependence. It used to be that the only time representatives of an anesthesia group met with their hospital administration was to renegotiate the contract. Today's healthcare market requires a collaborative partnership between anesthesia and administration. Most anesthesia practices understand this intuitively but still struggle making it a reality.

In her book *Confidence*, Rosa Moss Kantor identifies three qualities that make for confidence in a business relationship. She sees them as accountability, collaboration, and innovation. It is an especially relevant observation and framework for understanding the challenges facing today's group practices. The market expectation is that all providers and practices will be completely accountable for the consistency and quality of the care they provide; that has always been an implicit expectation, if not an objectively verifiable one. There is supposed to be a collaborative work environment in the OR, but the reality is that personality may often make it otherwise. More recently anesthesia is attempting to take the lead in its perioperative surgical home initiative, but there is still work to be done.

For years anesthesia providers tended to be viewed as very highly paid technicians whose knowledge of physiology and pharmacology made them indispensable to effective OR management. Most of today's anesthesia practices have more and better data in their billing computers about what actually happens in the OR and delivery suite than anyone else in the facility. And yet is any of this valuable data being used to effect meaningful changes in the way ORs are managed or staffed? This remains one of the great opportunities for the specialty. The training and insights of its practitioners should prove ripe for innovation but it does not. Even today most anesthesia providers see themselves as captive to a system over which they have no control. Such thinking and an unwillingness for self-promotion has defined the box in which most practices still operate.

There are many notable exceptions. Those with strategic vision talk of reclaiming control over the factors that determine their income and lifestyle. Most recognize that the relationship between anesthesia and administration is the critical factor. Simply said, the more partnership, the more potential for anesthesia. It is now widely accepted that regular involvement in hospital committees and administration is essential to long-term survival.

Without a doubt, though, the specialty of anesthesia is at a strategic crossroads. Practitioners must come to terms with their sacred cows. Times of rapid change force one to evaluate those core values that define your being and which should never be compromised. At the same time practices must assess the beliefs and strategies that were once so important but which no longer serve the organization. It is not an easy task. It is tough to let go of beliefs and practices that have worked so well like physician-only anesthesia or democratic group management.

Are anesthesia practices more challenged in the face of today's healthcare market changes than other specialists? Probably not, but every medical specialty has its own specific challenges and issues. The typical anesthesia group practice is still a work in progress, as old habits die hard. If we accept the importance of an effective and efficient OR suite in the profitability of a hospital, then the specialty of anesthesia and its potential to provide comprehensive perioperative management has an opportunity that no other specialty enjoys. If the primary customer is the surgeon then there is no other category of providers that has the same potential to influence and manage surgeon behavior. The question is always who will take this on and is the practice willing to pay its members for their nonclinical contributions.

More often than not a practice's history is its greatest obstacle to change. Despite the clinical risks that anesthesia providers manage so competently, most providers tend to be very risk-averse by nature, which shows up clearly in the organizations they form. There are exceptions to every rule. Some notable practices stand out as models of effective business

units, but most do not and the sad reality is that most will not survive.

Those of us who have been in this business for a long time, and my career goes back to 1982, have seen a dramatic transformation in the specialty over the past 35 years. The change has reflected a collective provider response to key developments in healthcare such as the expansion of managed care, the refinement of Medicare guidelines relative to medical direction, Medicare rate cuts, manpower shortages, hospital consolidations, the expansion of the role of anesthesia into perioperative care, and, most recently, healthcare reform. It has been an evolution from simplicity to complexity, where each new overlay of issues further complicates an already complex landscape. Good clinical outcomes used to be all that really mattered but now good outcomes are a given and taken for granted.

What has changed? Probably how hard it has become to make a good living as an anesthesia provider. Looking back we can see how virtually all practices have evolved through three very distinct phases or eras which are defined by the financial status of the practice. We can think of them as the fee-for-service, subsidy, and self-determination.

The Fee-for-Service Era

Charles Darwin would have found anesthesia a fascinating study in evolution. How the specialty appears now and how different each practice is today seems to have so little relationship to how the specialty looked even 30 years ago. Individual practices had to adapt to such a variety and diversity of market changes. The basic genetic make-up of the provider is still pretty much the same, although there have clearly been generational factors that have conditioned provider outlook, and yet every practice has had to adapt in its own way to the environment in which it is trying to exist. There have been so many practices and so many that have failed over the years and so many more that will fail in the next year or two. Can we describe the process as anything but the survival of the fittest?

If few go back far enough each of today's formal group practices was probably little more than a loose confederation of independent fee-for-service anesthesiologists. Such arrangements tended to be rather informal, which is to say that usually one person took control and managed the schedule in a way that he benefitted. There was never any documentation. The physicians somehow figured out how to meet the coverage requirements of the facility. While there were few guarantees and fewer legal protections to their practices there was no managed care and you could make as much as you wanted; it just depended how hard you wanted to work. In retrospect we can see the challenges clearly. There was definitely favoritism and cherry picking of cases by those with the most influence, usually the cardiovascular anesthesiologists. It was not easy to break into a good practice. Many practices in the West would let young physicians work as locums until a full-time slot opened up. You had to cover all your own expenses until your collections ramped up. It was all about performing billable services. There were lots of reasons why hospitals were so eager to see these groups form into more formal entities not the least of which was there was no real accountability.

Many of the values that still inform today's anesthesia practices go back to those early days. Those founding doctors prided themselves on their clinical skills. Having completed an anesthesia training program at a reputable training program, you were assumed to be qualified. No one was going to oversee or monitor the care you provided. That was one of the hallmarks of the specialty. An anesthesiologist sized up the circumstances of each case and defined his or her own solution; it was both art and science. Having privileges at a facility was viewed as a personal right, equal to having tenure at an academic center. There was great personal and professional pride in the service provided but you were really only as good as you said you were.

This type of practice and this way of thinking also defined how most anesthesiologists preferred to practice and what attracted physicians to the specialty. Anesthesiologists strove for a maximum of freedom and independence and a minimum of interference and oversight. Departmental decisions tended to either be made by the chief (or czar in some cases) or based on majority vote, which as we all know is the surest way to maintain the status quo. Even as formal group practices eventually started to be established in the 1980s and 1990s the governance was always based on a purely democratic model of decision making. Even today, many cite their democratic governance structure as one of their most important features. Usually a president or managing partner would either appoint himself or be picked by the group. In many cases this person held the position until he retired. Nobody ever thought about succession planning.

While it was not always easy for a young graduate to obtain an ideal position at a good hospital – one with busy ORs and a favorable payer mix – what made the system work so well was the potential for success. Anesthesiologists were becoming some of the highest paid physicians. With all the exciting developments taking place in the specialty with new technology, powerful pharmacology and diverse clinical opportunities the specialty started to attract the best and the brightest of American graduates. Up until the bottom fell out of the market in 1994, anesthesia was the place to be if you wanted to make money. The specialty was infused with a spirit that you could write your own ticket.

One of the historical ironies of the specialty is that there was nurse anesthesia before there was physician anesthesia and yet we think of it the other way around. Many hospitals, especially in the east, employed nurses to administer anesthesia. It is no accident Pennsylvania has always had the highest number of CRNAs in absolute terms of any state and also the highest number of CRNAs employed by hospitals. Physician anesthesiologists were gradually layered in as part of departments of surgery. Practices where there were nurse anesthetists tended to evolve into formal group practices first because a formal group structure was necessary for physicians and CRNAs to work together effectively. Physician-only practices, by contrast, were slow to accept the need for a formal group structure. This historical fact also explains why there are so many practices today where a private physician group manages a staff of hospital-employed CRNAs.

The unique history of the specialty resulted in five private practice models (nonacademic) across the country by the early 1990s. The status of university providers evolved in a completely different manner and is not particularly germane to our discussion here.

1. Some physicians, especially in the west, continued to practice as solo practitioners working in loose confederations.
2. Some hospitals employed anesthesiologists to medically direct employed CRNAs.
3. Some hospitals that employed CRNAs, encouraged the physician anesthesiologists to create group practices with which they contracted.
4. Other practices that employed CRNAs formed group practices as a logical means of managing physicians and nonphysician staff.
5. Many physician-only practices reluctantly gave in to the pressure to form a group practice.

This last category has proved the most interesting and diverse but probably the most illustrative. Given the inherent prejudice among independent anesthesiologists against employment by a group practice, there had to be a compelling reason to get the individual providers to sign on to a corporate entity. More often than not it was a hospital administration that had run out of patience dealing with multiple anesthesia providers many of whom were reluctant to agree to manage care contracts that were deemed to be strategically important to the facility. We still refer to the origin of many practices as "shot gun marriages." An enlightened few actually came to the conclusion on their own that there was strength in numbers and understood the strategic advantage a strong group structure would provide. The best example of this was the big group in San Diego, Anesthesia Services Medical Group, the oldest and largest group practice up until about 10 years ago.

Perhaps the most interesting example took place in Salt Lake City. By the mid-1990s the administration of LDS Hospital had made it very clear that it was tired of dealing with 35 individual physician practices and that they must merge into a single group. The physicians considered their options and hired two consultants from for San Diego, George Viglotti and Leslie Allison, who encouraged them to think bigger. The resulting entity, Mountain West Anesthesia was formed as the consolidation of anesthesiologists up and down the Wasatch front. Its initial membership was somewhere above 100 providers. One might suggest that the moral of the story is to be careful what you ask for; you just might get it. For a while the press referred to the group as the Mountain West Cartel. This was not an isolated example. All across the country anesthesiologists were struggling with the same strategic question: how do we gain some level of control over the factors that determine our income and lifestyle.

It is impossible to consider the history of anesthesia practice management without factoring in the role of managed care. So long as an anesthesiologist could simply bill patients for his fees life was simple and a physician could make a good living. In the premanaged care era many physicians even did their own billing or had their wives do it. Most people don't remember this today but the real impetus for the expansion of managed care was Medicare. It all started with the Medicare fee freeze in 1984. Medicare payment rates were frozen for 2 years and then they started to drop as HCFA (Health Care Finance Administration), which became CMS (Center for Medicare and Medicaid Services) under the second Bush administration, experimented with a variety of payment mechanisms the end result of which was the Resource-Based Relative Value System (RBRVS) that was implemented in 1992. By most estimates RBRVS reduced the average anesthesiologist's compensation by 30 percent for Medicare patients. To offset this impact most physicians started raising their rates to all non-Medicare patients. There was a period of time during with virtually all medical practices had two fee schedules: the Medicare fees and the non-Medicare fees. The push back came from commercial payers who introduced a variety of preferred provider organization (PPO) options. The basic concept was simple: with negotiation of a slightly reduced contracted rate, the check would come directly to the provider who would only have to bill patients for deductibles and copayments. Sounds simple, but the repercussions were dramatic. Instead of getting paid what they billed, all providers would only get paid based on the rates they had negotiated. This was a game changer.

As the percentage of patients covered by PPO and HMO plans increased, the challenge was to obtain competitive rates. Of course, you had to do this without any knowledge of what other groups were getting paid. Consider this example. Suppose an anesthesiologist was collecting an average of $40 per ASA unit billed. Typically a physician working alone would generate about 10,000 units per year. Let us suppose that 2,500 units were billed to Medicare and 500 to Medicaid. In 1984 with a Medicare rate frozen at $40 per unit and a Medicaid rate at $15 the remaining 7,000 units would have to generate at average yield of $41.25 to maintain practice collections at the same level. When the Medicare rate dropped to $30 per unit the offset average would have to be $45 per unit and by the time it reached the current rate of $20 per unit the average commercial and managed care yield would have to be $50 per unit and these are net yields after bad debt. This is why the concept of payer mix became so important. Being able to monitor and confirm the financial impact of each payer on the overall net yield to the practice was not just a good idea but an essential strategic tool. Ever since the mid-1980s practices in most parts of the country have been watching the percentage of low-paying Medicare and Medicaid patients increase meaning that the only way to maintain practice income was to aggressively negotiate higher managed care rates. We now refer to this critical indicator as the Public Payor Percentage.

If the key to effective negotiation is leverage, then individual providers have none. Small groups have some and mega-groups potentially have a lot. As anesthesiologists started to understand and appreciate the significance of managed care in their specific markets, and the impact varied dramatically from one part of the country to another, they started to consider strategies to gain leverage thinking that this was the key to their success and survival.

One of the interesting and enduring legacies of this period is that business strategies tended to focus only on one aspect of the practice: revenue generation, which can easily be a very short-sighted objective. If your only goal is to maximize your collections today you may be eroding your reputation for the future. Experience has shown that it is better to focus on customer service and quality of care because and the security of your franchise first because having a place to practice is far more important than just having good contract rates. There is also the legal argument. A large group of providers proposed a big group practice in Texas. Many of the potential providers touted the leverage this would provide to obtain better managed care contracts. Unfortunately, once the practice was operationalized there was an antitrust review in which these initial claims were cited as evidence of antitrust activity.

The 1990s was a period of great introspection and uncertainty in the specialty. The ASA hired ABT and Associates to assess anesthesia manpower needs. The conclusion of its report suggested there were too many providers which many providers took to heart and left anesthesia. A period of significant anesthesia manpower shortage ensued. In fact it took years for levels to recover.

It should also be noted that the ASA was so concerned about the changes taking place that it initiated an entirely new type of conference for its membership. The first ASA Conference on Practice Management was held in Phoenix in 1994. Each year since then this meeting consistently attracts more than 500 attendees to discuss key practice management trends. The general theme of each meeting have been quite consistent: what strategies will prove most effective in securing your practice for the future? Much of the discussion since the first meeting has focused on changing market conditions and threats to the status quo.

The fact is that most group practices exist to maintain a status quo. They are not intended to be vehicles for creative strategic thinking or quick responses to market changes; just the opposite. For all their ability to make 10-s life-and-death decisions in the OR, as business managers anesthesiologists tend to suffer from paralysis by analysis. More often than not, change comes slowly and only in response to significant and negative trends. Where there are issues and problems, physician managers tend to look for the quick fixes first.

As more anesthesia groups were formed, a simple reality became evident: ultimately security was recognized as far more important to the success of the organization than revenue. Those entities that were formed primarily as vehicles for contracting tended to be shaky and many did not survive whereas those that were designed to provide a better product and to ensure the security of the practice tended to survive and thrive. Historically the expectation has been that anesthesia is a very profitable specialty. Most providers have assumed their income would increase each year. Learning that collections are flat or declining can have a profound impact on group members. Many a group president or managing partner has been displaced as a result of poor collections performance.

Disappointing collections performance inevitably leads to a review of the billing solution, either in house or outsourced. This is entirely consistent with the prevailing belief of the day that all any practice needed was enough money and it would do fine. In the face of changing payer mix and contract challenges many anesthesia managers had to get a crash course in accounts receivable management. These were boom times for consultants whose experience in accounts receivable management was eagerly sought. These were also busy times for providers of outsourced billing and management solutions. Many in house billing offices were shut down as practices sought state of the art revenue cycle management and systems.

In many practices the discussion of the size of the revenue pie leads to a discussion of the best way to divide it up. It would appear that a group of anesthesiologists given the challenge of deciding how to pay its members has an almost unlimited capacity to make things complicated. A well-known practice manager and consultant, Linda Venters, was once quoted as saying, "If you have seen one anesthesia compensation plan, you have seen one anesthesia compensation plan."

How anesthesia practices pay themselves is significant and can have far reaching implications in its relationship to the administration and staff. The OR staff virtually always knows how the physicians get paid based on their behavior. It is always obvious what services they are motivated to perform and which they choose to avoid. In the early days the distinguishing feature was payer mix. In a true fee-for-service environment the patients with good commercial insurance were always preferred over those with Medicare and Medicaid. Most groups adopted a payer neutral system that paid providers on a common or neutral unit basis but this did not eliminate the reality of cherry picking. Smart anesthesiologists have a way of figuring out which rooms or which surgeons will allow them to generate the most units and the best incomes. One should never underestimate the impact of compensation in organizations that have basically been created as vehicles for income distribution. The two most contentious issues an anesthesia practice will ever face are those related to how the billing is done and how the income is distributed and once these decisions are made it is virtually impossible to unmake them.

The most significant aspect of this era was that anesthesia was a free good to most administrations. A commitment to customer service meant that pretty much whatever level of service a hospital asked for they got. The joke was if an anesthesia provider was asked to jump, he would respond, "how high?" The problem with scope creep is that eventually it becomes expensive and unsustainable. While many practices started to see the handwriting on the wall there was little they could do to push back on expanding administration expiectations. No one wanted to jeopardize the contractual relationship with the facility by saying no to a service request.

Many of the challenges and opportunities facing anesthesia practices in the current environment are a direct result of their history. Once a culture has been established it is very difficult to change it. Having carefully shielded their practices from any outside scrutiny or oversight by constructing very distinct firewalls between the group and the administration it has not been easy to admit that such a strategy was a self-limiting proposition. This is why the transition from a fee-for-service environment to a subsidy environment has proved to be so disruptive and challenging to so many practices; it required a paradigm shift that most were not ready to accept.

The Subsidy Era

In a fairly short period of time, from about the early 1990s to the end of the decade, the world of anesthesia was tipped upside down. Once proudly independent practices started to realize that they could not survive based on the revenue they were generating from the professional services they provided. This was more than just a financial challenge. It was structural and cultural challenge. Asking for money and being held accountable for anything other than clinical outcomes would require most practices to completely reinvent themselves. The ASA was starting to provide guidance and advice, but the real job of preparing for the future always fell to the individual practice.

By the end of the decade (1999) according to an Medical Group Management Association (MGMA) survey, 75 percent of all anesthesia practices were receiving some form of financial subsidy or support. While some of the arrangements were limited to a specific service, cardiac coverage, obstetrics, etc., many were comprehensive and substantial. In the current environment it is not uncommon to find practices where more than 30 percent of the cost of providing anesthesia comes directly from the facility. Many practices have spent tens of thousands dollars with consultants trying to determine and negotiate a level of support that will ensure their viability, at least in the short term. It is impossible to survey the current landscape without asking the following three questions:

- How did this happen?
- What is the solution?
- Why weren't practices more prepared?

In many ways the transition was a perfect storm and an unfortunate combination of market factors any one of which would not have been very significant but which, when taken together have resulted in a management challenge few could have envisioned. Medicare rate cuts and managed care contracting laid the foundation by creating downward pressure on practice income. The labor shortage of the mid-1990s created a staffing challenge that fueled income expectations. Competition in healthcare caused many hospitals to close and others to merge. Changes in how and where anesthesia services were being provided including the proliferation of ambulatory surgery centers dramatically increased the number of anesthetizing locations. Increasingly anesthesia providers were being viewed as perioperative management consultants. Little by little the number of anesthetizing locations that had to be covered outstripped the revenue generated.

The impact of the squeeze play was felt over time and the initial response was one of denial. Anesthesia had always been subject to peaks and valleys. The fact that the valleys started outnumbering the peaks did not trigger a serious response for a while. Anesthesiologists are used to doing what needed to be done, no matter how long it made their weeks. Eventually, though, the "bleeding" became so serious that it could not be ignored. This was when things got scary. Anesthesia groups had to start asking their primary facilities for financial support.

It is often said that doctors are not businessmen. The need to negotiate with hospital administrations brought this clearly to light. It was the rare anesthesia practice that could define the problem and craft an effective strategy without professional assistance. Part of the problem stemmed from the basic psyche of the anesthesia provider. The physician problem solver who prides himself on being able to diagnose complex clinical problems and make clinical corrections in a matter of seconds tends not to have the patience or discipline to strategize a significant financial request and think through all the dimensions of a comprehensisve stakeholder analysis. Anesthesia providers have been trained to work their way through clinical decision trees that they have been trained on. They think in terms of if-then statements, always looking for the best option. The difference is that in the OR, the anesthesia provider controls all the variables, which is not the case in the board room, where they may not control any of the variables.

The problem was simple in its essence, but the myriad of possible solutions was not always obvious or intuitive. While most anesthesiologists will have delivered thousands of anesthetics, they are likely to negotiate only one or two hospital contracts. When there is not enough revenue being collected from professional services provided to cover the cost of the staff and overhead necessary to provide the service one musts ask two basic questions. Is the problem that anesthesia salary and benefits requirements are unreasonably high? Or is the problem that hospital expectations for coverage and call are unrealistic given the revenue potential of the services provided and the payer mix at the facility? Addressing both of these questions in a way that can lead to a mutually agreeable solution is no small feat and one for which most practices were completely unprepared in the 1990s and even into the new millennium.

It is a basic premise of business that one cannot manage what one does not measure. Developing the necessary practice management tools became job one. Traditional practice management tended to focus only on one thing: revenue generation. A good month was defined by strong collections. Accountants would prepare financial statements that made little sense and which were of little relevance to the average shareholder. It was management by ATM card. There were good months and bad months. If collections were down, the standard response was to beat on the billing staff. Very few practices even prepared regular budgets and fewer still understood the arcane science of cost accounting.

A well-managed company with a CFO (Chief Financial Officer) and a controller should always know how profitable the business is. Financial reporting tools should help identify and distinguish lines of business based on their profitability. The problem with a hospital-based anesthesia practice is that there is not a clear or consistent definition of profitability. The group practice is essentially little more than a distribution mechanism for collections. There is only one practical benchmark: does the practice generate enough revenue to cover the cost of the providers necessary to meet the needs of the facility.

Herein lay one of the basic challenges. Most businesses staff for average levels of production and tend not to hire new employees until there is revenue to cover them. This is based on a strategy of aggressive cost management. Most anesthesia practices, by contrast, tend to staff for peak periods, which means that there is often excess staff. It is an effective strategy to meet the service requirements of the facility and the lifestyle expectations of the providers, but it is an expensive solution.

Those care team practices in which anesthesiologists managed CRNAs tended to have an advantage in cost management. With varying degrees of success these practices understood how to leverage the cost of physicians across less expensive nonphysician providers. Even so, it was the rare practice that knew what its real cost per anesthetizing location was. Staffing decisions tended to be made based on gut feel and intuition. Before long the largest and most aggressive management companies would develop detailed financial staffing models, but their application and use was not understood by the average practice.

An objective assessment of the cost of providing anesthesia services required an entirely new management model. These were boom times for qualified anesthesia consultants who could help practices make sense of their finances in a way that they could objectively benchmark their practices to determine whether their staffing level, compensation and benefits were in line with the market. Most anesthesia practices had had little need for MGMA survey data until they had to make their first subsidy request. The market was no longer defined by the specific facility, but rather by national trends.

Being able to package and present the finances of the practice in a cogent and compelling manner was an essential prerequisite for the preparation of a formal presentation to administration but it was only part of the picture. Maybe the administration was simply unrealistic in its coverage and call expectations. This was particularly challenging to a practice that had no tradition of saying no to an administration's requests for coverage.

Anesthesiologists tend to assume that hospital administrators understand the economics of the specialty, but nothing could be further from the truth. In fact, many simply assumed that most anesthesia practices were very profitable, which is why most anesthesiologists are so well paid. Getting the administration to understand and appreciate the correlation between the economics of anesthesia and that of the facility requires a clear and compelling educational strategy. The administration has to be objectively shown the problem and this requires a sharing of data, which tended to fly in the face of the anesthesia psyche.

Successful negotiations of a reasonable contract for professional services with some level of financial support have become a three-phase process. The practice must first define its requirements and develop a logical and compelling format to present them. There is an art and science to this process. It is impossible to identify the best approach without a careful review of the data, the perspective of the hospital and the relationship of the stakeholders. Anyone who thinks this is easy to accomplish is a terrible liar or a terrible negotiator.

The administration must then assess the request and subject it to appropriate due diligence. It is not uncommon for the hospital to bring in an independent consultant to perform a Fair Market Value assessment. Especially in the current environment, hospital administrations must meet rigorous inurement requirements, in other words they cannot be seen as paying above fair market value for anesthesia services.

Once a financial deal is agreed to, the terms of the contract must be hammered out. Exclusivity takes on an entirely new meaning when there are funds being exchanged. With money comes leverage. If the terms of the contract cannot be met hospitals want the ability and right to terminate the privileges of the anesthesia providers. Many a practice has agonized over such clean sweep provisions.

A professional services agreement between an anesthesia practice and a facility should meet at least three objectives.

1. The scope of expected services should be clearly defined and realistic given available resources. Compensation terms and any subsidy calculations should be structured so as to align the incentives of the group practice and the facility administration.
2. The agreement should represent an opportunity for a win–win relationship, which means that the terms would allow the practice and the facility to achieve and maintain financial viability.
3. Ideally, the entire agreement should not reflect a one-time fix but a creative and flexible solution that anticipates changing market conditions.

Too often the process of negotiating an agreement reflects a fast-track approach which glosses over key issues and potential challenges for the sake of stabilizing the practice today but which does not give adequate consideration to the dynamic nature of all the variables that must be considered for a long-term solution.

Balancing the economics of anesthesia, the strategic objectives of the administration, and the internal political and cultural considerations of the anesthesia practice is no mean feat and those practices that jump into the process without adequate preparation and planning often get it wrong, the result of which can even result in the loss of the franchise. Because every anesthesia practice is unique there is no universal playbook. There are standard and basic considerations but the unique circumstances of each anesthesia practice's history, culture and staffing must be assessed against the coverage requirements, financial constraints and customer service expectations of the administration. Anesthesia has established itself over time as the quintessential service specialty. Whatever the facility requested they generally got. While this has been a strategy that has served the specialty well over time it is now becoming a fundamental challenge in an era in which such value propositions must be defined in financial terms. As the number of anesthetizing locations continues to expand without a corresponding increase in revenue there is a consistent refrain that is being articulated with increasing frequency: "We are being asked to do more for less." No one wants hospitals or anesthesia practices to fail but continuing the same policies and strategies will not allow for viable arrangements in the face of changing market conditions.

The ideal hospital contract provides the structure and support for the anesthesia practice to remain financially viable once the contract is signed. Many contracts have met this fundamental requirement, but the reality is that many have not and there is the apocryphal anecdote about the practice that spends months negotiating an agreement only to determine a few months later that the terms are unsustainable. There is a saying among consultants that anyone can get the level of financial support right today but will it be appropriate tomorrow. That continues to be the fundamental challenge of negotiation.

There are probably as many variations to hospital contracts as there are hospitals but essentially they fall into three broad categories:

1. The limited service line agreement
2. A global fixed subsidy contract
3. A flexible, formula-driven arrangement

As a general proviso, hospitals always attempt to limit their exposure in the negotiation of contracts while anesthesia practices prefer to provide for maximum financial protection against vagaries of the market. Ultimately, the determining factor is the amount of financial risk assumed by each party.

Early subsidy arrangements tended to be very specific to a particular aspect of the full scope of services. This might be limited to a medical directorship, obstetric coverage or cardiac care. For the most part these were fixed fee arrangements in which the hospital agreed to pay a certain amount of money to the practice each year. Typically, the amount of financial support was a relatively small percentage of the total monies collected by the anesthesia practice.

Over time, however, it became clear that many practices needed much more than a band aid to cover the cost of the care. Hospitals have always had a preference for fixed funding arrangements because they fit well into the context of a budget-driven organization. What worked for the hospital, however, rarely worked for the practice. There are simply too many variables that determine the revenue potential of an anesthesia practice for one to be able to predict the amount of support that will be needed over a year's time.

These shortcomings of traditional approaches led to some very clever and creative options that were flexible and formula-driven. The simplest of these were based on FTEs employed by the practice. The objective was to ensure that the practice had enough revenue to employ the requisite number of physicians and CRNAs that had been agreed to. Another approach focused on the number of anesthetizing locations that had to be covered. A per anesthetizing revenue target would be agreed to. Each month the practice would report the number of locations covered multiplied by the contractual rate guarantee. The practice would subtract actual date of entry collections posted and invoice the hospital for the difference.

The subsidy era has changed the specialty of anesthesia in many profound ways. Practices have had to develop new practice management tools to measure and monitor the profitability of the agreement. Inevitably anesthesia practices have had to develop much closer and stronger relationships with their administrations. While there is still a focus on revenue potential what matters most is the cost of the service. The other thing most practices have come to appreciate that what worked in one negotiation might be woefully inadequate in subsequent negotiations. There was a lot of experimentation as practices struggled to find the formula and the methodology that worked best for their practice.

The other legacy of this era is the request for proposal (RFP). Prior to 2000 few people in the world of anesthesia knew anything about RFPs unless they had experience in business. In a fairly short period of time, however, the use of the RFP epitomized the dramatic changes taking place in medicine. Hospital administrators would threaten an intransigent practice with the prospect of soliciting bids from other entities to provide service. The generation of an RFP did not always spell the end of a practice but it clearly created a new administrative hurdle that few practices were prepared to handle. Any time a hospital negotiation appeared to stall the administration would play the RFP card. And because RFPs became so common, they inspired and facilitated the growth of a new industry: the anesthesia management company. Ultimately, one might just as easily refer to the subsidy era as the RFP era. What had been a pretty stable and predictable environment in which anesthesiologists and CRNAs worked was now a place of considerable uncertainty in which every relationship was in a constant state of renegotiation.

We can now see how hospital contracts have changed the specialty. In its essence a hospital contract provides a structure for accountability in terms of clinical care, customer service and financial viability. While these were all concepts people talked about, the acceptance of a legal contract made them significant realities. You could no longer just claim you were providing quality care and contributing to the effective management of the OR, now you had to show it. Increasingly, especially in recent years, contracts include extensive lists of specific performance measures and metrics. This has required a material rethinking of the management of the practice to meet the contractual obligations, which has proved to be a significant challenge to many practices.

The Self-Sufficiency Era

Darwin posited that those organisms would survive that adapted to the environment in which they lived. He seems to have predicted the future of anesthesia practice. We now understand and can see clearly how anesthesia has evolved. The early fee-for-service providers saw themselves as independent but they were actually quite dependent in that their income and lifestyle was clearly defined by the environment in which they worked. During the subsidy era practices felt they had become totally captive and dependent but actually there was a symbiosis: neither the practice nor the facility could succeed without the other. And now we are moving into the third era in which the entities that now provide anesthesia are becoming more like the gas company: not dependent on any one client practice for overall financial viability.

A new set of market factors has given rise to a new type of anesthesia practice. Over the past 30 years we have seen the prevalence of the mega-group, a practice with more than a hundred providers that competes aggressively in its regional market. Many of these mega-groups have migrated into very sophisticated management companies. And now the most significant phenomenon is the availability of venture capital

funds to buy and consolidate anesthesia practices. Anesthesia practices used to operate quietly in the shadows of the OR but now they are serious market players eager to use their size and market power to be market makers.

The extent of the consolidation of the anesthesia market cannot be overestimated. The following is a partial list of significant players who collectively employ a significant percentage of all anesthesia providers. While the particular focus and strategy of each may be different they all share a commitment to expansion either by winning contracts with facilities or by acquiring other anesthesia practices. While the reality of their service agreements may not always live up to the representations of their sales teams, there is no doubt about the impact these organizations have had on the market. Not only has the world of anesthesia become much more competitive, it has become considerably more sophisticated.

- North American Partners in Anesthesia, Roslyn, NY
- EmCare, Dallas, TX
- Sheridan Healthcare, Hollywood, FL
- Mednax, Inc., Fort Lauderdale, FL
- Somnia, White Plains, NY
- Northstar Anesthesia, Fort Worth, TX

The slick presentations and glossy brochures are designed to speak directly to the strategic objectives of the facility. What used to be a pro forma exercise is now something much more sophisticated. These organizations have invested heavily in marketing and market research. Their fundamental approach is to propose a collaborative partnership with the facility that will minimize subsidy requirements, enhance productivity and ensure consistency of quality.

There was a practice in the central valley of California that had been providing services to the same facility for 35 years. An RFP was generated. A bidding war ensued and the hospital decided it was time for a change and brought in a national company with limited experience in the state. The take away is that the national company proposed a value proposition that was more than just a service and a subsidy.

It is often said that the more big players are in a market the less room there is for the small players. Fundamentally, every anesthesia practice must now make a simple strategic decision. Either it is going to remain a niche practice dedicated to one facility or it is going to merge with a larger entity. In the current environment only the second option will provide any form of long-term security. This is to say that the small, single facility practice can compete with the national aggregator, but it is not easy. While hospitals once strove to simply balance their bottom line, what they are now seeing is a partnership that will improve their competitive position in the local market.

Final Thoughts

It is often said that the only constant in life is change. Certainly this is true of American healthcare. The current environment highlights the enormous frustration and stress so many anesthesia practices are experiencing. It is clear that the actual service provided to the patient is less important than how it is documented and what statisticians can do with that information to improve the quality and reduce the cost of healthcare. We have entered into an era of meaningful use. The basically Byzantine record-keeping of the specialty is having to leap-frog into the twenty-first century. It is now clear that if you do not meet the technology requirements of today's healthcare environment, you will not survive.

What ultimately defines the value of an anesthesia service and why is it so hard to determine? It used to be easy: just get the number right. Assessing the revenue potential and minimizing the cost of the care are now essential requirements but they do not completely answer the question. Every aspect of the financial management process must be clearly delineated. Are your managed care contract rates competitive? Is your billing operation effective? Is management monitoring Accounts Receivable closely and interacting with the billing operation? Is the practice staffed appropriately for the scope of services provided? Are compensation packages consistent with market norms? Have you aligned the incentives of the anesthesia providers with those of the customers? Who is at risk for downturns in volume and payer mix? It is no longer acceptable to manage the practice intuitively; cost accounting is an essential prerequisite, especially in a subsidy environment, but it is no less critical if the goal is to avoid a subsidy.

But even that is not enough anymore. Anesthesia can no longer be viewed as just a service. It must be a collaborative partnership with the facility. The definition of the customer has changed. There was a point in time when it was the patient. Then the focus was on the surgeon. Now it is the facility. Healthcare is

now so competitive that the goal of every practice is to partner with the horse that will go the course, which may mean partnering in a way that ensures that the horse goes the course. The successful practice cannot just understand and be addressing the economics of the specialty, it must understand and be proactive in managing the economics of healthcare.

If you want to know what are the biggest changes that have affected the specialty of anesthesia over the past 35 years they can be summarized in three words: customer, competition, and consolidation; and they are interrelated. If you do not have a strategy for each one, you will be left behind. Today's healthcare environment is all about the customer. Every practice must clearly define who its customers are and, more importantly, what their expectations are. This used to be simple, but now it is not. If you are not familiar with stakeholder analysis, it is time to get up to speed. In trying to anticipate the needs and expectations of patients, surgeons and hospitals, the anesthesia practice must often reconcile seemingly contradictory requirements. It is no longer as simple as ability, affability, and availability; today's market requires that it also be affordable.

It used to be that there was little or no competition in the provision of anesthesia services. It used to be that the contract memorialized a relationship. Now it has become the objective of a competitive bidding process that is no longer defined by a local market or historical precedent. When an RFP is sent out, bidders may respond from all over the country. This has been a game changer. Now the local practice must compete against the most qualified national option. This has raised the bar for small practices focused on one or two facilities. The local niche practice does not always lose to the big national player but they must compete on the same playing field. This has made it essential to rely on consultants and national practice management options to craft an effective proposal.

And finally, it is safe to say the number of provider entities is shrinking as large mega-groups and management companies continue their aggressive consolidation of the market. Venture capital never used to be an option in anesthesia and now it is redefining the specialty. In light of this, there is a tendency to suggest that the game is over, that the days of the small, private anesthesia practice entering into a contract with a single facility are over. This may be the perception but it is not always the reality. But let us not lose sight of what got us here: competition. When you consider where the specialty has been and how it has evolved we may be heading back to where we started: swifter, quicker, nimbler may still be the better option if it can be executed competently and consistently.

Suggested Reading

Abouleish A, Prough DS, Whitten CW, et al. Comparing clinical productivity of anesthesiology groups. *Anesthesiology* 2002; 97(3).

Fisher R, Ury WL. *Getting to Yes: Negotiating Agreement Without Giving In*. Random House Business Books, 2011.

Hedman L. Compensation is major when anesthesia groups merge. *Anesthesiology News* 2010.

Kantor RM. *Confidence: How Winning and Losing Streaks Begin and End*. Three Rivers Press, 2006.

Lanier W. Changing trends in the U.S. anesthesiology workforce, with a focus on geographic regions and gender. *Anesthesiology* 2015.

Linder H. The disparity factor: How to improve anesthesia managed care contracts. *Becker's Hospital Review* 2013.

Locke JA, Greenfield H. Strategy and adaptability in a competitive market: Lessons from the nation's largest anesthesia organizations. *ABC Communique* 2017.

Mira T. Managing compensation for anesthesiologists, CRNAs and AAs. *ABC Communique* 2012.

Szokol J, Stead S. The changing anesthesia economic landscape: Emergence of large multi-specialty practices and accountable care organizations. *Current Opinion in Anesthesiology* 2014.

Chapter

22

Anesthesia Billing, Coding, and Compliance

Devona Slater

Overview of Coding Systems

Providers are required to use a variety of coding systems to translate services into reimbursement. Understanding these systems is critical, not only for correct reimbursement but also for compliance and maintaining your medical license.

Coding is defined as the process of translating a service, a supply, or a patient condition into a numeric or alphanumeric code, using only those codes in a mandated code set so that a third party can understand what happened to the patient and why. For a code to be considered correct, it must be supported in the official medical record and legally accurate, and that it will not mislead the recipient into a false belief about the services performed.

Many confuse the difference between correct coding and reimbursement rules. While both are extremely important to providers, correct coding rules establish how a service must be represented so that it is properly understood. It incorporates interpretations from the American Medical Association (AMA) and the National Correct Coding Initiative (NCCI) to properly report services. Reimbursement rules on the other hand, establish whether the service reported, which is correctly coded, is covered and payable under an insurance benefit contract. A service may be correctly coded yet not paid due to insurance coverage policies.

The first set of codes providers need to become familiar with is known as CPT. The AMA established

the Physicians' Current Procedural Terminology (CPT) coding as a consistent method of describing services performed by providers. The CPT codes are updated annually with new codes added and established codes reviewed for revisions or deletions to reflect the ongoing changes in medical technology. CPT lists descriptive terms and assigns numerical codes to the most commonly performed diagnostic and therapeutic procedures. Included with CPT codes is the concept of modifiers that help explain additional circumstances that may occur with the code. Examples of modifiers may include increased services, separate and distinct services or in the case of anesthesia, physical status. It is important to understand that not all payers recognize CPT modifiers.

ICD-10-CM is the second set of codes providers must be aware of. The WHO established the *International Classification of Diseases* (ICD-CM) to aid in the collection of morbidity statistics. ICD-10-CM codes refer to specific diagnoses for the condition for which the patient is receiving treatment. ICD-CM codes must be linked appropriately to the CPT code to establish the medical necessity for the services provided. Thus, all providers are responsible for reporting why they are seeing or treating the patient. Reimbursement may hinge on whether or not medical necessity is established based on the ICD-10-CM code(s) selected.

The Healthcare Common Procedure Coding System (HCPCS) is the third published code set that is universally used to identify drugs, supplies, special procedures and products that may be covered by insurance. These codes are easily identified because they begin with an alpha character followed by four numerical digits. The codes primarily represent items and nonphysician services used in the office or ambulatory surgery center/outpatient facility. HCPCS codes also contain modifiers which are two-position codes and descriptors that alter the original code by some specific circumstance but do not change the definition of the code. Again, the goal in using HCPCS is uniform reporting of supplies, products and services within the office or ambulatory surgery center/outpatient setting.

Some additional systems that providers must be familiar with to understand coding and reimbursement systems are those that have been generated by the federal government. Resource-Based Relative Value System (RBRVS), implemented in 1992 by Medicare, is the most widely used standardized system for reimbursement of physician services. Simply put, payment for services is determined by the resource costs needed to provide a service. In RBRVS the cost of providing each service is divided into three components: physician work, practice expense, and professional liability insurance. Reimbursement is calculated by multiplying the combined costs of the service by a conversion factor (which is adjusted by geographic region in the country). Annual updates are mandated and involve the AMA and national medical specialty societies known as the RVS Update Committee. Every CPT code must be reevaluated every 5 years.

NCCI was developed by Health Care Finance Administration in 1996 as part of an effort to reduce coding errors and the inappropriate payments resulting from those errors. NCCI edits focus on what is known as "unbundling of procedures" by providing definition of the anesthesia and global surgery rules. These rules define all procedures/services necessary to accomplish a given procedure to be included (bundled) in the description of that procedure. The edits are two tables that coders must consider in appropriate code selection; the mutually exclusive table, which matches codes for services that cannot reasonably be performed together based on code definitions or anatomic considerations and the comprehensive/component table which identifies component parts of a CPT code. The component code reflects the integral procedure or service when reported with another code. The integral code in certain circumstances can be separately billed with a modifier; the modifier would signify the component code is separate and distinct or performed at a different time in order for the procedure not to be included with the primary (comprehensive) service. NCCI edits change quarterly and coders should check the complete listing from the Centers for Medicare and Medicaid Services (CMS) web site prior to assigning codes.

The final system anesthesia providers must be familiar with is the ASA Relative Value Guide (RVG) and the ASA Crosswalk for anesthesia coding. Published by the ASA, these books are not intended to suggest any monetary value; they are designed and nationally recognized as a uniform fee schedule for anesthesia services. The RVG is best used in conjunction with the ASA Crosswalk. The ASA Crosswalk links each surgical CPT code to an appropriate anesthesia code. Alternate anesthesia codes are given for certain circumstances where the RVG may need to be consulted. Both guides are updated annually by the ASA and providers should only use the most current edition when assigning codes.

In today's environment, understanding coding systems is as important as documenting the services that are delivered. Basic principles of documentation and the appropriate coding of services lay the foundation for reimbursement. Accurate coding provides a picture of the "work" that was performed. Many debate whether coding should be done by a coding professional or by the providers themselves. It is important to keep in mind that even if a professional coder performs the assignment of codes for the services performed, it is the provider that is held responsible for any coding errors. Coding must be assigned based on the written, legible, documentation that exists in the patient's medical record. The goal of correct coding is twofold: (1) to ensure proper payment from government and third-party payers; and (2) to reduce the provider's chance of an audit.

Anesthesia Services

Anesthesia services include all types of sedation. Typically there is no separate payment for local/topical anesthetic. It is included in the surgeon's global fee and cannot be charged separately.

The next level of services is moderate (conscious) sedation. Sedation services are billed with CPT codes

99143–99150 depending on whether the surgeon is overseeing a trained third-party observer (99151-99153) or whether a separate physician is providing the moderate sedation (99155-99157). Moderate (conscious) sedation is a drug-induced state of consciousness where patients can respond purposefully to verbal commands, either alone or by light stimulation. Interventions are not required to maintain a patent airway and spontaneous ventilation is adequate. Moderate sedation requires recording of intraservice time, defined as continuous face-to-face attendance with start defined as indicating administration of the sedation and end time defined as the conclusion of the personal service of the physician providing or overseeing the sedation.

Monitored anesthesia care (MAC) is a billable anesthesia service and involves intraoperative monitoring by a physician or qualified anesthesia professional. While MAC may or may not include the administration of drugs, it differs from moderate sedation in that the anesthesia provider must be prepared and qualified to convert to a general anesthetic when necessary. While payment for MAC is equal to that of a general or regional anesthetic and requires all the same level of documentation, specific modifiers are required when filing claim forms to denote MAC services. The following modifiers denote MAC services for Medicare claims:

QS – designates MAC

G8 – designates the MAC services are necessary because the procedure is noted as deep, complex, complicated or markedly invasive

G9 – designates the MAC services are necessary because the patient has a personal history of cardiopulmonary disease

Other third-party payers may or may not require the above modifiers for the identification of MAC services. Payer policies should be closely reviewed before appending modifiers.

The importance of the anesthesia preevaluation cannot be over emphasized to support MAC. Many carriers have requirements for payment that reference specific diagnosis to support the medical necessity for an anesthesia provider. Documenting physical conditions and comorbidities that place the patient at risk are to be explained on the claim form with supplemental diagnosis.

Regional anesthesia care includes many types of blocks. The main purpose of a regional technique is to anesthetize only one area of the body, such as an arm, leg or lower extremities in order to perform an operation. Regional anesthesia care is compensated exactly the same as a general anesthetic, and unlike MAC services, does not require any special modifiers to denote the service. It requires all of the same elements in documentation such as the preanesthesia evaluation, administration of anesthesia agents, and monitoring intraoperatively and postanesthesia care.

General anesthesia is the final level of anesthesia compensated. General anesthesia is a state of unconsciousness where the patient loses protective reflexes resulting from the administration of drugs. A physician, a certified registered nurse anesthetist or an anesthesiologist assistant under the medical direction of an anesthesiologist may be reimbursed for anesthesia services.

Billing Anesthesia Services

Billing for all types of anesthesia services must take into consideration base units, time units, physical status and qualifying circumstances.

The base unit is defined by the ASA RVG. Base units take into account the complexity, risk, and skill required to perform the service. The base units include all of the value for normal and usual anesthesia services except for time factors and what is known as modifying factors. The base value specifically includes the anesthesia preevaluation service where the physician must document an evaluation, a physical exam, an anesthesia plan and discuss the risks with the patient. It also includes the administration of fluids and blood products that may be incidental to the anesthesia care as well as any noninvasive monitoring. The final element included in the base unit value is the postoperative visits. Anesthesia billing is different than other specialties in that only one anesthesia code is reported no matter how many procedures are performed. When multiple procedures are performed during a single anesthetic encounter, only report the anesthesia code with the highest base unit value.

Added to base units are time units. Anesthesia time is defined as the period of time which an anesthesia practitioner is present with the patient. It begins when the anesthesia provider begins to prepare the patient for anesthesia services in the operating room (OR) or an equivalent area and ends when the anesthesia provider may safely place the patient with postoperative care personnel. Anesthesia time is a continuous time period. Medicare does recognize the concept of discontinuous anesthesia time, where a provider may add blocks of time around a break in anesthesia time as long as the provider is furnishing continuous anesthesia care within the time periods around the interruption. An easy example of discontinuous time occurs in regional anesthesia techniques. Since the regional block is the mode of anesthesia for the case, the anesthesia time could start while the provider is placing the block. The first recorded time would be the amount of time it takes to place the block. Recognizing that it may take several minutes for the block to take effect, the anesthesia provider may step away from the patient and during that time the documentation indicates a break in anesthesia care. The time would start again when the patient was rolled into the OR for the surgery. While the ASA states that time units may be calculated as to what is customary in the local area, most carriers pay in exact minutes or 15-min blocks of time to equal one unit.

Modifying units come in two specific categories. First we have physical status modifiers which are designed with the initial P followed by a single digit. These modifiers distinguish between different levels of complexity of anesthesia service provided, depending on the patient's circumstances, and are consistent with the ASA ranking of the patient's physical status. Carriers may or may not pay for physical status modifiers based on payment policies. The second category of modifying units is qualifying circumstances (99100–99140). These are conditions that significantly impact the anesthetic service provided. Again, these are separate line item charges that are added to the anesthesia service. Qualifying circumstance codes may or may not be covered based on payer reimbursement policies.

Key Documentation Elements

Documentation is the cornerstone for billing. As the saying goes, "if it is not documented, it did not happen." Only written entries in the official medical record can be used in the coding and billing process. Many practices use a charge ticket to summarize billing information, but the actual documentation of the service must be supported in the medical record because the charge ticket is not part of the medical record and cannot be relied upon for support in an audit situation.

There are key items that are reviewed for documentation in billing anesthesia services. The anesthesia preevaluation is the first item reviewed. From a billing viewpoint, the preoperative evaluation would include an appropriate anesthesia evaluation and exam, discussion of risk with the patient and an anesthesia plan. From the preevaluation, billing personnel look for justification of the ASA physical status and MAC to add diagnosis for support in ICD-10 coding on the claim form.

On the anesthesia record, there are several important things that coders and billers verify before billing. First, the record should identify the facility and the place of service. This is important because each claim must identify the facility and whether services were performed in an outpatient, inpatient, ambulatory surgery, or office setting. Services should clearly reflect the patient name, date of service, and the type of anesthesia administered. In addition, the anesthesia provider should record all procedures performed by the surgeon and the postoperative diagnosis so that correct coding can be ascertained. Anesthesia start and end time should be taken directly from the anesthesia record. Many times coders will need to look at the monitoring on the time line to verify the time reported or to support the time charged. It is best if monitoring occurs within five minutes of anesthesia start time and continues up until the time the patient leaves the room. While this will not necessarily prove medical necessity of the services, it does provide documentation of constant attendance with the patient. Other key services that may be pulled from the record are the delivery of ancillary lines or postoperative pain services.

From a billing standpoint, there is little to review on the post anesthesia care record. Currently, only the hospital conditions of participation have requirements regarding the elements of a postoperative anesthesia visit within a certain timeframe. Anesthesia providers are required to be available to treat postoperative complication in the post anesthesia care unit but no specific documentation of availability is reviewed on an individual record.

Concurrency

Involved in anesthesia time is the Medicare definition of concurrency. Concurrency is simply the reference to how many services an anesthesiologist is involved with at any one time. While concurrency was originally a government term, most third-party payers have jumped on the bandwagon and actually now have some type of concurrency modifiers. These anesthesia-specific modifiers tell payers how anesthesia services are delivered in the OR. Providers must pay close attention to their times because starting and ending on the same minute will cause the two cases to be concurrent. Concurrency is the reason why so many billing professionals harp on documentation of relief services. Anesthesia providers are to file under the provider who has the most time on the case so tracking who is where and when plays a large component in anesthesia billing. The only exception in provider reporting is in the teaching rules where Medicare has instructed to bill under the provider who starts the case.

The medical direction modifiers are as follows:

- AA – anesthesia services performed personally by an anesthesiologist
- QY – medically directed by a physician: one CRNA
- QK – medically directed by a physician: two, three, or four CRNAs
- AD – supervision by a physician: more than four CRNAs
- QX – CRNA with medical direction by a physician
- QZ – non–medically directed CRNA

You cannot determine concurrency without looking at the elements of medical direction. Medical direction requirements are made clear in the *Medicare Carriers Manual*, MCM 15018.C. These requirements detail seven specific steps that an anesthesiologist must meet in order to file the claim as medically directed. These seven steps are:

1. Perform a preanesthesia examination and evaluation
2. Prescribe the anesthesia plan
3. Take part personally in the most demanding procedures of the anesthesia plan, including induction and emergence
4. Ensure that any procedures in the anesthesia plan that he/she does not perform are performed by qualified anesthesia personnel
5. Monitor the course of the anesthesia administration at intervals
6. Be physically present and available for immediate diagnosis and treatment of emergencies

7. Provide the postanesthesia care indicated

The government never makes a rule without creating a few exceptions and the medical direction rules have six. While medically directing, a physician may:

1. Address an emergency of short duration in the immediate area
2. Administer an epidural or caudal anesthetic to ease labor pain
3. Perform periodic, rather than continuous, monitoring of an obstetrical patient
4. Receive patients entering the operating suite for the next surgery
5. Check on or discharge patients from the recovery room
6. Coordinate scheduling matters

The government believes that none of these exceptions substantially diminishes the scope of control exercised by a physician in directing the administration of anesthesia to surgical patients. Many carriers have added other items, like placing invasive lines or postoperative pain blocks to these exceptions but again you must check with your individual carrier to see if there are additional services allowed in your state.

Many people mistakenly use the words medical direction and supervision interchangeably. In anesthesia reimbursement, the two have very different meanings. Supervision specifically refers to an anesthesia provider who is involved in more than four concurrent procedures. Medical direction means that the anesthesia provider is involved with one, two, three or four concurrent procedures.

If these seven steps are documented on the anesthesia record and the concurrency calculation is below four or less cases, the medical direction modifier QK or QY can be assigned to physician claims. Payers differ as to how they want claims submitted when the seven steps are not complete. Currently there is much controversy over this issues. Some require the case to be billed as a CRNA service alone (QZ modifier) while others allow the physician to claim supervision (AD modifier) for their work in the case. Every practice should check with their own state and local carriers before determining how to submit claims of incomplete medical direction.

In working with AAs, SRNAs and residents, you must always document the steps of medical direction to qualify for payment. The teaching rules were amended for dates of service on or after January 1, 2010 to allow the AA modifier to be used when teaching two residents, which allows 100 percent reimbursement for each case. All services that involve residents must be identified with an additional modifier, GC. While medical direction is allowed in cases involving residents of three or four concurrent cases, you will only be reimbursed for the physician portion (50% of the allowable) of the case. With SRNAs you are not allowed to medically direct more than two at any one time and the QK modifier is appended which would only allow the physician payment as the SRNA services are not billable.

Important Documentation Factors

Appropriate anesthesia coding starts with the anesthesia provider documenting the procedure on the anesthesia record with a goal of matching the surgeon's postoperative procedure. Providers should think about location, site, position, approach and technique used in providing enough information to code for anesthesia services. The next step in coding is to select the CPT procedure code (10021–99174) that most accurately describes the documented procedure. At this point the procedure code is cross-walked to the anesthesia code (00100–01999). Selection of the anesthesia code can be a bit tricky as the procedure code can link to multiple anesthesia codes which are identified under "Alternate(s)." For example, code 20680 (removal implant; deep) links to 13 different anesthesia codes. This is why detailed documentation by the provider is crucial to accurate billing and reimbursement.

In the above example the provider needs to indicate the specific site where the implant was removed to select the correct alternate; which has been pointed out by italicized comments under the alternate codes. Base units for procedures on bones can vary depending on: (1) an open or closed procedure; (2) the site and location of the repair (i.e., humerus upper, shaft or lower end); (3) a diagnostic or surgical arthroscopy; and/or (4) documentation of radical procedure. If the surgeon also performs an artery repair while repairing the fracture, this can increase the units by 1 unit or as much as 5 units depending on the site of the fracture.

The documented site and position can also alter the anesthesia code and base units in the integumentary system. Procedures performed on the head, neck, and posterior trunk have a base unit value of 5, but 3 units are assigned for extremities, anterior trunk, and perineum. Position is helpful to support coding of

the service as anterior versus posterior. It also helps support the RVG instruction that position other than supine or lithotomy is assigned 5 units regardless of a lesser base value.

Italicized comments are included in both ASA guides to help simplify assignment of alternate codes. Under procedure codes for mediastinoscopy, diagnostic thoracoscopy and surgical thoracotomy procedures comments are included to "consider single or double lung ventilation." Documentation by the anesthesia provider should include under the procedure to clearly document one lung ventilation for support of the additional 3 unit valuation. Reporting abbreviation can cause misunderstanding which could lead to over or under reporting of services. Only approved abbreviations should be used.

One example of an abbreviation that lead to under reporting of the base unit is "CABG OP." CABG (coronary artery bypass graft) codes have three alternates: 00566 without pump oxygenator (25 units), 00567 with pump oxygenator (18 units), or 00562 with pump for reoperation for coronary bypass more than 1 month after original operation (20 units). The coder thought the code "OP" meant "on pump," but the provider intended the abbreviation as "off pump," which caused a loss of 7 units. If the coder had a copy of the anesthesia record, they could have checked the graph line to verify on/off pump; that is, if they had been trained in how to read an anesthesia record. As for the third alternate, to determine "1 month after original operation" the anesthesia providers would have to be a mind readers or ask the surgeon. This information can be easily overlooked by an anesthesia provider and disregarded by coding if not documented on the anesthesia record.

Other common and not-so-common examples of documentation that caused a loss in base units based on the ASA Crosswalk 2016 are presented in Table 22.1.

These examples are provided to help physicians understand the importance of documentation and understanding correct code selection. While these examples imply a loss in revenue by insufficient documentation, coders can easily over report services from misunderstanding of abbreviation or new technology. Providers should have at a minimum, a common working knowledge of anesthesia coding to understand the documentation needed to help facilitate correct coding, billing and payment of services provided.

Table 22.1 Other Common and Not-So-Common Examples of Documentation That Caused a Loss in Base Units

Procedure documented by anesthesia	Alternate choices of anesthesia coding	ASA codes	Base units
Cysto	Transurethral urethrocystoscopy	00910	3
	With manipulate and/or removal ureteral stone	00918	5
	Removal of stone in upper one-third of ureter or kidney	00862	7
Abdominal wound closure	Integumentary system anterior trunk	00400	3
	Intraperitoneal procedure in lower abdomen	00840	6
	Intraperitoneal procedure in upper abdomen	00790	7
	Management of liver hemorrhage	00792	13
THR	Total hip arthroplasty	01214	8
	Total hip revision	01215	10
TAH	Intraperitoneal procedure in lower abdomen	00840	6
	TAH, S&O, omentectomy, lymphadenectomy	00846	8
Epigastric hernia	Hernia repairs upper abdomen	00750	4
	Strangulated epigastric hernia	00790	7
Placement interstitial radioelement prostate	Placement of needles, integumentary system	00400	3
	Perineum	00902	5
	Transrectal approach		
Anterior lumbar interbody fusion	Open procedures in lumbar region	00630	8
	ALIF with pins at L3, L4, L5	00670	13
	Use 00670 if performed with spinal instrumentation or on multiple vertebral levels		

Based on the ASA Crosswalk 2016.

Ancillary Services

In addition to the anesthetic, the providers place arterial, central venous, and pulmonary artery catheters. These services are not included in the basic unit value. Medicare and other carriers allow separate payment for invasive monitoring lines as long as they are not routinely inserted during anesthesia time. Per the Payment for Anesthesiology Services (Chapter 12, Section 50, F. Rev. 1859; Issued: 11-20-2009; Effective Date: For services furnished on or after 1-1-10; Implementation Date: 1-4-10),

> Payment may be made under the fee schedule for specific medical and surgical services furnished by the anesthesiologist as long as these services are reasonable and medically necessary or provided that other rebundling provisions (see subsection 30 and Chapter 23) do not preclude separate payment. These services may be furnished in conjunction with the anesthesia procedure to the patient or may be furnished as single services, e.g., during the day of or the day before the anesthesia service.

The anesthesia provider is responsible for documenting the insertion of the invasive monitoring lines in the patient's medical record. These are considered to be "surgical procedures" and a procedure note needs to include: (1) description of the nature, (2) extent and need of the procedure for the patient's condition; (3) medical assessment for the procedure; (4) method/technique utilized; (5) drugs and dosage; (6) time involved; (7) effort; and (8) the equipment necessary. Radiology guidance is sometimes needed to assist in line placements. Ultrasound guidance for vascular access can be reported in addition to a CVP placement when guidance is utilized. The code descriptor indicates the service requires the provider to indicate ultrasound evaluation of potential access sites, documentation of selected vessel patency, concurrent real-time ultrasound visualization of vascular needle entry with permanent recording and reporting. Use of a simple hand-held or other Doppler device that does not produce a hard copy is considered part of the examination of the vascular system and should not be reported separately. Ultrasound utilized only to identify a vein, mark a skin entry point or proceed with nonguided puncture should not be reported separately.

Transesophageal echocardiography (TEE) is also sometimes perceived as an extra ancillary service. Per the NCCI Policy (Revision Date: 1/1/16, Chapter 2 (B) (6)),

> Transesophageal echocardiography when utilized for *monitoring purposes*" is considered part of bundled services. "However, when performed for diagnostic purposes with documentation including a formal report, this service may be considered a significant, separately identifiable, and separately reportable service.

It would be inappropriate to bill for TEE services that are for monitoring purposes. There is one exception regarding the placement of a TEE. Pursuant to Medicare TEE National Coverage Policy Pub.100–4, Ch. 12, §30.4,

> Diagnostic intra-operative TEE is indicated when the surgical procedure is expected to alter the anatomy or function of the cardiac or thoracic structures: 1. If the evaluation of cardiac function and/or thoracic structures is necessary for the safe conduct of anesthesia or surgery. 2. If the surgical technique will be affected by the intra-operative TEE findings, thus assisting in surgical management decision. 3. If thoracic structures and/or cardiac function were not adequately evaluated pre-operatively AND the information is necessary for the safe conduct of anesthesia and surgery.

It is the government's intent to require the surgical technique to be affected by the intraoperative TEE findings, thus assisting in surgical management decisions. TEE is only billable during surgery when the surgeon requests the TEE for a specific diagnostic reason, (determination of proper valve placement, assessment of the adequacy of valvuloplasty, placement of shunts or other devices, assessment of ventricular function, assessment of vascular integrity or detection of intravascular air). Documentation should include a complete interpretation and report by the performing physician. The anesthesia provider may only be asked by the surgeon to place the probe and documentation would, in this instance, only include the placement.

Many individuals have questioned whether ancillary lines should be included in anesthesia time. The only guidance we have on this issue comes from the *CPT Assistant*, 17(5), May 2007, "Reporting Post-Operative Pain Procedures in Conjunction with Anesthesia":

- If the service is conducted PRIOR to induction of the anesthesia for a surgical procedure being performed by another provider, the line is separately reportable, but should not be part of the anesthesia time.
- Sedation for placement of the line does not qualify as an event that starts anesthesia time.
- When lines are placed or performed AFTER anesthesia has been induced, the time spent performing these procedures does not need to be deducted from the anesthesia time.

Providers should take reasonable care in documenting start and end times in placing invasive lines and post-operative pain blocks so that documentation can demonstrate that the services were done outside of anesthesia start time or done after the induction of anesthesia.

Acute Pain Management

Anesthesiologists are allowed to bill for postoperative pain services if the sole purpose of the service is management of postoperative pain. Per the NCCI Policy (Revision Date: 1/1/16, Chapter 2 (B) (3)),

> Postoperative pain management services are generally provided by the surgeon who is reimbursed under a global payment policy related to the procedure and shall not be reported by the anesthesia practitioner unless separate, medically necessary services are required that cannot be rendered by the surgeon. The surgeon is responsible to document in the medical record the reason care is being referred to the anesthesia practitioner.

Modifier 59 is appended to the surgical CPT code to denote that the service was distinct and separate from the anesthesia service performed on the same day. Postoperative pain services are to be billed under the provider who placed the block.

Because these services normally fall under the surgeon's global package, it is important to document the request for the service from the surgeon. These services are considered surgical procedures and a procedure note needs to include: (1) description of the nature, extent and need of the procedure for the patient's condition; (2) medical assessment for the procedure; (3) method/technique utilized; (4) drugs and dosage; (5) placement time; (6) effort; and (7) equipment necessary. Needle placement performed under ultrasound guidance can be reported in addition to the surgical procedure, if documentation supports imaging supervision and interpretation. Written documentation should include that a hard copy of the image was taken. If fluoroscopic guidance is utilized, it can also be separately reported and also must include written documentation. These blocks are never done within anesthesia time as they are billed as separate and distinct surgical services.

Daily management of an epidural catheter has a special code that is not subject to evaluation and management documentation guidelines. CPT code 01996 represents follow-up care of an epidural catheter. There are no published requirements for documentation of 01996 other than there must be a catheter in place. Providers should consider supporting the service by documenting: (1) current regimen; (2) reported pain scale and pain relief; (3) current activity functions; (4) inspection of the catheter site; and (5) any side effects. Supporting documentation should include a medical plan such as continuing the epidural, removal and/or transferring to oral analgesics. Other continuous catheter follow-up services should be billed with the subsequent hospital visit codes. Visit codes must meet documentation guidelines of evaluation and management services.

ICD-10-CM includes several acute pain diagnosis codes specific to postoperative pain. When postoperative pain services are provided, individual carrier guidelines for appropriate diagnosis reporting should be followed.

While acute pain management is an important part of anesthesia services, documentation should be very clear that the block is not being used as part of a combine technique for the case. If used as a combine technique, no separate billing for the block is allowed and the time it takes to provide the regional technique for the case is then added to the case time (discontinuous anesthesia time) for billing.

Obstetric Anesthesia

Obstetric services continue to be an issue in the billing arena. The ASA 2016 RVG states:

"Unlike operative anesthesia services, there is no single, widely accepted method of accounting for time for neuraxial labor analgesia. Professional charges and payment policies should reasonably reflect the costs of providing labor analgesia as well as the intensity and time involved in performing and monitoring any neuraxial labor analgesic." Methods to determine professional charges consistent with these principles include:

A. Base units plus time reported in minutes (insertion through delivery), subject to a *reasonable cap*. Delivery may include related services such as delivery of placenta or episiotomy/laceration repair.

B. Base units plus one unit per hour (time unit defined by local standards and time reported in minutes) for neuraxial analgesia management plus direct patient contact time (insertion, management of adverse events, delivery, and removal).

C. Incremental time-based fees (e.g., 0<2 h, 2–6 h, >6 h).

D. Single fee.

The phrase "costs of providing labor analgesia" guides anesthesia practices to analyze their professional time, work, etc. for providing neuraxial labor analgesia. Labor services should be assessed to determine appropriate charges, especially since Medicaid and third-party carriers may differ in their requirements for reporting labor time and the appropriate methodology for payment. Without a specific labor time policy, a carrier may hold providers accountable to the anesthesia time definition to include constant attendance. Research of all local payer policies is a must to stay compliant in billing for obstetric anesthesia specifically paying close attention to the definition of anesthesia time.

Physician Quality Report System

Physician Quality Report System (PQRS) quality data code reporting, established by the CMS, is a statutory program that creates a financial incentive/penalty for eligible professionals who volunteer in this quality reporting program. Successful reporting of the identified quality measures may earn a bonus payment up until 2014 and after that date a reduction of the fee will be applied to the total allowed charges for covered services.

Currently in 2016, anesthesia providers can elect to report on seven specific anesthesia measures. It should be noted that only Measure 76, Prevention of Catheter-Related Bloodstream Infections, can be claims- or registry-reported. All of the other measures must be reported via a qualified registry. See Table 22.2.

In addition, if anesthesia providers bill for services that are deemed face-to-face encounters, evaluation and management codes, they will also need to choose a crosscutting measure to report. There are many cross cutting measures that might apply as

Table 22.2 Anesthesia-Specific PQRS Measures

PQRS #	Measure title	MAV clinical cluster	NQS domain	Measure type	Reporting method
44	Coronary artery bypass graft: preoperative beta-blocker	Registry cluster: CABG care requires reporting measure 44 when measures 43 and 164 are submitted	Effective clinical care	Process	Registry; CABG measures group
76	Prevention of catheter-related bloodstream infections	Not included within a cluster	Patient safety	Process	Claims or registry
404	Anesthesiology smoking abstinence	Not included within a cluster	Effective clinical care	Intermediate outcome	Registry
424	Perioperative temperature management	Registry cluster: anesthesiology care report measures 426, 427, and 430 to avoid MAV penalty process	Patient safety	Outcome	Registry
426	Postanesthesia transfer of care measure (PACU)	Registry cluster: anesthesiology care report measures 424, 427, and 430 to avoid MAV penalty process	Communication and care coordination	Process	Registry
427	Postanesthesia transfer of care measure (ICU)	Registry cluster: anesthesiology care report measures 424, 426, and 430 to avoid MAV penalty process	Communication and care coordination	Process	Registry
430	Prevention of postoperative nausea and vomiting	Registry cluster: anesthesiology care report measures 424, 426, and 427 to avoid MAV penalty process	Patient safety	Process	Registry

they are designed to be situations that apply to a variety of specialties across many clinical settings. All reference information for the PQRS data collection program can be found by going to www.cms.hhs.gov/PQRS.

It is important to realize that the ASA or surgical CPT code itself is the identifier to CMS that a provider is eligible for reporting the measure(s). Each measure has a set of CPT codes to report along with possible modifiers. The other key element to understand is that the bonus/penalty payment is for reporting, not in the performance of the measure.

Accurate reporting requires an understanding of PQRS modifiers. Modifier 1P indicates the measure was not met due to medical reasons; modifier 8P indicates the measure was not met due to reasons not otherwise specified.

PQRS is set to be eliminated and will be replaced by the Merit-Based Incentive Payment System (MIPS), which will start in CY 2017. This system combines four performance categories into a "MIPS score" that will then apply either an incentive or penalty to the provider's reimbursement during a payment year. It basically takes the current programs of meaningful use, PQRS and EHR and combines them into one program. Twenty-five percent of the MIPS score will be tied to meaningful use measures, thirty percent to quality, thirty percent to cost and finally fifteen percent to clinical practice improvement. The way it is currently explained in the regulations is that each performance year CMS will set a performance threshold (PT) which defines at which point a provider will receive a zero percent adjustment. So, for example, if the PT is set at 50 points, then a provider earning 51 points and above would receive an incentive payment, and those at 49 points and below would be penalized. The farther away from the set PT, the greater the incentive or penalty will be. The entire program is designed to be budget neutral so if there are many providers with lower scores that create penalties, the higher scored providers could reap substantial financial rewards because of the bucket of money created from the providers scoring below the PT is distributed to those above the PT. In addition, the provider MIPS score will be available on the Physician Compare website so that consumers can see how their providers compare to other providers and score against the PT set by CMS.

Alternative Payment Systems

At the time of this writing there is a huge transformation occurring in healthcare. It is the goal of the CMS to move the system towards value-based purchasing and away from the traditional fee for service. CMS plans over the next few years to increase accountability for both quality and total cost of care and to have a greater focus on population health management. CMS plans to have 90 percent of payments linked to quality in some sort of alternative payment model by 2018.

All alternative payment models have the goal to deliver better care at a lower cost. Providers should realize to be successful they must make fundamental changes in their day to day operations, CMS believes that making these operational changes will only be effective if the process is adopted by a critical mass of payers and are therefore encouraging the same payment methodologies described below to any plans who offer Medicare replacement plans or Medicaid services. If these alternative payment models show the amount of savings represented in the target, providers can expect that the traditional commercial market will move at a rapid pace to duplicate these payment models.

There are two overall categories of payment methodologies at this time with over 66 different programs specifically listed on the CMS website. The first general category is called Accountable Care Organizations (ACOs). ACOs are groups of doctors, hospitals, and other healthcare professionals who come together voluntarily to give coordinated high quality care to Medicare patients. This coordinated care is to ensure that patients, especially those with chronic diseases, get the right care at the right time,

avoiding duplication of services and expensive trips to the emergency room while preventing medical errors. Specific performance standards are set and the goal is for all providers of service to work together in improving care and lowering costs.

The second methodology is called the Bundled Payments for Care Improvement and links payments for all services received during a single episode of care. There are several models under this methodology with the significant difference being whether the payment is a retrospective bundle or a prospective bundled payment.

In the retrospective bundled payment arrangement, all providers of care submit their actual expenditures which are then reconciled against a target price for an episode of care. Different models include different time frames but most have a preoperative or planning phase, an inpatient stay in a hospital plus all related services for up to 90 days after the hospital discharge are included in the bundle. Under these retrospective models, Medicare makes the fee for service payments and then the total expenditures are reconciled against the target price determined by Medicare. If the bundled exceeds the target price, a recoupment amount would then assessed from Medicare. The time frames differ as to when this actual recoupment occurs but several of the models have a greater than twelve month period to evaluate these expenditures and recoup the revenue.

In the prospective bundled payment arrangement, CMS makes a single payment to the hospital that is to encompass all services furnished by the hospital, physicians, and other practitioners during the defined episode of care. The providers submit "No-Pay" claims to Medicare and are paid by the hospital out of the bundled payment received. These "No-Pay" claims are used to identify patients so quality and patient satisfaction can be monitored.

In both models, the beneficiaries retain the full freedom of choice to choose services and providers. As part of the monitoring system, both quality and patient assessment tools will be used to evaluate the care experience and health outcomes of the beneficiary. All models work under the premise that by implementing process improvements, specific changes in outcomes will occur and reductions in expenditures will produce significant savings.

While it is impossible to predict how successful these models will be, it is evident that the reimbursement in the near future will undergo a massive change and what we know as the traditional provider fee for service payments will slowly become obsolete.

Measurement of Key Billing Benchmarks

The billing process is the heart of the revenue cycle and must be monitored consistently. Anesthesia groups should develop a business office scorecard to provide a foundation of measurements to ensure processes and resources are aligned to achieve business goals. There are several business measures that should be calculated and measured in the billing cycle process. Below are suggestions of measurements that should be monitored.

Gross collection ratio is the amount paid to the practice divided by the total charges billed. This does not include any write-offs or adjustments. This ratio varies based on the practice and the payer mix. For example, a payer mix consisting of a larger percentage of Medicaid and Medicare may result in a lower gross collection ratio. Therefore, this would not be a dependable metric to use for comparison to other practices. If this metric is used for comparison it is best to compare practices that are similar in nature and when seeing large shifts tells providers to immediately review the payer mix to see why the change is occurring.

Net collection ratio is the amount paid to the practice divided by the total charges after the adjustments due to contractual write offs. Controllable adjustments (i.e., small balance write offs, bad debt write offs to outside collections) should not be included in these adjustments. This ratio basically measures what was collected versus what should be collected. For a high level of performance, this ratio is typically over 90 percent. A drop in this number would indicate a problem within the billing process.

Days in accounts receivable is the time elapsed between billing the charge and collecting the payment. This is an important metric to evaluate efficiency of a billing office/service. The number of days it takes to collect a bill varies by specialty and can be affected by timely follow up with the payer and quick rectification of any issues that may arise. The lower the number of days in accounts receivable demonstrates the efficiency in the process. A good number of days in accounts receivable would be somewhere between 35 and 45 days.

Accounts receivable aging tracks past due accounts. The billing office/service should report this as a number and percent of accounts that are current, 30, 60, 90, 120+ days past due. It should have an effective analysis process to troubleshoot the reasons for accounts falling in past due status. A highly performing billing office/service should constantly improve upon its processes to reduce the aging of accounts. Ranges for accounts receivable breakdown in aging categories in general is: current 50–55 percent; 30 days 12–15 percent ; 60 days 8–12 percent ; 90 days 4–7 percent ; and 120+ days 15–18 percent.

The average charge per case is the total charges billed divided by the number of cases in the month. This metric should be reported and reviewed on a monthly basis to determine trends that impact the practice. A shift in this number would indicate volume problems within the OR and should be addressed with the facility.

The average collection per case is the amount paid to the practice divided by the number of cases. Collection per case indicates actual money paid and the collection efforts of the practice. A decrease in this number would indicate problems within the billing process. Reviewing this metric monthly is important to determine collection trends that impact the practice.

The average collection per unit is the amount paid to the practice divided by the total number of units billed. This metric should be reported and compared on a monthly basis for the current year, and to the previous year's monthly average. Fluctuations in this metric may be an indication of a shift in payer mix and should be analyzed to determine the cause(s). The average charge per case, average collection per case and number of cases should be used in conjunction to provide a clearer picture of trends within the practice.

Compliance

In today's environment one cannot discuss billing and coding without compliance. No matter what continues to unfold in healthcare, the government's activities indicate continued recoupment of monies that have been paid inappropriately. Every physician should realize that the government has a tremendous return on fraud and abuse dollars and as keeper of the purse; it will continue to scrutinize services. Physicians can be penalized monetarily or in some cases where fraud is involved, jail time, a loss of medical licensure or exclusion from the government programs may prevail. It is for this reason all anesthesia groups should understand it is critical to have an active compliance program.

The implementation of a compliance program can be a challenge, as many physicians are still unclear as to "What makes an effective compliance program?" The most effective programs will have integrated the compliance activities into the day to day operations of the group and will incorporate the seven federal sentencing guidelines.

The first of the sentencing guidelines require written policies and procedures. The policies and procedures that have been written for the program need to be understood by all members of the group. How to complete the anesthesia record, definitions of anesthesia start and end time and specific types of anesthesia delivered would all be examples of policies an anesthesia group might have. It is important that employees have guidance in understanding the basic concepts discussed in the plan. It is recommended that plan policies be tested and results kept in personnel files to assure that everyone knows the commitment of the group to the compliance program and the intention to only bill for services that are appropriately documented.

The second of the federal sentencing guidelines specifically asks that a compliance officer be designated for the group. The group must evaluate the performance of the compliance officer and while the compliance officer does not necessarily have to be a physician, it does have to be someone who has the absolute authority to hire and fire personnel. The Board should assess whether the compliance officer has sufficient knowledge and education to deal with the assigned responsibilities. It would be important for them to judge whether appropriate auditing and education is being carried out to fulfill the requirements of compliance. Compliance committee minutes and processes of handling any reported violations should be reviewed to ensure all issues have been dealt with and recorded as to corrective action.

Education and training of all levels of employees must be done according to the third step in the sentencing guidelines. Courses and educational materials should reflect the important aspects of the group's compliance program. Ongoing training and demonstration of evaluation of knowledge should be recorded. Keeping accurate records of content, frequency and attendees are very important in order to demonstrate educational efforts.

The fourth sentencing guideline stresses open communication and it is considered an essential element in active compliance programs. You must have a way to receive feedback from employees on issues and concerns that they might have regarding activities within the group. A plan is not considered effective if the program receives minimal or no feedback from employees. Simply recording that there have not been any violations reported would not be enough to qualify as open communication. A record of questions regarding policies, and any guidance given or research done by the compliance officer or committee members should be documented to show open lines of communication.

The fifth key component of the sentencing guidelines stresses ongoing monitoring and auditing. Auditing, both internal and external, is critical to a successful compliance program. The frequency and the extent of the audit function will vary depending on the size and issues identified by the group. Audits must not discriminate between providers and must address issues that are considered "hot spots" in the specialty. Things such as anesthesia time, postoperative pain, ancillary line placements and medical direction would all be appropriate topics for audits. Audits should ensure that elements set forth in the compliance plan are being monitored and that auditing techniques are valid and conducted by objective reviewers. For example, we know that postoperative rounding for acute pain services use the evaluation and management coding guidelines to bill for services. A compliance professional would want to audit these services based on the billing guidelines to see if they meet the criteria for billing. Medical direction elements would be another example of a focused audit that may be done evaluating the documentation of the seven required elements.

The sixth element of the federal sentencing guidelines requires suspected violations to be thoroughly investigated. In doing so, groups must also assure that there is no retaliation to those who report violations. When a compliance officer learns of an issue, it is important to contact legal counsel to properly handle and circumvent any exposure to the group. Placing the audit under "attorney-client privilege" helps to maintain control of the investigation and documentation until a determination can be made regarding the errors. If evidence exists that misconduct has occurred, counsel will be needed to work through the process of self-disclosure.

Finally, the seventh factor that makes up the key ingredient to the federal sentencing guidelines is discipline. Disciplinary action must be taken for those employees who fail to adhere to the group's standards set forth in the compliance program. Discipline must be applied consistently among employees regardless of the employee's level in the corporation. Senior management must demonstrate a serious commitment to foster a climate that will require adherence to all federal and state regulations.

In summary, compliance must be an activity that is incorporated into the day-to-day practices of the anesthesia group. Government investigations will continue. All new healthcare legislation mentions the need for continued efforts to fight fraud and abuse. The best protection for an anesthesia group is an active compliance program.

Suggested Reading

American Medical Association. *CPT 2011 Professional Edition*. Chicago, IL: American Medical Association, 2011.

Blount LL. *Mastering the Reimbursement Process*, 3rd ed. Chicago: American Medical Association, 2001.

Buck CJ. *2011 HCPCS Level II*. St. Louis, MO: Elsevier/ Saunders, 2011.

Buck CJ. *2011 ICD-9-CM, Volumes 1 & 2 for Physicians*. St. Louis, MO: Elsevier/Saunders, 2011.

Centers for Medicare and Medicaid Services. Anesthesiologists Center. July 19, 2011. www.cms.gov/ center/anesth.asp

Centers for Medicare and Medicaid Services. National Correct Coding Initiative edits. July 19, 2011. www .cms.gov/NationalCorrectCodInitEd/NCCIEP/ list.asp.

Centers for Medicare and Medicaid Services. Physician quality reporting system. July 19, 2011. www.cms.hhs .gov/PQRS.

Keegan DW, Woodcock EW, Larch SM. *The Physician Billing Process: 12 Potholes to Avoid in the Road to Getting Paid*, 2nd ed. Englewood, CO: Medical Group Management Association, 2008.

Stead SW. *2011 Crosswalk*. Park Ridge, IL: American Society of Anesthesiologists, 2010.

Stead SW. *2011 Relative Value Guide*. Park Ridge, IL: American Society of Anesthesiologists, 2011.

Troklus D, Warner G. *Compliance 101 Second Edition*. Minneapolis, MN: Health Care Compliance Association, 2006.

Chapter

23

Postanesthesia Care Unit Management
Building a Safe and Efficient Service

Henry Liu, Longqiu Yang, Michael Green, and Alan David Kaye

Quality perioperative care of surgical patients takes comprehensive and integrated approaches, which may involve many functional departments and specialized teams. Surgeons, anesthesiologists, operating room (OR) nurses, postanesthesia care unit (PACU) nurses, and nurses in the surgical ICUs and regular wards, all must work together to assure the very best care of surgical patients. In general, identification of a director of the PACU, an anesthesiologist, can effectively communicate with all stakeholders as to policy, systems, compliance, and ongoing improvements. In this regard, a nurse director of the PACU can implement these ongoing activities and further enhance communication when problems arise.

PACU, therefore, refers to those all activities undertaken to manage patients after the completion of a surgical procedure and the concomitant primary anesthetic. PACU is a critical care unit where the patient's vital signs are closely observed, pain management begins, temperature is corrected, and fluids are given as needed. The nursing staff is skilled in recognizing and managing problems in patients after they have received anesthesia [1]. PACU nurses play an important role in the postsurgical period; they affect not only the patient's continuing emergence from general anesthesia and the recovery of cognitive, sensory, and motor functions following anesthesia, but also the turnover rate of ORs and ambulatory surgery clinics or outpatient surgery, the patient's length of hospital stay, gate-keeping the discharge of ambulatory patients, and the overall efficiency of surgical services of a modern medical facility [1, 2]. PACU may ultimately affect the profitability of a hospital and overall patient satisfaction in a medical facility [1, 2].

Phases of Postanesthesia Recovery

The concept of recovery phases from general anesthesia was initially developed for ambulatory surgery. Nowadays, some of the concepts are gradually being adopted for hospital-based surgical procedures. Hospital-based anesthesiologists usually focus primarily on the initial recovery phases in PACU, while the ambulatory anesthesia providers will have to plan for, to observe, and to manage patients' extended recovery and their readiness to be discharged from PACU to return home [3]. This three-phase concept has not only helped surgeons, nursing staff, and anesthesia service providers to better understand the importance of the surgical patient's step-by-step postoperative care, but also their continual recovering process, to dedicate more time, resources, and efforts to the patient's recovery, and to better prepare patients for their discharge from the PACU. By realizing that patient recovery from anesthesia is a continual process, there will be some overlapping between the arbitrary recovery phases.

Phase I recovery, or early recovery, is the transition from the care mainly provided by anesthesia providers to that predominantly provided by PACU nurses. This phase spans from the discontinuation of anesthesia to the point at which the patient recovers from their mental cognitive ability, respiratory function, and protective air-way reflexes. The patient usually undergoes a return of basic physiological functions with in this period of postsurgical time. In addition, during this phase of recovery, patients will demand a significant amount of attention from PACU nurses, and potentially from anesthesia or surgery providers as well. Indeed, the intensity of care of this phase is

Table 23.1 The Original Aldrete Scores [4]

	2 points	1 point	0 point
Activity	Move four extremities	Move two extremities	Cannot move
Respiration	Able to breathe deeply and cough freely	Limited breathing, dyspnea	Apneic
Circulation	BP changes within 20% of baseline level	BP changes in 20–50% of baseline level	BP changes over 50% of baseline
Consciousness	Fully awake	Arousable on calling	Not responding
Color	Pink	Pale, dusky, blotchy, jaundiced	Cyanotic

almost equivalent to ICU care and requires similar monitoring equipment as ASA standard care in the OR, except for gas spectrometry. The PACU phase I monitoring includes at least electrocardiogram (EKG), noninvasive blood pressure, pulse oximetry, temperature, and urine output.

Patients in phase I are likely to begin responding to verbal stimulations when alveolar anesthetic concentrations are decreased to about 0.5 minimum alveolar concentration (MAC) or less for the volatile anesthetic drug (MAC awake) if not impeded by other factors. The MAC is defined as the concentration of an inhalational anesthetic in pulmonary alveoli in which 50 percent of patients will not move in response to surgical stimulation. Increased ventilation results in a more rapid decline in alveolar anesthetic concentration, which hastens recovery, provided that the arterial carbon dioxide pressure is not so low that it may decrease cerebral blood flow and slow down the removal of anesthetic agent from the central nervous system. Recovery from neuromuscular blockade may need to be monitored by peripheral nerve stimulation and by clinical indices. Recovery from intravenous opioids and hypnotics may be more variable and difficult to quantify than recovery from inhalation anesthesia and neuromuscular blocking agents.

The most common practice in most institutions in determining whether to have a postanesthetic patient to the ICU or not is consensus between the surgery team and the anesthesia team, based on patient's pathophysiological conditions. Often times it may be also determined by ICU bed availability. Commonly agreed criteria for admitting a patient to ICU include, but are not limited to, the following: (1) unstable hemodynamic parameters, which require meticulous monitoring and pharmacological intervention(s); (2) expecting prolonged intubation and mechanical ventilation; (3) long surgery time, significant intraoperative blood loss, and a large quantity of fluid shifts; (4) multiple invasive monitoring and multiple inotrope/vasoactive medications.

Phase II recovery, or intermediate recovery, is the phase of anesthesia recovery needed to get the surgical patient ready to be discharged from the medical facilities. Many different scoring systems have been used to evaluate the patient's recovery status in this phase. The Aldrete Score is a 10-point scale based on extremity movement, respiration, blood pressure, consciousness, and oxygen saturation (Table 23.1) [4]. Originally published in 1970, the Aldrete Score has been widely used as a guideline for PACU care for many years. However, the original Aldrete Score is not an ideal guideline for postoperative patient recovery, especially for the ambulatory surgery patient, because the Aldrete Score ignores the importance of postoperative pain and postoperative nausea and vomiting (PONV). Thus the modified version of the Aldrete Score (1995) is probably the most commonly used scoring system, with a score of 9 or higher required for patient discharge [5]. In the modified Aldrete Score, a patient who is able to maintain oxygen saturation above 92 percent on room air scores 2 points, a patient needing oxygen inhalation to maintain oxygen saturation above 90 percent scores 1 point, and a patient with oxygen saturation less than 90 percent even with oxygen supplementation scores 0 point. The modified Aldrete Score seems to work better than the original Aldrete Score for the recovery from phase I to phase II.

Other also widely accepted scoring systems are the postanesthesia discharge scoring system (PADSS) and the White–Song score [6, 7]. The PADSS serves as the scoring system getting the patient ready to be discharged home (Table 23.2). The White–Song score, which was published in 1999 (Table 23.3), was designed to qualify patients to bypass phase I recovery

Table 23.2 The Postanesthesia Discharge Scoring System for Home Readiness [6]

	2 points	1 point	0 point
Vital signs	BP and SpO$_2$ change <20%	BP and SpO$_2$ change 20–40%	BP and SpO$_2$ change >40%
Activity	Steady gait, no dizziness, meets preop level	Requires assistance	Unable to ambulate
Nausea and vomiting	Minimal, treated with p.o. medication	Moderate, treated with parental medication	Severe, continue despite treatment
Pain	Controlled with p.o. medication and acceptable to patient; yes = 2	No = 1	
Surgical bleeding	Minimal, no dressing change	Moderate, up to two dressing changes required	Severe, three or more dressing changes

SpO$_2$, transcutaneous pulse oximetry; p.o., per os.

Table 23.3 The White-Song Recovery Scores [7]

	2 points	1 point	0 point
Mental status	Awake	Arousable	Unresponsive
Motor	Move all extremities	Some weakness	No movement
Blood pressure	Within 15% of baseline	15–130%	>30%
Respiration	Deep breathing	Tachypnea	Dyspnea
Pulse oximetry	>90% room air	Requires O$_2$	SpO$_2$<90 with O$_2$
Pain	No pain	Moderate pain	Severe pain
PONV	No to mild nausea	Transient vomiting	Persistent vomiting

and be discharged from the OR directly to the less intensive phase II recovery area. The PADSS uses five parameters with a score of 0–10, while the White–Song score includes seven parameters with a total score of 0–14 and takes into account of PONV [8]. These two scoring system and the PADSS seem to be more acceptable than many other scoring techniques published in the last decade.

However, there continue to be many controversies regarding the currently used scoring systems and discharge criteria. For example, requiring patients to take oral fluid before discharge may not be necessary according to some recent observations. Eliminating drinking as a requirement before discharge can slightly shorten the phase II recovery without convincing evidence of significant adverse effects, and there are studies supporting this practice [9, 10]. If a practice can reach universal agreement, recovery room nurses should be educated to remove the drinking requirement before discharging patients home. Another controversy is whether the ability to void is truly necessary before discharge. Several studies have demonstrated that even patients at high risk

of urinary retention can be discharged before they have voided in the recovery room [11]. Eliminating the voiding requirement before discharge can significantly shorten recovery room stay without adding a negative impact to the clinical outcome.

Phase III recovery, or late recovery, and psychological recovery extend from the discharge from hospital or ambulatory surgery center to full psychological, physical, and social recovery and return to work. This phase of recovery can have significant individual variations due to various factors. Phase III recovery usually occurs outside the medical facility.

PACU Admission, Fast-Tracking, and Discharge

ASA guidelines state that all patients who have received general anesthesia, regional anesthesia, or monitored anesthesia care, should receive appropriate postanesthesia management in a PACU, where intense monitoring almost equivalent to ICU care is offered [1], with the potential exceptions of following patients: all open heart surgery patients, who will generally be transported to ICU directly from the OR after surgery; all patients who have undergone major surgical procedures (prolonged intubation and mechanical ventilation, large quantity of volume resuscitation, delicate hemodynamic maneuvering, such as liver transplantation patients) and patients with significant vital organ dysfunction who will potentially need a longer period of ICU care; and patients who had obstetric procedures, cardiac special procedures, gastroenterological procedures; these patients will usually be transferred to their own PACU-equivalent recovery area, where PACU guidelines generally apply [1]. There are recent studies showing that even cardiac surgery patients can be safely recovered in PACU [12].

Fast-track/PACU bypass refers to discharging a patient from the OR to phase II recovery directly, bypassing phase I recovery. According to the White–Song scoring system, the criteria for a patient to be a candidate for fast track or PACU bypass is a score of 12 or higher (Table 23.3) [7].

The following procedures are generally considered to be qualified for fast tracking [13]:

- Most eye procedures
- Some cesarean sections
- Some cardiac catheterizations
- Most gastroenterological endoscopy
- Most radiological special procedures with monitored anesthesia care
- Most patients with regional block as surgical anesthesia for their procedures
- Some surgical patients with local anesthetic infiltration under minimal intravenous sedation

There are institutional variations in criteria for discharging patients from the PACU.

Criteria to discharge patients from PACU can depend upon where the patients are discharged, patient age, and coexisting medical conditions. Box 23.1 shows the acceptable criteria for PACU discharge [14]. These criteria can be used alone or in combination with the PADSS, to enhance patient safety during discharge from phase II to phase III recovery.

The criteria for discharging a patient from the PACU to the hospital ward can be slightly different from discharging a patient to home. The patient does not need to be able to ambulate, void, or prove oral fluid intake. It is much safer to send a patient to the hospital ward than to discharge the patient home for recovery. Also, the criteria can be different for the pediatric

> **Box 23.1. Clinical Criteria for PACU Discharge [14]**
>
> - Stable vital signs for at least 1 h
> - Alert and oriented to time, place, and person
> - No excessive pain, bleeding, or nausea
> - Ability to dress and walk with assistance
> - Discharged home with a vested adult who will remain with the patient overnight
> - Written and verbal instructions outlining diet, activity, medications, and follow-up appointments provided
> - A contact person and circumstances that warrant seeking the assistance of a healthcare professional clearly outlined
> - Voiding before discharge not mandatory, unless specifically noted by physician (i.e., urological procedure, rectal surgery, history of urinary retention)
> - Tolerating oral fluids not mandatory, unless specified by physician (i.e., patient is diabetic, frail, and/or elderly; not able to tolerate an extended period of NPO status)

patient population and the geriatric population. In Europe, the International Association for Ambulatory Surgery adopts the following guidelines [15].

Essential invariant criteria for patient discharge:

- Stable vital signs
- Oriented to preoperative stage
- Minimal nausea and vomiting
- Controlled pain
- Without significant bleeding related to the procedure(s)
- Variable criteria for discharging patient from PACU
- Micturition prior to discharge; essential following epidural or spinal anesthesia; may be deemed essential following certain surgical procedures
- Fixed length of stay in day unit following surgery; plays no part in the generality of surgical procedures; may be deemed necessary after certain procedures to minimize the risk of reactionary hemorrhage at home, e.g., tonsillectomy, thyroidectomy
- Individual for certain specific procedures

There are many strategies to minimize PACU stay time. These should be considered whenever the opportunity avails itself. Decreased PACU stay time will lead to a lower requirement for PACU beds. These strategies should include PONV prevention and prompt treatment, multimodal pain management, choice of shorter-acting anesthetic agent, nurse reeducation [16], etc. Delays in discharge from the PACU due to systems errors should be kept to a minimum. In addition, fast track should be considered whenever possible.

PACU Design and Staffing

Many factors need to be taken into consideration in designing a PACU. The design, equipment and staffing of the PACU shall meet requirements of the facility's accrediting and licensing bodies.

- **Functionality:** Most PACUs are responsible for the recovery of postsurgical patients and discharge them either to home or to general wards. Some PACUs are used strictly for phase I and early phase II recovery. Other PACUs function as the patient's room throughout his or her stay for the day, beginning as a preoperative assessment room, then becoming the phase I recovery room, and progressing through phase II and early phase III until the patient is discharged, and either home or to the floor. In addition, some hospitals have specialized PACUs for general surgical patients, pediatric patients, interventional radiology patients, gastroenterological patients etc.

For the convenience of transportation of patients, OR and PACU are generally located on the same floor of the hospital. Automatic doors should be installed for the ease of transferring patients. PACU should have indirect lighting, soundproof ceiling, noise control mechanisms, and walls and ceiling painted in soft, pleasing colors. The precise recommendations on the design of the PACU are still lacking, unfortunately.

- **Beds:** The number of PACU beds is determined by the hospital's surgical volume and the nature of its surgical procedures. The generally accepted ratio of PACU beds–OR is 1.5–2:1.

This recommended ratio of PACU beds to ORs is not clearly defined [17]. Patient demographics and types of surgical cases affect those needs. Surgical procedures with quicker turnover will require more PACU beds due to greater number of patients admitted into the PACU over a shorter period of time. And generally longer and more extensive surgical procedures will decrease the PACU admission rate and thus decrease the PACU bed requirement, while increasing ICU admission. On the other hand, sicker patients admitted into PACU will have the potential of requiring greater nursing care and a longer stay in PACU than relatively healthier patients, resulting in greater bed requirements. Obviously simpler surgeries should require less postoperative care routinely than complicated surgeries, which should decrease the PACU bed needs. In one study with unlimited resources available for the PACU patients, the required PACU bed to OR ratio came to less than 1:1 [17]. However, this result was from a simulated situation with unlimited resources, which is far from the reality in which most practitioners find themselves.

- Size: Physical size or area of PACU depend upon the number of beds, equipment to be installed, and any special needs like isolation room etc.
- Equipment: Basic equipment requirement should include monitors for respiration (SpO2, respiratory rate), circulation (BP, EKG, HR), temperature, urine output and voiding, neuromuscular function, etc.

Adequate PACU nurse staffing is undoubtedly critical to quality and safe patient care. The American Society of Perianesthesia Nurses (ASPAN) offers Standards of PACU Nursing Practice. ASPAN recommends staffing ratios that correlate to the level of care required in PACU phase I, phase II, and extended observation settings [18]. In addition, ASPAN has established minimum staffing guidelines to provide a safe environment for patients during nonpeak hours, as well as a "position statement on on-call/work schedule" to address issues related to nursing fatigue and patient safety: ASPAN recommends that one nurse can only safely care for up to two healthy, adult, conscious patients not requiring frequent cardiopulmonary intervention [19]. These recommended staffing ratios are based on the best available expert opinion and consensus. Although the nursing literature claimed evidence on the relationship between nurse staffing ratios and nursing-sensitive outcomes, there was a paucity of scientific postanesthesia evidence that related to safe staffing ratios or nursing-sensitive indicators specific to the specialty practice [20].

Precise calculation of adequate PACU nursing staffing is very difficult. Whereas other hospital units (ICU, regular wards, and emergency department) have relatively consistent daily patient census, PACU should start and end the day with a census of zero while throughout the day PACU may have a large variation in the census. The best way to figure out proper staffing level for each PACU may be through computer modeling and historical data [21]. Many other factors may potentially affect PACU staffing requirements. One of these is the sequence of surgical cases. Proper surgical sequencing should bring more predictable staffing requirements in PACU. Small facilities with just a few ORs will generally benefit proper surgical case sequencing, while in larger PACUs, the benefits of case sequencing are unclear when compared with the good performance of adjusting staffing and beds to match workload using statistical optimization [22].

Other factors may also affect PACU nursing staffing requirements. Delays in patient flow before and after PACU may subsequently change PACU staffing. These delays can be due to system errors, such as receiving units not ready, patients awaiting radiological imaging and/or interpretation, unevaluated patients waiting for anesthesia assessment [23]. Process engineering and corrections of these systems errors should potentially decrease PACU staffing requirement and lead to a smoother flow of patients throughout the postsurgical period.

Financial Considerations in the PACU

To cut health expenses, all institutions must reduce their human and financial costs. The evaluation of costs is an essential part of medicoeconomic analysis. The PACU is a major component of perioperative patient flow. As reimbursement for surgical procedures continues to decline, the costs of perioperative services continue to increase. Efforts to improve the profitability in perioperative services depend on improving efficiencies in each perioperative component. Many strategies have been applied to decrease costs in the PACU [24]. The effect of these strategies on fixed costs versus variable costs varies considerably. Fixed costs refer to those that do not vary in relation to the surgical volume (e.g., capital equipment, physical plant, salaried personnel); variable costs include those costs that vary directly with the surgical volume (e.g., disposable supplies, pharmaceuticals, laboratory tests, and hourly personnel). The strategies for decreasing the PACU costs include following [24]:

1. OR scheduling changes to decrease the daily PACU peak number of patients admitted from the ORs

2. Improvement of PACU nurse productivities by optimizing nurse working hours and shift adjustment, i.e., increasing patient care hours without increasing work hours

3. Cost-reducing interventions, such as modifying the medical practice patterns to reduce PACU length of stay, cutting variable costs, etc.

4. Use of short-acting anesthetic agents or drugs with favorable pharmacology, including multimodal management of PONV and postoperative pain

5. Fast-tracking patients whenever possible by bypassing PACU or discharging patients home directly from the PACU

6. OR patients bypassing the phase I recovery being directly admitted to phase II PACU

7. Improving phase I PACU process and inpatient bed availability

8. Timely transporting patient out of PACU

9. Optimizing PACU discharge criteria or hospital policies

10. Avoiding communication problems

Numerous studies and computer models were attempted to predict or suggest the effect of cost-cutting strategies for decreasing the PACU costs. The applicability and success of these strategies may vary greatly in different institutions and practice environments (i.e., ambulatory surgical centers, specialty surgery centers, tertiary care facilities, low-volume or high-volume facilities). The largest portion of the PACU costs is nursing staff wages. Nurse staffing level is primarily dependent upon the daily peak number of patients admitted to the PACU from the OR [25]. Therefore, the most effective strategies in decreasing the PACU costs involve those that decrease the amount of nurse staffing (i.e., FTEs) either directly or indirectly. The standards set by ASPAN state the number of patients that each nurse can simultaneously care for (i.e., one nurse per intubated patient or per two extubated patients) may prevent or decrease the ability to maximize nursing productivity in facilities with frequent high patient acuity levels [24, 26].

Other factors affecting productivity include the increasing use of the PACU as an overflow location for ICU, step-down care, and patient wards. Ziser et al. prospectively studied patient overflow admission to the PACU over a 33-month period and found that lack of an available bed was the most common reason for PACU stay (85.5%) [27]. This undoubtedly results in variable acuity needs and can interrupt patient flow from OR to PACU, contributing to inefficiencies in surgical services and increased pertinent costs [28]. The ASPAN statement on overflow patients in the PACU raises additional staffing concerns regarding maintenance of appropriate competencies for the patient population, maintenance of patient safety, coordination of OR scheduling, and appropriate staff utilization, further complicating this recurrent problem in some facilities [29]. Dexter et al. have suggested use of computer optimization methods to determine staffing level for phase I recovery because of the complexity of staffing, especially when variability in patient acuity occurs [26].

PACU nursing staff wages generally fall into four categories [24]: hourly employees with no minimum numbers of hours worked each week; "full-time" salaried employees (no overtime pay); "full-time" hourly (not salaried) employees with no minimum number of hours of work each day; "full-time" hourly (not salaried) employees with frequent overtime.

Creative and flexible scheduling of PACU nurses in proportion to the predicted daily peak number of patients admitted to the PACU may allow some cost savings by reductions in staff hours during low admission periods [30]. However, the practice environment may not be conducive to the needed flexibility and creative scheduling that may be required for a given nursing staff wage category. Avoidance of frequent overtime and use of hourly employees with no minimum number of work hours may improve efficiencies. Other strategies may include the use of a combination of more than one wage category in a particular PACU staffing model to add flexibility in scheduling. Improvements in surgical sequencing of cases, the sequence in which surgeons perform their cases in an OR on one day, may also result in reduced PACU staffing needs [30]. Unfortunately surgeons may not be agreeable to loss of control over the order of their cases [24]. Waddle et al. studied medically appropriate PACU length of stay (LOS), defined as the time required achieving a medically stable condition for safe PACU discharge, compared to actual LOS in 340 patients [31]. They revealed the actual LOS to be >30 min longer than the medically appropriate LOS in 20 percent of patients. The most frequent causes of prolonged LOS were waiting for physician release or waiting for laboratory or study results (i.e., radiograph and laboratory results). Some studies have

implicated PACU nurses being too busy, lack of transport, procedures performed in PACU, postoperative monitoring, pain management, bed availability, and PONV as additional causes of increased LOS [32, 33]. Improvements in the efficiencies in the administrative issues that have resulted increased LOS may lead to significant cost reductions. However, because of difficulty in scheduling full-time PACU nursing staff and wide variability in increased LOS, it is very difficult to fully assess the benefit of any single intervention aimed at decreasing LOS [24, 25, 34].

Some studies suggested that strategies such as use of short-acting drugs, multimodal antiemetics, and regional anesthesia, fast-tracking of patient discharge directly from the PACU or bypassing of phase I PACU to phase II PACU, may directly or indirectly decrease PACU costs [34–36]. Regional anesthesia techniques have been shown to reduce costs in the ambulatory setting as a result of reduced postoperative complications, fewer unintended hospital admissions, and earlier home readiness of the patients [37]. However, the effectiveness of these strategies may vary significantly with the practice environment and PACU staffing needs. It is often difficult to measure the true costs of implementation (i.e., drug, equipment, and staffing costs) when evaluating presumed cost savings [36–39].

Use of standard operating procedures and alternative definitions of discharge criteria may reduce surveillance time and improve fast-tracking and bypassing of phase I recovery, resulting in cost savings [40, 41]. Many discharge criteria and policies (i.e., oral fluid intake, voiding, awaiting full return of motor function after regional block) may be modified based on outcome studies or planned location of discharge (i.e., inpatient versus home) [23, 40].

In summary, this chapter emphasizes the key players in an effective PACU, the three phases of postanesthesia recovery, criteria of PACU discharge, PACU design, and staffing-related issues. The financial implications of the PACU, especially those involving cost savings, are complicated and mostly a function of nurse staffing, owing to its overwhelming proportion of cost in PACU operation. Leadership in the PACU at the level of the physician rests solely on the shoulders of the Anesthesiology Department. When anesthesia training and rotations are designed in the PACU, a curriculum and didactics will strengthen a learning atmosphere. A weekly or monthly conference of stakeholders can be beneficial in many aspects, much like Morbidity and Mortality/Grand Rounds conferences are invaluable for an OR or ICU team. Finally, many strategies to decrease costs may have potential benefits, especially if they result in improved OR process flow efficiencies. Future strategies to decrease PACU costs will probably require incorporation of the total OR process flow. It will be important that these strategies also incorporate maintenance of patient safety and good quality outcomes.

References

1. American Society of Anesthesiologists. Postanesthesia care standards for 2014. www.asahq.org/quality-and-practice-management/standards-and-guidelines

2. F. Dexter, A. Macario, P. J. Manberg, D. A. Lubarsky. Computer simulation to determine how rapid anesthetic recovery protocols to decrease the time for emergence or increase the phase I postanesthesia care unit bypass rate affect staffing of an ambulatory surgery center. *Anesth Analg* 1999; 88: 1053–63.

3. J. Boncyk, J. Fitzpatrick. Discharge criteria. In: S. R. Springman, ed. *Ambulatory Anesthesia: The Requisites in Anesthesiology*. Philadelphia: Mosby Elsevier, 2006: 109–17.

4. J. A. Aldrete, D. Kroulik. A post anesthetic recovery score. *Anesth Analg* 1970; 49: 924–34.

5. J. A. Aldrete. The post anesthesia recovery score revisited [letter]. *J Clin Anesth* 1995; 7: 89–91.

6. F. Chung, V. Chan, D. Ong. A post anaesthetic discharge scoring system for home readiness after ambulatory surgery. *J Clin Anesth* 1995; 7: 500–6.

7. P. White, D. Song. New criteria for fast-tracking after outpatient anesthesia: A comparison with the Modified Aldrete's scoring system. *Anesth Analg* 1999; 88: 1069–72.

8. M. S. Schreiner, S. C. Nicholson, T. Martin, et al. Should children drink before discharge from day surgery? *Anesthesiology* 1992; 76: 528–33.

9. W. T. Fritz, L. George, N. Krull, J. Krug. Utilization of a home nursing protocol allows ambulatory surgery patients to be discharged prior to voiding [abstract]. *Anesth Analg* 1997; 84: S6.

10. F. L. Jin, A. Norris, F. Chung, T. Ganeshram. Should adult patients drink fluids before discharge from ambulatory surgery? *Can J Anaesth* 1998; 87: 306–11.

11. H. Ead. From Aldrete to PADSS: Reviewing discharge criteria after ambulatory surgery. *J Perianesth Nurs* 2006; 21: 259–67.

12. J. Ender, M. A. Borger, M. Scholz, et al. Cardiac surgery fast-track treatment in a postanesthetic care unit: Six-month results of the Leipzig fast-track concept. *Anesthesiology* 2008; 109(1): 61–6.

13. M. Yarborough, H. Liu, S. Bent. Management of PACU. In: A. D. Kaye, C. J. Fox, III, R. D. Urman, eds. *Operating Room Leadership and Management*. Cambridge University Press, 2012.

14. K. Korttila. Recovery from outpatient anesthesia: Factors affecting outcome. *Anesthesia* 1995; 50(suppl): 22–8.

15. International Association for Ambulatory Surgery. Discharge criteria following day surgery. www.iaas-med.com/index.php/recommendations/discharge-criteria

16. J. M. McLaren, J. A. Reynolds, M. M. Cox, et al. Decreasing the length of stay in phase I postanesthesia care unit: An evidence-based approach. *J Perianesth Nurs* 2015; 30(2): 116–23.

17. E. Marcon, S. Kharraja, N. Smolski, et al. Determining the number of beds in the postanesthesia care unit: A computer simulation flow approach. *Anesth Analg* 2003; 96: 1415–23.

18. American Society of PeriAnesthesia Nurses. Practice recommendation 1: Patient classification/recommended staffing guidelines, 2010–2012. www.aspan.org/ClinicalPractice/PatientClassification/tabid/4191/Default.aspx (accessed May 10, 2012).

19. F. Dexter, H. Rittenmeyer. Measuring productivity of the phase I postanesthesia care unit. *J Perianesth Nurs* 1997; 12: 7–11.

20. M. E. Mamaril, E. Sullivan, T. L. Clifford, et al. Safe staffing for the post anesthesia care unit: Weighing the evidence and identifying the gaps. *J Perianesth Nurs* 2007; 22: 393–9.

21. F. Dexter. Why calculating PACU staffing is so hard and why/how operations research specialists can help. *J Perianesth Nurs* 2007; 22; 357–9.

22. E. Marcon, F. Dexter. An observational study of surgeons' sequencing of cases and its impact on postanesthesia care unit and holding area staffing requirements at hospitals. *Anesth Analg* 2007; 105: 119–26.

23. M. J. Tessler, L. Mitmaker, R. M Wahba, C. R. Covert. Patient flow in the post anesthesia care unit: An observational study. *Can J Anesth* 1999; 46(4): 348–51.

24. A. Macario, D. Glenn, F. Dexter. What can the postanesthesia care unit manager do to decrease costs in the postanesthesia care unit? *J Perianesth Nurs* 1999; 14: 284–93.

25. F. Dexter, J. H. Tinker. Analysis of strategies to decrease postanesthesia care unit costs. *Anesthesiology* 1995; 82: 92–101.

26. F. Dexter, R. E. Wachtel, R. H. Epstein. Impact of average patient acuity on staffing of the phase I PACU. *J Perianesth Nurs* 2006; 21: 303–10.

27. A. Ziser, M. Alkobi, R. Markovits, B. Rozenberg. The postanaesthesia care unit as a temporary admission location due to intensive care and ward overflow. *Br J Anaesth* 2002; 88: 577–9.

28. M. F. Watcha, P. F. White. Economics of anesthetic practice. *Anesthesiology* 1997; 86: 1170–96.

29. American Society of PeriAnesthesia Nurses. A position statement for medical-surgical overflow patients in the PACU and ambulatory care unit. *J Perianesth Nurs* 2003; 18: 301–2.

30. E. Marcon, F. Dexter. Impact of surgical sequencing on postanesthesia care unit staffing. *Health Care Manage Sci* 2006; 9: 87–98.

31. J. P. Waddle, A. S. Evers, J. F. Piccirillo. Postanesthesia care unit length of stay: Quantifying and assessing dependent factors. *Anesth Analg* 1998; 87: 628–33.

32. P. Saastamoinen, M. Piispa, M. M. Niskanen. Use of postanesthesia care unit for purposes other than postanesthesia observation. *J Perianesth Nurs* 2007; 22: 102–7.

33. K. Samad, M. Khan, Hameedullah, et al. Unplanned prolonged postanesthesia care unit length of stay and factors affecting it. *J Pak Med Assoc* 2006; 56; 108–12.

34. F. Dexter, D. H. Penning, R. D. Traub. Statistical analysis by Monte-Carlo simulation of the impact of administrative and medical delays in discharge from the postanesthesia care unit on total patient care hours. *Anesth Analg* 2001; 92: 1222–5.

35. B. A. Williams, M. L. Kentor, M. T. Vogt, et al. Economics of nerve block pain management after anterior cruciate ligament reconstruction. *Anesthesiology* 2004; 100: 697–706.

36. W. S. Sandberg, T. Canty, S. M. Sokal, et al. Financial and operational impact of a direct-from-PACU discharge pathway for laparoscopic cholecystectomy patients. *Surgery* 2006; 140: 372–8.

37. M. Schuster, T. Standl. Cost drivers in anesthesia: Manpower, technique and other factors. *Curr Opin Anaesthesiol* 2006; 19: 177–84.

38. D. Song, F. Chung, M. Ronayne, et al. Fast-tracking (bypassing the PACU) does not reduce nursing workload after ambulatory surgery. *Br J Anaesth* 2004; 93: 768–74.

39. F. Dexter, A. Macario, P. J. Manberg, D. A. Lubarsky. Computer simulation to determine how rapid anesthetic recovery protocols to decrease the time for emergence or increase the phase I postanesthesia care unit bypass rate affect staffing of an ambulatory surgery center. *Anesth Analg* 1999; 88: 1053–63.

40. F. Chung. Discharge criteria – A new trend. *Can J Anaesth* 1995; 42: 1056–8.

41. R. I. Patel, S. T. Verghese, R. S. Hannallah, et al. Fast-tracking children after ambulatory surgery. *Anesth Analg* 2001; 92: 918–22.

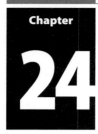

Chapter

24

Pain Practice Management

Steven Waldman

Contents

Introduction

Over the past several years, there has been considerable interest in expanding the role of the pain management specialist as an integral member of the healthcare team. This interest has been stimulated in part by the increased availability of healthcare professionals with a special interest and advanced training in pain medicine and in part by the unprecedented economic pressures of our rapidly evolving healthcare system. These economic pressures have forced many pain management specialists to explore new avenues of revenue generation as well as to examine new strategies to help improve the efficiency and cost-effectiveness of the care they provide.

The purpose of this chapter is to serve as a guide for the pain management specialist who may be considering setting up a pain treatment center or expanding the scope of services currently offered. Although many of the concepts presented in this chapter are basic, failure to take them into consideration may lead to high levels of professional frustration and dissatisfaction, damage to the professional image of the pain management specialist, economic loss, and increased exposure to malpractice liability.

Basic Considerations

Should Pain Management Services Be Offered?

There is no question that there is a huge demand for quality pain management services. The most recent National Insitutes of Health report on pain reveals that an estimated 126.1 million adults reported suffering from pain within the last three months of the study period, with 25.3 million adults reporting chronic daily pain [1]. From these data, it is obvious that there is a huge number of patients who could potentially benefit from quality pain management services, and equally obvious is the fact that our specialty continues to have a problem with recognition and identity.

Interfacing Pain Management Services with Existing Services

The first question that must be asked when considering the implementation or addition of new pain management services is how the addition of this new service will interface with existing professional activities. One must take into account the impact of such new services on existing care. The addition or expansion of pain management services requires a high level of commitment from *all* members of the healthcare team. Even if additional professional members of staff are added to provide pain management services, consideration must be given to such issues as call responsibilities, vacation coverage, etc.

As with all healthcare endeavors, there must be sufficient expertise to provide an ongoing level of quality care. One would not implement an open-heart surgery program or start a burn unit without adequate expertise and/or additional training. Pain management requires the same level of training, expertise, and commitment. In addition to the clinical expertise required to provide quality pain management services, there must be the administrative expertise if the endeavor is to be economically viable. This is especially important when setting up a pain treatment facility under the managed care paradigm [2].

Are There Adequate Personnel to Provide Quality Care?

It is extremely important when setting up a pain treatment facility that the pain management specialist recognize the high level of commitment in terms of the time and energy essential to provide quality pain management services. For this reason, the pain management specialist must insure that there are adequate personnel to provide high-quality coverage for any new services that are contemplated or to cover the expansion of existing services.

There is a common misconception that pain management can be done at the convenience of the pain management specialist. This is simply not the case. This approach can only lead to high levels of dissatisfaction from both patients and referring physicians. Today's patient, or what has become affectionately known as today's "healthcare consumer," is unwilling to wait for extended periods of time in order to receive care. The proliferation and success of urgent care centers and walk-in clinics staffed by physician extenders attest to this fact. During implementation of a new pain management facility or expansion of an existing one, a realistic appraisal of the time required to provide the proposed care must be undertaken to assure the provision of care in a timely manner. Just as there must be an adequate number of healthcare professionals to provide high-quality pain management services, there must also be a high level of motivation in order for the pain facility to ultimately succeed [3]. *All* members of the healthcare team must be committed to quality and compassionate provision of pain management services. A lone pain management specialist, no matter how motivated and caring, can do little to make up for the disinterest and lack of support of the remainder of the pain management team. This statement applies not only to the clinical personnel but to the administrative personnel as well.

Is the Support Staff Adequate?

When setting up a pain treatment facility, care must be taken to be sure that the practice infrastructure is adequate to support a busy and growing pain management service. If the pain management specialist's existing billing office is unable to keep up with the volume of work generated from existing activities, the addition of billings from new or expanded pain management service may throw the entire office into disarray and adversely affect cash flow. Additional help can be added to alleviate this situation, but this should be done in a prospective manner [4].

Services Offered

Prior to setting up a new pain treatment facility, the first decision that needs to be made is the decision as to which specific services (e.g., evaluation, neural blockade, behavioral interventions, drug management, and detoxification, etc.) should be offered. In order to delineate these services adequately, pain management specialists must take into account their existing expertise, experience, and preferences as well as those of other healthcare professionals providing pain management services within the group practice. The availability of support services such as physical therapy, occupational therapy, psychiatry, and radiology support services such as computerized tomography scanning, magnetic resonance imaging, ultrasound, and biplanar fluoroscopy must also be considered. Under the managed care paradigm, some services may not be reimbursed at levels adequate to justify their use from a purely economic viewpoint and may have to be subsidized from more profitable product lines.

It is very important to define clearly to patients as well as referring physician what a new pain treatment facility can and cannot offer. Too often pain management specialists with limited experience and training tries to hold themselves out as specialists in all areas of pain management. This is not only academically dishonest but often leads to high levels of patient and referring physician dissatisfaction [5]. It may also place pain management specialists and those with whom they practices in a potentially serious medicolegal situation. Services should not be advertised that are not available or cannot be provided with sufficient expertise to keep complications to a minimum. A clear policy regarding whether specialists will prescribe controlled substances for chronic nonmalignant pain is mandatory to avoid upsetting patients and referring physicians.

Types of Patients Seen

The second decision that needs to be made is delineating the types of patients that pain management specialists feel are appropriate for the scope of pain management services they have chosen to offer at the new pain treatment facility. The pain management specialists should determine whether they are comfortable treating cancer pain, headache and facial pain, chemical dependence problems, and acute and postoperative pain, etc. They must also determine whether they will accept patients who are involved in workers' compensation claims and patients who are involved in litigation. Third, pain management specialists must decide whether they will accept self-referred patients or will require patients to be evaluated and then referred by another physician (see below). Finally, pain management specialists will also have to decide whether they will accept primary responsibility for patients who are admitted to the hospital. This decision has specific implications that must be carefully thought out from a quality of care viewpoint, because some pain management specialists may be incapable or unwilling to deal with the many medical problems that may occur while the patient is hospitalized under their care. Political issues as to the appropriateness of pain management specialists providing primary care may also have to be addressed [6, 7].

Financial Considerations

The following issues must be handled according to each pain management specialist's existing financial situation, current policies, prior contractual agreements with the hospital and/or third-party carriers, and philosophical and ethical viewpoints on providing indigent care. To ignore these variables when starting a pain treatment facility is to insure economic disaster.

In order for the pain management service to remain on a strong economic footing in this period of ever-decreasing revenues, financial considerations must be carefully considered [8]. Some pain management specialists have chosen to provide pain management services on a cash-only basis. Although this may work in some affluent communities, by and large, in view of the high cost of many of the modalities offered, this represents an impractical approach for most pain management specialists.

A decision must be made as to the desirability of accepting Medicare assignment as well as other third-party assignments of insurance benefits. Participation in managed care plans should also be carefully weighed [2]. Obviously local factors have to dictate the variables to be taken into account when making this decision. Pain management specialists must also decide what provisions will be made for indigent patients who have Medicaid or who are solely responsible for the payment of their healthcare costs. Pain management specialists are likely to be approached by attorneys who desire care to be rendered on a contingency basis. The economic impact of these decisions cannot be overstated.

Availability

It has been said that there are three "A's" of a successful practice of pain management: ability, amiability, and availability. From a patient care viewpoint, ability is the most important issue. However, from a practice management viewpoint, there is no question that availability is the most important. When a pain treatment center is started, it is imperative that the clinical and administrative staff all agree on the appropriate levels of availability if the facility is to succeed. Most patients expect to see the same physician at each visit, and this fact has a specific impact on call schedule issues such as days off after call, vacation scheduling, afternoons off, etc. If *all* members of the pain management care team are not motivated to facilitate the provision of quality pain management services, it is impossible for a single member of the team to make the pain management service successful. This statement also applies to the administrative staff. If the administrative staff refuse to factor in additional patients, or limit the hours of operation of the pain treatment facility, adverse economic consequences will often result.

Additional issues that need to be determined when setting up a pain treatment facility include the hours of operation for the pain management center. The availability of evening hours has become more and more important and is increasingly expected by the healthcare consumer in today's competitive market. Weekend and holiday coverage must also be clearly defined for both the patient and referring physician. Expectations of the pain management specialist who is covering these periods should also be delineated to avoid friction between members of a group pain management practice and to assure appropriate availability from *all* members of the pain management care team. A clear protocol for how emergency referrals will be handled is mandatory in order to assure quality, compassionate care with a high level of satisfaction for both patient and referring physician.

How patient phone calls are handled will also impact the ultimate success of the pain management specialist. Calls from referring physicians, the pharmacy, and patients, as well as support services including laboratory, radiology, physical therapy, and occupational therapy are the rule rather than the exception. Again, it must be clearly defined as to how these calls will be handled by all members of the pain management care team in order to provide consistent, quality care and avoid lost revenues through missed consults or unavailability. The use of answering machines and voice mail as a way to evade dealing with patients and referring physicians is to be avoided and may require careful monitoring by the pain treatment facility management team.

Coupled with the need for the prompt returning of phone calls is the timeliness in which outpatient appointments and inpatient consultations are handled. Although specific times may vary from community to community, seeing inpatient consults (other than emergencies) within 24 h of being called works well in most situations. Any consult requested on an emergency basis should be seen as soon as possible. Seeing all routine consults that are received before 16:00 h on that same day (this includes Saturdays, Sundays, and holidays) projects a very strong message that the pain patient will not suffer needlessly while waiting for the pain management service to be implemented. The same reasoning applies to the availability of outpatient consultation. When a pain treatment facility is set up, immediate appointments should be available on a same-day basis for patients with acute pain problems and pain emergencies. Such appointments should allow appropriate screening and triage for such patients without disrupting the flow of previously scheduled patients.

This approach also makes good sense from a time management viewpoint. As the pain treatment facility grows busier, if inpatient and outpatient consultations are put off, a large backlog of patients waiting to be seen may result. Given the competitive nature of pain management services in most geographic areas, such delays will result in significant lost revenues and high levels of patient and referring physician dissatisfaction.

Support Staff Availability

Tandem to the issue of physician availability is the issue of support staff availability. How consultations and phone messages for the pain management service are to be handled is of paramount importance to the ultimate success of the pain practitioner. In many hospital-based pain treatment facilities, all scheduling activities have been made the responsibility of the hospital secretarial staff. Often this simply does not work, in terms of both efficiency and motivation,

when applied to the pain management service. Hospital employees may not be willing or able to provide prompt and courteous handling of phone calls from referring physicians as well as patients. Messages may get misplaced or lost. Generally the 07:00 to 15:30 h staffing patterns of the hospital does not meet the needs of referring physicians, who are often in their office until 17:00 or 17:30 h. For this reason it is desirable as well as cost-effective to hire a high-quality secretary whose prime responsibilities are the administrative aspects of the pain management service. This will insure that the phone is answered courteously and promptly, that phone messages are handled appropriately, that patient records are readily available, and that there is an appropriate level of motivation to work in add-on and emergency patients.

The pain management support staff must be available during regular clinic hours. The overuse of answering machines or voice mail is strongly discouraged, as most busy referring physicians are unwilling to make several phone calls trying to reach the pain management physician to discuss or schedule a patient. Provisions for phone coverage during lunch and break periods by the pain management support staff are mandatory.

Physician-Referred versus Self-Referred Patients

Pain management specialists have traditionally felt that physician-referred patients are desirable. In fact, many practitioners will not accept self-referred patients. There are distinct advantages and disadvantages to this philosophical viewpoint, as outlined in Boxes 24.1 and 24.2.

The physician-referred patient *may* be appropriately worked up and carry a correct diagnosis; however, the pain specialist has limited control over the appropriateness and quality of the evaluation and treatment of the physician-referred patient; the patient may be inadequately or inappropriately evaluated, which puts tremendous medicolegal responsibilities on the pain management physician to complete the evaluation. These problems can be magnified under the managed care paradigm, as the managed care plan may want to save money by limiting diagnostic testing. Furthermore, the patient referral may not be appropriate for the services and expertise available at the pain treatment facility chosen by the referring physician or managed care plan.

Advantages of the self-referred patient include the fact that the pain management specialist maintain

---

Box 24.1. Physician-Referred Patients

Advantages

1. The patient *may* be appropriately worked up.

2. The patient *may* be appropriately diagnosed.

3. The patient *may* be familiar with pain management services and the reason that they have been sent to the pain center.

4. The referral *may* be appropriate for the services and expertise of the pain center.

5. Patient acquisition is low cost relative to advertising for self-referred patients.

Disadvantages

1. The pain specialist has limited control over the appropriateness of the evaluation and treatment.

2. The patient may be inadequately worked up, which puts tremendous medicolegal responsibilities on the pain management physician to complete the evaluation.

3. The patient may be sent to the pain management specialist carrying the wrong diagnosis.

4. The patient may be an inappropriate referral to the pain clinic relative to the services being offered.

5. The pain management physician may inherit a patient who has been inappropriately treated by a referring physician and assume significant medical liability if he or she continues this treatment.

Box 24.2. Self-Referred Patients

Advantages

1. The pain management specialist may control the evaluation and treatment.

2. The pain management specialist may choose consultants needed to help him or her make the diagnosis that are of a higher quality than those chosen by the referring physician.

3. The pain management specialist has control over treatment and the use of prescription medication (especially controlled substances).

4. The pain management physician may exercise a choice in diagnostic imaging facilities or for hospitals should admission for further evaluation be necessary.

Disadvantages

1. The pain management specialist has sole responsibility for the evaluation and treatment.

2. The pain management specialist assumes the role of primary care physician.

3. Once the patient is under the care of the pain management specialist, transfer of the patient to a more appropriate specialist may be difficult should a problem arise.

4. Cost of patient acquisition is high relative to physician-referred patients if advertising is used.

---

control over the evaluation and treatment and may choose consultants necessary to help him or her make the diagnosis who may be of a higher quality than those utilized by some referring physicians. The pain management specialist has control over treatment and the use of prescription medication (especially controlled substances) when providing care for the self-referred patients. Furthermore, the pain management specialist may exercise a choice in diagnostic imaging facilities or for hospitals, should admission for further evaluation be necessary. As an increasing number of patients under managed care have out-of-network or point-of-service benefits as part of their managed care contract, such patients can choose the pain management physician and/or pain treatment facility in spite of the dictates of the managed care plan [9, 10]. Such patients can represent a significant source of revenue for a pain treatment facility, and care should be taken to identify patients with such benefits before assuming they cannot be seen at a pain treatment facility.

Disadvantages of self-referred patients include the fact that the pain management specialist and pain treatment facility has sole responsibility for the evaluation and treatment, essentially assuming the role of primary care physician. Once the patient is under the care of the pain management specialist and facility, transfer of the patient to a more appropriate specialist or facility may be difficult, should a problem arise.

The pain management specialist and the pain treatment facility must weigh these variables to determine the best course to follow. Should a pain management specialist decide to accept self-referred patients, he or she must recognize that in essence one is assuming the role of primary care physician. Incumbent to this role is an increase in responsibility with its attendant nighttime phone calls, emergencies, talking with family members, etc. Regardless of the pain management specialist's ultimate decision, it is my strong belief that the physician-referred patient requires the same level of vigilance and quality of evaluation that a self-referred patient does, especially under the managed care paradigm.

Hospital-Based Versus Free-Standing Facilities

As hospital administrators, government, managed care plans, and third-party payers seek to exert greater control over hospital-based physicians, pain management specialists have sought to limit their vulnerability to this situation, e.g., by opening of surgical centers, affiliating with rehabilitation centers, etc. [11]. An additional option is the development of a free-standing pain treatment facility. By developing such a facility, the pain management specialist may avoid the "label" associated with a given hospital. This can be good or bad, depending on the public perception of the specific hospital. It should be remembered that these perceptions can change over time, and what may be a desirable hospital to practice in at one point in time may represent a negative practice location at another.

An additional advantage of starting a free-standing pain treatment facility is that the pain management specialist may choose its geographic location. This is advantageous if the pain management specialist's primary hospital practice is located in a less desirable geographic area of the city [12].

In some localities, it is possible for the pain management specialist to bill not only for his or her professional fees but also for the drugs, trays, radiology services, laboratory services, block room, and recovery room charges. Some third-party carriers in specific geographic locations in the United States, e.g., the east coast, allow the pain management specialist to charge 150 percent of his or her professional fee to cover the cost of drugs, trays, and room charges. In other areas, local or state law as well as policies of the third-party carriers may require that the facility be licensed and accredited as an ambulatory surgery center in order for a facility fee to be paid. Medicare pays the pain management physician a higher professional fee if he or she provides care in an office setting rather than an ambulatory surgical center or hospital-based pain treatment facility. Changes in this policy may lead to a shift in where pain management services are provided in the future.

In the free-standing pain treatment facility, the pain management specialist will have greater control of the space, staffing, hours of operation, capital expenditures, and utilization review/quality assurance activities. Obviously with this added control and flexibility, there comes an added measure of responsibility and risk [13].

The major disadvantage of the free-standing pain treatment facility is cost. The pain management specialist can anticipate a large capital expenditure to provide adequate space, equipment, and personnel to implement pain management services at a free-standing location. In addition, the pain management specialist assumes the added liability and cost of malpractice insurance of the facility as well as the liability for professional services offered. The pain management specialist also inherits the liability for the actions of his or her staff. The advantages and disadvantages of the hospital-based pain management practice versus the free-standing pain center are summarized in Box 24.3.

Box 24.3. Hospital-Based Pain Center

Advantages

1. The rent is free.
2. The personnel are free.
3. The equipment is free.
4. There is high visibility to referring physicians.
5. There is a high level of convenience for inpatients.
6. There is excellent emergency support should problems arise.
7. There is high-tech equipment readily available.
8. Support services such as physical therapy, occupational therapy, etc. are available.

Disadvantages

1. There may be a lack of adequate designated space.
2. The pain management specialist does not have control of staffing.
3. The hospital administration may be very unwilling to provide the capital expenditure necessary to provide appropriate diagnostic and therapeutic equipment.
4. If the hospital develops a negative perception in the community, this will be carried over to the pain management services.
5. The pain management specialist will be subject to hospital utilization review and quality assurance activities.
6. The pain management specialist is subject to medical staff rules, which may limit his or her ability to use operating room facilities, admit patients, etc.
7. The pain management specialist receives no portion of the revenues from the facility, lab, radiology, and support service fees generated.

Summary

Starting a pain treatment facility is a significant undertaking, in terms of both time and tangible expense. Although the risks are great, so can be the rewards if done properly. By addressing the above-mentioned issues as an integral part of the planning process, the pain management specialist will be better able to determine whether setting up a pain treatment facility is the right decision.

References

1. R. L. Nahin. Estimates of pain prevalence and severity in adults: United States. *J Pain* 2015; 8: 769–80.

2. D. H. Gesne, M. Wiseman. How to negotiate with health care plans. *J Oncol Pract* 2010; 64: 220–22.

3. S. D. Waldman. Motivating the pain center employee. *Am J Pain Manag* 1993; 3: 114–17.

4. S. D. Waldman. Hiring employees for the pain center. *Am J Pain Manag* 1992; 2: 164–6.

5. S. D. Waldman. Total quality management for the pain center – An idea whose time has come. *Am J Pain Manag* 1993; 3: 38–41.

6. S. D. Waldman. The antitrust implications of medical staff credentialling – Part I. *Am J Pain Manag* 1997; 7: 22–7.

7. S. D. Waldman. The antitrust implications of medical staff credentialling – Part II. *Am J Pain Manag* 1997; 7: 66–9.

8. J. Mathew, T. Wagner. Pain management in 2017: Tips for thriving dispite challenges. *Becker's ASC Rev* 2017; 9: 1–2.

9. P. Barros, X. Martinez-Giralt. Selecting health care providers: "Any willing provider" vs. negotiation. *Eur J Polit Econ* 2008; 24: 402–14.

10. S. D. Waldman. Any willing provider laws – Paradox or panacea, part II. *Am J Pain Manag* 1996; 6: 93–6.

11. S. D. Waldman, N. A. Ford. Selling your medical practice – Part I. *Am J Pain Manag* 1998; 8: 23–8.

12. E. Rabinowitz. Successful strategies when selling your medical practice. *MD Mag* 2016; 9: 1–2.

13. B. A. Fiedler. Challenges of new technology: Securing medical devices and their software for HIPPA compliance. In *Managing medical devices within a regulatory framework*, edited by Beth Ann Fiedler. Elsevier, 2017, 315–29.

Chapter

25

Office-Based Surgery Practice

Jonathan P. Eskander, Cory Roberts, and Charles J. Fox

Contents

Introduction to Office-Based Surgery

Office-based surgery, a subset of ambulatory surgery, has been the mainstay for certain medical fields like dentistry and dermatology. Potential advantages afforded by office-based surgery include greater privacy for the patient, consistency of personnel, leaner and more efficient systems, as well as added physician control over facility processes. However, while the number of surgical procedures performed in office-based settings has increased, the outcomes of procedures in this setting continue to be investigated.

The shift in office-based surgeries versus hospital-based procedures is based generally on four main factors: advancements of medical technology and new surgical and anesthetic techniques, changes in policy, comparatively leaner management systems, and cost-competitive options for patient care.

With the advancements in surgical techniques and technology as well as favorable economic conditions, complex procedures once thought only possible in a traditional hospital settings, began to migrate to office-based facilities. In the mid-1990s, primarily due to the expansion of non-hospital-based surgical procedures by Medicare, ambulatory surgical centers (ASCs) proliferated. However, current policy changes will again continue to significantly impact office-based surgery.

Hospitals continue to evolve into increasingly complex entities. Many place procedure block time limits for "new" surgeons or possess service lines that necessitate emergent operating room (OR) time. This may result in OR inefficiency and inconvenience for patients and surgeons in need of a hospital OR. Healthcare costs have also escalated significantly in recent years; and, with many elective procedures left uncovered by conventional insurance carriers, patients have gravitated to the more cost-competitive options offered by office-based surgery. Therefore, more patients undergo procedures in an office-based facility.

However, office-based practice has inherent challenges in regard to safety. A lack of early state and federal regulations allowed rapid unchecked expansion of the office-based practice. With an absence of governance, reporting adverse and sentinel events was not mandated. While pushing the limits of ambulatory surgery, several highly publicized poor outcomes necessitated an immediate need for regulation and guideline development. Task forces were created to improve patient safety. Yet, insufficient research and data were available, partly due to the lack of adverse event reporting. This has added to the difficulty in implementing universal standards for such a wide range of procedures with varying complexity and sedation requirements.

In order to ensure the safety of their patients, healthcare providers must be knowledgeable and up-to-date with current practices and policies. Therefore, the aim of this chapter is to discuss the foundations in providing safe office-based practices by, first, discussing necessary accreditation and licensing, second, detailing practice management and oversight strategies; and, lastly, highlighting pertinent clinical considerations for those practicing in an office-based surgical setting.

Guidelines, Accreditation, and Licensing

Individualized guidelines have been made available by the leading societies of the various medical specialties that partake in office-based surgery. While one should be familiar with the guidelines and advisories made by his or her respective field; the foundation of these guidelines are the safety recommendations for ambulatory anesthesia and surgery drafted by the American Society of Anesthesiologists (ASA). The ASA stresses that patient safety should serve as the cornerstone for crafting actions, and it would be prudent to be familiar with their guidelines as well. Over several years, the topics that have been addressed include the types of procedures performed in the office-based facility, patient selection, and perioperative pain management, among others. These guidelines were not developed with the intention to be legal standards of medical care, but rather, a strategy highlighting patient care based on recommendations from relevant and current medical literature.

There are numerous qualifications and standards that the surgeon and organization must achieve before opening an office-based facility. In some states, the above-noted guidelines for office-based surgery have been adapted into law. An example of state that has heavy government oversight is New York, and it is worth reviewing their detailed clinical guidelines for office-based surgery (www.health.ny.gov/professionals/office-based_surgery/obs_faq.htm). However, these laws are not applicable universally, and requirements for licensing of the physician, accreditation of facility, and adverse event reporting vary widely from state to state. If accreditation is required, it may be obtained

through the Joint Commission, Accreditation for Ambulatory Health Care, or American Association for Accreditation of Ambulatory Surgery Facilities (AAAASF). Accrediting agencies address the facility layout, patient records, personnel records, peer review, quality assurance, OR personnel, equipment, operations and management, and environmental safety. Although the AAAASF is the only accrediting body that requires mandatory reporting of adverse events, all three organizations are working to create standardized definitions of adverse events.

The facility should have a medical director or governing body that establishes policy and is responsible for the activities of the facility and staff for ensuring that facilities and personnel are adequate and that all applicable local, state, and federal laws, codes, and regulations are observed. All healthcare practitioners and nurses should hold a valid license or certificate to perform their assigned duties. The surgeons performing the operation should have hospital privileges for that procedure and either board certification or qualifications leading to board certification by a surgical specialty board recognized by the American Board of Medical Specialties. The supervising operating practitioner or other licensed physician should be specifically trained in the office-based surgery being performed as well as sedation, anesthesia, and rescue techniques appropriate to the type of sedation being provided. It is critical that anesthesiologists and surgeons practicing in an office-based setting maintain current advanced cardiac life support with hands-on airway training.

All patient records must be kept on file and available for review. Preoperative and postoperative evaluations must be documented in the patient record. All medical information must be maintained in a fashion that is compliant with the Health Insurance Portability and Accountability Act (HIPAA). The list of forms that may be required is shown in Box 25.1.

Office-based anesthesia practices should have a written quality improvement plan in place to continually assess, document, and improve outcome. The quality improvement plan should utilize peer reviews, benchmarking, and risk management strategies. The quality improvement plan should also include review of morbidity and "adverse" or "sentinel" events (Table 25.1). The review of quality indicators should also include measures of patient satisfaction.

Outcomes-based accountability practitioners, generally anesthesiologists, will often get asked to help in

Box 25.1. Suggested Forms

Patient demographics	Pregnancy disclaimer	Notice of privacy practices
Medical records release	Preoperative instructions	NPO instructions
Preoperative checklist	Surgery consent	Anesthesia record
PACU record	Postoperative instructions	Intraoperative record
Health history questionnaire	Blood-borne pathogen testing release	Patient satisfaction survey
Photo release	Acknowledgement of preoperative instructions	Universal protocol verification
PACU orders		

Table 25.1 Adverse and Sentinel Events Suggested for Review

Death	Cardiac arrest	Respiratory arrest
Unplanned reintubation	Central nervous system deficit within 2 days of anesthesia	Peripheral nervous system deficit within 2 days of anesthesia
Myocardial infarction within 2 days of anesthesia	Pulmonary edema within 1 day of anesthesia	Aspiration pneumonia
Anaphylaxis or adverse drug reaction	Postdural puncture headache within 4 days of neuraxial anesthesia	Dental injury
Eye injury	Surgical infection	Excessive blood loss
Unplanned admission to a hospital or acute care facility	Drug error	Wrong surgical or regional block site
Wrong procedure or patient		

facility operations, such as scheduling, equipment and supply ordering, medical directorships, and accreditation. It is usually advantageous to be involved in facility operations, but it should be viewed more as consultative role with contractual arrangements made with facilities for anesthesiologists to serve in that capacity. Such services must be provided at fair market value by the practitioner, and must not be construed as a "bonus" service, which can be considered a kickback.

A federal law, known as Stark II, prohibits certain physician self-referrals for "designated health services" and prohibits physicians from making referrals for such designated health services to an entity in which the physicians or their immediate family members have financial interest, either by way of ownership or compensation, unless an exception applies.

The federal anti-kickback law prohibits offering, paying, soliciting, or receiving any "remuneration" to induce referrals of items or services that are reimbursable by federal healthcare programs. Because it is a criminal statute, it requires proof of intent, unlike Stark II. Situations involving the provision of drugs and supplies may raise concerns for potential anti-kickback law violations, and individual providers should seek legal counsel if questions arise regarding anti-kickback laws. Because of the current lack of oversight in the office-based setting, individual providers may find themselves in questionable ethical situations. Direct employment relationships may jeopardize the autonomy of office-based practices if economics influence medical judgment.

Insurance Coverage

Insurance providers do not discriminate against office-based practitioners, but because office-based practices are an emerging concept, insurers may lack many of the traditional tools utilized to establish rates and plans. Insurers may lack an established peer-review structure to examine the quality of the exclusively office-based practitioner and a facility accreditation system to assess risk related to adequacy of the equipment, supplies and protocols and procedures.

257

Box 25.2. Professional Liability Insurance Agents Requirements

Clinic ownership and practitioner list	Assurance that all patients will be discharged in the care of a responsible adult
Policy and procedure manual for routine and emergency situations	Assurance of adherence to all applicable ASA standards and guidelines
Policy and procedure manual for record review	Presence of a defibrillator if general anesthesia, regional anesthesia, or parenteral sedation/analgesia is to be administered
Policy and procedure manual for outcome analysis	On-site inspection by the company's consultant anesthesiologist
Types of anesthesia to be administered	Compliance with all applicable federal and state statutes
Description of equipment and monitoring capabilities	Any voluntary accreditation obtained
Evidence that all patients give informed consent to the surgeon and anesthesiologist	Procedures for resuscitation and arrangements for transport to an emergency facility in a timely manner
Evidence of adherence to a formal credentialing policy	

Underwriting calculations are complicated because providers often work in an office-based setting only part time, at multiple sites, or across state lines.

Individual practitioners should be familiar with all practice guidelines. Insurance providers will cite standards and guidelines and require adherence to these as a condition of coverage. For example, pulse oximetry, electrocardiogram, end-tidal CO_2 and blood pressure measurement are considered standard monitors, and noncompliance with these standards may void coverage and payment. Requirements for obtaining professional liability insurance are listed in Box 25.2.

Practitioners should also understand the concept of vicarious liability, which is the legal liability that may exist for the actions of others involved in the same incident. Individual practitioners should personally examine all liability insurance policies for limitations or restrictions on the type of surgery to be performed and inquire of the state medical board about any limitations placed on the operating surgeon's license. Individual practitioners should also compare coverage limits with those of the other practitioners. A wide disparity in coverage could invite disproportionate accusations of liability (i.e., the "deep-pocket" phenomenon). It is vital that practitioners in an office be absolutely certain of the license status, training qualifications for the procedures performed, and professional liability insurance of the operating surgeon and all assisting personnel.

Reimbursement

A variety of unique payment plans may be created for office-based procedures. Patients may make direct cash payments to the provider for purely elective cases or may make hybrid insurance/cash payments for combined procedures that are both medically necessary and elective (ventral herniorraphy and abdominoplasty). Medicare pays only for covered services that are medically necessary, and often pays less than one's standard fee for covered services. Because it is illegal to bill Medicare patients directly to cover the difference, it is very important to get an accurate picture of the payer mix during the initial negotiation phase.

Although commercial third-party payers have higher reimbursement rates, there are additional complexities to understand. Office-based providers must decide whether or not to become a participating provider in a particular insurance plan. Provider participation with CMS or any insurance company is strictly voluntary, although some hospitals or facilities may require an anesthesiologist to participate. Surgeons and/or the facility would prefer an upfront agreement that all anesthesia providers must be a participating provider with all contracted insurance plans of the facility.

Anesthesiologists must consider many factors before accepting such an upfront agreement. In the office-based setting, insurers do not have to pay the traditional facility fee, and otherwise poor insurance plans are often able to lure surgeons with an additional nonprofessional fee that is paid to surgeons who perform procedures in the office-based setting. Every effort should be made to insert language such as "agree to negotiate in good faith with all insurance companies" into the contract, in order to protect from being bound to participate in undesirable insurance plans.

If the anesthesiologist is not a participating provider, often the insurance company will send the payment directly to the patient, who then pays the anesthesiologist his or her fee. This can result in delays at best and total nonpayment at worst. Patients are often charged an "out-of-network" fee when the anesthesiologist is a nonparticipating provider, and this frequently causes lots of complaints from patients and surgeons.

When considering becoming a participating provider, first compare the rates of the third-party payer with the rates charged by anesthesia providers. Analyze the payer mix. Compare the rates paid by the third-party payer for participating providers with the rates paid for nonparticipating providers. Determine if the patient is billed an "out-of-network" fee for non-participating providers.

Billing Methodology

Billing for services should be clear to all participating parties during negotiations to provide services. Anesthesia providers may perform their own billing, engage a billing service, or have the facility/owner(s) collect anesthesia fees and pay the anesthesia provider in a prearranged fashion. If anesthesia providers choose not to perform their own billing, it is important to understand that the anesthesiologist is responsible for all claims submitted in his or her name.

Individual anesthesiologists or practices must set their own fees for services, because coordination of charges among groups can be viewed as illegal price fixing. A methodology must be established for charging for services. Anesthesiologists typically bill by base time with added modifier units, case type, or hourly.

Billing by base time with modifier units is an accepted methodology and generally used when billing third-party payers and insurance companies. However, when billing the patient or facility directly, practices may choose to bill by hour, by case, or by an all-inclusive "package fee" to provide additional convenience to the patient. Providers must negotiate their global and professional fees in advance when billing the patient by hour, case, or package fee. Providers should be familiar with their state legislation regarding billing HMO patients. Providers should be prepared to accommodate insurance companies that require preauthorization for both surgery and anesthesia.

Facility Considerations

Office-based facilities are typically constructed differently. The OR environment has a high degree of occupational hazard risk, and currently most of the safeguards and redundancies designed to protect patients and providers do not exist in the office-based setting.

Evacuation Plan

Office-based practices should be compliant with the National Fire Protection Association (NFPA) 99 Healthcare Facilities document, which details the requirements for healthcare facilities. Because most office buildings are built with the assumption of an ambulatory population, office-based practices must have a plan for evacuating patients who may be under the effects of anesthesia during an emergency. An office-based practice's policy and procedures manual must include a plan for transporting an artificially ventilated patient, either because of a medical necessity or because the building must be evacuated. For example, the elevators must have the capacity to carry a supine, artificially ventilated patient for transport out of the office.

Medical Gases

The logistics of using volatile anesthetics and/or nitrous oxide introduce an additional level of complexity for many office-based practices, most of which do not have the level 1 medical piped gas systems found in hospitals. If the anesthesiologist plans on using volatile anesthetics for general anesthesia, a system must be developed to access and then eliminate these gases. Many office-based practices use portable tanks; if such tanks are used, storage must conform to NFPA guidelines and an adequate volume of gas must be on hand to meet the day's needs. The Compressed Gas Association and the Department of Transportation provide the information and regulations that address the transportation of compressed or liquefied gases. The NFPA standards for eliminating medical gases are not required in the office setting unless the accrediting organization requires it. Most office-based facilities do not have the capability to actively vacuum and pipe gases or passively direct gases into the facility ventilation exhaust system, so an office-based practice may run an exhaust hose to an outside window, but must insure that the gases do not reenter or contaminate another commercial or residential space. As a result, many office-based practices opt for total intravenous techniques to eliminate the need for medical gas waste systems.

Backup Power and Electrical Wiring

The backup power in most medical or commercial office buildings is only required to allow a safe and orderly exit from the building, but appropriate backup power should be in place for life support equipment. A minimum of two independent sources of power is required. When general anesthesia and electrical life support systems are used, a type I essential electrical system is typically required. The Joint Commission recommends that the generator should be tested 12 times a year for at least 30 min under a dynamic load of at least 30 percent of the nameplate rating on the generator. In the absence of line-isolation monitors, the use of ground fault circuit interrupters should be used to limit the shock hazard.

Anesthesia and Life Support Equipment

All anesthesia and life support equipment should be fully factory supported and include current factory technical support, parts availability, and continued factory service training. A biomedical technician or equivalent should annually inspect all of the equipment. The manufacturer's specifications and requirements are kept in an organized file. All equipment should be on a preventative maintenance schedule. A biomedical technician or equivalent should perform all equipment repairs and changes. Anesthesia machines should not be obsolete.

Infection Control

Practices should adhere to the Centers for Disease Control and Prevention Standard Precautions for Infection Control, which summarizes methods for body substance isolation (B81) and universal precautions to prevent transmission of a variety of organisms.

The office-based practice should have policy and procedure for sterilization of surgical equipment, cleaning and disinfecting procedure rooms, and managing patients with multidrug-resistant organisms.

Box 25.3. Infection Control: Suggested Policy and Procedure

Sterilization of surgical equipment and supplies

Managing patients with multidrug-resistant organisms

Cleaning and disinfecting procedure rooms

Occupational health and blood-borne pathogens standard

Protective clothing appropriate to the procedure

Safe injection practices and appropriate aseptic techniques

Box 25.3 shows a suggested infection policy and procedure. Lastly, employees should be compliant with all Occupational Safety and Health Administration standards.

Controlled Substances

Policy and procedures are required to comply with laws and regulations pertaining to controlled drug supply, storage, and administration. The Federal Drug Enforcement Administration (DEA) requires separate registration certificates for manufacturing, distributing, and dispensing and administering controlled medications, and a separate state-controlled drug registration may also be required. Office-based practices probably do not need a registration certificate for manufacturing, but some practices may choose to function as a distributor. Controlled substances may be supplied by the office location or by the anesthesiologist. If the office supplies the controlled substances, the site will have a DEA 223 registration number and will order controlled Substances with their DEA 222 order form. If the anesthesiologist provides the medication at different locations under the practitioner's DEA license, a separate DEA registration for each site is not needed. Narcotics must be stored in a double-locked box. Any person or place acting as a "dispenser" of controlled drugs must take an inventory on the date of DEA registration and every 2 years thereafter.

A daily drug use inventory must be maintained that accounts for the use and wastage of all controlled medications on each patient for each date. The recording method and any backup media should be specified and records are subject to DEA inspection. Loss or theft of a DEA Controlled Drug Order Form 222 must be reported immediately. Expired drugs

Box 25.4. List of DEA Forms

DEA Form 222	Schedule I and II drug order form
DEA Form 223	The DEA Controlled Substances Certificate of Registration issued to the practitioner or entity
DEA Form 224	Application for registration; renewed every 3 years on Form 224a. The address on the form is important. DEA registrations are issued for principle place of business or professional practice where controlled substances are distributed or dispensed
DEA Form 106	Report of Theft or Loss of Controlled Substances Form
DEA Form 41	Request to Dispose of Stocked Controlled Substances Form

can be disposed of by filing a form 41 with the DEA. Important DEA forms are shown in Box 25.4.

Mobile Anesthesia

Mobile anesthesia may be defined as a practice in which the anesthesiologist transports all anesthesia equipment from office site to office site. A site visit should be conducted before the start of mobile anesthesia services. Mobile anesthesia practices are considering accrediting themselves as a separate entity, as a means of enhancing the credibility and value of the anesthesia practice. Mobile anesthesia providers cannot bill a facility fee or share a facility fee, but may recoup the costs of durable and disposable equipment/supplies provided by the practitioner. Many anesthesia machines are not meant for frequent transport, and many calibrations may be invalidated by spillage of gases. The Food and Drug Administration has approval for anesthesia machines that are suitable for "mobile" anesthesia use.

Patient Selection and Testing

Once reserved for young healthy patients, out of hospital procedures are now being offered to a patient population with significant comorbidities, including those necessitating corrective procedures in the office because they were deemed "unfit for surgery." Each office should establish patient selection guidelines based on the patient's medical status, stability of medical status, psychological status, social support

system, postprocedure monitoring, and risk of deep vein thrombosis/pulmonary embolism (DVT/PE) (Table 25.2). Generally, ASA physical status I and II patients can proceed by protocol, but ASA III and IV must have a direct consultation and the conditions must be medically optimized (Box 25.5). The history and physical should be within 30 days of the procedure and reassessed on the day of surgery. Ideally, every office-based surgery should begin with a thorough preoperative visit where careful preparation and planning can take place. In addition, an appropriate fasting protocol and specific perioperative medication instructions should be clearly explained to the patient. This visit should be conducted by a member of the anesthesia team if sedation is to be used and be in accordance with the 2012 ASA Guidelines for Preanesthetic Evaluation. The goal of the preoperative history and physical examination is to allow the medical staff to select the appropriate time and facility for the patient's procedure. Also, it should identify risk factors and establish baseline preoperative values that will be used by the staff when caring for the patient perioperatively. Since, it is not uncommon for significant comorbidities to be discovered in the preoperative period that warrant further investigation by medical specialists, the optimal time for the preoperative visit to take place is the same day that the decision to operate is made.

A vital part of patient selection is the ability to identify those comorbidities preoperatively which may affect the procedure planned or increase the incidence of perioperative complications for the patient. It has been determined that office-based surgeries entail their own inherent risks on top of those specific to the procedure and sedation. Therefore, it is important to consider how management of potential complications from the patient's identified comorbidities may be affected by the proposed surgical setting.

The preoperative history and physical exam should include age, body mass index (BMI) determination and careful questioning and examination of the cardiac and pulmonary systems. In addition, a history of diabetes mellitus or risk factors for thromboembolism should be ascertained.

Although there is no prohibitive age for office-based surgery, those patients over the age of sixty are at increased risk for cardiac events, other complications, and unanticipated admissions. They can have their procedure at an office-based setting, but this determination depends on a multitude of factors, such as

Table 25.2 Risk Factors for PE

Age >40	Venous insufficiency	Factor V leiden mutation
History of PE or DVT	Elevated factor VIIIc	Protein C deficiency
Protein S deficiency	Hypercoagulable states	Lupus anticoagulant
Polycythemia	Oral contraceptives	Postmenopausal HRT
History of >3 pregnancies	Previous miscarriage	Current pregnancy
Chronic heart failure	Malignancy	Obesity
Trauma	Bedbound	Radiation therapy to pelvis
Infectious disease	Abdominoplasty	Recent long-distance travel
Use of general anesthesia		

Adapted from: Iverson RE, and the ASPS Task Force on Patient Safety in Office-based Surgery Facilities. Procedures in the office-based surgery setting. *Plast Reconstr Surg* 2002; **110**: 1337–42.

Abbreviations: PE, pulmonary embolism; DVT, deep venous thrombosis.

Box 25.5. Medical Conditions Requiring Additional Consideration

Difficult airway	Morbid obesity	Obstructive sleep apnea
Hx anesthetic complications	Malignant hyperthermia	Anaphylactic drug allergy
Latex allergy	Inadequate NPO status	Alcohol abuse
Substance abuse	Inadequate social support	

---

type of procedure planned, anticipated length of surgery, and availability of equipment for perioperative monitoring.

Those considered obese (with a BMI >30) are at increased risk for intra- and postoperative complications. Because of this, some of these patients should not have their surgery performed outside the hospital setting. However, it is strongly advised by the ASPS task force that all patients with a BMI >35 have their procedure performed in a hospital.

Managing those patients with obstructive sleep apnea (OSA) can prove to be extremely challenging; and, because of this, certain factors should be weighed preoperatively. The factors include, but are not limited to, severity of their sleep apnea, presence of other comorbidities, type of surgery, type of anesthesia, need for postoperative narcotics, and resources of the office-based facility. These patients may need an extended postoperative recovery time, sophisticated respiratory care, or extensive postoperative pain management. Obviously, these needs are met most easily in a hospital. For those patients with a suspected but unconfirmed diagnosis of OSA, careful questioning of them and family members should take place preoperatively. A history of loud and frequent snoring, airway obstruction during sleep, daytime somnolence, or falling asleep in a nonstimulating environment should raise suspicion for OSA. These patients warrant further investigation before proceeding with surgery.

Based on the preoperative history and physical examination, and taking into consideration for the procedure planned, additional preoperative testing may be warranted. It is generally acceptable to use results of tests obtained from the medical record within 6 months of surgery, as long as the patient's medical history has not changed substantially. Unfortunately, despite remaining common practice in some locations, the use of "routine" preoperative tests should be avoided. Common labs and studies include complete blood count (CBC), basic metabolic profile (BMP), chest radiographs, and ECG. The CBC should be strongly considered in those with anemia or at risk for significant blood loss. Patients with diabetes or those with hypertension taking certain medications, such as diuretics, should have preoperative BMP lab evaluation. The ECG is not indicated simply due to advanced age. However, it is indicated for patients of any age with known or suspected cardiac disease. Lastly, the procedure being performed may dictate other specific lab evaluations to establish baseline values.

Once the preoperative physical examination, history, and test results are completed, the patient should be assigned an ASA code. Box 25.6 lists the ASA physical classification system. Patients classified as ASA physical status I or II are the best candidates for office-based surgery. Patients classified as ASA physical status III can have their procedure performed in the office-based facility if the surgery can be performed using local anesthesia with or without sedation. Patients classified as ASA physical status IV can have their procedure in an office-based surgery facility if the surgery can be performed using local anesthesia only.

Objectifying the Severity and Risk of a Procedure

Many times the healthcare practitioners themselves establish written policies governing the specific surgical procedures that may be performed in the office. Classifications are usually delineated based on a combination of the complexity of surgical procedure as well as the level of anesthesia required for the given office-based procedure.

All surgical procedures produce physiologic stress for the patient. The degree of stress seems more linked to the severity of the physiologic derangement rather than the procedure. Rather than excluding certain surgical procedures from being done in the office-based setting, surgeons should base the degree of surgical involvement on the facility's resources. Hypothermia, blood loss, and duration of surgery have been acknowledged as factors that should be considered when selecting the appropriate facility. Any procedures involving significant blood loss (>500 cc); major intraabdominal, intrathoracic, or intracranial cavities; significant postoperative pain; or elevated risk of postoperative nausea and vomiting are not appropriate for the office-based setting. Qualifying procedures with high complexity levels should be scheduled early in the day, because they may require longer recovery periods. Procedures should last no longer than 6 h to allow for adequate recovery and discharge.

Sedation is recognized on a continuum from anxiolysis, moderate sedation/analgesia (conscious sedation), deep sedation/analgesia (MAC), to general anesthesia. Patients under conscious sedation respond purposefully to verbal commands or light tactile stimulation and require no airway support. Patients under deep sedation respond purposefully

---

Box 25.6. ASA Physical Status Classification System

ASA physical status I – a normal healthy patient

ASA physical status II – a patient with mild systemic disease

ASA physical status III – a patient with severe systemic disease

ASA physical status IV – a patient with severe systemic disease that is a constant threat to life

ASA physical status V – a moribund patient who is not expected to survive without the operation

ASA physical status VI – a declared brain-dead patient whose organs are being removed for donor purposes.

---

to painful stimulation and may require assistance in maintaining a patent airway. Patients under general anesthesia cannot be aroused and may require respiratory and cardiovascular support.

The anesthesiologist should focus on providing an anesthetic that will give the patient a rapid recovery to normal function, with minimal postoperative pain, nausea, and other side effects. The intraoperative record must document anesthetic agents, medications, and supplemental oxygen used, vital signs, oxygen saturation, ECG interpretation, end-tidal CO_2, inspired oxygen, and temperature measurements when required. Pain should be managed proactively. Multiple modalities should be used to manage pain, including nonsteroidal anti-inflammatory drugs (NSAIDs), opioids, local anesthetics, acetaminophen, gabapentin or pregabalin, and regional or neuraxial anesthesia.

Avoiding Intraoperative Complications

Hypothermia and blood loss are two common intraoperative issues faced by surgeons. The body's protective thermoregulatory measures to conserve heat loss are blocked by regional or general anesthesia. Combined with the colder temperatures common to most ORs, these factors increase the patient's risk of developing hypothermia. Because of this, the surgical facility should have forced air warming blankets and intravenous fluid warmers. The OR should have the equipment and ability to monitor and regulate room temperature. Surgery, without the use of hypothermia prevention measures, should be of short duration (1–2 h) and not involve more than 20 percent of the patient's body surface area.

When a general or regional anesthetic is planned, the patient should be actively prewarmed and core temperature should be measured throughout the procedure. In addition, one should cover as much body surface area as possible with blankets or drapes to minimize radiant or convective heat loss during the procedure. If large volumes of irrigating or infiltrating fluids are used, they should be warmed. Postoperative shivering should be aggressively treated with forced air warming or resistive heating blankets and pharmacologic intervention if needed.

Surgical blood loss occurs to varying degrees, depending on the type and duration of each procedure. For the average-sized adult, anticipated blood loss of 500 ml or more may necessitate blood and blood component replacement. So when scheduling the procedure the surgeon should select a facility with this capability.

Thromboprophylaxis

Indeed, most patients presenting for office-based surgery have a small chance of developing a DVT/PE; but the significance of such an event postoperatively either in the office or worse, after the patient has been discharged home, led to development of guidelines for the office-based setting. The guidelines should help physicians when evaluating the patient preoperatively. Numerous studies have identified risk factors thought to predispose patients to developing DVT/PE (see Table 25.2). One should try to uncover subtle clues of past DVT/PE or identify risk factors associated with their development. For example, a history of dyspnea, syncope, or pleurisy may indicate a past PE, whereas a history of calf pain or leg swelling may indicate past DVT. A detailed list of medications, past and present, should be ascertained preoperatively. Close attention should be paid to those patients found to be taking anticoagulants, oral contraceptives, or hormone replacement therapy. A detailed family history may uncover valuable clues concerning past thrombotic events or hypercoagulable states that may require further investigation before proceeding with surgery. When present on the physical exam, finding such as leg swelling, calf pain, and skin discoloration/ulceration may warrant further analysis.

The information gathered from the history and physical examination allows patients to be assigned to predefined risk classifications for developing a DVT or PE, and a thromboprophylaxis strategy based on the risk classification should be determined. Low-risk patients are usually under 40 years of age and have no risk factors. For these patients, thromboprophylaxis

may include positioning the lower extremity in a comfortable position with knees slightly flexed and avoiding constriction or external compression of the lower extremity. Optional therapy for these patients includes the use of graduated compression stockings at home.

Patients categorized as moderate risk are 40 years of age or older undergoing procedures longer than 30 min. Patients taking oral contraceptives or on hormone replacement therapy are also found to be at moderate risk. Prophylaxis for this group includes the use of lower extremity pneumatic compression devices for the calf and ankle, which should start before the induction of general anesthesia and continue until the patient is awake and active postoperatively, along with those recommendations used for lower-risk patients. These patients should also qualify for pre- and postoperative chemoprophylaxis with low-molecular-weight heparin continued until fully ambulatory.

High-risk patients include those over 40 years of age with one risk factor who are undergoing surgical procedures lasting longer than 30 min. Thromboprophylaxis for these patients should include those advised for low- and moderate-risk patients as well as a preoperative hematology consultation and preoperative and postoperative antithrombotic drug therapy. Chemoprophylaxis for this group may be warranted for up to ten days postoperatively.

Very-high-risk patients include those over 40 years of age with more than one risk factor who are undergoing procedures lasting longer than 30 min. These patients should have the same thromboprophylaxis as the high-risk group. In addition, they may require longer prophylaxis with agents such as warfarin. This may necessitate anticoagulation monitoring using the blood test for International Normalized Ratio.

Avoiding Postoperative Complications

The Standards for Postoperative Care and Guidelines for Ambulatory Anesthesia and Surgery on the ASA website apply to all anesthesia services; but, in the office-based setting, providers must recognize that differences in the facility structure and/or support services may present unique challenges to successful post anesthesia care. In many office-based practices, patients recover in the surgical room or procedure room without transport to a PACU. Oxygenation, ventilation, circulation, and temperature should

Box 25.7. Combined Modified Aldrete Score and Fast-Tracking Criteria

Moves all extremities voluntarily

Breathes deeply and coughs freely

Blood pressure within 20 mm of preanesthetic level

Fully awake

Pulse oximetry of >92 percent on room air

Postoperative pain: none or mild discomfort (VAS <3)

Postoperative emetic symptoms: none or mild nausea with no active vomiting

Data from White PF, Song D. White PF, Song D. New criteria for fast-tracking after outpatient anesthesia: a comparison with the modified Aldrete's scoring system. *Anesth Analg* 1999; **88**: 1069.

be monitored on all patients, including a quantitative method of assessing oxygenation (pulse oximetry). The anesthesiologist should be immediately available until the patient has been discharged from anesthesia care. If the patient remains in the facility after discharge from anesthesia, personnel trained in basic life support/advanced cardiac life support should be present until the person leaves. Office-based practices do not have to have a designated area for recovery and the modified Aldrete score and fast-tracking criteria are often combined (Box 25.7). Postoperative discharge instructions should include the procedure performed, information about potential complications, telephone numbers and names of medical providers, instructions for any medications, instructions for pain management, date, time, and location of the follow-up or return visit, and predetermined places to go for treatment in the event of an emergency.

Two frequent reasons for postoperative hospital admission after office-based surgery are failure to control postoperative pain or nausea and vomiting. Therefore, prevention of these two factors is vitally important to physicians treating patients in the office-based facility. Prevention and treatment of these disorders starts preoperatively. A thorough preoperative history will uncover factors such as: a history of motion sickness, previous postsurgical nausea and vomiting, or allergies and/or reactions to certain analgesics. Also, an adequate explanation of pain management and postoperative pain management expectations allows the patient to understand the process better, which decreases postoperative anxiety. Patients are frequently fearful of becoming addicted

to postoperative narcotics. Because of this, they should be counseled on the appropriate need and use of postoperative narcotics at this visit.

On the day of the procedure, in addition to efficient intraoperative management and atraumatic surgical technique, there are a number of strategies that should be employed to combat postoperative complications. Those patients with a prior history of motion sickness or postoperative nausea and vomiting will require a multimodal pharmacologic plan for prevention, and this can be initiated upon the patient's arrival. Avoidance of fentanyl and nitrous oxide further decreases the overall incidence of postoperative nausea and vomiting. Using a combination of both NSAIDs and opiates lowers the total narcotic requirements and helps to ensure a timely discharge by avoiding their side effects. The use of local anesthetics, either locally infiltrated by the surgeon or as a regional technique by the anesthesiologist, aids in reducing postoperative pain. If present, despite having used preventative measures, postoperative pain and/or nausea and vomiting are treated quickest with intravenous medications. Home management of pain and postoperative nausea and vomiting must be discussed with the patient and a capable adult before discharge.

Office-Based Dental Procedures

Office-based procedures have been the mainstay of dentists for many years. Because of this, the practice of dentistry has had involvement with the administration of sedation and general anesthesia. In the 1840s, nitrous oxide was first used by the Hartford dentist Horace Wells. His student, William Morton, revolutionized surgery by unveiling the anesthetic capabilities of ether. Today dentistry continues to build on this rich foundation. The American Dental Association has multiple venues where dentists can train to become knowledgeable and adept at the delivery of sedation and/or general anesthesia.

Dentists and oromaxillofacial surgeons realized the need for specialization training in anesthesiology many years ago. A large number of the patients presenting for procedures were either pediatric or physically and/or mentally challenged. These patients traditionally had trouble accessing the standard hospital OR. Today dental anesthesiologists provide anesthetic services for a multitude of patients undergoing dental procedures. They undergo two years of postdoctoral anesthesiology training at one of ten recognized training programs in North America. During their training, the majority of their training time is spent in hospital OR anesthesiology rotations. In addition, they spend the remainder of their time in ambulatory centers caring for medical and dental patients undergoing various procedures. They have an ongoing dialogue with the ASA and share their views concerning delivery of anesthesia and sedation in the office-based facility.

Affordable Healthcare Act and the Future

Since its implementation in 2010, the Affordable Care Act (ACA) continues to be a significant driver of change in healthcare. For example, an influx of newly insured Americans under the ACA may over-load capacity at certain hospitals. Therefore, ASCs could anticipate an increased patient volume since they tend to provide lower cost alternatives and a more streamlined and efficient service. While still too early to accurately predict how the ACA will change office-based surgery practice, further investigation of outcomes related to office-based procedures may determine the fitness of higher-risk procedures in

this setting. However, if history serves as an indicator for the future, medical advancements will allow for a wider array of procedures to be safely performed in the ambulatory setting.

Suggested Reading

ASA. Office-based anesthesia – Considerations for anesthesiologists in setting up and maintaining a safe office anesthesia environment. 2nd ed. November 2008.

www.asahq.org/quality-and-practice-management/ standards-and-guidelines

American College of Surgeons. Guidelines for optimal ambulatory surgical care and office-based surgery. www.facs.org

www.plasticsurgery.org/for-medical-professionals/ advocacy/key-issues/office-based-surgery.html

www.aaahc.org/en/news/Federal-and-State-Regulations/ State-Laws-and-Regulations/

www.health.ny.gov/professionals/office-based_surgery/ obs_faq.htm

www.samba.org

www.asda.org

Shapiro FE, Punwani N, Rosenberg NM, Valedon A, Twersky R, Urman RD. Office-based anesthesia: safety and outcomes. Anesth Analg. 2014 Aug;119(2):276–85.

Chapter

26

The Future of Perioperative Medicine

Michael R. Hicks and Laurie Saletnik

Introduction

Surgical care has historically been provided to patients in heavily siloed work areas much like inventory moving down an assembly line in a manufacturing process designed to create a quasi-made-to-order industrial product. Initial referrals by primary care providers to surgeons, decisions for referrals for imaging, labs, medical screening and preparation, scheduling and facility registration, the procedure itself, and postoperative pain management and rehabilitation in this model are all essentially treated as separate workstations along the surgical assembly line. While the care delivered at each individual step certainly has some individualization seldom is the care delivered within the intent of promoting or maximizing the overall experience and value for the patient or for the healthcare system. This organizational structure, designed to meet and even optimize the workflow at each station, typically produces an overall experience not focused on the patient, inadequate for its intended purpose of maximizing patient safety and experience, wasteful of resources, and confusing to patients and their family members.

It is our contention that the primary goal of perioperative medicine should be to create an optimal environment for all stakeholders – patients, families, surgeons, and the many other contributors involved in creating the surgical experience. Optimizing health, minimizing risk, streamlining processes, creating an easy to engage workflow, and doing so in a

cost-effective manner should always be the goal in creating patient flow in all aspects of healthcare. This certainly should be true as well in the perioperative continuum. Modern management science has successfully addressed similar issues in other industries. In healthcare, however, we have been slow to embrace this science, often with a dismissive argument that healthcare is different from other industries and therefore not appropriate for management strategies proven to work elsewhere. Not surprisingly, we believe otherwise.

Fortunately, increasing numbers of clinicians and administrators are adding management expertise and experience to their clinical abilities. Clinicians in particular are in an ideal position to best understand the clinical and financial needs of direct care provision and must have a voice in the decision-making process. A collaborative team with an extensive and diverse skill set is essential to lead the changes necessary as healthcare evolves. This chapter explores integrative options for improving and redesigning the surgical patient experience for the future.

As with all aspects of American healthcare, the structure in which surgical care has been provided has been largely driven by the volume-based fee-for-service payment system. This payment methodology, rewarding more for doing more, focuses wrongly on the needs and incentives of individual contributors and not on the overall performance of the system and the care delivered to the patient. Since payment has been directed at what one does to the patient instead of on the total process itself, it is not surprising that little attention has historically been given to the functioning of the system as a whole and to the culture in which patients receive care.

In our view, organizational culture is inextricably linked to behaviors and in ideal circumstances should serve to reinforce each other in a virtuous circle. The culture of American medicine, however, has been for physicians to focus attention primarily on the care and services that a patient needs at any given moment in time (the behaviors) and not on the activities that comprise the patient's journey through a continuum of care with the patient at its center and with all activities focused on the patient (the culture). While those of us working in perioperative medicine are familiar with a team-based approach inside of the operating room (OR), once outside of this environment the degree and extent of collaboration begins to decline markedly. Preoperative preparation, if it occurs at all, is frequently seen as distinct from intraoperative care and postoperative recovery and rehabilitation. This is driven not only by financial disincentives to care coordination but also by the trend for increasing levels of subspecialization across both medicine and nursing. Unfortunately, it is the exception rather than the rule that a patient's care is coordinated across all areas in the American healthcare experience. This is as true for the perioperative experience as it is for care across other domains of medicine and healthcare.

Similarly, the current reimbursement system – and its attendant system of incentives, intended or not – is responsible for the lack of anesthesiologist involvement in the care of the surgical patient at points temporally distant from the actual surgical procedure and the OR. With little personal financial incentive otherwise, anesthesiologists and CRNAs have left the perioperative management of patients to others, outside of course the actual provision of the actual anesthetic itself. These non-anesthesiology-trained physicians and nurses are compensated for services that anesthesiologists typically are not (for example, physician E&M codes as opposed to American Society of Anesthesiologists [ASA] base units plus time) and generally have differing skill sets, training, and clinical interests than anesthesiologists.

The Perioperative System

A discussion of the future of perioperative medicine requires exploration of many subtexts for completeness. Clinicians tend to focus primarily on the delivery and quality of clinical care that they personally provide with some consideration to the quality of the patient experience while the patient is in front of them. Whether explicitly stated or not, clinical workflow is typically oriented to maximize the efficiency of the healthcare workforce in that particular phase of the care continuum. In maximizing individual or departmental efficiency, minimal attention is typically given to basic operating and global throughput measures and to the surgical experience as a whole. Efficiency and effectiveness measures such as frequency of unnecessary testing, case cancellation rates, OR start and turnover times, as well as overall customer satisfaction have been typically secondary concerns at best. Even if given consideration, however, these items are only partial reflections of the quality of the overall system of perioperative care.

Counterintuitively, focusing just on the individual aspects of the process will not necessarily result in the optimization of any system. This is true for the comprehensive surgical ecosystem as well. This requires coordination of surgical care across the entire continuum by a collaborative team working together on each step of patient care delivery with a constant appreciation of the effects that individual decisions have on the overall system. A more holistic approach to the analysis and management of the perioperative delivery system is needed if we are to truly meet the expectations of consumers and payers for increased quality, safety, efficiency and effectiveness. Understanding clinical delivery as a system and thinking strategically and globally, beyond the individual successes, will lead to more sustained programmatic success. Most importantly, from a patient satisfaction and safety perspective our currently heavily siloed model does not place patients where they rightfully belong, at the center of the delivery system. Moving toward patient-centered care will refocus our efforts and assure that we are individualizing our care by incorporating each patient's values, preferences and decisions.

Largely because of the reimbursement system and its inherent incentives, both explicit as well as implicit, perioperative clinicians and managers have focused upon optimizing their own particular subsystems (e.g., preoperative testing, admitting, preoperative holding, the OR, PACU, etc.) and have given minimal thought to how these subsystems interact with each other, particularly from the perspective of the patient.

The resulting effect of this, called suboptimization in systems theory [1], is that the system is designed to maximize the efficiency for those providing care in the various silos and not for improving the patient experience or enhancing the system's performance or value.

Current System

In planning for surgery, activities are scheduled for the convenience of the surgeon, other consultants, the preoperative clinic (if one exists), and finally time availability in an OR, usually, again, around the schedule of the surgeon. In this model each provider segment, or subsystem, can and frequently does optimize workflow for its own self-benefit. Issues such as office and clinic hours, staff compensation including overtime, and equipment availability all require consideration. While resource constraints are real issues in all systems [2], this approach unfortunately makes little sense for patients in terms of ease of use or clarity of purpose. Likewise, insurers and employers paying for the services often subsidize inefficiencies at a system level that result from this desire to achieve optimization at the subsystem level. When viewed as a whole, this approach to managing perioperative care is generally inefficient and results in decreased satisfaction, wasted efforts, decreased quality, increased risk, ineffective use of resources, and increased cost at the macrolevel. As societal resources continue to shrink, appropriate and efficient utilization become more critical.

System Theory Research

Fortunately, there is heightened interest in better coordination and creating value in surgical care. More perioperative medicine clinicians are gaining knowledge and experience in operations management and system theory and the body of knowledge in this space continues to grow. Familiarity with the work of pioneers like Shewhart and Deming in quality improvement and statistical process control are allowing many healthcare organizations to improve their processes in substantial and significant ways [3, 4]. Tools such as Lean, Six Sigma, Continuous Quality Improvement, Toyota Production System, and statistical process control that have driven advances in other industries are now proving their value in the healthcare environment. Examples of this in healthcare are now increasingly common and the evidence is strong that sound clinical care is the result of a well-managed perioperative process [5].

Blurring and Expansion of Specialty Lines

A primary issue in the evolution of perioperative medicine is the question of how care is provided, where, by whom and with what level of coordination. Historically, surgeons have taken responsibility for directing the preoperative and postoperative care, either directly or through consultation, and anesthesiologists and CRNAs have controlled the process from the time immediately prior to the surgical procedure through the PACU experience or admission to a critical care unit. Even here, however, there has been great disparity as to the role of the anesthesia providers' involvement after leaving the OR despite long-standing suggestions that anesthesiologists will play a bigger role in perioperative care [6].

However, other than possibly the anesthetic care itself, the bulk of patient care is delivered by nurses who have assumed specialized roles throughout the system. Adoption of team-based care across throughout the healthcare system continues to grow and it is not surprising that this is true for perioperative care as well. According to the Institute of Medicine report on the Future of Nursing, as healthcare reform brings more people into the healthcare system, it needs to bring to bear all of the high-quality practitioners available. Nurses are the largest component of the healthcare workforce. They spend the most time with patients making them an essential partner in transforming the way that Americans receive healthcare. Nurses will require new competencies to deliver high quality care such as leadership, health policy, system improvement, research, and evidence-based practice, teamwork, and collaboration. Nurses, as well as other disciplines, should be given the opportunity to further develop their leadership skills and competencies. It is important to focus on making sure nurses have multiple pathways to advanced degrees that are affordable and accessible. Having enough nurses with the right kind of skills will contribute to the overall safety and quality of a transformed healthcare system. Currently business and management training for nursing and others are acquired on the job. A more educated workforce would be better equipped to meet the demands of an evolving healthcare system. Focus should expand beyond those in system leadership positions and include many additional clinicians who are managing programs and service lines on a daily basis.

As clinical care progresses, clinicians themselves must adapt by changing their skill sets to meet the demands of evolving clinical practice. In addition, clinical leaders will need to expand their leadership and operations management skills if they are going to remain relevant in setting the future strategic agenda in operations. At the same time, assuring that the workload is delegated to the appropriate level of healthcare worker will be required to assure that the demands can be met. *Training must continue to be transformed to include the multidisciplinary team and to incorporate simulation experiences.*

There has been historical reluctance for anesthesiologists to engage significantly in the preoperative care of surgical patients. As previously mentioned, one of the key drivers of this reticence is the compensation methodology for anesthesia services. Additional barriers that contribute to the lack of anesthesiologist involvement in patient preparation include the fear of malpractice litigation as well as concerns about the adequacy of anesthesia training in terms of managing chronic medical conditions outside of the OR.

The ASA has embraced a concept of a multidisciplinary care team model led by physician anesthesiologists which it calls the perioperative surgical home (PSH). In the PSH model, a clinical team led by an anesthesiologist prepares the patient for the surgical experience through evaluation, education and care coordination. The focus is on creating a care plan that optimizes the patient's readiness for the procedure and the subsequent recovery process that follows. Risk stratification, treatment interventions and appropriate resource planning are hallmarks of this approach. While there is evidence that the PSH model provides some benefit to both patients and the healthcare system, it remains to be seen if the model as currently espoused becomes a standard part of the surgical workflow.

In all likelihood, the PSH model will represent a broad conceptual model with many different forms of implementation all centered on the goal of active management of the surgical patient across the care continuum. Variations as to team leadership (e.g., anesthesiologist, surgeon, hospitalist, or other clinician) and composition will likely be common. Formal training in perioperative systems and design thinking is largely lacking in the historically surgical care-oriented clinical disciplines at the undergraduate and graduate medical education levels and so expertise in system design and implementation from experts in other industries may be necessary. Obstacles to further adoption of the PSH model by anesthesiologists include disincentives related to legacy fee-for-service and fragmented payment methodologies, questions about ownership, liability, and adequacy of education and training in the clinical aspects of the PSH process and resistance to changing current roles, responsibilities, and workflows [7, 8].

Given the reluctance of many anesthesia clinicians to expand beyond the confines of the OR it is not surprisingly that other medical and nursing specialties continue to fill the voids created in perioperative care. Emergency medicine physicians, gastroenterologists, and registered nurses continue to expand their roles in performing sedation analgesia that was previously the domain of anesthesia professionals. Even more striking is the degree of similarity between the care offered in intensive care units by critical care nurses working under the direction of intensivists and the care delivered in the OR by anesthesiologists and CRNAs. In many respects the care provided, and the physiologic effect on the patient, is indistinguishable from that offered in the OR except for the training of the provider and the location in which it is offered.

Aside from the actual administration of anesthetic and sedation agents, primary care providers, especially hospital medicine specialists, now play a major role in the care of perioperative patients. The Society of Hospital Medicine, for example, offers educational programming to address the role played by hospitalists in caring for surgical patients. In addition, primary care physicians have developed novel approaches to the care of the surgical patient [9]. Several well-known healthcare systems, such as the Cleveland Clinic with its Internal Medicine Preoperative Assessment Consultation and Treatment Center, have formal preoperative clinics that are managed and staffed by hospitalists. Likewise, hospitalists now increasingly "co-manage" surgical patients along with the surgeons. This type of collaborative approach allows surgeons to focus on surgical issues while hospitalists and, to a lesser extent anesthesiologists, manage medical issues, the patient's transition through the hospital experience, postoperative pain control, as well as the nonsurgical discharge planning and follow-up [10, 11].

Management of the OR will continue to require clear structure, strong leadership, and interdisciplinary communication and collaboration. This often means negotiating between competing agendas of clinicians and the institution. The growing list of quality and regulatory expectations demands constant oversight and engagement of the key stakeholders. Provision of accurate data that is received in a timely manner will allow for appropriate data analysis so that evaluating progress and changing course when necessary can be done in real time.

Technology

Indeed, the future evolution of perioperative medicine depends on developing and enhancing collaborative care and expanding care from a single provider to an integrated healthcare team [12]. For collaborative and coordinated care to reach its maximum potential, a robust interoperable health information management system is required. Access to relevant, accurate, timely and actionable information is required so that appropriate clinical and process decisions can be made. Decision support systems, both clinical and managerial, allow decision-makers to collect and analyze data prospectively and make meaningful interventions to enhance care, safety, and throughput. An important component of this is the ability to monitor clinical performance (both intermediate process inputs such as imaging and lab results as well as final outcomes like overall quality of care and satisfaction) at a level allowing for the immediate feedback needed for a robust continuous quality improvement process. In addition, health information management systems must promote adherence to evidence-based treatment protocols by providing relevant information for clinical decision making and the ability to track deviations from the protocols as well as clinical outcomes. More individualized patient care will be the result of emerging technologies aimed at optimizing patient care.

Clinicians should be engaged to work with developers and manufacturers in design, development, purchase, implementation and evaluation of medical and health devices and health IT products. Sharing clinical expertise and outlining current challenges during the design phase of development assures a more relevant product that meets the needs of patients and healthcare providers. The healthcare evolution and constantly changing technology will require all clinicians to commit to lifelong learning. As the complexity of the technology increases, other specialized roles may be added to support the environment and the multidisciplinary team.

Technology will continue to advance and move more and more procedures to minimally invasive approaches. This will be aided by enhanced imaging procedures and computer technologies. These advances will require more specialized training for the healthcare team [13].

Telehealth and Telemedicine

Perioperative medicine, much like medical and nursing practice, is replete with treatment practices of questionable value that are based on personal anecdote and tradition and not on formal controlled clinical studies. Wide spread adoption of electronic health records as part of wholesale adoption of health information technology initiatives will illuminate some of the variability in perioperative practices as well as remove some of the mystique that accompanies the surgical patient's passage through the OR.

Rapid advances in machine learning, artificial intelligence, augmented reality, and data science will change the nature of perioperative and even intraoperative surgical care. With current estimates of the amount of medical knowledge doubling every 75 to 90 days [14], it is impossible for clinicians to remain current without assistance from curated and intelligent databases. In addition, advances in machine learning and data science are enhancing and in some cases supplanting the abilities of human clinicians to synthesize relevant patient data into diagnoses and treatment interventions. Data science will play an increasing role in perioperative medicine advancement. Large data sets drawn from across all the perioperative continuum will allow the continued development of correlative risk and predictive scoring systems that will be useful in patient optimization, selection, and postoperative recovery.

Advances in telemedicine capabilities in areas such as e-ICUs and field medicine in the military, combined with telemetric sensor capabilities currently available or under development, will likely transform the way anesthesia services are delivered. When viewed in the context of projecting knowledge and experience over a distance, telemedicine may radically change the practice of anesthesiology and perioperative medicine. Telemedicine, clinical decision support tools, and machine learning may profoundly modify the roles and responsibilities of the clinical workforce in terms of how and where they work. For example, advances in technology may result in fewer anesthesiologists providing more care to greater numbers of patients over larger geographic areas.

In fact, only the physical or technical component of anesthesia administration requires the actual presence of a caregiver with the patient. The cognitive or intellectual component, with the appropriate technology, can be provided from practically anywhere in the world. There are several potentially striking aspects of the ability to place-shift expertise across the continuum. First, it could lead to the use of nontraditional caregivers to physically provide the care heretofore requiring the presence of an anesthesiologist or CRNA. This could serve to mitigate the feared shortage of anesthesiologists that has long been predicted [15].

Second, patient care that currently requires transfer to facilities offering more specialized or sophisticated care may be unnecessary if someone on site has the capability to perform relatively routine functions such as vascular access placement and airway control or to physically manipulate diagnostic equipment such as ultrasound or other imaging technologies. For example, most emergency medicine physicians have the requisite skill set to establish a controlled airway and place invasive monitoring lines. The expertise of a critical care physician such as an anesthesiologist at some distant site could provide the necessary fund of knowledge and experience to direct the patient's care and remove the need for transfer.

Third, advances in surgical technology, when combined with the continuing advances in pharmacology and monitoring, will accelerate the existing outmigration of procedures from hospitals to other locations such as ambulatory surgery centers and even physician offices. This migration continues to accelerate and will continue to redefine the nature of surgery and perioperative medicine not only in terms of location but also in terms of the skill set needed to provide safe care. This will continue to challenge the historical reticence for anesthesia providers to leave the safety of the traditional OR and may result in other types of providers assuming the responsibility for providing this care.

Finally, many aspects of the preoperative experience can be performed over distance with the widespread availability of broadband Internet [16]. Several web platforms utilizing HIPAA-compliant web tools currently exist for collecting and aggregating patient information and several are now incorporating clinical decision support and risk stratification capabilities. Information gleaned from these tools is allowing clinicians to perform more comprehensive reviews of patients' readiness for surgical care at earlier points in the continuum. With appropriate changes in preprocedure workflows clinicians can then make more timely and informed decisions concerning potential optimization interventions such as targeted laboratory testing, specialty consultations and in-person preoperative clinic assessments. With continued advances in wearable health monitoring systems perioperative clinicians will have additional continuous clinical data collected over long intervals that is likely to be more representative of true physiologic status than the static values derived from a typical clinic or preoperative visit.

In general, the workflow for perioperative care follows the same pattern as in other areas of patient care; there is a data-gathering phase, an analytical and interpretive phase, and then ultimately a decision or intervention treatment phase. In a technologically enhanced workflow model much of the intellectual effort can be place- and time-shifted to maximize benefit to both the patient and to the clinician. Despite technology capabilities that can largely already allow this to occur there remain significant instances to widespread adoption. These include reluctance to change traditional workflows and clinical roles, lack of adequate compensation methodologies to endurance adoption, and persistent regulatory and legal barriers to implementation.

Similarly, much of the routine care of the postoperative patient, using existing telemetric capabilities, can be shifted out of the acute care hospital setting to environments that are more patient and family friendly as well as potentially less problematic from a risk perspective. Combined with the ability to dispatch multidisciplinary care teams into homes for short term or intermittent low acuity intervention perioperative telemedicine may lead to a higher acceptance rate among patients and surgeons of the value of preoperative anesthesia consultation by the elimination of an additional clinic or office visit.

Implications of Payment Reform

Finally, many policy makers continue to predict the decline of fee-for-service medicine, if not its elimination completely. While the fate of the Patient Protection and Affordable Care Act (PPACA) and any replacement legislation remains unclear at the time of this writing, it appears that the movement to value-based care will continue as it is unlikely that continued pressure for pricing and quality transparency will abate. The current system of reimbursement continues to encourage higher resource consumption and the financial burden on the US economy and on many individuals and families has continued to increase despite changes mandated by PPACA. The effect of continuing healthcare reform and changing levels of insurance coverage on the utilization rate of surgical procedures remains to be seen. However, changes in payment methodologies are already underway. The most likely mechanisms to date are payments for episodes of care or other payment bundling programs in which a total payment is issued for a procedure and all related care and continued migration of surgical care to sites with lower cost structures. Regardless of payment methodology or site of care payments must reward quality and value and be adequate to cover all costs and be inclusive of all services if perioperative care models are going to be sustainable.

Regardless of type of reimbursement the healthcare system will demand a perioperative medicine program that is streamlined, efficient, cost-effective and quantifiable. Classic business concepts such as strategic and financial planning as well as return on investment analysis will be required skills. Currently, expertise in these areas is still largely lacking in healthcare management [17]. However this deficiency offers opportunities for current leaders in perioperative medicine to provide creative and constructive solutions for the future. Organizational commitment, both in terms of time and financial support, to the development and refinement of these skills will assure sustainable progress toward the future of the healthcare environment.

Summary

As healthcare becomes more patient centered with greater emphasis on, and reimbursement for, an episode of care rather than individual services, a new skill set, as well as updated tools to enhance decision making will be required. This transformation does not stop at the OR doors, but rather encompasses the perioperative environment. Appropriate decisions regarding resource acquisition and allocations,

including individual members of the healthcare team, will become even more critical to assure quality healthcare is delivered.

This will require engagement and development of not only the multidisciplinary leadership team, but inclusive of frontline clinicians. As more surgical procedures move to the outpatient setting, patients and their families will become more actively involved in their own care. A more holistic approach to the analysis and management of the perioperative delivery system with broader collaboration, extending beyond the immediate care setting, is what will be required of future leaders. Recruitment and retention of qualified healthcare team members will be a challenge and require investment and constant attention. Investment in these healthcare team members will assure a successful transformation to meet the requirements for the future of healthcare.

References

1. B. Ronen, J. S. Pliskin, S. Pass. *Focused Operations Management for Health Services Organizations* (1st ed.). Jossey-Bass, 2006.

2. E. Goldratt, J. Cox. *The Goal* (2nd ed.). Gower, 1996.

3. W. A. Shewhart. *Economic Control of Quality of Manufactured Product*. American Society for Quality Control, 1980.

4. W. E. Deming. *Out of the Crisis*. MIT Press, 2000.

5. J. Toussaint. *On the Mend: Revolutionizing Healthcare to Save Lives and Transform the Industry* (1st ed.). Lean Enterprise Institute, 2010.

6. P. Rock. The future of anesthesiology is perioperative medicine. *Anesthesiol Clin North America* 2000, 18(3), 495–513.

7. T. R. Vetter, L. A. Goeddel, A. M. Boudreaux, T. R. Hunt, K. A. Jones, J. F. Pittet. The perioperative surgical home: How can it make the case so everyone wins? *BMC Anesthesiology* 2013, 13(6).

8. Z. N. Kahn, S. Vakharia, L. Garson.(2014). The perioperative surgical home as a future perioperative practice model. *Anesth Analg* 2014, 118(5),1126–30.

9. D. G. Silverman, S. H. Rosenbaum. Integrated assessment and consultation for the preoperative patient. *Anesthesiol Clin* 2009, 27(4), 617–31.

10. M. Magallanes. The perioperative medicine service: An innovative practice at Kaiser Bellflower Medical Center. *Permanente Journal* 2002, 6, 13–16.

11. K. Hinami, C. T. Whelan, R. T. Konetzka, D. O. Meltzer. Provider expectations and experiences of comanagement. *J Hosp Med* 2011, 6, 401–4.

12. B. Vaida. For super-utilizers, integrated care offers a new path. *Health Affairs* 2017, 36(3), 394–7.

13. K. Putnam. The future of perioperative practice. *AORN J* 2017, 105(2), P6–15.

14. P. Densen. Challenges and opportunities facing medical education. *Trans Am Clin Climatol Assoc* 2011, 122, 48–58.

15. L. Daugherty, R. Fonseca, K. B. Kumar, P. C. Michaud. *An Analysis of the Labor Markets for Anesthesiology.* RAND Corporation, 2010.

16. J. A. Galvez, M. A. Rehman. Telemedicine in anesthesia: An update. *Curr Opin Anaesthesiol* 2011, 24, 459–62.

17. P. H. Song, J. Robbins, A. S. McAlearney. High-performance work systems in health care, Part 3: The role of the business case. *Health Care Manage Rev* 2012, 37, 110–21.

Chapter

27

Operating Room Metrics

Todd Brown

The operating room (OR) is a complex and dynamic environment that is difficult to manage and almost impossible to control. Increasing the efficiency and effectiveness of an OR seems to be every hospital's goals with administration and surgeons supplying ample motivation to be striving for constant improvement. One of the more interesting aspects of measuring OR performance is determining which metrics to use when creating your operational dashboard. When you look at the metrics and dashboards used to measure performance, there is considerable variance in which metrics hospitals use to measure performance. When determining the metrics to include on a dashboard, there seem to be several key assumptions that must be met to make the dashboard meaningful in the decision-making process. These assumptions include that the data should be available in an information system, be meaningful to the key stakeholders, use standard definitions whenever possible, not be qualitative and be detailed enough to be actionable in performance improvement.

The requirement to have the data in an OR information system meets the criteria to have easily extractable data that can be reported on consistently in a timely manner. Manual accumulation of data is useful, but often by the time the data is accumulated and reported, the data is stale and cannot lead to clear meaningful timely action. By using extractable data, the dashboard can be assured to be accurate, reliable and repeatable with limited opportunities for data manipulation.

A dashboard must be meaningful to key stakeholders to be relevant in the decision-making process. Key stakeholders can include surgeons, administration, anesthesia and the management team. For example, the turnover time (TOT) is a key measure of efficiency. The TOT that may be meaningful to the management team may be prior patient out of the room to subsequent patient in the room (wheels in to wheels out) while the surgeon may want

to measure TOT from incision closure to ready to be draped. By including the metrics that are meaningful to the key stakeholders the dashboard becomes a way for the OR managers to communicate performance by continually infusing the conversation with accurate data. For example, in an OR committee the TOT was challenged by a surgeon. The surgeon stated his TOT was not anywhere near the presented time. The ability to immediately drill down to the surgeon's cases and review the TOT defused the situation and validated the data presented. The power of data cannot be understated.

Using standard definitions is critical if the OR chooses to benchmark themselves against an outside organization. Using nonstandard definitions can undermine the credibility of data making external benchmarking less than meaningful. Although benchmarking against external competitors is useful in determining OR performance; best practice is to be using internal benchmarks to strive for continual improvement.

The use of qualitative data can be useful for the internal benchmarking of the customer satisfaction of both the surgeon and patient. These are important measures but should not be confused with more quantitative measures. Because of the wide variation in questions and processes used to collect qualitative data, external benchmarking can be problematic. The recommendation is to stick to quantitative metrics for measuring operational efficiency.

An operational dashboard can be a great opportunity to measure and present the performance of the OR. But without the ability to make decisions and analyze the data in a detailed manner, the management team can measure performance but have a difficult time impacting operations. For instance, if first case on time starts (FCOTS) begin to decrease, the ability to localize the process that is causing the late starts can be difficult to track down. Detailed documentation of the reasons for variances is critical to drive meaningful change in performance improvement. Remember, when you use detailed analysis to drive change it is more often a process problem than a person problem. This should not be a punitive process or the blame game will take over your documentation.

What are some of the top metrics to measure on your operational dashboard? FCOTS, TOT, same day case cancellations, block utilization, prime time room utilization, and case volumes (number of cases over a defined date range, number of case minutes over a defined range and number of procedures performed).

FCOTS is defined as the first scheduled case of the day starting at the scheduled time. This simply means the first scheduled patient of the day is in the room at the scheduled time. The literature suggests most organizations allow a grace period anywhere from zero to fifteen minutes with most suggesting a 6–7-min grace period. FCOTS is one area that a detailed reason for delays can contribute extensively to improving on time performance. One area that has a significant impact on FCOTS is preadmission screenings. Hospitals that offer 100 percent of their patient's preadmission screenings have 10 percent higher FCOTS than those that do not [1]. Benchmarks suggest the median score is 64.3 percent with the 90th percentile at 88.3 percent [1]. Keep in mind that a first case delay affects every case for the remainder of the day.

Some organizations will also measure second or subsequent cases on-time starts. There are so many variables that can affect second or subsequent on-time starts that I do not find this is an actionable or useful metric to place on the OR dashboard.

TOT is a measure of the time from the prior case patient out of the room to the subsequent patient into the room [2]. Many clinicians will refer to this time as wheels in to wheels out. Most organizations will only measure the TOT for the same surgeon following him- or herself or same surgeon back to back to keep the data set as clean as possible. The literature suggests most organizations will exclude scheduled gaps in the surgery schedule. This is accomplished in several manners including excluding any TOT greater than 60 min. Like FCOTS detailed tracking of the reasons for delays is critical for process improvement. What is a good TOT? There is not a consistent recommendation for TOT. There are so many variables from ambulatory surgery to an academic medical center that it is difficult to set a clear benchmark. I usually strive for a 25-min TOT but strive for an incremental decrease

until the goal is attained. The key is to show improvement and set attainable internal benchmarks as the internal benchmark is incrementally decreased. This allows the staff a series of wins as we work together to reach the benchmark. Keep in mind the balance between efficiency and quality when TOT is measured to assure high quality care is not sacrificed to increase efficiency.

Same day case cancellations are a measure of the number of cases cancelled on the same day as scheduled. Unfortunately, this is another case where the literature suggests the definitions "same day" differ from organization to organization. The most common definition of "same day" appears to be from the time the schedule closes the day prior to the cancelled case. The documentation of the reasons for cancellations is critical to process improvement. Same day case cancellations can have a significant impact on OR prime time utilization leading to underutilization of prime OR time. The benchmarks for same day cancellations are as varied as the organizations. For example, hospitals in urban areas experience a much higher same day case cancellation rate than those in more rural areas [1]. Like so many of the OR metrics, the key is to set measurable goals for internal benchmarks with continual performance improvement.

Block time utilization is defined as the actual room time used by the surgeon or group assigned by the actual block time available. Block time usually is assigned to an individual surgeon but can be assigned to a group or service. Block time is neither a good nor a bad thing, but too much allocated block time can decrease flexibility and frustrate the ability to add new surgeons. Managing block utilization can be a significant challenge so a strong policy is a must with clear definitions of the process used for calculating, adding, or subtraction of block time. Recommendations for managing block time can be to include TOT in the actual room time used for calculation, develop a block committee to manage block time with a strong surgeon champion to chair it, only allow blocks of eight hours or more and follow the policy without exception. However, controversial block release should not be an across the board decision because different services typically schedule with different lead times. Automatic block releases should be set to assure there is time to schedule as much as possible in underutilized block times. Benchmarks for block time utilization can vary between 65 to 85 percent with the inclusion or exclusion of TOT having a significant impact on the block utilization goal.

Prime time utilization measures the percentage of total available operating time between 7:00 a.m. and 3:00 p.m. against the total amount of actual case time including TOT. Prime time may vary among organizations depending on the operating start time. Typically, the higher the prime time utilization, the better for the organization but when prime utilization becomes too high it can be a key indicator of the need to expand facilities. Prime time utilization can be measured by day of the week with a target of 75–85 percent utilization.

Case volume is another critical measure of operational efficiency. Of all the other metrics, volume is a key quantitative indicator of surgeon satisfaction. Generally, when surgeon satisfaction is high, volume increases. Case volume can be broken down into three distinct types of volume. Case volume or number of cases completed in the OR, procedures completed (a case can have multiple procedures) and the minutes of surgery completed. Each type of volume should be further analyzed by service and surgeon. Volume can be analyzed by month year over year to account for seasonality and year to date to measure performance. Anytime there is a decrease in volume, it is a perfect time to show your surgeons you appreciate their business. If there is a decrease in volume, it takes only a moment to draft a quick email to the surgeons and let them know you noticed a decrease in volume. This allows you to let them know you appreciate their business and want to follow up and ensure that there are no significant reasons for the decrease. Most of the time there is a vacation, conference or some other reason for the decrease but almost all the time the surgeons appreciate that you noticed. Occasionally you will get feedback for areas of opportunity which gives you the opportunity to respond with a plan for improvement. This opens communication and shows your surgeons you appreciate them and the business they bring to the OR.

There are many more metrics that can and should be monitored in the OR. We have not even begun to touch on the financial cost and reimbursements metrics that can be measured. But from an operational standpoint with these six-metrics, operational efficiency can be measured and more importantly acted upon to drive operational improvement.

References

1. T. Foster (Ed.). (2012). Data for bench marking your OR's performance. *OR Manager*, 28(1).
2. S. D. Boggs, M. H. Tsai, R. D. Urman, Association of Anesthesia Clinical Directors. (2018). The Association of Anesthesia Clinical Directors (AACD) glossary of times used for scheduling and monitoring of diagnostic and therapeutic procedures. *J Med Syst*, Aug 10;42(9):171.

Chapter

28

Operating Room Staffing Guidelines

Todd Brown

Contents

The operating room (OR) is a complex and dynamic environment where the only constant seems to be change. Staffing the OR to meet the needs of the environment is a daunting task that is equally complex and dynamic. A difficult task has become even more challenging with the changing generational demographics of the OR, rising labor costs and decreasing reimbursement placing more emphasis on resource utilization including human capital.

As a new manager, I distinctly recall the sense of panic when attempting to develop the first staffing grid or plan to staff the OR while remaining within budget. Over the years the panic has become less although it has never gotten easier. This chapter is not intended to be a how to guide with clear standards and recommendations but rather guidelines that may be useful in trying to meet the staffing needs of a complex and dynamic environment.

The foundation upon which any staffing plan should be built is the core belief that all staff and patients deserve a safe environment. The AORN Position Statement on Perioperative Safe Staffing and On-Call Practices (2014) states "AORN believes that patient and workforce safety must be the foundation for all staffing plans." Key factors must be considered such as the complexity of cases and staff fatigue. For example, 36 h in a week may not seem excessive but 3 consecutive days in a complex work environment combined with covering call may be cause for concern. Knowing your staff, knowing the specialty they are working in and factoring in the call schedule are important factors to be considered. Recommendations for placing limits on staff work schedules should include scheduling no more than

12 h a day, no more than 3 consecutive days of 12-h shifts or 60 h a week.

When working to determine OR staffing, we will divide the process into direct (core staffing) and indirect staffing. Core staffing or direct staffing will be considered those staff members who are directly staffing the OR suites.

Direct Staffing

Case volume is a key consideration when building a staffing grid. Rooms in progress by hour of the day can be a key indicator for building the core staffing. In many ORs, breaking the cases into rooms in progress by hour of the day by day of the week is necessary because of the differences in block schedules or case volume. See Figure 28.1. In this example based on a 10-bed OR using historical ORs in progress by day and OR scheduling guidelines we will staff the following rooms.

Monday–Friday

10 rooms	7:00 a.m.–3:00 p.m.
7 rooms	3:00 p.m.–5:00 p.m.
5 rooms	5:00 p.m.–7:00 p.m.
4 rooms	7:00 p.m.–9:00 p.m.
1 room	9:00 p.m.–7:00 a.m.

Saturday

2 rooms	7:00 a.m.–5:00 p.m.
1 room	5:00 p.m.–7:00 a.m.

Sunday

1 room	7:00 a.m.–7:00 a.m.

Recommendations for core staffing include one RN for circulating and one scrub person. This equates to

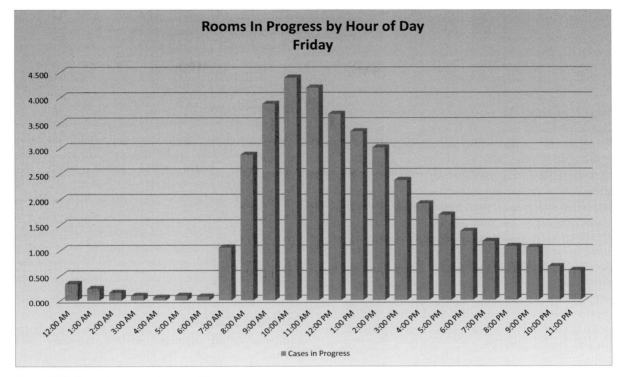

Figure 28.1 Rooms in progress by hour of day.

2.5 staff per room per hour. In many nonacademic settings scrub assistants are not supplied, so an additional scrub person is required. This equates to 3.75 staff per room per hour for cases requiring an assistant.

Rooms in progress	RN staff	RN break/ lunch	Scrub	Scrub break/ lunch	Total personnel
1	1	+.25	1	+.25	2.5

In the example in Figure 28.1, direct or core staffing would consist of the following.

Monday–Friday	RN	Scrub	Hours × rooms × staff hours
7:00 a.m.–3:00 p.m.	100	100	8 × 10 × 1.25
3:00 p.m.–5:00 p.m.	17.5	17.5	2 × 7 × 1.25
5:00 p.m.–7:00 p.m.	12.5	12.5	2 × 5 × 1.25
7:00 p.m.–9:00 p.m.	10.0	10.0	2 × 4 × 1.25
9:00 p.m.–7:00 a.m.	12.5	12.5	10 × 1 × 1.25
Total worked hours	152.5	152.5	

Saturday	RN	Scrub	Hours × rooms × staff hours
7:00 a.m.–5:00 p.m.	25	25	10 × 2 × 1.25
5:00 p.m.–7:00 a.m.	17.5	17.5	14 × 1 × 1.25
Total worked hours	42.5		

Sunday	RN	Scrub	Hours × rooms × staff hours
7:00 a.m.–7:00 a.m.	30	30	10 × 2 × 1.25

Holiday	RN	Scrub	Hours × rooms × staff hours
7:00 a.m.–7:00 p.m.	30	30	10 × 2 × 1.25

Annually this would equate to:

	RN	Scrub	Days		Hours
Monday– Friday	38,888	38,888	255	×	152.5
Saturday	2,210	2,210	52	×	42.5

	RN	Scrub	Days		Hours
Sunday	1,560	1,560	52	×	30
Holiday	1,560	180	6	×	30
Total	42,838	42,838			

After calculating the number of direct or core staffing hours, it is necessary to calculate the number of replacement hours or the replacement factor. The replacement hours are the number of hours necessary to replace core staffing while they are on sick time, education, or other paid time off. The quickest and most accurate method to determine the replacement factor is to ask your payroll department for the total hours paid and worked. You will then divide the hours paid by the hours worked (paid hours/worked hours). This will give you a replacement factor. You will then take the replacement factor and multiply it by the number of calculated direct or core staffing hours. This will give you the total number of hours paid required to staff the direct or core staffing, including paid time off.

	RN	Scrub
Total worked	42,838	42,838
Replacement factor	1.136	1.136
Total paid hours	48,680	48,680

After calculating the number of hours required to staff the OR, it is necessary to convert the hours into full-time equivalents (FTEs). FTEs are calculated by taking the total number of annual hours divided by 2080. (Some organizations may use 2085 or 2088).

	RN	Scrub
Total paid hours	48,680	48,680
FTE hours	2,080	2,080
Total direct FTEs	23.4	23.4

Calculating the hours of core staffing or direct care staff is relatively easy. The challenge is converting direct care hours into a staff schedule incorporating full-time, part-time, and per diem staff. When calculating the mix of full-time and part-time/per diem mix, developing the right mix to allow the flexibility of scheduling and meet departmental needs is an important consideration. Recommendations for

staffing seem to consistently fall within the range of 80–90 percent full-time and part-time/per diem making up the remainder. ORs in areas with seasonality highly impacting volume may want to increase the percent of per diem staff while those with consistent case volume may want to decrease the percent of per diem staff.

Traditionally ORs have relied on a staffing mix of 8 and 12-h shifts. As pressure to expand OR hours of operation while increasing staff utilization have increased many operating managers and directors have increased the types of available shifts to 6, 8, 10 and 12-h shifts. Often the idea of being able to fill a 6-h shift was expected to be difficult if not impossible to fill but when posted was surprisingly easy. As the demographics of the OR have shifted to a more tenured staff, developing nontraditional ways of staffing the OR will be critical to retain experienced staff.

Indirect Staffing

Indirect staffing includes all the ancillary staff necessary to support the direct patient caregivers. Calculating indirect staff can be more art than science. These positions can include the team leaders, charge nurse, director surgical services, managers, schedulers and other indirect caregivers.

To many providers, the surgery case scheduler is their first customer service interaction with an OR. One of the many concerns expressed by surgeons or their office is the difficulty scheduling a case. Efforts have been made to reduce costs by allowing surgeons or their office to schedule their own cases. This effort is either highly successful or very frustrating for providers. Many times, the best answer is a hybrid approach. Offer access to self-scheduling to providers who prefer to self-schedule while having a scheduler readily available for those who do not. Taking a hybrid approach still leaves unanswered the question of how much scheduling staff is enough. Often the recommendations for calculating scheduling hours include 10–15 min per scheduler case scheduled. In the examples reviewed thus far we have looked at a 10-bed OR. In the following example, we will look at a 10-bed OR that offers self-scheduling in addition to a centralized surgery scheduling center. The case volumes are approximately 12,500 cases annually with 22 percent being self-scheduled. To determine the scheduler hours to budget, consider the following example.

Cases scheduled		Percent call center scheduled		Call center cases scheduled		Average scheduling time		Convert to hours		Worked hours
12,500	×	.78	=	9,750	×	12.5/		60	=	2031

Remembering to include replacement factor:

	Scheduler
Total worked	2,031
Replacement factor	1.136
Total paid hours	2,307

Calculating FTEs

	Scheduler
Total paid hours	2,307
FTE hours	2,080
Total scheduler FTEs	1.11

The surgery liaison is another position that has oftentimes been replaced through automation. If you walk into many waiting rooms, you will be greeted by a giant screen that is supposed to keep a family informed. Recognizing the isolation and loss of control many families feel while interacting with the healthcare community, the faceless monitor seems to place one more barrier to human interaction and the assurance a voice you begin to recognize can bring. Consequently, the small cost of a surgery liaison returns outsized customer service and is one position worth fighting for. The recommendation is a minimum of one surgery liaison.

The position of clinical assistant (CA) has as many job titles as there are hospitals. This position assists with turning over rooms, running specimens, gathering supplies, transportation and other critical tasks. The most important function a CA supports is the ability of the circulating nurse to stay in the room focused on his or her patient. Recommendation is one CA every 4–5 rooms.

	CA	Hours × rooms × staff hours
Monday–Friday		
7:00 a.m.–3:00 p.m.	16	8 × 10 × .2
3:00 p.m.–11:00 p.m.	8	8 × 5 × .2
Saturday		
7:00 a.m.–3:00 p.m.	8*	8 × 2 × .2

*Minimum of 1 CA.

Annually this would equate to:

	CA	Days × hours
Monday–Friday	6,120	255 × 24
Saturday	416	52 × 8
Sunday	0	52 × 0
Holiday	0	6 × 0
Total	6,536	

Remembering to include replacement factor

	CA
Total worked	6,536
Replacement factor	1.136
Total paid hours	7,424

Calculating FTEs

	Scheduler
Total paid hours	7,424
FTE hours	2,080
Total CA FTEs	3.57

Span of control is the number of staff a manager is directly responsible for. Outside of healthcare, the span of control is determined by the complexity of the work the subordinate is responsible for. For routine work, 20 is considered the maximum number of direct reports a manager can manage without losing effectiveness. Healthcare tries to mitigate this by assigning charge nurses and team leaders. Recommendation is one charge nurse per shift per operating location not included in core staffing, anytime more than one room is routinely in use.

Monday–Friday	Charge RN
7:00 a.m.–3:00 p.m.	8
3:00 p.m.–11:00 p.m.	8
Saturday	
7:00 a.m.–3:00 p.m.	8

	Charge RN	Days × hours
Monday–Friday	4,080	255 × 16
Saturday	416	52 × 8
Sunday	0*	52 × 0
Holiday	0*	6 × 0
Total	4,496	

* Included in core staff

Remembering to include replacement factor:

	CA
Total worked	4,496
Replacement factor	1.136
Total paid hours	5,107

Calculating FTEs

	Scheduler
Total paid hours	5,1074
FTE hours	2,080
Total charge RN FTEs	2.45

Clinical nurse coordinators/supervisors/team leaders/service leaders are also positions that assist with the mitigation of the high span of control found in ORs. The key role this position can play is to assist with the management of surgeon specialties or service lines. Assuring preference cards are updated, surgeon special requests and equipment are prepared for individual cases and managing the flow of the surgery schedule are critical skills to assure surgeon satisfaction. Recommendation is no more than two to three major surgical specialties per clinical nurse coordinator. In this example, there are six major surgical specialties.

Total clinical nurse coordinator FTEs, 3.00

Total OR manager FTEs, 1.00

Total surgical services director FTEs, 1.00

Equipment specialist, administrative assistants, unit secretaries and other miscellaneous positions are largely going by the wayside. When revenue is decreasing and expenses increase many managers are having to make choices between clinical staff positions and support personnel.

One area many ORs are not budgeting for is the turnover of staff. With the national average for surgical services turnover rates hovering around 17 percent [1] and a 4–6-month orientation training period for OR staff; failing to plan can lead to failure such as excess overtime, use of agency staff and closed OR suites. With a long training period, ORs are particularly at risk as nurses with less than 2 years' experience account for 51.4 percent of staff turnover [1]. This can lead to the loss of a 6 months' investment in human capital leaving with minimal return. Recommendation is to account for expected or historical turnover in key core staffing positions. In this example using 17 percent this would mean planning for almost eight positions turning over in a year. With 6 months of orientation four FTEs would need to be budgeted for to account for the high rate of turnover.

Strategies for decreasing turnover need to be developed to try to mitigate the high losses through turnover. The following are some examples of methods to reduce employee turnover.

1. Provide continual feedback and encouragement. The OR orientation process is a long and often discouraging process. Particularly when our new orientees compare themselves to highly tenured staff.
2. Remain as flexible as possible with scheduling. Multiple different shift opportunities and self-scheduling is an incentive to build loyalty to the organization.
3. Recognize individual high achievers and develop mentorship programs so employees can see opportunities as they grow.
4. Involve staff in departmental operations where possible. Shared governance and collaborative practices can assist with employee engagement.

As revenues decrease and expenses increase, pressure is continually exerted on operating staffing models. Regardless of the model or method used to develop staffing, the focus should remain on offering a safe environment for both patients and staff. Developing core staffing should be based upon the OR scheduling guidelines and actual utilization. Developing a strong indirect staffing model to support the direct caregivers is critical to operating a safe and effective OR. Decisions for ancillary or indirect staffing should be based on clear cost benefit analysis. Turnover continues to rise within the surgical services and is a clear threat to OR staffing. Methods to manage expected turnover as well as strategies to reduce turnover should be developed and implemented.

Reference

1. Brian Colosi, ed. *2016 National Healthcare Retention & RN Staffing Report*. Nursing Solutions, 2016, 1–13.

Resource Management

29

Todd Brown

The operating room (OR) in many instances is the highest revenue-generating service line in the hospital. As reimbursement has declined expenses have been increasing, driving an accompanying decrease in profits. With the OR often accounting for greater than 50 percent of total supply costs in a hospital, the decrease in profits can make the OR a target for supply side savings [1]. The opportunity for savings can be great but the challenges can be even greater. Surgeon preferences, vendor management, diverse number of specialties, preference card management, lack of standardization and a lack of an inventory control system often lead to poor data and inefficient supply management. When a revenue center like the OR begins to look like a cost center, a sense of urgency begins to develop to better manage supply costs. As clinicians, our focus was most often on assuring we had the products we needed to care for our patients with virtually no knowledge in regards to the cost. The purpose of this chapter is to explore the ways we can better understand and manage supply costs. Several questions must be answered before embarking on a supply management initiative; among them are the following. Can OR supply expenses be controlled without sacrificing quality? How can we balance the cost quality ratio?

Surgeon preference items and standardization can often be a real challenge to the management of supply side costs. Surgeon preferences often begin to develop during training, many times without any clinical or quality data to support the choices made. This may be true even before things like vendor relationships come into play. Other items may have clinical benefits for the surgeon, including just having familiarity with the function of the item chosen. Recognizing that the surgeon is a customer, how do we work towards standardization and cost savings while still showing the customer appreciation and respect for their preferences? One thing to note is you will frequently see the words surgeon and customer used interchangeably. The surgeon as customer is a concept that is critical to supply side management. Increasing standardization is one area a surgeon can help, but for those preference items surgeons determine are necessary to supply quality care to their patients, surgeons can assist with cost as well. Working with surgeons to clearly communicate with the vendor that the price must be reduced can have the largest impact on preference item cost. One hospital in the Midwest was having a significant challenge with spine implants. One surgeon insisted on using a noncontract vendor as the surgeon believed the patient outcomes were much better. The challenge for the hospital was the implants were almost thirty percent higher than the contract vendor. The hospital met with the vendor and they were unable to come to agreement to reduce the cost of the implants. The hospital shared the cost data with the surgeon and the surgeon was shocked at the cost disparity. The hospital and the surgeon met with the vendor and again they were unable to come to agreement to reduce the cost of the implants. The surgeon left the meeting and called the surgery scheduling department and changed all the surgeon's cases to the contract vendor. By the end of the day the hospital had an agreement in principle with the vendor.

The first step in any supply side initiative is to gain the support or buy-in of administration for the initiative. There will be difficulties encountered throughout the journey but without administrative buy-in, the one-offs for commodity type items like drapes can sink the process before it begins. With administrative buy-in, the development of a multidisciplinary team can begin. As a clinical perioperative leader, admittedly I have often viewed materials management initiatives as a bureaucratic, heavy method of controlling supplies without regard to clinical needs and customer service. One challenge we must overcome is this reluctance of clinical leaders to engage with materials management. We need to develop the same sense of urgency the clinical team brings to the table within the materials department. We need to move the supporting materials department staff out of the basement and into the OR department to begin to develop the relationships that are the foundations of trust. The clinical team must support materials in designing a method with control but also the flexibility to trial or receive surgeon preference items in a timely manner. Equally important is for the surgeons, our customers, to see a response to their requests, to see that the desire to not just reduce costs but to assure that quality outcomes are at the forefront of any decisions. As in so many projects in the hospital, a multidisciplinary approach is a must. This can and must include such diverse groups as information technology, infection control, surgeons, materials, reimbursement and clinical leaders.

Next the multidisciplinary team must develop a surgeon champion. Surgeons almost always respond better when it is a peer-to-peer conversation preferably from a surgeon who is in a senior position. Having a surgeon champion is critical but having a surgeon champion who is supported with data is even more effective. One effective strategy is to share cost comparison data by surgeon. OR cost dashboards can be a significant tool in managing operating supply expenses. Many experts advocate publishing the surgeon's names with the cost comparison data to ignite a competitive spirit. My personal preference is to publish the data without names, for example, surgeon A, B, C etc. It does not take long for the surgeons to figure out who is who and you do not run the risk of embarrassing or alienating your customers. In a recent study, hospitals that used a cost dashboard saw an average decrease in per case cost of 6.4 percent while those that did not saw an increase in cost [2].

Once the team is formed and data is accumulated, it is time to begin to develop the process. Often choosing commodity type items can be a good place to start. The first couple of initiatives should be chosen to assure successes to bring the team together and garner a quick win. Sharing the success with the team is important but sharing the success with the surgical committee is equally important to facilitate continued cooperation. One method often used is to show the savings with some tangible method used to enhance the OR. Next the team must keep the initiatives moving. There should be a continual process of evaluation, trial, and sharing of success. After the first initiative, it is critical that this process becomes integrated into the day-to-day operation of the OR.

A value analysis committee is another method used to limit, manage, and control the introduction of new products into the hospital. The benefit is the ability to manage and control the introduction of new products into the hospital. The cost is if the committee is so rigid it impacts the ability to react to new products in the OR delaying cases and frustrating surgeons. The key to a successful value analysis committee is to have rigidity to control the introduction of new products without impacting the ability to conduct operations. Several successful value analysis committees have a short form for immediate clinical needs with a retrospective review of the product.

A cost accounting system is another important tool in managing surgeon preference items and standardization. Having the ability to discuss costs and reimbursement at the procedure level can be a real advantage in gaining surgeon trust and support in supply management. Many times, the difference between a surgeon's perception and the actual cost and reimbursement for a procedure is substantial. Having the ability to have this data at your fingertips assists with the conversation in reducing supply costs and increasing standardization. A cost accounting system is also critical to the development of a cost dashboard.

Another item that is often overlooked in supply side management is vendor access and management in managing supplies. Putting policies and procedures in place that put the onus on the vendor is critical to vendor management. A vendor management system is the first step in managing vendor access. Vendor policies should address the following at a minimum.

1. Vendors should be signed in and wear time-limited identification at all times.
2. Verify the documentation of education and training in Health Insurance Portability and Accountability Act (HIPAA) compliance, appropriate conduct and attire in the OR, aseptic principles and sterile techniques, infectious disease and blood borne pathogens, occupational safety and operation-applicable practices for the Health Care Industry Representatives (HCIR).
3. Vendors shall have all required immunizations up to date.

There many policies that address vendors in the OR. I would like to introduce just a few. The first is new products requested for products or trials. New products or trial requests should be required to come from the surgeon in a written form such as an email. If the hospital has a value analysis committee requests should through the value analysis committee except patient specific items. This is to assure only items the surgeon wants to trial are going to be introduced into the OR. Frequently vendors will drop by, suggesting the surgeon would like to try a new widget. After following up with the surgeon, it is noted the surgeon has no desire to try the product. Requiring written requests facilitates limiting the trials to only those the surgeon wants to trial. The vendor should then work with the value analysis committee to schedule a trial. Working with the value analysis committee assures that the contracts necessary for compliance are in place to protect the hospital. The price of the current item as well as the cost of the trial item should be shared with the surgeon to assure informed decisions are made. Many surgeons express dismay when they find out the cost of the new product and will work with the hospital to reduce the cost of the item to be trialed. Sharing the cost data also begins to develop the trust necessary to work together to reduce supply costs. In most instances the goal should be to assure the item trialed is at or below the current vendors cost. One of the key initiatives to control new vendor items is to clearly state in the policy that any new item introduced into the OR without written preapproval will not be paid for. Equally important to the vendor process is to assure that items invoiced are charged for. One process frequently used is case specific invoices. The invoice, implant log, and patient charges should all be verified before any vendor invoice is signed or paid. This is frequently completed by the OR business manager.

When dealing with implants, consignment can be a valuable tool to reduce costs. Many surgeons prefer a vendor which can cause several vendor's products to be on the shelf, making purchasing the implants cost prohibitive. Consignment can assist with reducing the cost of implants while mitigating the impact of the risk of obsolescence.

Preference cards often are one of the easiest but often overlooked methods to control costs. Many times preference cards are not updated or do not reflect the items the surgeon prefers to have opened. Open unused items increase costs without bringing any value to the surgeon, patient, or facility. Having surgeons review the preference card, with emphasis on the open or hold columns of the card, can derive significant savings. This takes a coordinated effort between surgical staff and physicians to update the cards. One challenge to this approach that cannot be overstated is when staff do not use the preference cards but rely on past practice. This can derail the most diligent process to update preference cards.

Of all the challenges faced by supply management, we often think of surgeon preferences as the largest challenge to overcome. I would argue that the lack of meaningful, reliable data is the largest challenge, including a cost accounting and inventory control system. Being able to produce reliable, verifiable and repeatable data is key to gaining the buy-in of the stakeholders in the inventory management team.

An inventory control system is also a must in supply management. One of the challenges to implementing an inventory control system is the significant upfront costs with a limited ability to show a true return on investment. But having the ability to produce reports showing the duplication of inventory, inventory turns, Periodic Automatic Replenishment (PAR) levels, inventory consignment are all critical tools in managing inventory. Having the ability to automate inventory control can reduce stock outs, rush or overnight orders and helps to increase the efficiency of the purchasing process. One of the key areas automation assists with is allowing the clinicians to take care of the patients instead of managing inventory. Other areas automation helps with is the auditing of charge capture, management of implants, and assuring charges are correct. One additional area an inventory control system assists with is managing redundancy in supplies. Many items are stocked in multiple locations without any person having a clear idea of all the locations in which inventory is stored. Other area redundancy impacts are when multiple types of items are kept in stock for the same purpose. An inventory control system can make it possible to locate items in the same class across the organization.

New surgeons being introduced to the organization is one area of opportunity to begin the customer service experience and facilitate the management of new preferences. You only get one opportunity to make a first impression. Making that first impression will set the stage for future discussions around the supply side management. I have included a process for all new surgeons to manage the supply side of their experience while introducing them to the OR.

Objective: To prepare the OR to the degree possible, so the surgeon has a smooth transition into their new OR. The surgeon should be viewed as our customer. Their first impression is critical to forming a long-term relationship with the organization.

1. Introduction

    a. Contact surgeon and introduce yourself, emphasizing your goal is to make their transition as smooth as possible

    b. Request the following items

        i. Copies of preference cards

        ii. Special instrument sets

        iii. Preferred implants/vendors

        iv. Preferred equipment

        v. Order sets (Usually surgeon will share a contact at current hospital)

        vi. Any other special requests

        vii. A meeting time to review available block or surgery schedule time

2. Preparation

    a. Build preference cards, noting any items or equipment that vary from surgeon preference or may impact ancillary services such as anesthesia

        i. Contact surgeon and ask if he or she would like to review preference cards prior to arrival

        ii. Notify surgeon of items on preference cards that may vary from surgeon's preference.

            • Determine which items are preference or which are must-have items

            • Develop list of must-have items

    b. Request special instrument set lists. Surgeon may give you hospital contact person

        i. Determine if you have similar sets

            • If not, add to must-have items list

        ii. If you have similar sets, notify surgeon to determine if similar sets are acceptable

            • If not acceptable, add item to must-have items list

    c. Develop list of preferred vendor/implants

        i. Work with materials to determine if vendor is on contract list

            • If on vendor contract list, notify vendor of new surgeon. Usually surgeon's current vendor will have already contacted local vendor

            • If vendor is not on contract list, contact surgeon with the hospital contract vendor. If contract vendor is not acceptable, add to must-have items list

    d. Develop list of preferred equipment

        i. Compare preferred equipment against current in-house equipment

        ii. Contact surgeon with any equipment you do not have or if significantly different than requested. If current equipment not acceptable or if equipment is not available, add to must-have items list

    e. With surgeon's permission, contact current hospital and request current order sets.

        i. Contact hospital coordinator in charge of order sets and share copies of order sets

        ii. Share surgeon's contact information for questions or clarification

    f. Review any other special requests

        i. Determine if what is available is acceptable. If not, add to must-have items list

    g. Review scheduling guidelines

        i. Review scheduling policy

        ii. Review block time policy

        iii. Review available times, noting preferences

3. Follow-up

    a. Review must-have list

        i. Contact purchasing to collect quotes for must-have items

        ii. Divide into operational and capital items

            • Capital

                • Prioritize capital items with surgeon and department chair

                • Review with administration and develop plan and timelines

                • Inform surgeon and clarify expectations for capital equipment lists

            • Operational

                • Prioritize operational items with surgeon and department chair

- Review with administration and develop plan and timelines
- Inform surgeon and clarify expectations for operational items
- Noncontract vendor items
  - Prioritize noncontract vendor items with surgeon and chair
  - Review with purchasing and administration. Develop plan and timelines
  - Inform surgeon and clarify expectations for noncontract items
  - Block time requests
  - Surgeon requests for block time should be taken to OR committee for approval
  - Inform surgeon and clarify expectations for block time or alternatively open scheduling time

4. Final preparations
   a. Coordinate time with surgeon to meet in the OR
      i. Introduce surgeon to scheduler and review scheduling process
         - Be sure to give surgeon copy of scheduling guidelines again
         - Introduce surgeon to management team and share contact information
         - Introduce surgeon to team leader
         - Introduce surgeon to charge nurse
      ii. Review preparations status
         - Share with surgeon progress list with dates and timeline of incomplete items
      iii. Coordinate meeting with surgeon's office staff

- Review scheduling guidelines including contact information for scheduling office
- Review process for scheduling cases
- Share management contact information with surgeon's office staff

      iv. Give surgeon tour of the area

5. Day of first procedure
   a. Contact surgeon day prior to case to assure all preparations are complete
   b. Stop into OR prior to first case to assure staff and equipment are ready
   c. Contact surgeon postop to verify expectations were met
   d. Send follow up email to surgeon with any identified areas of opportunity and the plan to remedy

With the OR many times being the highest revenue-generating service line in the hospital, controlling costs can be a critical factor in managing the razor thin profit margins of the hospital. There are many challenges such as surgeon preferences, vendor management, diverse number of specialties, preference card management, lack of standardization, and a lack of an inventory control system but with proper planning and a diligent team effort supply costs can be managed.

References

1. Profit opportunities still exist . . . in the operating room. (2002). *Healthcare Financial Management*, 56(10).

2. OR cost scorecards help reduce healthcare supply chain costs. (2016, December 9). Retrieved from http://revcycleintelligence.com/news/or-cost-scorecards-help-reduce-healthcare-supply-chain-costs

Chapter

30

The Joint Commission, CMS, and Other Standards

Shermeen B. Vakharia and Zeev Kain

Contents

The operating rooms (ORs) are subject to several standards set by governmental and private not-for-profit agencies. Accreditation by these agencies is a way through which a healthcare organization is recognized as offering quality healthcare that meets established standards. This chapter provides a brief history of Centers for Medicare and Medicaid Services (CMS) and The Joint Commission (TJC) and the influence of their standards on the perioperative arena.

The Joint Commission

Almost a century ago in 1919, minimum standards for hospitals were developed by the American College of Surgeons (ACS), as a result of Dr. Earnest A. Codman's vision for standardization based on "end result" of treatment. Over the next 30 years, the quality of care in the hospitals improved, and more than 3,200 US hospitals approved and embraced these standards. In 1951, ACS collaborated with the American College of Physicians, American Medical Association, America Hospital Association and the Canadian Medical Association to form the Joint Commission on Accreditation of Hospitals (JCAH). In 1952, ACS formally transferred their Hospital Standardization Program to JCAH and accreditation process began in 1953. As the scope of JCAH expanded, it was renamed in 1987 as the Joint Commission for Accreditation of Health Care Organizations (JCAHO), which was then shortened to The Joint Commission in 2007 [1].

In 1965, the Congress passed the Social Security Amendments with a provision that hospitals accredited by JCAH were "deemed" to be in compliance with most of the Medicare Conditions of Participation for Hospitals. This gave the commission authority and power to determine whether a healthcare organization would be eligible to receive Medicare reimbursement. Over the years, TJC standards have improved and expanded to hold hospitals to optimal standards rather than minimal standards. All TJC standards are compiled in the Comprehensive Accreditation Manual for Hospitals (CAMH) [2]. There are more than 250 standards that pertain to patient safety and quality of care. These standards are divided into chapters for each accreditation program, for example the Hospital Accreditation program has 19 chapters. TJC assesses both processes and outcomes during their inspection, the philosophy being that good processes lead to favorable outcomes and not all outcomes are easily measurable. TJC surveys are random and unannounced and held at least once every 39 months.

The Centers for Medicare and Medicaid Services

In 1965, President Lyndon Johnson signed the Social Security Act, and Medicare and Medicaid were enacted as Title XVIII and Title XIX of this act. As a result health coverage was extended to almost all Americans aged 65 or older, low-income children deprived of parental support, the elderly, the blind, and individuals with disabilities. In 1966 when Medicare was implemented and more than 19 million individuals enrolled. In 1977, the government established Health Care Financing Administration (HCFA) which was responsible for the Coordination of Medicare and Medicaid. In 2001, HCFA was renamed Centers for Medicare and Medicaid Services to reflect increased emphasis on responsiveness to beneficiaries and providers, and on improving the quality of care that the beneficiaries received [3].

CMS establishes Conditions of Participation (CoP) for all facilities that participate in the Medicare and Medicaid programs. CoPs are first published in the Federal register and subsequently the standards with interpretive guidelines and survey procedures are published in the State Operations Manual (SOM) for certification of hospitals [4].

All facilities participating in the Medicare and Medicaid programs are required to undergo an initial CMS inspection, followed by surveys on a regular basis to ensure compliance with Federal health and safety standards. CMS contracts with state agencies to conduct these inspections. If any deficiencies are found during the initial certification or recertification process, the facility has to bear the full cost of a revisit survey to ascertain that corrective action has been implemented. Initially, TJC was given authority by Congress to determine whether hospitals met the requirements for Medicare reimbursement. In 2008, this automatic authority was eliminated. Since July 2010, TJC's accreditation program is required to meet all CMS standards.

With a few exceptions, the majority of the CMS and TJC standards apply directly or indirectly to the OR. The OR managers have to familiarize themselves with these standards and establish policies and procedures to ingrain these standards into the daily practice and culture of the OR environment. Discussion of all applicable standards is beyond the scope of this chapter. Instead, chapter gives a broad overview of some of the standards as they apply to the OR suite. The reader is encouraged to look up the SOM and the CAMH for details and also be aware that the standards and interpretive guidelines are subject to periodic change and updates [5].

CMS and TJC Standards in the OR

Patient Rights

CMS and TJC have standards that protect and promote patients' rights. Many of these standards apply throughout the perioperative period including the right to privacy, confidentiality of medical records, the right to participate in decisions about their care, treatment and services, and the right to receive safe care (CMS §482.13; TJC RI.01.01.01, EC.01.01.01-EP3,EP4, IM.02.01.01). Informed consent process is a right that the patients or their representatives may need to exercise after receiving adequate information and disclosures about anticipated benefits, risks and alternative therapies. Federal and state laws or regulations set minimum requirements for informed consent (CMS §482.24(c)(2)(v)). Hospitals are required to have policies and procedures that also protect the patient's right to request or refuse a procedure or treatment.

Per CMS and TJC standards, Medical staff is responsible for determining which procedures or treatments require informed consent. Due to the procedural nature of the OR, the physicians and staff taking care of operative patients should be aware of the policies that apply when documenting various forms of informed consent particularly, consent for surgery and anesthesia, consent for transfusion of blood or blood products, consent for producing images or recordings of the procedure for purposes other than patient care, consent for participation in perioperative research and clinical trials. TJC and CMS inspections of the perioperative area include determining the proper execution of informed consent.

Although not directly applicable to the OR, restraints are used on rare occasions in the postanesthesia care unit (PACU). CMS and TJC require that hospitals have policies regarding the use of restraints including documenting the rationale for use, using least restrictive interventions, age specific monitoring, early discontinuation, staff training and reporting requirements (CMS §482.13(e); TJC PC.03.05). The PACU staff must be appropriately trained and be aware of the policies and procedures that apply to the use of restraints.

Surgical Services

Scope and Standards for Surgical Services

CMS recommends ACS definition of surgery and requires that the hospitals have appropriate organization, equipment and qualified personnel to ensure the health and safety of the patient (CMS §482.51; TJC LD.03.06.01, IC.01.01.01). Accreditation survey generally includes observation of practices in the inpatient and outpatient OR suites for adherence to acceptable standards of practice. Acceptable standards of practice include recommendations by nationally recognized professional organizations (ACS, American Medical Association, American Society of Anesthesiologists, Association of Operating Room Nurses, etc.), federal agencies and state regulations. The needs of the population should guide the types surgical services provided directly or through referral and agreements (CMS §482.51(b); TJC LD.04.03.01). Policies governing surgical care, including postoperative care (CMS §482.51(b)(4)) should be designed to achieve the highest standard of clinical practice. CMS interpretive guidelines for standard §482.51(b) in SOM provides a comprehensive list of policies governing surgical care which OR staff could be asked about during survey.

Provider Qualifications and Scope of Practice

Per CMS, the OR supervisor has to be a Registered Nurse, Doctor of Medicine, or Doctor of Osteopathy. Both TJC and CMS require that the hospital determines the appropriate qualifications for OR supervisors and is able to provide surveyors with a position description with required qualifications (CMS §482.51(a)(1), TJC HR.01.02.01). Per CMS regulations, all scrub and circulatory duties performed by technologists or licensed practical nurses must be supervised by a qualified registered nurse (CMS §482.51(a)(2), §482.51(a)(3); TJCPC.03.01.01-EP5).

The process of privileging and credentialing of all practitioners including surgeons, is a function of organized medical staff and is subject to surveyor review (TJC MS.03.01.01, MS.06.01.07, MS.06.01.09). TJC requires that information from ongoing professional practice evaluation be factored into the decision to maintain privileges (TJC MS.08.01.03). A current roster of each practitioner's privileges must be maintained in the OR suite and at the request of the surveyors, the OR staff must be able to demonstrate how to check a practitioner's privileges (CMS §482.51(a)(4)).

Patient Assessment and Documentation Requirements

This section pertains to CMS standard §482.51(b)(1). TJC standards also reflect CMS requirements for patient assessment and documentation (PC.01.02.03-EP4 and EP5, MS.03.01.01-EP6, RC.01.03.01-EP3 and EP4). According to these standards, prior to surgery or administration of anesthesia, a medical history and physical exam must be completed and documented and should be timed and dated no more than 30 days before or 24 h after admission (or registration). If the medical history and physical exam is completed and documented within 30 days prior to admission, an updated physical exam must be completed and documented within 24 h of admission. These standards apply to all cases even if surgery occurs within 24 h of admission the only exception being emergencies. Survey procedures include a review of patient's medical records to confirm compliance with these standards.

TJC requires that the operative report written or dictated before the patient leaves the operative suite for the next level of care, unless accompanied by the practitioner to the next area of care where it can be completed. It is common practice for surgeons to write a brief operative summary immediately after the surgery, in which case a detailed report can be completed and authenticated in a timeframe specified by the hospital (CMS §482.51(b)(6)), RC.02.01.03-EP 5 and EP 6). The surgeons should be aware of the minimum requirements of an operative report. Generally a review of approximately six surgical reports is performed during CMS surveys to verify it includes specified information and is signed and dated by the surgeon. These standards were prevalent when this chapter was written and the reader is advised to look for the most recent updates.

Informed Consent for Surgery

CMS and TJC specify minimal requirements for informed consent policy (CMS §482.51(b)(2), TJC RI.01.03.01). A properly executed surgical consent is required to be patient's medical record prior to surgery. The only exception to this regulation is emergency surgery to save a patient's life or limb. Appropriate documentation in the patient's medical record by the surgeon is considered acceptable under most circumstances, however different approaches may be used depending on the local regulations and hospital policy.

Since most surgeries are performed under anesthesia, CMS recommends that the hospitals extend their surgical consent policy to include anesthesia. CMS and TJC recommend that hospitals have policies for handling Do-Not-Resuscitate (DNR) in the perioperative period. Since survival and functional outcome of resuscitation in the OR differs greatly from resuscitation on the hospital wards, and automatic upholding or discontinuation of DNR is no longer practiced. American Society of Anesthesiologists' *Ethical Guidelines for the Anesthesia Care of Patients with Do-Not-Resuscitate Orders or Other Directives That Limit Treatment* recommend that a discussion should transpire before surgery and that DNR orders be revised to allow intubation and resuscitation that would constitute a part of administering anesthesia (ACS and AORN guidelines formulated later also reflect ASA standards) [6]. Any modification to existing DNR order should be made in accordance to the patient's goals and values and documented in the patient's medical record.

Anesthesia Services

Scope and Standard of Anesthesia Services

Standards on anesthesia services are perhaps among the most complex and controvertible, and the interpretive guidelines have undergone several updates. The scope of anesthesia services was expanded in December 2009 into two categories: (1) anesthesia including general, regional, and monitored anesthesia care, and (2) analgesia and sedation with increased emphasis being on ability to rescue if level of sedation became deeper than intended. CMS requires that anesthesia services throughout the hospital, including all off-site locations, be organized into a single service under the direction of a doctor of medicine or doctor of osteopathy (CMS §482.52). Services provided should be consistent with the needs of the hospital. Anesthesia services policies must designed to ensure the delivery of care is consistent with recognized standards (for example, ASA standards) and address important issues pertaining to staff responsibilities, documentation and reporting requirements, protocol for supportive life functions, patient safety and consent issues.

Qualifications and Scope of Practice

The hospital's policies and procedures must define the circumstances when a nonanesthesiologist MD or DO can administer or supervise anesthesia services, for example procedural sedation as determined by the state scope of practice law. Medical staff bylaws must specify criteria for obtaining and maintaining sedation privileges. The type and complexity of procedures for which each individual practitioner who may administer anesthesia must be specified in his or her privileges (CMS §482. 22(c)(6), TJC MS.03.01.01-EP 2). Providers with sedation privileges should have credentials for rescuing patients from various levels of sedation (TJC MS.06.01.01-EP1). CMS requires supervision of anesthesiologist's assistants and certified registered nurse anesthetists while providing anesthesia services, by an anesthesiologist who is available to furnish assistance and direction (or supervision in case of a CRNA) throughout the performance of the procedure (CMS §482.52 (a), TJC PC.03.01.01). CRNA supervision by an anesthesiologist is not obligatory in states that have opted out of the CRNA supervision requirement (CMS §482.52 (a)(c)).

Patient Assessment and Documentation Requirements

In February 2011, Anesthesia CoPs were updated to align preoperative assessment and documentation with standards for surgical services. According to these standards, prior to administration of anesthesia, a preanesthesia evaluation must be completed and documented no more than 30 days prior to procedure requiring anesthesia; however, certain elements of the history, risk assessment, physical exam and discussion of risks and benefits have to be completed within a 48-h time frame before administering anesthesia (CMS §482.52(b)(1), TJC PC.03.01.03-EP8 and EP 18). Per CMS standards, preanesthesia evaluation can only be performed by a practitioners qualified to administer anesthesia (CMS §482. 52(a)).

Postoperative evaluation should be performed by a practitioner qualified to administer anesthesia, and completed within 48 h of the patient being moved to the designated recovery area. The postoperative evaluation is performed after the patient has sufficiently recovered from anesthesia (CMS §482.52(b), TJC PC.03.01.07-EP1, EP2, EP7, EP8). The 48-h timeframe for postoperative evaluation also applies to outpatients unless state law and hospital policy specify more stringent standards. CMS, TJC, and the American Society of Anesthesiologists specify minimal requirements for preanesthesia evaluation, anesthesia intraoperative documentation and postanesthesia evaluation [7]. Accreditation surveys generally include review of anesthesia records to verify that current documentation standards are met. Due to frequent updates to anesthesia standards, the reader is advised to check for latest updates.

TJC's National Patient Safety Goal

The National Patient Safety Goal (NPSG) was developed by the Patient Safety Advisory Group of TJC in 2002. The goal was to help accredited hospitals address most challenging patient safety issues. The NPSG that apply to the perioperative environment are summarized below. Where CMS or TJC has corresponding or related standards, a reference is to the standard is provided. NPSG is revised annually and new goals may be added.

Identify patients correctly

NPSG.01.01.01: *Use at least two patient identifiers when providing care, treatment, and services.* This also applies to labeling of blood samples and specimens.

NPSG.01.03.01: *Eliminate transfusion errors related to patient misidentification.* This NPSG requires two-person (qualified per hospital policy and state law) verification that the blood component matches to the order and patient, with one verifier being the transfusionist.

Improve communication

NPSG.02.03.01: *Report critical results of tests and diagnostic procedures on a timely basis.* This is important during the perioperative period when patient's condition can change rapidly and handoffs also occur during the episode of care.

Safe use of medication

NPSG.03.04.01: *Label all medications, medication containers, and other solutions on and off the sterile field in perioperative and other procedural settings.* Recommendations for labeling include medication name, strength, quantity, diluent and volume (if not apparent from the container), expiration date when not used within 24 h expiration time or when expiration occurs in less than 24 h. Two-person verification is required when the medication is not prepared by the person administering it. This safety goal also requires that medications be reviewed by entering and exiting staff.

NPSG.03.05.01: *Reduce the likelihood of patient harm associated with the use of anticoagulant therapy.* Perioperatively, this standard requires use of approved protocols for the initiation, maintenance and monitoring of anticoagulant therapy and use of infusion pump when heparin is administered continuously.

NPSG.03.06.01: *Maintain and communicate accurate patient medication information.* Transferring accurate medication information is critical in the perioperative period where several handoffs can occur during the episode of care.

Other medication safety standards in the OR are discussed under a separate section in this chapter.

Alarm System Safety

NPSG.06.01.01: *Improve the safety of clinical alarm systems.* This standard requires the use of clinically appropriate alarms and set parameters to improve patient safety. Policies and procedures should be established for alarm management and should address issues like designating authority to change alarm parameters, periodic checking of alarm settings and alarm function.

Prevent infection

NPSG.07.01.01: *Comply with either the current CDC hand hygiene guidelines or the current WHO hand hygiene guidelines.* The standard requires implementation of a hospital-wide goal-based hand hygiene improvement program (TJC IC.01.04.01-EP5, IC.03.01.01-EP3).

NPSG.07.03.01: *Implement evidence-based practices to prevent healthcare-associated infections due to multidrug-resistant organisms in acute care hospitals.* The standard requires implementation of policies and practices that apply organization-wide as well as to the perioperative environment, aimed at reducing the risk of transmitting multidrug-resistant organisms. This includes targeted risk assessment, surveillance programs, provider and patient's family education, and reporting outcome data to stakeholders.

NPSG.07.04.01: *Implement evidence-based practices to prevent central line-associated bloodstream infections.* Per this standard, the policies and practices aimed at reducing the risk of central line-associated bloodstream infections must be implemented and complied with. These policies and practices must be aligned with state and national regulatory requirements and professional organization guidelines. Some provisions in this NPSG are the use of standardized supply cart or kit that contains all necessary components for the insertion of central lines, use of standardized protocol for hand hygiene, aseptic skin prep and sterile barrier precautions, use of a standardized protocol to disinfect catheter hubs and injection ports before accessing them, and avoiding femoral vein for central line insertion unless other sites are unavailable.

NPSG.07.05.01: *Implement evidence-based practices for preventing surgical site infections.* Elements of performance include implementation of educational, preventive and surveillance strategies. This goal requires measurement of surgical site infection rates for up to 30 or 90 days following surgical procedures based on National Healthcare Safety Network procedural codes.

CMS condition of participation §482.42 on Infection control, requires that healthcare-associated infection prevention be a part of the hospital-wide infection control program. Hospitals that employ alcohol-based skin preparations in anesthetizing locations are required to have appropriate policies and procedures to reduce the associated risk of fire. Failure to implement appropriate measures to reduce the risk of fires associated with the use of alcohol-based skin preparations in anesthetizing locations is considered a condition-level noncompliance.

NPSG.07.05.01: *Prevent indwelling catheter-associated urinary tract infections.* This goal applies to adult patients only and requires using evidence-based criteria for perioperative placement of indwelling urinary catheters. Examples include critically ill patients who need accurate urinary output measurements, prolonged duration of surgery, patients anticipated to receive large volume infusions, and patients undergoing urologic surgery of the genitourinary tract.

Universal Protocol

The Universal Protocol focuses on eliminating all wrong-person, wrong-site, and wrong-procedure events with the consistent use of a standardized checklist type protocol. It applies to all surgical as well nonsurgical invasive procedures that expose patients to more than minimal risk. It includes the following three standards.

UP.01.01.01: *Conduct a preprocedure verification process.* This NPSG requires implementation of a preprocedure protocol to verify the correct procedure, for the correct patient, at the correct site, with patient involvement if possible. Use of a standardized list to verify at a minimum relevant documentation (for example, history and physical, signed procedure consent form, nursing assessment, and preanesthesia assessment), diagnostic and radiology test results, and any special requirements, matched to the patient.

UP.01.02.01: *Mark the procedure site.* The standard requires marking of procedure site, side and level if applicable, before the procedure is performed, and with patient involvement if possible. Marking should preferably be done by a licensed practitioner who is accountable for the procedure and will be present when the procedure is performed. If hospital policy allows, a designated qualified practitioner may perform site marking to meet this standard. The mark should be visible after skin prep and draping. Exceptions for site marking include mucosal surfaces, perineum, teeth, premature infants and patient refusal.

UP.01.03.01: *A time-out is performed before the procedure.* This requires performing a standardized time out immediately before the procedure, initiated by a designated member of the team. The members of the procedural team should agree on at least three elements: correct patient, correct site, procedure to be done. The completion of the time out should be documented.

Medication Safety

Medication safety presents a unique challenge in the OR environment. Medication errors are amongst the most common errors in anesthesia because of the practice where an anesthesia provider orders, dispenses and administers a drug, and monitors the patient in the absence of double checks and other safety measures taken when medications are ordered and administered on the hospital wards. Twelve out of 20 medications categories designated as "high-alert medications" by Institute for Safe Medication Practices are commonly stocked in anesthesia carts [8]. Appropriate safeguards must be in place to prevent errors with the use of risky medications especially ones that are in look-alike containers, are highly concentrated and those that may need dilution before administration (TJC MM 01.02.01). ASA statement on *Labeling of Pharmaceuticals for the Use in Anesthesiology* recommends color coded, legible labels consistent with American Society for Testing and Materials International and the International Organization for Standardization. The purpose is to enhance visual features in accordance with human factors to prevent errors of syringe swaps [9].

CMS and TJC standards require all noncontrolled medications to be locked when a patient care procedural area is not staffed by a healthcare professional (CMS §482.25(b)(2)) [10]. Medications listed in Schedules II–V of the Comprehensive Drug Abuse Prevention and Control Act of 1970 must be locked and accurate records of the disposition of all controlled substances must be maintained (CMS §482.25(b)(2)(ii), §482.25(a)(3), TJC MM.01.01.03) by the hospital pharmacy. The hospitals are required to have policy and procedures for reporting diversion, managing recalls and expired drugs, and reporting errors and adverse reactions through a hospital-wide medication safety program (CMS §482.25(b) (6)(7)(8), TJC MM.07.01.03). The professional staff must have access to Information relating to drug indications, interactions, side effects, toxicology, dosage, and routes of administration 24 h a day, 7 days a week (CMS §482.25(b)(8), TJC IM.03.01.01).

In the PACU, verbal orders must be minimized to avoid medication errors, and should be authenticated promptly according to state law or hospital policy (CMS§482.24(c)(1)(iii), TJC RC.02.03.07-EP4).

Environmental and Occupational Safety

Physical Environment and Facilities

Most standards in CMS CoP §482.41 Physical Environment apply to the OR environment and pertain not only to physical construction and planning of the perioperative areas but also to emergency preparedness plans and capabilities to ensure patient safety and well-being (TJC Life Safety Standards). All hospitals participating in Medicare are required to comply with Life Safety Code requirements of the National Fire Protection Association (NPFA), unless State fire and safety codes are more stringent and protect patients adequately (CMS §482.41(b), TJC EC.02.03.01). Operating and recovery rooms are required to have emergency power and lighting (CMS§482.41(a) (1), TJC EC.02.05.03, NPFA 101, 2000 edition). The OR must have a fire response and evacuation plan as a part of the larger hospital plan (CMS §482.41(b)(7) TJC EC.02.05.07). All new staff must be oriented to fire safety and must know how to contain fire, use the fire extinguisher and evacuate safely. The staff should be able to describe the key safety steps if asked by TJC surveyor.

Infection Control and Occupational Safety

CDDC has published extensive guidelines for infection control in case of both nosocomial and occupational acquired infections [11, 12]. Occupational Safety and Health Administration in section IV off its manual addresses several occupational hazards in healthcare facilities and recommends preventive measures [13]. Exposure to blood-borne pathogens, laser use and laser smoke, multidrug resistant organisms, surgical instruments/equipment and anesthesia equipment in the OR make it a unique and high-risk environment for infection control. American Society of Anesthesiologists' recommendations for infection control and AORN guidelines are specifically directed to the Perioperative environment [14, 15].

Quality Assurance and Performance Improvement

TJC and CMS identify the OR as a high-risk area and require that the anesthesia and surgical services be a part of the organization-wide quality assurance performance improvement program (QA/PI). QA/PI activities that apply to the perioperative environment are broadly categorized below.

Data Collection

Leaders are the motivating force behind quality driven organizations and CMS requires hospital leaders (governing body) to set priorities and determine the detail and frequency of data collection for performance improvement activities. Data collection sources can include a variety of sources like patient charts, staff, observation, interviews etc. to identify vulnerable areas and direct performance improvement activities. Priority is given to high-volume, high-risk, or problem-prone processes, perioperative processes being amongst them (TJC PI. 01.01.01). Participation in Medicare requires data collection in the following procedural areas:

- Surgery and other procedures that place patients at risk of disability or death
- Significant discrepancies between preoperative and postoperative diagnoses
- Adverse events related to using moderate or deep sedation or anesthesia.
- The use of blood and blood components
- All reported and confirmed transfusion reactions
- Results of resuscitation
- Significant medication errors
- Significant adverse drug reactions
- Patient perception of the safety and quality of care, treatment, and services

TJC also recommends data collection on staff opinions and needs, staff perceptions of risk to individuals, their suggestions for improving patient safety and willingness to report adverse events.

Data Compilation and Analysis

Statistical analysis and display of data helps in trending and identification of opportunities for improvement. TJC requires that any undesirable trends or variation should include staffing analysis (TJC recommends use of National Quality Forum Nursing Sensitive Measures). Organization-wide safety programs must establish a method of communicating critical information to hospital leaders, so that prompt actions can be taken to resolve any problems identified (Box 30.1).

Ongoing Performance Improvement

As quality measures evolve, healthcare organizations need to be able to adapt and prioritize performance improvement opportunities. CMS and TJC in particular, evaluate healthcare facilities' care processes that enhance safety and produce the best outcomes for their patients. Ever since TJC adopted the its mission of "continuously improve healthcare for the public, in collaboration with other stakeholders, by evaluating healthcare organizations and inspiring them to excel in providing safe and effective care of the highest

---

Box 30.1. Emergency Management Standards by JCAHO

1. Develop a management plan that addresses emergency management. Four phases of emergency management are:

   mitigation

   preparedness

   response

   recovery

2. Perform a health vulnerability analysis

   Establish emergency procedures in response to a hazard vulnerability analysis

   Define the organization's roles with other community agencies

   Notify external authorities

   Notify hospital personnel when emergency procedures initiated

   Assign available personnel to cover necessary positions

   The following activities must be managed:

   . . . patient/resident activities;

   . . . staff activities.

   Staff /family support

   Logistics of critical supplies

   Security

   Evacuation of facility, if necessary

   Establish internal/external communications

   Establish orientation/education programs

   Monitor ongoing drills and real emergencies

   Determine how an annual evaluation will occur

   Provide alternate means of meeting essential building and utility needs

   Identify radioactive and biological isolation decontamination needs

   Clarify alternate responsibility of personnel

3. Involve community-wide response

4. Reestablish and continue operations after disaster

---

quality and value," the cramming mentality before an inspection has become a phenomenon of the past. Instead, TJC standards set benchmarks that accredited institutions must meet or exceed on a continued basis. Creating a culture of safety through leadership involvement, organization-wide safety programs, education of the staff, effective communication of changes and safety tips to frontline providers and visible evidence of safe practices through posters and pocket cards can help achieve and maintain accreditation.

References

1. Facts about The Joint Commission. www.iom .edu/~/media/Files/Activity%20Files/Workforce/ ResidentDutyHours/PaulSchyveTestimonyFactsaboutt heJointCommission.pdf

2. Joint Commission Resources Inc. *Comprehensive accreditation manual for hospitals.* jcrinc.com.

3. Key milestones in CMS programs. www.cms.gov/ History/downloads/CMSProgramKeyMilestones.pdf

4. State Operations Manual (SOM) Appendix A. Revision 151, November 20, 2015.

5. 2016 Joint Commission and CMS Crosswalk, Comparing hospital standards and CoPs. jointcommissioninternational.org

6. American Society of Anesthesiologists. Ethical guidelines for the anesthesia care of patients with do-not-resuscitate orders or other directives that limit treatment. October 16, 2013.

7. American Society of Anesthesiologists. Statement on documentation of anesthesia care. October 28, 2015.

8. Institute for Safe Medication Practices. ISPM list of high alert medication in acute care settings. ispm.org

9. American Society of Anesthesiologists. Statement on creating labels of pharmaceuticals for use in anesthesiology. October 28, 2105.

10. American Society of Anesthesiologists. Statement on security of medications in the operating room. October 16, 2106.

11. Center for Disease Control and Prevention. Guidelines for isolation precaution: Preventing transmission of infectious agents in health care setting. 2007.

12. Center for Disease Control and Prevention. Guidelines for environmental infection control in health-care facilities. June 6, 2003/52(RR10), 1–42.

13. Occupational Safety and Health Administration. *OSHA technical manual*, Section VI, osha.gov.

14. American Society of Anesthesiologists. *Recommendations for infection control for the practice of anesthesiology*, 3rd ed. 2011.

15. Association of periOperative Registered Nurses, Inc. *Guidelines for perioperative practice*. 2016 edition.

Chapter 31

Procedural Sedation
Clinical and Safety Considerations

Ann Bui and Richard D. Urman

Contents

Introduction

As healthcare and technology progress, the need for anesthesia services escalates both in and out of the operating room (OR). Ideally, individuals with the most training and experience with sedation would administer it. Owing to the high volume of cases that require sedation, however, many nonanesthesiologists are providing this service. Today, sedation is administered by both anesthesia professionals (anesthesiologists, certified registered nurse anesthetists, and anesthesiologist assistants) and nonanesthesia professionals (physicians, dentists, registered nurses, physician assistants, etc.). Generally, sedation is optimal for procedures that are quick and/or noninvasive (Table 31.1). Although general anesthesia can be performed for every procedure that could otherwise be done with sedation, sedation is preferred by many patients and healthcare providers. Depending on the knowledge and experience of the person providing sedation, sedation may offer a quicker recovery time and may be less invasive compared with general anesthesia.

Advances in interventional medicine have allowed procedures, which typically took place in the OR, to be performed outside of the OR (OOOR). Nowadays procedures done with sedation, both in the OR and OOOR, are increasing in complexity, and the patients

receiving these procedures are having more comorbidities. Despite this, many patients receiving sedation do not necessarily require the presence of an anesthesiologist. The American Society of Anesthesiologists' (ASA) Statement on Granting Privileges for Administration of Moderate Sedation to Practitioners Who Are Not Anesthesia Professionals states that "only physicians, dentists, or podiatrists who are qualified by education, training, and licensure to administer moderate sedation should supervise the administration of moderate sedation." The ASA Statement on Granting Privileges to Nonanesthesiologist Supervising Deep Sedation by Individuals Who Are Not Anesthesia Professionals states that "due to a significant risk that patients who receive deep sedation may enter a state of general anesthesia, privileges to administer deep sedation should be granted only to practitioners who are qualified to administer general anesthesia or to appropriately supervise anesthesia professionals." The aforementioned ASA statements address education, training, licensure, supervision, performance evaluation, and improvement requirements for a sedation program involving nonanesthesia providers [1–3]. Although the ASA guidelines are generally supported by most regulatory agencies, there are many other professional societies that have their own standards and guidelines on procedural sedation (see Appendix: Professional Guidelines and Standards).

Table 31.1 Examples of Procedures Performed under Moderate Sedation Under the Direction of Non-Anesthesia Practitioners

Head and neck	Superficial thoracic	Extremity procedures	Gastrointestinal/ abdominal	Vascular	Gynecologic/urologic	Emergency department/ radiology
Dental extractions	Breast augmentation	Carpal tunnel release	Endoscopic retrograde cholangiopancreatography	Hemodialysis access placement	Dilatation and curettage	Reduction of dislocation or fracture
Blepharoplasty	Breast biopsy	Trigger finger release	Colonoscopy	Pacemaker insertion	Fulguration of vaginal lesions	Complex suturing
Rhytidoplasty	Bronchoscopy	Removal of pins/wires/ screws	Endoscopic ultrasound	Angiography	Fulguration of anal lesions	Insertion of elective chest tube
Rhinoplasty	Chest tube insertion	Closed reduction	Gastroscopy	Cardiac catheterization	Cystoscopy	MRI
Laceration				Radiofrequency ablation	Incision and drainage of Bartholin's cyst	Arteriograms
Cataract				Electrophysiologic testing	Vasectomy	Liver biopsy

Source: Adapted from E. E. Whitaker, A. Mukherjee, T. Liu, B. Hong, E. S. Heitmiller. Introduction to moderate and deep sedation. In: R. Urman, A. D. Kaye. *Moderate and Deep Sedation in Clinical Practice*, 1st edn. Cambridge University Press, 2012. Chapter 1, pp. 1–7, Table 1.1.

Table 31.2 Continuum of Depth of Sedation: Definition of General Anesthesia and Levels of Sedation/Analgesia

	Minimal sedation	Moderate sedation/analgesia (conscious sedation)	Deep sedation/ analgesia	General anesthesia
Responsiveness	Normal	Purposeful[a] response to verbal or tactile stimulation	Purposeful[a] response after repeated or painful stimulation	Unarousable even with painful stimulus
Airway	Unaffected	No intervention required	Intervention may be required	Intervention often required
Spontaneous ventilation	Unaffected	Adequate	May be inadequate	Frequently inadequate
Cardiovascular function	Unaffected	Usually maintained	Usually maintained	May be impaired

[a] Reflex withdrawal from a painful stimulus is not considered a purposeful response.

Source: American Society of Anesthesiologists. Contiuum of Depth of Sedation. Definition of General Anesthesia and Levels of Sedation/Analgesia. Available at: http://www.asahq.org/quality-and-practice-management/standards-guidelines-and-related-resources/continuum-of-depth-of-sedation-definition-of-general-anesthesia-and-levels-of-sedation-analgesia (accessed August 20, 2018).

For example, the American Nurses Association's Procedural Sedation Consensus Statement states that procedural sedation medications can be administered by a Registered Nurse (RN) only in the presence of a physician, advanced practiced registered nurse or other healthcare professional qualified and trained for procedural sedation.

Definitions of Sedation

It is important to realize that sedation and general anesthesia are on a continuum. There are different levels of sedation, but they can easily blend with one another and evolve into general anesthesia. Each patient responds differently to sedation medications, and thus, even if the healthcare practitioner intended on delivering moderate sedation, a deep sedation or even a general anesthetic can occur. The ASA defines sedation levels according to responsiveness, airway, spontaneous ventilation, and cardiovascular function (Table 31.2). According to the ASA, there are three levels of sedation, which culminate in general anesthesia [4].

- **Minimal sedation** – this is primarily done for anxiolysis. Patients respond normally to verbal commands, are able to maintain a patent airway, are spontaneously breathing and have an unchanged cardiovascular system.
- **Moderate sedation** – this was previously known as "conscious sedation." It is a drug-induced state in which there is a depression of consciousness. However, patients still have a purposeful response to verbal commands, plus or minus light tactile stimulation. Patients continue to maintain a

patent airway without any intervention and have adequate spontaneous ventilation. The cardiovascular system is usually unchanged.
- **Deep sedation** – consciousness is depressed significantly and patients require repeated or painful stimuli to evoke a purposeful response. An intervention may be required for patients to maintain a patent airway and spontaneous ventilation may be inadequate. Cardiovascular function is usually unchanged.
- **General anesthesia** – consciousness is lost and patients are unarousable even to painful stimulation. Patients often need assistance in maintaining a patent airway and with ventilation, as this is frequently inadequate. Positive pressure ventilation may be required because of depressed spontaneous ventilation or drug-induced depression of neuromuscular function. Cardiovascular function may be impaired.

Clinically there is not a clear distinction between the levels of sedation and because the levels of sedation can quickly progress into general anesthesia, the ASA standard is that healthcare providers should be able to rescue patients from any level of sedation and return them to the original intended level of sedation.

Preprocedure Evaluation

Before the procedure, it is imperative to review the patient's medical history, preprocedure labs, diagnostic tests and physically examine the patient. This includes reviewing nil per os status, medications and

Box 31.1. ASA Physical Status Classification System

ASA physical status I	A normal healthy patient
ASA physical status II	A patient with mild systemic disease
ASA physical status III	A patient with severe systemic disease
ASA physical status IV	A patient with severe systemic disease that is a constant threat to life
ASA physical status V	A moribund patient who is not expected to survive without the operation
ASA physical status VI	A declared brain-dead patient whose organs are being removed for donor purposes

Box 31.2. Equipment Needed for Moderate and Deep Sedation

Oxygen source

Airway equipment – including a self-inflating oxygen delivery system capable of delivering 100 percent oxygen

Suction source with suction catheters

Pulse oximeter with audible alarms

Cardiac monitor with audible alarms

Blood pressure device and stethoscope

Capnography

Emergency cart and defibrillator

Medications to be used for the procedure and their reversal agents

Fluid bags of either 0.9 percent normal saline or lactated Ringer's solution

Source: Adapted from L. Caperelli-White. Nursing considerations for sedation. In: R. Urman, A. D. Kaye. *Moderate and Deep Sedation in Clinical Practice*, 1st edn. Cambridge University Press, 2012. Chapter 8, pp. 103–4.

drug allergies, previous anesthesia and/or sedation experiences, and health problems. It is critical to recognize the comorbidities that place a patient at higher risk for sedation; these comorbidities include, but are not limited to, morbid obesity, extremes of age, sleep apnea, and an anticipated difficult airway. Patients with multiple systemic comorbidities (ASA physical status III–V; see Box 31.1) also are at an increased risk for complications (Table 31.3). The presence of these factors should prompt an anesthesiology consult. The physical examination portion should include obtaining the patient's height, weight, and baseline vital signs along with assessing the airway. The ability to identify a potentially difficult airway is essential. Lastly, before giving any sedation medications, one must ensure that appropriate consents have been completed.

Monitors and Equipment

Once sedation has started, proper monitoring of the patient's oxygenation, ventilation, circulation, and level of consciousness must be continually assessed; therefore, it is necessary for the person administering sedation to be present throughout the entire procedure and to have no other responsibilities. Oxygenation is monitored via continuous pulse oximetry, and every patient should receive supplemental oxygen. Supplemental oxygen along with pulse oximetry can prevent and detect hypoxemia, but neither is ideal for the identification of hypoventilation, airway obstruction, or apnea. In fact, supplemental oxygen can mask problems with ventilation. Ventilation is monitored by continuously observing patient chest movement, evaluating airway patency, and auscultating breath sounds. The ASA Standards for Basic Anesthetic Monitoring state that "During moderate and deep sedation the adequacy of ventilation shall be evaluated by continual observation of qualitative clinical signs and monitoring for the presence of exhaled carbon dioxide unless precluded or invalidated by the nature of the patient, procedure, or equipment" [5]. Capnography can significantly aid in monitoring ventilation and alerts sedation providers to hypoventilation/apnea much more quickly than clinical observation alone. Evaluation of circulation is done via continuous electrocardiogram and measuring blood pressure at least every 5 min; circulation can also be assessed by palpating pulses and auscultating heart sounds. A patient's level of consciousness is easily monitored by talking to and/or stimulating the patient. The ASA Standards for Basic Anesthetic Monitoring also state that, "Every patient receiving anesthesia shall have temperature monitored when clinically significant changes in body temperature are intended, anticipated or suspected" [5]. Although not every procedure done with sedation will require the monitoring of temperature, sedation providers should be cognizant of when it is needed. Before every procedure, it is necessary to ensure the availability of monitors and equipment and that they are functioning correctly (Box 31.2). Despite this, monitors can malfunction at any time during the procedure; thus, no monitor is more valuable than the vigilant healthcare provider.

Medications

An important aspect of safely providing sedation is knowing the pharmacologic profiles of the common medications used. Although a plethora of medications exist that will provide sedation and/or analgesia, the agents most commonly used are benzodiazepines and opioids (Table 31.3). Both are easily titratable and their actions can be mitigated by reversal agents. Because benzodiazepines and opioids are commonly given together, one must acknowledge that their actions and side effects are synergistic and must be careful to avoid oversedation and/or respiratory depression. Although benzodiazepines lack analgesic properties, they are anxiolytics, anticonvulsants, sedatives, and amnestics.

Of the benzodiazepines, midazolam is very popular because of its quick onset, short duration of action, and favorable hemodynamic profile. In situations of oversedation, flumazenil is the reversal agent for benzodiazepines. It is usually given in increments of 0.2 mg and is titrated to effect (i.e., desired level of consciousness). It has a quick onset and a half-life shorter than most benzodiazepines; thus, to avoid resedation, flumazenil may have to be administered more than once.

Unlike benzodiazepines, opioids are primarily analgesics. Opioids are administered to prevent and alleviate pain and as an adjunct to sedatives/hypnotics, such as benzodiazepines. Of the opioids, fentanyl is very popular because of its quick onset, short duration of action, and favorable hemodynamic profile. In situations of undesired respiratory depression or excessive sedation, naloxone is the reversal agent for opioids. It is usually given in increments of 0.04 mg and is titrated to effect (i.e., respiratory rate over eight breaths per minute). In cases in which long-acting opioids have been given, it may be necessary to readminister naloxone to avoid repeated respiratory depression.

Recovery and Discharge

After receiving sedation, patients should continue to be monitored in a postsedation recovery area until time of discharge. This is because many complications can occur during the postoperative period, with respiratory depression and aspiration being the most common. How long patients must spend in the recovery area and how frequent their vital signs should be monitored and recorded are dependent on the institution, but commonly, vital signs are recorded every 10 min for a minimum of 30 min. Before being discharged, patients must meet certain criteria. These criteria are also dependent on the institution, but generally include adequate oxygenation and ventilation, hemodynamic stability, and return to baseline level of consciousness. The Aldrete scoring system [6] was one of the first sets of objective discharge criteria used (Box 31.3); a minimum score of 9 out of 10 allowed for discharge. Along with the appropriate monitors, the recovery area must also have the same equipment that was available during the time of sedation in case a patient was to require resuscitation. Many complications occur during the recovery period because of inadequate monitoring, equipment, and personnel training. If a patient is being discharged home, the patient must receive both verbal and written discharge instructions. It is optimal that the person taking the patient home also be present for these instructions, as the patient may not remember everything. Instructions usually include any activity or diet restrictions specific to the procedure performed and any problems the patient should anticipate.

Regulation

Unlike the Center for Medicare and Medicaid Services (CMS), which is a federal agency, the Joint Commission is "an independent not-for-profit organization" (About The Joint Commission, 2012). Although they each have their own regulations and standards, they also operate together to ensure patient safety at an institutional level. The Joint Commission audits and accredits institutions to ensure that they hold up to the regulations and standards put forth by the Joint Commission and CMS. According to the CMS Condition of Participation, "If the hospital furnishes anesthesia services, [the services] must be provided in a well-organized manner under the direction of a qualified doctor of medicine or osteopathy. The [hospital's anesthesiology department] is responsible for all anesthesia administered in the hospital" [7], whether it was administered by anesthesia providers or nonanesthesia providers. The CMS and The Joint Commission dictate anesthesia/sedation care preoperatively, intraoperatively, and postoperatively (Box 31.4). The CMS orders that patients must be

Table 31.3 Medication Chart

Drug	Sedational amnesia	Anxiolysis	Analgesia	Route/dose	Onset (min)	Peak (min)	Duration (min)	Comments
Sedative/hypnotics*								
Midazolam (Versed)	Yes	Yes	No	IV: 0.5–1 mg (titrate to effect up to 5–10 mg/h)	0.5–1	3–5	10–30	Minimal cardiorespiratory depression
				IM: 0.08 mg/kg	10–15	20–45	60–120	Reduce dose when used in combination with opioids
								Midazolam is benzodiazepine of choice for short procedures
								Antagonist: flumazenil
Diazepam (Valium)	Yes	Yes	No	IV: 2–3 mg (titrate to effect up to 15 mg)	1–2	8–15	15–45	
				PO: 5–10 mg	30–60	45–60	60–100	
Lorazepam (Ativan)	Yes	Yes	No	IV: 0.25 mg (titrate to effect up to 2 mg)	1–2	15–20	60–120	
				PO: 2–4 mg	60–120	120	>480	
Opioids*								
Fentanyl	No	No	Yes	IV: 28–50 µg intermittent boluses	1–2	5	30–40	Respiratory depression decreased
Meperidine (Demerol)	No	No	Yes	IV: 2.5–75 mg	3–5	5–7	63–180	Response to hypercarbia and hypoxia
								Synergistic sedative and respiratory depressant effects (reduce dose with sedatives)
								Nausea, vomiting
								Meperidine: histamine release
								Antagonist: naloxone

(continued)

Table 31.3 (*Cont.*)

Drug	Sedational amnesia	Anxiolysis	Analgesia	Route/dose	Onset (min)	Peak (min)	Duration (min)	Comments
Reversal agents (antagonists)								
Flumazenil (Anexate)	No	No	No	IV: 0.1–0.2 mg (titrate to effect to max of 5 mg)	1–2	5–10	45–90	Short-acting, repeat doses may be required Avoid in patients receiving benzodiazepines for seizure control Caution with chronic benzodiazepine therapy (withdrawal effect) or with tricyclic antidepressants
Naloxome (Narcan)	No	No	No	IV: 0.02–1.04 mg (titrate to effect)	1–2	2–3	30–60	Short-acting, repeat doses may be required May cause hypertension and tachycardia Pulmonary edema reported

* Alterations in dosing may be indicated based upon the clinical situation and the practitioner's experience with these agents. Individual dosages may vary depending on age and coexistent diseases. Doses should be reduced for sicker patients and in the elderly. When using drug combinations, the potential for significant respiratory impairment and airway obstruction is increased. Drugs should be titrated to achieve optimal effect, and sufficient time for dose effect should be allowed before administering an additional dose or another medication.

Source: Taken from J. Metzner, K. B. Domino. Anesthesia and sedation outside of the operating room: outcomes, regulation, and quality improvement. In: R. Urman, W. Gross, B. K. Philip. *Anesthesia Outside of the Operating Room*, 1st edn. Oxford University Press, 2011. Chapter 8, pp. 62–73.

Box 31.3. Aldrete Scoring System

Respiration

　　Able to take deep breath and cough = 2

　　Dyspnea/shallow breathing = 1

　　Apnea = 0

Oxygen saturation

　　SaO_2 >95 percent on room air = 2

　　SaO_2 >90–95 percent on room air = 1

　　SaO_2 <90 percent even with supplemental O_2 = 0

Consciousness

　　Fully awake = 2

　　Arousable on calling = 1

　　Not responding = 0

Circulation

　　BP ±20 mm Hg baseline = 2

　　BP ±20–50 mm Hg baseline = 1

　　BP ±50 mm Hg baseline = 0

Activity

　　Able to move 4 extremities = 2

　　Able to move 2 extremities = 1

　　Able to move 0 extremities = 0

Note: Monitoring may be discontinued and patient discharged to home or appropriate unit when Aldrete score is 9 or greater.

Sources: D. E. Morrison, K. Dorn Hare. Patient evaluation and procedure selection, In: R. Urman, A. D. Kaye. *Moderate and Deep Sedation in Clinical Practice*, 2nd edn. Cambridge University Press, 2017. Chapter 4, pp. 47–59. Data from: J. A. Aldrete. The post-anesthesia recovery score revisited. *J Clin Anesth* 1995; 7: 89–91.

Box 31.4. Summary of the Joint Commission Standards for Moderate Sedation

1.　Moderate sedation must be administered by a qualified provider.

2.　Patients who will receive moderate sedation must be assessed prior to sedation/procedure.

3.　The provider must discuss risks and options with the patient or his/her family prior to sedation/procedure.

4.　The provider must reassess the patient immediately before the sedation is initiated.

5.　Monitoring of the patient's oxygenation, ventilation, and circulation during sedation is mandatory.

6.　Postsedation assessment in the recovery area is necessary before the patient is discharged.

7.　A qualified provider must discharge the patient from the postsedation recovery area or discharge must be based on established criteria.

Source: M. T. Antonelli, D. E. Seaver. Quality, legal, and risk management considerations: ensuring program excellence. In: R. Urman, A. D. Kaye. *Moderate and Deep Sedation in Clinical Practice*, 2nd edn. Cambridge University Press, 2017. Chapter 7, pp. 85–105.

assessed within 48 h of receiving sedation, monitored intraoperatively with proper documentation as proof, and appropriately cared for postoperatively.

Credentialing and Competency

Although on a national level, The Joint Commission requires all institutions to verify a practitioner's state license, Drug Enforcement Administration number, and education and training prior to granting the privilege of administrating sedation, the specific credentialing and training one must possess is determined by individual institutions. The ASA has set forth different requirements for practitioners administrating moderate versus deep sedation, which may be viewed in entirety on their website. Owing to the high potential for deep sedation to evolve into general anesthesia, the ASA states that practitioners administrating deep sedation should also be able to provide general anesthesia safely. The CMS additionally adds that only anesthesia providers (anesthesiologists, nurse anesthetists, and anesthesiology assistants), physicians, dentists, oral surgeons, and podiatrists should be granted the privilege of providing deep sedation. A practitioner providing deep sedation must be trained in advanced cardiac life support and/or pediatric advanced life support, depending on the patient population receiving deep sedation. A physician, dentist, oral surgeon, and podiatrist must be present to supervise moderate sedation, which can be administered by the aforementioned, in addition to anesthesia providers, registered nurses, and physician assistants. A practitioner administrating any level of sedation should possess the skills to rescue a patient in case the patient enters a deeper level of sedation than intended and return the patient to the intended level of sedation. Hence, it is absolutely crucial that the practitioner performing the procedure and the practitioner administering sedation are separate individuals, with the latter solely focused on monitoring the patient and immediately available in case cardiopulmonary compromise were to occur. Generally, "the Joint Commission requires that sedation providers have adequate training to administer the sedative drugs effectively and safely, the skills to monitor the patient's response to the medications given, and the expertise needed to manage all potential complications" [8]. In addition, practitioners should be able to identify the varying levels of sedation, which will allow them to intervene appropriately when the patient is being under- or oversedated. Not only should the practitioner have comprehensive knowledge about the sedative drugs, but also about the available reversal agents. Anticipating and recognizing patients' varying response to medications is needed and allows the practitioner to maintain patient hemodynamic stability. Understanding the physiology of oxygenation and ventilation and the ability to differentiate between normal and abnormal vital signs and cardiac rhythms and then relate them to the patient's current state is a necessary skill. Also, practitioners providing all levels of sedation should be competent in assessing and managing the airway and be able to determine when an anesthesiology consultation is needed.

Education

To ensure practitioners have the essential knowledge and skills that are crucial to being a competent sedation provider, institutions must develop educational programs that identify and assess these knowledge and skills. Traditionally, knowledge is obtained via lectures and assessed via written tests. Although this method facilitates basic science knowledge, it is not proficient at teaching and validating clinical skills, reasoning, and decision-making behavior. The latter can be done with simulation-based education, which creates real-life clinical scenarios. No matter the method taken, the institution is obligated to routinely validate and assess the knowledge and skills required, as the responsibilities of sedation practitioners change due to the emergence of new technology and procedures.

Quality Improvement and Risk Assessment

Internally, institutions need a process to address quality improvement and risk assessment to ensure the institution's policies and practices are at the best clinical standard to minimize potential risks of injury. This process provides the ultimate goal of delivering patient safety. Through review and evaluation of institutional policies, quality of care, and patient outcomes, the quality improvement processes improve the practice of sedation. This confirms adherence to standards of care and can systematically be done by regularly reviewing charts chosen at random, and by direct observation of care. The risk assessment processes are responsible for analyzing situations in which an adverse patient outcome has occurred or almost occurred. By investigating all the factors that contributed to or caused an adverse patient outcome, changes can be made to prevent such events in the future. The Joint Commission mandates that all sentinel events (i.e., wrong-site or wrong-patient surgery) be reviewed with a root cause analysis.

"The University of HealthSystem Consortium (UHC), an alliance of academic medical centers and affiliated hospitals that focus on excellence in quality, safety, and cost-effectiveness, recommends the following . . . patient outcomes" be monitored and documented: deaths, aspirations, reversal agent used, unplanned transfer to higher level of care, cardiac/respiratory arrest, medications administered other than those approved, inability to complete procedure as planned, and emergency procedures without a licensed independent practitioner present [7].

Outcomes

Examining the ASA Closed Claims Project data on procedures performed with sedation or monitored anesthesia care, the most common etiology of death or permanent brain damage is respiratory depression due to oversedation [9, 10]. The use of propofol in combination with benzodiazepines and/or opioids increased the incidence of respiratory depression. Most of these events were deemed preventable either by better monitoring techniques, in particular capnography, or enhanced vigilance by the sedation provider. As a result, the ASA considers capnography a standard monitor.

Controversies

Because the use of propofol increases the risk of moderate sedation slipping into deep sedation or even general anesthesia, the ASA Statement on Safe Use of Propofol [11] says that when propofol is administered, patients "should receive care consistent with that required for deep sedation" and that the nonanesthesia provider "should be qualified to rescue patients whose level of sedation becomes deeper than initially intended and who enter, if briefly, a state of general anesthesia." Whether or not propofol can safely be administered by nonanesthesia providers remains a topic of controversy. The studies that have been done on propofol administration by nonanesthesia providers have not shown an increased incidence of severe adverse patient outcome, such as airway compromise requiring bag mask ventilation and/or endotracheal intubation, but these studies do not take into account the incidence and magnitude of respiratory obstruction, hypoventilation, or hemodynamic compromise [12–17]. Future studies that completely investigate the safety of propofol administration by nonanesthesia providers are needed.

Future of Sedation

Increasing patient safety during procedural sedation may lie in the use of new medications and new medication delivery techniques. Fospropofol, the prodrug of propofol, has been approved by the Food and Drug Administration (FDA) for the sedation of adults. The slower onset and longer duration of action of fospropofol make it possibly advantageous in minimizing the risk of oversedation. The pharmacokinetic profile of fospropofol is still in progress, but its use as a sedative drug is promising. Because fospropofol gets converted to propofol, its package insert also says that it "should be administered only by persons trained in the administration of general anesthesia and not involved in the conduct of the diagnostic or therapeutic procedure" (Lusedra Warnings and Precautions).

Similar to patient-controlled analgesia, patient-controlled sedation/analgesia (PCSA) enables patients to control how much sedation/analgesia they receives and when. With the push of a button, patients can have medications (i.e., midazolam, fentanyl) delivered; and with the lockout interval, bolus doses, and maximum infusion rate set by the healthcare provider, the risk of oversedation is minimized. Such PCSA offers high patient satisfaction, and patients tend to use less medication compared with healthcare provider administration of sedation/analgesia.

Computer-assisted personalized sedation (CAPS) is a program that monitors a patient's vital signs and level of responsiveness and then determines if and when a patient receives sedation medications. If a patient is being oversedated, as determined by vital signs and lack of responsiveness, then the delivery of sedation medications will be paused or stopped and the delivery of oxygen will increase. The CAPS is not meant to replace the sedation provider, but instead aid in providing sedation; it has not been approved by the FDA at this time.

Summary

In conclusion, it is important for sedation providers to realize that there are distinctly different levels of sedation, but that clinically it may be difficult to differentiate between them. Each institution offering sedation services must follow the federal and state regulations on moderate and deep sedation, and sedation providers must have the appropriate qualifications [18]. The specific education and training required of sedation providers differs between institutions. Although most institutions adopt the ASA guidelines and standards, each professional society also has its own set of guidelines. In the end, whether sedation is administered by an anesthesia or nonanesthesia provider, patient safety is of utmost concern.

Appendix: Professional Guidelines and Standards (the following organizations have guidelines that pertain to the administration of procedural sedation. Please visit their individual websites for up-to-date information)

American Academy of Pediatrics and American Academy of Pediatric Dentistry
American Association of Critical-Care Nurses
American Association of Nurse Anesthetists
American Association of Oral and Maxillofacial Surgeons
American College of Cardiology and American Heart Association
American College of Emergency Physicians
American College of Radiology and Society of Interventional Radiology
American Dental Association
American Nurses Association

American Society for Gastrointestinal Endoscopy
American Society of Anesthesiologists
Association of Perioperative Registered Nurses
Centers for Medicare and Medicaid Services
Society of Critical Care Medicine
The Joint Commission
University Health System Consortium

References

1. American Society of Anesthesiologists. Practice guidelines for moderate procedural sedation and analgesia 2018: A Report by the American Society of Anesthesiologists Task Force on Moderate Procedural Sedation and Analgesia, the American Association of Oral and Maxillofacial Surgeons, American College of Radiology, American Dental Association, American Society of Dentist Anesthesiologists, and Society of Interventional Radiology. *Anesthesiology* 2018 Mar;128(3):437–479.

2. American Society of Anesthesiologists. (2017). Advisory on granting privileges for deep sedation to non-anesthesiologist sedation practitioners. Available at: http://www.asahq.org/quality-and-practice-management/standards-guidelines-and-related-resources/advisory-on-granting-privileges-for-deep-sedation-to-non-anesthesiologist-physicians (accessed August 20, 2018).

3. American Society of Anesthesiologists. (2017). Statement on granting privileges to non-anesthesiologist practitioners for personally administering deep sedation or supervising deep sedation by individuals who are not anesthesia professionals. Available at: http://www.asahq.org/quality-and-practice-management/standards-guidelines-and-related-resources/statement-on-granting-privileges-to-nonanesthesiologist-supervising-deep-sedation (accessed August 20, 2018).

4. American Society of Anesthesiologists. (2014). Continuum of depth of sedation: Definition of general anesthesia and levels of sedation/analgesia Available at: http://www.asahq.org/quality-and-practice-management/standards-guidelines-and-related-resources/continuum-of-depth-of-sedation-definition-of-general-anesthesia-and-levels-of-sedation-analgesia (accessed August 20, 2018).

5. American Society of Anesthesiologists. Standards for basic anesthetic monitoring (2014). Available at: http://www.asahq.org/quality-and-practice-management/standards-guidelines-and-related-resources/standards-for-basic-anesthetic-monitoring (accessed August 20, 2018).

6. J. A. Aldrete. The post-anesthesia recovery score revisited. *J Clin Anesth* 1995; 7: 89–91.

7. M. T. Antonelli, D. E. Seaver. Quality, legal, and risk management considerations: Chapter 7. Ensuring program excellence. In: R. Urman, A. D. Kaye. *Moderate and Deep Sedation in Clinical Practice*, 2nd edn. Cambridge University Press, 2017.

8. The Joint Commission. Standards Interpretation. Available at: https://www.jointcommission.org/standards_information/jcfaq.aspx (accessed August 20, 2018).

9. J. Metzner, K. L. Posner, K. B. Domino. The risk and safety of anesthesia at remote locations: The US closed claims analysis. *Curr Opin Anaesthesiol* 2009; 22: 502–8.

10. S. M. Bhananker, K. L. Posner, F. W. Cheney, et al. Injury and liability associated with monitored anesthesia care: A closed claims analysis. *Anesthesiology* 2006; 104: 228–34.

11. American Society of Anesthesiologists. (2014). Statement on safe use of propofol. Available at: http://www.asahq.org/quality-and-practice-management/standards-guidelines-and-related-resources/statement-on-safe-use-of-propofol (accessed August 20, 2018).

12. A. H. Bui, R. D. Urman. Clinical and safety considerations for moderate and deep sedation. *J Med Pract Manage* 2013;29(1):35–41.

13. M. T. Antonelli, D. Seaver, R. D. Urman. Procedural sedation and implications for quality and risk management. *J Healthc Risk Manag* 2013;33(2):3–10.

14. A. J. Pisansky, S. S. Beutler, R. D. Urman. Education and training for nonanesthesia providers performing deep sedation. *Curr Opin Anaesthesiol* 2016.

15. L. Caperelli-White, R. D. Urman. Developing a moderate sedation policy: Essential elements and evidence-based considerations. *AORN J* 2014;99(3):416–30.

16. D. Schilling, A. Rosenbaum, S. Schweizer, et al. Sedation with propofol for interventional endoscopy by trained nurses in high-risk octogenarians: A prospective, randomized, controlled study. *Endoscopy* 2009;41:295–8.

17. K. R. McQuaid, L. Laine. A systematic review and meta-analysis of randomized, controlled trials of moderate sedation for routine endoscopic procedures. *Gastrointest Endosc* 2008;67:910–23.

18. M. R. Jones, S. Karamnov, R. D. Urman. Characteristics of reported adverse events during moderate procedural sedation: An update. *Jt Comm J Qual Patient Saf* 2018 Jul 27.

Chapter 32

Medical Informatics in the Perioperative Period

Ori Gottlieb and Keith J. Ruskin

Contents

Introduction

Although many healthcare providers are familiar with an electronic health record (EHR) and use it routinely, anesthesiologists have a unique understanding of how information is used throughout the perioperative period. Anesthesiologists are responsible for knowing all aspects of the patient's medical history, and therefore review all relevant sections of the patient's chart. Most other medical specialties work with only one portion of the record, review notes and laboratory data and then write a series of recommendations. Radiologists may view the patient's admitting data, read an x-ray, and then dictate a note into the chart. Anesthesiology, however, is one of the most information-intense medical specialties. Anesthesiologists also produce a highly detailed record of the intraoperative course, which may include imaging (from a cardiac echocardiogram or fluoroscopic images of a nerve block), laboratory data (e.g., arterial blood gas analysis), and consultations.

Health information technology is a broad topic, and anesthesia informatics is the subject of large textbooks. However, it is possible to summarize key points of health information technology as they pertain to management of the perioperative suite. This chapter discusses anesthesia information management systems (AIMS) and operating room (OR) information systems, with special attention to benefits, implementation, and obstacles to deployment. It also discusses the Health Insurance Portability and Accountability Act (HIPAA) and Health Information Technology for Economic and Clinical Health (HITECH) regulations and how they impact medical care. Lastly, a brief discussion of communication in the perioperative environment explains how technology can facilitate transmission of important information.

Medical Information Systems

For many years, the medical profession was slow to adopt information technology. While most other industries used computers to track inventory, schedule workers, and bill for products and services, physicians relied on handwritten notes and slips of paper glued into charts. Computers were used mainly for billing and transmitting laboratory results. The first anesthesia information management systems were developed by physicians who were also computer enthusiasts. These early systems were designed for the needs of a specific practice, usually only interfaced with one type of physiologic monitor, and were little more than a record generator. The primary advantages of these early systems were that they relieved the anesthesia provider of the task of writing vital signs down every few minutes and they created a legible replacement of a paper record.

Healthcare professionals and institutions are now rapidly incorporating computer systems into every aspect of medical practice. Information technology is now being rapidly embraced as an aid to OR management. AIMS create a comprehensive, legible record of the patient's course throughout the perioperative period. Scheduling systems are used to manage the flow of patients through the OR, postanesthesia care unit (PACU), and ICUs. Radiofrequency identification technology is used to track patients, equipment, instruments, pharmaceuticals, and blood products.

Medical information systems can provide critical information at the point of care, facilitate communication between healthcare providers, and track outcomes – all of which have the potential to increase efficiency while making patients safer. OR information systems can also integrate information such as guidelines and protocols with patient information, affecting clinician behavior by making specific recommendations. Clinical decision support extends the physician's knowledge base by placing information into context with regard to a specific patient.

Anesthesia Information Management Systems

AIMS are a specialized form of an EHR that automatically collect, store, and present patient data that are gathered during the perioperative period. Modern AIMS are composed of an integrated suite of hardware and software that can interface with a variety of physiologic monitors and anesthesia machines. These systems can usually be interfaced with other hospital information systems, such as a laboratory information systems and the patient's EHR, bringing the comprehensive medical record to the point of care within the perioperative suite. Although most of the functionality of an AIMS involves collecting and storing data from the perioperative period, many systems include a preoperative evaluation module, automated paging capabilities, and many other features.

Benefits of AIMS

The promise of AIMS is to improve patient safety and the quality of care, and these benefits are beginning to be realized. The Anesthesia Patient Safety Foundation stated over a decade ago that the Foundation "endorses and advocates the use of automated record keeping in the perioperative period and the subsequent retrieval and analysis of the data to improve patient safety" [1]. Although AIMS are costly and complex to implement and maintain, their advantages are rapidly becoming apparent and these systems are likely, with financial "encouragement" from government agencies, to become a de facto standard of care.

The adoption of AIMS has been accelerating over the past several years. Although fewer than 10 percent of ORs were estimated to have an AIMS installed in 2007 [2], a more recent survey reveals that 24 percent of ORs had installed a system by 2010, with 13 percent in the process of installation and another 13 percent actively evaluating a system [3]. There are several reasons for this rapid growth in the number of planned and installed AIMS, including patient safety, quality management, economic factors, research facilitation, education, and compliance with government regulations. Given the density of information generated by modern physiologic monitors, AIMS are the only practical way to collect and interpret all of the data generated during the perioperative period.

National organizations whose purpose is to analyze perioperative data to detect ways to improve quality and outcomes, such as the National Surgical Quality Improvement Program, Multicenter Perioperative Outcomes Group, and the Anesthesia Quality Institute (AQI), depend upon receiving data in digital form. This information, as well as that analyzed by institutional QI committees, can help to identify areas in which patient care can be improved. This information can also be used for maintenance of board certification: The American Board of Anesthesiology offers credit as part of its MOCA 2.0 program to physicians who develop and implement an improvement plan based on data from national quality data registries or patient feedback surveys.

Benefits to individual patients include an accessible and legible record that is integrated into the EHR and available to the care team at the point of care. Dexter et al. were able to significantly reduce waiting and nil per os times of children undergoing endoscopic procedures by analyzing information from an OR information system and applying a statistical model for case scheduling [4].

The AIMS can provide decision support and enhance compliance with guidelines such as those of the Surgical Care Improvement Project and pay-for-performance measures [5]. In an outpatient surgery center, a new antibiotic prophylaxis form combined with prebuilt order sets improved compliance with timely antibiotic administration to over 90 percent while saving an estimated $8,500 per year in pharmacy costs [6]. An AIMS developed by the Massachusetts General Hospital and Vanderbilt University, and General Electric's Centricity, incorporates modules that prompt users to administer an antibiotic prior to surgical incision and then document compliance [7], which has been shown to decrease surgical infection rate [8]. In addition, AIMS can generate alerts for drug interactions or patient allergies, decreasing the possibility of an adverse event. Lastly, a recent study suggests that automated reminders can reduce the frequency of prolonged gaps in blood pressure management during surgical procedures [9]. Economics is an important factor in the decision to implement perioperative information management systems, and in many cases, drives the choice of a specific product. The OR is one of the largest revenue streams within most healthcare institutions, and managers can use information generated from AIMS and OR information systems to track outcomes, scheduling and operational efficiency, and, and formulate strategic plans. Most payers now require electronic documentation of patient encounters as a condition of reimbursement for healthcare services, a significant motivator in the decision to purchase an AIMS.

The primary financial benefits of an AIMS include a reduction in drug costs, improved charge capture, reduced staffing costs, and improved OR and scheduling efficiency. The AIMS probably do not decrease anesthesia time [10], but they can improve OR turnover and scheduling efficiency. Epstein et al. were able to infer a patient's correct room location using vital signs transmitted from a monitor to the AIMS, something that could not be done using an AIMS or OR information management system alone. This enabled them to efficiently track patients as they moved, for example, from a block room to the OR for an orthopedic procedure [9]. By analyzing aggregate data, it is possible to determine actual mean procedure durations for specific surgeons, which can make scheduling ORs more efficient. In one novel application of real-time data analysis, a group of electrical engineers was able to interpret multichannel audio and video recordings to detect the specific phase of surgery. The authors postulate that their technique may be used to automatically detect adverse events [11]. Although this technique remains to be validated and implemented, the use of real-time data analysis is an intriguing possibility.

An AIMS has the potential to offer a significant return on investment through increased payments (and avoidance of withheld payments) from Physician Quality Reporting System initiatives, improved charge capture, and better documentation. At the University of Chicago, the procedural team and anesthesia team automatically receive a page when the preoperative workup is complete and the room is ready to receive the patient. The AIMS can also automatically search for missing documentation and alert the appropriate provider. At the Massachusetts General Hospital, customized software written for the AIMS automatically identifies missing procedure attestations and alerts the appropriate provider. This system has significantly increased collection of appropriate physician fees for services that had previously not been reimbursed [12].

An AIMS can facilitate clinical research through a large patient database that can be queried in order to find ways to improve clinical practice. Many healthcare payers are beginning to offer incentives to institutions that benchmark their care to determine the incidence of complications and the quality of their patient outcomes. This process will likely become a de facto requirement within the next few years. The AQI is a nonprofit foundation that was created by the American Society of Anesthesiologists to maintain a comprehensive, national clinical outcomes registry. The AQI relies on AIMS to provide the clinical information needed to objectively evaluate anesthesia practice patterns and ultimately improve patient care. At the present time, the AQI is using this information to provide benchmarking information to participating practices.

Implementation of an AIMS

Despite their benefits, there are significant obstacles to the adoption of an AIMS. Specific challenges include adapting preexisting workflows to the new system, training providers, device integration, creating downtime procedures, and tracking errors in charting and billing that may occur during the transition. Many healthcare professionals view the implementation of information technology as a goal in and of itself, but successful adaption of an EHR or other information system requires a fundamentally different approach. Information systems should be viewed as a solution to a specific problem or as a way to meet a defined goal. Before choosing a system, it is critically important to identify the problems that must be solved or the needs that must be met. This will make it possible to identify a solution that meets these exact needs.

The cost of installing and maintaining a system is substantial, and includes the "upfront" charges for hardware and software, the costs of customizing the product, and ongoing support and maintenance. This cost has been estimated to be as high as $4,000–6,000 per OR and between $14,000 and $45,000 for installation of a server [13]. The return on investment depends upon the financial and management practices at each institution, but usually includes improvements in scheduling, decreased drug costs, improved charge capture, and improved coding.

Because of the high cost of installation, a healthcare institution may choose an AIMS as part of the purchase of a larger information system. The benefits to the institution of choosing such a system include compatibility with other parts of the EHR, and possibly a discounted price. The system chosen by the hospital may, however, not be the ideal one for the practice model. Often, a hospital may choose a particular EHR to purchase and implement without considering the capabilities of that system's anesthesia module. The anesthesiologists who will be using the system must therefore be involved with all aspects of the purchase and implementation. An AIMS does not simply replace a paper chart with an electronic one; successful adoption of this complex system requires substantial changes in workflow.

During the purchase process, the initial focus is almost exclusively on clinical implementation, but it is essential to plan for how the product will be used, which types of reports are required, and how the existing workflow integrates with the system. Consideration should be given to the functionality that will be required (e.g., preoperative evaluation or postanesthesia care unit documentation), the variety of anesthetizing locations at which workstations must be installed, support services that will be provided after the initial deployment, and initial and ongoing training for users. Maintenance and system upgrades should also be considered, as should backups of the data and the purchase of redundant hardware to minimize downtime in the event of a system failure.

It is important for the anesthesia department to identify a clinical champion who will work with the vendor during the initial design and customization. The champion should have a background in both clinical anesthesia and information technology and work with the vendor and healthcare institution information services personnel to facilitate all stages of implementation [14]. S/he should create a committee of advisors and super users representing the different interests and sections of the department. A comprehensive plan should be outlined and distributed to all members of the department well in advance of the scheduled implementation. This plan should include the strategy that will be used for the "go-live" ("Big Bang" or a phased implementation), as well as a training schedule and a contingency plan that will be implemented in the event of a system failure [13].

If the goal of purchasing an AIMS is to produce a paper printout of an anesthesia record at the end of an anesthetic, this functionality is likely to be available "out of the box." Reports that have been built into the software are usually generic in nature, however, and generally do not include custom elements have been added to the database. If the goal of implementing an AIMS is to archive electronic medical records, push and pull information to and from an institutional EHR, track drug usage, or create customized reports, then additional resources and planning will be required, and this will incur additional planning, time, and costs. It is not uncommon to discover that the system does not produce reports that the physicians or institution consider to be essential. Technical or licensing restrictions may not even permit the data to be directly accessible. It is therefore imperative that all of the anticipated requirements be carefully thought out and clearly specified in the request for proposal. Additional items that should be considered include "paging modules" that will allow staff to be notified at specific milestones, integration with hospital, laboratory, pharmacy, and staffing systems, and the ability to interface with a billing system.

The new system and changes in workflow are a distraction that may temporarily impede patient care. Moreover, the presence of a computer on the anesthesia gas machine may tempt personnel to use it for online shopping, catching up on email, or other extraneous purposes during periods of low workload. Although there are no studies of how computer use affects anesthesia care in the OR, a recent study may provide clues. Observers found that anesthesia providers read books or magazines during periods of low workload in 35 percent of cases. Although vigilance did not appear to be impaired, performance of manual tasks, record keeping, and interacting with others was decreased [15]. It seems logical that implementing a new, unfamiliar system would have a similar effect. In addition, texting, calling, browsing, and other nonmedical use of digital technology can be tracked and would be deemed discoverable and admissible in a legal complaint. Inappropriate use can be minimized through the implementation of "appropriate use" policies, content filters, and education.

Security and Patient Confidentiality

HIPAA and HITECH

The HIPAA of 1996 was enacted to protect workers and their families from losing healthcare insurance coverage when they change or lose a job. Title

II of HIPAA required the establishment of national standards for exchanging healthcare information and for the creation of a national identifier for healthcare providers, institutions, and insurers. The HIPAA also established sweeping requirements for the security and privacy of health information. These requirements are meant to improve the efficiency of healthcare by facilitating electronic data interchange between healthcare providers, payers, and governmental agencies. Although HIPAA has fundamentally changed the healthcare infrastructure in the United States, most physicians are aware of HIPAA because of the Privacy Rule.

The HIPAA Privacy and Security Rules define protected health information (PHI) as any information that is held by a healthcare provider, a payer, or their business associates that concerns health status, medical treatment, or insurance payments and that can be linked to a specific individual. This has been broadly interpreted to cover a patient's entire medical record. The Security Rule describes three types of safeguards that must be put into place by "covered entities." *Administrative safeguards* describe how a covered entity will comply with the rules and include policies and procedures that govern the protection and use of PHI. These policies are developed and enforced by a privacy officer. *Physical safeguards* cover all aspects of the hardware and software used to store PHI. These rules mandate that access to computers be limited only to authorized personnel and that access be closely monitored and controlled. Computers or devices (such as a laptop or tablet computer) that store PHI must be protected against unauthorized use. In general, storing PHI on a personal device should be discouraged because of the possibility that it could be lost or stolen. *Technical safeguards* cover the security of PHI as it is transmitted from one entity to another. Health information must be encrypted when transmitted over an open network (e.g., the Internet). Before information is transmitted, both parties must authenticate each other, either by a password system (if computers are used) or by a telephone call-back (for a conversation).

HITECH was enacted as part of the 2009 American Recovery and Reinvestment Act and gives the US Department of Health and Human Services the authority to establish a set of programs, incentives, and penalties for adoption and use of certified EHR systems (see www.cms.gov/EHRIncentivePrograms/). The requirements of HITECH build upon the HIPAA regulations, which deal primarily with electronic data interchange, security, and privacy. The HITECH regulations cover content of the record, quality management, and transmission of health information. The Centers for Medicare and Medicaid Services (CMS) has proposed a set of requirements for "meaningful use" of electronic records in five areas under HITECH:

- improve quality, safety, and efficiency, and reduce health disparities
- engage patients and families in their healthcare
- improve care coordination
- improve population and public health
- insure adequate privacy and security of health information

The CMS defines a "meaningful EHR user" as a healthcare provider who uses a "certified" EHR for purposes such as order entry or e-prescribing; uses electronic transmission of data for the purposes of healthcare coordination; and submits clinical quality measures to an approved government agency. Healthcare providers who comply with these requirements through 2015 receive a small incentive payment, whereas providers who fail to meet the 2015 deadline for implementation may receive a reduction in Medicare payment as a penalty.

Although no AIMS have been certified as meeting "meaningful use" criteria, many of these systems fulfill the functions required in HITECH. For example, many AIMS offer decision support for items such as perioperative antibiotic administration. In addition, AIMS have the potential to automatically report disease conditions for which registries exist (e.g., malignant hyperthermia). They also meet many of the goals for quality, safety, and efficiency. Those AIMS that use accepted standards, such as SNOMED or HL-7, may allow devices to communicate with each other and with other AIMS. An AIMS can record vascular access or regional anesthesia techniques performed using ultrasound guidance, or transesophageal echocardiography utilized during cardiac surgery. The Epic EHR (Epic, Verona, Wisconsin, USA) has a feature called "Care Everywhere," which allows a healthcare provider to access patient records that were created at other institutions that use Epic.

Communication in the OR

Anesthesiologists work in a dynamic environment in which information critical to patient care must be quickly and accurately exchanged. Cellular telephones, tablets, laptops, and other electronic tools can improve patient care by providing rapid access to vital information from any location. Effective communication has been shown to be a critical component of safety in high-risk environments. Failure to convey information quickly and accurately has been shown to be a root cause of medical errors; one study found that communication failures were the second most prevalent cause of medical errors [16]. Reliable information technology tools are critical to patient safety in the perioperative environment. Ideally, a core communication infrastructure should be created that is compatible with new devices. In many cases, such a system can be installed using readily available equipment.

Voice Communication

A variety of options are available to facilitate voice communication within a hospital or other healthcare institution. Besides cell phone signal repeaters making intrahospital use possible, WiFi networks can be used to carry voice conversations. Voice-over Internet Protocol has become a common alternative to traditional telephone service. Either generic or specialized systems can be installed in the healthcare environment. These advantages, combined with the low cost and wide availability of WiFi equipment, make this technology well suited for many healthcare applications.

Paging and Text Messaging

Many communications experts recommend that healthcare institutions retain paging systems to transmit extremely urgent information. Despite their "one-way," asynchronous nature, paging systems do offer several advantages: they allow a simple message (e.g., a "Code Blue" page) to be conveyed simultaneously to a group of people. If the paging transmitter is in the hospital, messages can be sent very quickly. If, however, a commercial paging service is used, the latency period is specified in the terms of service and may allow up to an hour for a message to be sent out.

Some OR management systems include modules that can automatically alert specific members of the care team when certain milestones are reached, sending a message to the transport service to bring the next patient to the OR when the previous patient is transferred to the PACU, for example. This has the potential to improve OR efficiency. In one study, an AIMS automatically paged the attending

anesthesiologist if allergy information had not been entered into the medical record. This significantly decreased the incidence of incomplete charts [17]. Clinical alerting systems that automatically send laboratory results to alphanumeric pagers have been shown to improve patient care and are installed in a growing number of hospitals [18]. Epstein et al. have developed an automated staff recall system that uses short text messages and is accessible from an AIMS. In the event of a mass casualty incident, such a system can potentially reduce the amount of time required for a hospital to mount a response [19].

Advanced Communication Tools

The advent of low-cost tablet computers combined with high-speed WiFi networks has resulted in the development of systems that provide unprecedented access to information. The Department of Anesthesiology at Vanderbilt University has designed a comprehensive information management and documentation suite called the Vanderbilt Perioperative Information Management System. This system integrates data from physiologic monitors, the hospital information system, and in-room video cameras. This information is presented to anesthesiologists throughout the institution and can be accessed from laptop computers, desktop computers, display boards in the perioperative suite, and tablet computers [20].

Summary

Implementation of a comprehensive information technology program in the OR can improve patient care while maximizing efficiency and helping to capture reimbursement for services. Anesthesiologists have a unique understanding of how information flows through the hospital, and have historically been at the forefront of initiatives to improve patient safety. Using an AIMS in the perioperative period can facilitate efficient scheduling, improve patient care by providing access to critical information, and create a legible record that is available throughout the healthcare institution. Ever more widespread is the ability to make these records available to perioperative physicians at whichever care center the patient chooses (or finds him/herself needing care). A well-thought-out communication infrastructure can also improve patient safety by allowing patient information, reference materials, or clinical guidelines to be sent to the point of care. Modern communication tools also allow anesthesiologists to convey information to each other without leaving the patient's bedside. The discipline of anesthesia informatics is relatively new, but it has the potential to make dramatic improvements to the practice of perioperative medicine.

References

1. *American Patient Safety Foundation Newsletter* 2001; 16: 49.

2. R. H. Epstein, M. M. Vigoda, D. M. Feinstein. Anesthesia information management systems: A survey of current implementation policies and practices. *Anesth Analg* 2007; 105: 405–11.

3. T. L. Trentman, J. T. Mueller, K. J. Ruskin, B. N. Noble, C. A. Doyle. Adoption of anesthesia information management systems by US anesthesiologists. *J Clin Monit Comput* 2011; 25: 129–35.

4. B. Smallman, F. Dexter. Optimizing the arrival, waiting, and NPO times of children on the day of pediatric endoscopy procedures. *Anesth Analg* 2010; 110: 879–87.

5. D. B. Wax, Y. Beilin, M. Levin, N. Chadha, M. Krol, D. L. Reich. The effect of an interactive visual reminder in an anesthesia information management system on timeliness of prophylactic antibiotic administration. *Anesth Analg* 2007; 104: 1462–6, table of contents.

6. C. C. Braxton, P. A. Gerstenberger, G. G. Cox. Improving antibiotic stewardship: Order set implementation to improve prophylactic antimicrobial prescribing in the outpatient surgical setting. *J Ambul Care Manage* 2010; 33: 131–40.

7. B. Rothman, W. S. Sandberg, P. St Jacques. Using information technology to improve quality in the OR. *Anesthesiol Clin* 2011; 29: 29–55.

8. J. J. Stulberg, C. P. Delaney, D. V. Neuhauser, D. C. Aron, P. Fu, S. M. Koroukian. Adherence to surgical care improvement project measures and the association with postoperative infections. *JAMA* 2010; 303: 2479–85.

9. J. M. Ehrenfeld, R. H. Epstein, S. Bader, S. Kheterpal, W. S. Sandberg. Automatic notifications mediated by anesthesia information management systems reduce the frequency of prolonged gaps in blood pressure documentation. *Anesth Analg* 2011; 113: 356–63.

10. J. Balust, A. Macario. Can anesthesia information management systems improve quality in the surgical suite? *Curr Opin Anaesthesiol* 2009; 22: 215–22.

11. T. Suzuki, Y. Sakurai, K. Yoshimitsu, K. Nambu, Y. Muragaki, H. Iseki. Intraoperative multichannel audio-visual information recording and automatic surgical phase and incident detection. *Conf Proc IEEE Eng Med Biol Soc* 2010; 2010: 1190–3.

12. S. F. Spring, W. S. Sandberg, S. Anupama, J. L. Walsh, W. D. Driscoll, D. E. Raines. Automated documentation error detection and notification improves anesthesia billing performance. *Anesthesiology* 2007; 106: 157–63.

13. J. M. Ehrenfeld, M. A. Rehman. Anesthesia information management systems: A review of functionality and installation considerations. *J Clin Monit Comput* 2011; 25: 71–9.

14. W. S. Sandberg. Anesthesia information management systems: Almost there. *Anesth Analg* 2008; 107: 1100–2.

15. J. M. Slagle, M. B. Weinger. Effects of intraoperative reading on vigilance and workload during anesthesia care in an academic medical center. *Anesthesiology* 2009; 110: 275–83.

16. M. T. Kluger, M. F. Bullock. Recovery room incidents: A review of 419 reports from the Anaesthetic Incident Monitoring Study (AIMS). *Anaesthesia* 2002; 57: 1060–6.

17. W. S. Sandberg, E. H. Sandberg, A. R. Seim, et al. Real-time checking of electronic anesthesia records for documentation errors and automatically text messaging clinicians improves quality of documentation. *Anesth Analg* 2008; 106: 192–201, table of contents.

18. E. G. Poon, G. J. Kuperman, J. Fiskio, D. W. Bates. Real-time notification of laboratory data requested by users through alphanumeric pagers. *J Am Med Inform Assoc* 2002; 9: 217–22.

19. R. H. Epstein, A. Ekbatani, J. Kaplan, R. Shechter, Z. Grunwald. Development of a staff recall system for mass casualty incidents using cell phone text messaging. *Anesth Analg* 2010; 110: 871–8.

20. P. St Jacques, B. Rothman. Enhancing point of care vigilance using computers. *Anesthesiol Clin* 2011; 29: 505–19.

33

Simulation as a Tool to Improve Patient Safety

Valeriy Kozmenko, Lyubov Kozmenko, Melvin Wyche III, and Alan David Kaye

Patient safety is one of the most pressing challenges of the modern healthcare system. According to the Agency for Healthcare Research and Quality (AHRQ) report, "as many as 44,000 to 98,000 people die in U.S. hospitals each year as the result of lapses in patient safety" [1]. Patient safety is a multifactorial problem that requires attention on multiple levels including individual, team, unit/section, and the organization as a whole. Procedural skills competency, critical thinking and effective team communication are the important contributing factors that affect quality of patient care and safety in the clinical environment. As many other complex behaviors, these skills are best learned in the immersive clinical environment. Simulation is an ideal tool to teach clinical skills since it does not put a real patient to danger, allows for simulation of frequently occurring and rare conditions, and provides standardized teaching and learning experience in a reliable and repeatable manner. There are multiple simulation modalities, such as high-fidelity simulation (HFS), skills, standardized patient, virtual reality, combined and hybrid, and screen-based simulation, that can be used to identify patient safety gaps in healthcare delivery system and effectively address the problem. Simulation training can be conducted either in the real clinical environment (in situ simulation) or at the simulation center. Both methods are acceptable and have their advantages and disadvantages.

In situ simulation creates what is called mixed-reality immersive environment where real medical equipment can be used in conjunction with high fidelity and other simulation modalities. Since the trainees operate in the accustomed environment, they are quickly immersed into the scenario and engaged in a dynamic interaction with each other and the simulator. Conducting in situ HFS could reveal organizational breaches in patient safety. For example, when Louisiana State University Health Sciences Center in New Orleans conducted a series of team training sessions at a rural hospital, running a malignant hyperthermia scenario revealed the fact that there was not a designated freezer with cold IV fluids that must be used in that life-threatening medical condition [2]. Having training done at the site of daily work makes trainee scheduling easier; however, it creates a challenge of making clinical space available for the activity that does not involve real patient care. Transportation of simulation equipment to the site of training is another challenge. Also, bringing simulated clinical equipment such as defibrillators, patient monitors, as well as simulated medications to the point of patient care can potentially compromise patient safety if erroneously used in place of the real ones. Thus, all simulated equipment and supplies should be properly marked and stored if used for in situ training.

Conducting simulation in the setting of a simulation center has its own advantages such as no need to move simulation equipment, the possibility of using higher fidelity stationary simulators such as Medical Education Technologies Human Patient Simulator than its portable versions that have lower realism, the availability of the AV equipment for recording trainings with it following use during debriefing, etc. Since the training is done outside of the busy clinical environment, it is easier to schedule as many simulation sessions as needed. Usually, simulation centers have designated space for debriefing. On the other side, some trainees might find the simulation center setting quite different from the real clinical environment with different brands of mechanical lung ventilators, anesthesia machines, and surgical and other equipment, which can make translation of newly learned skills from simulated classroom to real life patient care more difficult. Several studies have shown that clinical experts are less prone to distraction by physical appearance of the simulator and adjust more easily to different training environments by more effective sorting out relevant and irrelevant

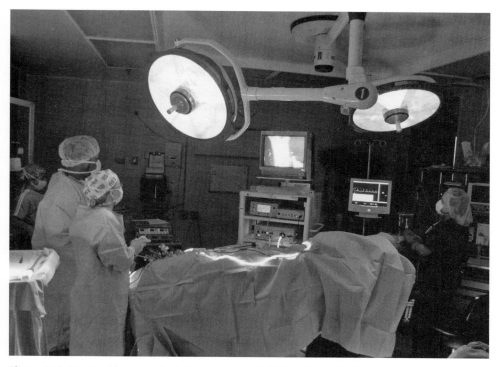

Figure 33.1 Simulated laparoscopic cholecystectomy at Earl K. Long Hospital in Baton Rouge, Louisiana.

information than novices. They more easily translate newly learned skills and acquired knowledge from simulated to clinical environment. Less experienced participants usually go through the initial subconscious rejection as a defense mechanism to justify their less than optimal performance during simulation. Developing teaching and learning objectives and setting simulation training requires taking into account the participants' level of expertise to ensure that the training is effective and well received. Immersing participants into a challenging clinical scenario without putting their self-esteem under stress makes their engagement easier and helps with suspending disbelief.

Regardless, whether the training is performed at the point of the patient care or in the academic environment, each simulation session should have clearly defined learning objectives and critical performance indicators that would allow to measure outcomes. They will help with the evaluation of the trainees' performances and gauge whether the skills have been learned and successfully used. For example, Louisiana State University Health Sciences Center has created and successfully conducted multiple team training

courses and has received several grants funded by the AHRQ and the National League of Nursing to train practicing operating room (OR) staff, medical and nursing students, and residents from different fields of healthcare on how to effectively communicate in a stressful dynamic clinical environment. See Figure 33.1.

All simulation courses were administered in the same fashion. Each training session started with a brief introduction, setting ground rules for the course and providing an orientation on how to interact with the simulator. The trainees were instructed to treat the simulator as a real patient and act as they would act in a real life situation. Using an LSU-patented proprietary technology, called "Clinical Model," greatly enhanced the realism of the simulation. See Figure 33.2.

To administer training, after the 10 to 15-min orientation, the first 40–45-min scenario was conducted and followed with a focused facilitated debriefing. Participants were encouraged to reflect on the events of the simulation and their relation to relevant individual and team behaviors and actions. These reflections were then linked to specific teamwork competencies. Video replay was used during

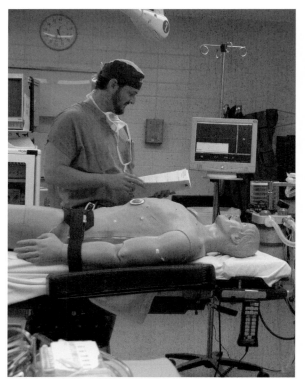

Figure 33.2 Patient interview before the surgical procedure in the OR at Earl K. Long Hospital in Baton Rouge, Louisiana.

the debriefing to illustrate key concepts and to promote team discussion. During the debriefing, the instructor facilitated the discussion in such a way that the following principles of an effective team communication were learned:

1. Flattened hierarchy to encourage sharing information between the team members
2. Role clarity
3. Cross monitoring
4. Anticipatory response
5. Closed loop communication
6. Situational awareness
7. Shared mental model
8. Mental rehearsal
9. Open communication

The authors' data collected during AHRQ-funded 2-year-long simulation training course demonstrated that the trainees perceived HFS training as highly realistic and useful (Table 33.1).

All other team training courses to improve patient safety were conducted in a similar fashion and collected data confirmed that this method of training was highly effective regardless of the trainee's level of clinical expertise.

Multiple studies have shown the ability of simulation to improve participants' knowledge and skills immediately after training but they would not be retained for more than six months if training was not repeated. Multiple exposures to the problem and training are required to enhance retention. Busy clinician's schedules and high cost of HFS [3] are the limiting factors in using HFS as a method to improve skills retention. Screen-based simulators, such as "Anesthesia Simulator" (Anesoft Inc) developed by Dr. Howard Schwid [4], can be repeatedly used after mannequin-based simulation and prevent knowledge and skills degradation over time. See Figure 33.3.

Maintaining healthcare providers' procedural competencies with the use of simulation is another way to improve patient safety. The University of South Dakota Sanford School of Medicine in conjunction with Sanford Children's Boekelhide Intensive Care Unit conducted a study to evaluate neonatal nurse practitioners' procedural skills [5]. During the study, the investigators examined correlation between the actual procedural competencies assessed with validated checklists and the subjective "perceived competencies" evaluated with the 360-degree surveys. The study demonstrated no correlation between providers' "perceived competencies" (i.e., how the providers and their peers subjectively perceive their competency in performing given procedural skills) and their actual performances. This emphasizes the need for and importance of objective evaluation of the healthcare providers' skills with the use of validated tools rather than relying on the results of the self-confidence surveys.

Summary

Simulation appears to be a useful tool for identifying and closing gaps in patient safety. It can help with team building, teaching effective communication skills, validating competencies for various procedural skills and education for potentially life-threatening situations. With appropriate session design, simulation will be perceived by participants as realistic and will ensure

Table 33.1 System for Teamwork Effectiveness and Patient Safety Training Module Questionnaire

Item	Post-training questions			
	Response	Frequency/ percentage	Mean	SD
Training features				
The training session was conducted in a setting that was convenient for me	1	0/0	5.553	.829
	2	1 / 2.1		
	3	1 /2.1		
	4	1 /2.1		
	5	12 / 25.5		
	6	32/ 68.1		
The training module fit well within my regular workday schedule	1	0/0	5.319	1.044
	2	2 /4.3		
	3	1 /2.1		
	4	5 /10.6		
	5	11 /23.4		
	6	28 / 59.6		
Authenticity of the training environment and simulation scenarios				
The physical setting of the training was realistic	1	0/0	5.425	.773
	2	0/0		
	3	1 /2.1		
	4	5/10.6		
	5	14/ 29.8		
	6	27/57.4		
Patient scenarios reflected realistic situations that teams might face in the OR	1	0/0	5.59	.717
	2	0/0		
	3	1/ 2.1		
	4	3/6.4		
	5	10/21.3		
	6	32/70.2		
Scenarios were effective for examining teamwork and patient safety practices	1	0/0	5.744	.440
	2	0/0		
	3	0/0		
	4	0/0		
	5	12/25.5		
	6	35/74.5		
During scenarios, I momentarily forgot about simulation and acted as if the situation were real	1	2/ 4.3	4.936	1.186
	2	0/0		
	3	2/4.3		
	4	8/17.0		
	5	18/38.3		
	6	17/36.2		

(continued)

Table 31.1 (*Cont.*)

Item	Post-training questions			
	Response	Frequency/ percentage	Mean	SD
The composition of the OR team reflected what I experience in the real life setting	1	0/0	5.55	.717
	2	0/0		
	3	0/0		
	4	6/12.8		
	5	9/19.1		
	6	32/66.7		
Training effectiveness				
I would benefit from participating in future training like today's session	1	0/0	5.48	.804
	2	0/0		
	3	0/0		
	4	9/19.1		
	5	6/12.8		
	6	32/68.1		

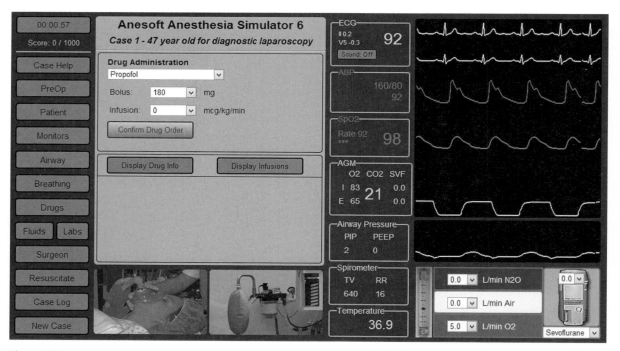

Figure 33.3 Anesthesia simulator.

Image courtesy of Anesoft, Inc., with permission to use.

translation of the knowledge and skills from simulated environment to patient care.

References

1. Patient safety. www.nlm.nih.gov/medlineplus/patientsafety.html

2. Evaluation of the System for Teamwork Effectiveness and Patient Safety (STEPS), S. W. Chauvin, Principal Investigator. (2006). Agency for Healthcare Research and Quality, Grant # U18 HS016680-01.

3. Gaba D, McIntosh C (2006). Simulation: What does it really cost? International Meeting for Society in Simulation in Healthcare.

4. Anesthesia Simulator 6. http://anesoft.com/shop.aspx?p=13862&k=Anesthesia-Simulator-6

5. Kozmenko V, Lubbers L, Messier S (2017). Clinical skills validation through simulation to improve patient safety, International Congress of Health Workforce Education and Research, Porto, Portugal.

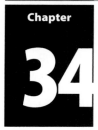

Chapter

34

Education in Operating Room Management

Sanjana Vig, Steven D. Boggs, Richard D. Urman, and Mitchell H. Tsai

Introduction

Operating rooms (ORs) are the most cost intensive area of a hospital system. They also provide the largest source of hospital income and profitability. With the current changes in healthcare – diminished reimbursement, tighter margins, a movement toward accountable care organizations and value-based outcomes – it is imperative that these areas be well managed. Consequently, OR management will assume even greater importance for many institutions.

Ensuring efficiency, maximizing productivity, resolving scheduling conflicts and adapting to last minute changes for clinical and resource demands are all crucial parts of day-to-day OR workflows. OR managers who have practiced for many years will have their clinical experience to draw upon. However, most residents finishing training will be unprepared for all aspects of managing an OR. In truth, there is a growing body of information that both experienced and new anesthesiologists can study to improve their managerial and leadership skills in the OR.

Anesthesia education is regulated by multiple entities. The Accreditation Council for Graduate Medical Education (ACGME) oversees all residency programs and periodically reviews each program before it is recredentialed. The American Society of Anesthesiologists (ASA) has been instrumental in developing new educational content for both anesthesiology trainees and practicing physicians. It is at the forefront of developing new models of care

and tools for anesthesiologists to succeed in their practices. The American Board of Anesthesiologists (ABA) regulates anesthesia training, certification and the overall core curriculum content required residency completion. While the ABA has incorporated some elements of OR and practice management into required training competencies, to date, it has not included a specific curriculum that addresses the required components needed to build a solid foundation in the organizational and business aspects of anesthesia [1].

In this chapter, we review current OR practices and future anticipated changes, and present the need for management education. We propose a series of didactics and a sample experiential curriculum, including suggested methods of implementation and assessment of progress, which is aimed toward preparing future anesthesiologists for leadership roles.

While not all residents may choose to become administrators or clinical directors, it is important that they have some exposure to these principles during residency. In much the same way that many do not choose careers in cardiac, obstetric, pediatric, or other subspecialties, exposure and training in those areas is imperative to a well-rounded anesthetic experience. Even without a career in management, understanding the underlying management principles for the entire perioperative process can help all anesthesiologists communicate effectively within, and outside of, the specialty.

Current OR Workflow

OR workflow includes several factors that are triggered days, or even weeks, before a patient actually comes to the hospital or ambulatory surgery center for surgery. It begins when a patient visits a surgeon, interventionalist or proceduralist. During this encounter, both the healthcare provider and patient agree that they need an intervention. The physician can then either book the procedure directly or – depending on institutional arrangements – refer the patient to an anesthesia preoperative clinic (APC). If an APC exists, patients are interviewed there to determine past medical, surgical and anesthetic histories, review medications and allergies, and order appropriate laboratory work and testing. Patients are also given instructions for the day of surgery including medication adjustments, how long to fast, and what time to arrive. This process serves to educate patients about all possible surgical and anesthetic outcomes, including potential complications [2, 3].

Patients are generally scheduled according to various models. In some instances, surgeons have a specific block of time allocated for their cases during the week. This allocation is determined by a surgeon's own utilization history, practice burden, average time needed for each specific case and other historical data. Another model would be open posting [4]. However, this decreases predictability for both surgeons and staff. At most institutions, OR managers employ a mixture of open and block allocations to facilitate patient care.

Nursing or ancillary staff usually calls patients the day prior to remind patients of their preoperative instructions. The day of surgery itself involves checking a patient into the preoperative, or holding area; nursing, anesthesia and surgeon assessment; then, coordinating the activities of the rest of the OR team, namely surgical scrub technicians and OR nurses, in order to determine when the OR is ready to receive the patient and begin care. Coordination of all these processes involves communication across multiple departments, including nursing, anesthesia, surgery, and ancillary staff, usually though a scheduling information technology system. As cases are scheduled they appear on a master list, which can be accessed by all of the appropriate managers. Information is also passed along organically, through phone calls, meetings, and emails.

Parallel to these processes is the OR preparation that occurs behind the scenes. As soon as a case is booked, operating case carts are prepared for each procedure. These carts have all the surgical instruments needed, along with surgeon and case specific tools required for successful completion of a particular procedure. Furthermore, vendors may need to be informed to bring in special equipment/implants.

Anesthesia setup prior to a procedure is also required, including the assessment of anesthesia machine function, the presence of airway equipment specific to each patient, appropriate medications for induction and maintenance of anesthesia, and adequate anesthesia staffing. In private outpatient surgery centers, there is typically one anesthesia provider per room. In academic hospitals, one anesthesia attending may either work in one room by him- or herself, or oversee multiple rooms. When the attending is working with an anesthesia trainee, the coverage ratio is usually one attending to two residents (or two-room supervision); with nurse anesthetists the ratio may go up to 1:4. In addition to providing oversight, the attending is also responsible for teaching residents and assessing their learning on a day-to-day, case-by-case basis. In private practice settings where the anesthesia care team model is used, it is very common to see supervision ratios of anesthesiologist:nurse anesthetist of 1:2 to 1:3 earlier in the day, with 1:4 as the day progresses.

Depending on the institution, current OR managers are anesthesiologists, surgeons or nurses. Anesthesiologists already take part in many areas of perioperative medicine, running preoperative clinics and overseeing postoperative care units (PACU). As a result, they are already familiar with standards of care in each of these environments and also the many roadblocks to process improvement, which may exist in each area [5]. Recent research has shown that OR governance structures change as OR size increases, transitioning from nurse-managed to anesthesia-managed, and ultimately to shared governance in very large departments.

The Future of the OR

Future changes in healthcare involve managed care and bundled payments. In the short term, OR managers will have to do more with presumably fewer resources. This scenario is not dissimilar to the current consolidation in the anesthesiology industry [6, 7]. Ultimately, long-term, sustainable adjustments in perioperative services will have to include increasing patient throughput, optimizing resources, reducing costs, balancing patient safety, and maintaining high quality outcomes [8].

The ASA and other stakeholders have proposed the perioperative surgical home (PSH) as a model [9] to address these changes [10]. The PSH aims to integrate the three phases surrounding surgical care: preoperative, intraoperative, and postoperative, and positions the anesthesiologist at the nexus of this integrative effort. This initiative will serve to broaden the scope of an anesthesiologists practice, encouraging standardization and shared decision making [9]. Per current literature in OR management, the PSH has identified two primary areas of cost reduction, including eliminating unnecessary interventions (e.g., preoperative lab studies; anesthetic medication waste) and optimizing staffing assignments and case scheduling [10].

This integration could mean more nonclinical, or non-OR time for anesthesiologists to allow them to manage the different PSH care pathways. As a consequence, attending anesthesiologists may find themselves with more administrative responsibilities including participating in committee meetings, developing and validating QA/QI processes, and establishing means of effective communication. In essence, the role of an anesthesiologist will shift from clinical decision making to management. Anesthesiologists will no longer be able to claim that basic financial accounting or organizational development and corporate stewardship fall outside of their role. Anesthesiologists will need the administrative know-how of which care points will affect reimbursement and how to optimize those parameters as they are essential to maintaining efficiency and OR operations.

Are We Preparing Residents for These Changes?

According to the ACGME, all programs must clearly delineate educational goals for residents and make these available to all trainees. For example, patient care responsibilities must be clearly outlined, and residents must continually demonstrate the ability to handle patient-centered decisions at an increasingly advanced level as they progress through training. Resident education must include regular didactics and competency based objectives must be achieved [11]. Educational goals must culminate in the ability

Table 34.1 ACGME Core Competencies [11]

Skill	Example
Appropriate patient care and procedural skills	
Experience and exposure to different subspecialty patient care	• Pediatrics • Cardiothoracic anesthesia • Obstetrics • Pain management, etc.

Sufficient medical knowledge, including that related to clinical anesthesia	• Practice-based learning improvement
	• Interpersonal and communication skills
	• Professionalism
	• Systems-based practice
	  • Contract negotiations; billing arrangements
	  • Professional liability
	  • Legislative and regulatory issues;
	  • Fiscal stewardship of health services delivery

Completion of various patient related procedures	• Central lines • Epidurals

of the resident to effectively make clinical decisions and display sound clinical judgment regarding safe and appropriate patient care. Table 34.1 lists specific ACGME required competency skills that residents must attain by the end of their training period.

Per the ACGME listed requirements, at the end of training, residents also "must demonstrate an awareness of and responsiveness to the larger context and system of healthcare, as well as the ability to call effectively on other resources in the system to provide optimal health care" [11]. In an effort to afford residents this broader context of healthcare, rotations of at least two weeks each are required in preoperative medicine and PACUs. In addition, there must be some exposure to diagnostic and therapeutic anesthesia procedures that occur outside of the surgical suite.

There are multiple teaching and learning modalities in residency programs today to help accomplish these core requirements. These include regularly scheduled, training level specific, didactic sessions; simulation laboratory sessions; journal clubs; daily teaching in the OR; and self-guided learning. Progress is assessed at different intervals. For example, upon initially entering clinical anesthesia year one, residents are given an anesthesia knowledge test at day zero (AKT 0) and then again at day thirty (AKT 30). Resident scholarly activities, such as preparing grand round presentations, writing review articles or book chapters, or participating in clinical or scientific investigations, also help with learning assessment. [11]. In addition, all residents are evaluated annually via the anesthesia in-training exam and then upon finishing residency all residents must pass both written and oral board examinations to achieve final certification.

What Does OR Management Entail?

Management/Leadership

There are many differences between management and leadership. In *Sense of Urgency*, Kotter clearly delineates the responsibilities and tasks for managers and leadership. Managers are responsible for concrete tasks of planning, budgeting, staffing, organizing, and problem solving with the goal of creating predictable and stable processes. Leaders, on the other hand, have the more abstract task of maintaining company values, motivating staff, and inspiring change.

This distinction is important to make. Physicians may have good managerial skills (e.g., being organized, solving problems) which they learned during medical training, yet have poor leadership skills. Anesthesiologists involved in creating change should appreciate that both skill sets are necessary and that the key to being an effective manager/leader is the ability to decide when to use each skill set.

Managing an OR requires effort and coordination from various departments in a way that allows efficient, safe and cost-effective surgical procedures to occur. As a result of ongoing healthcare changes, many surgery centers have seen an upswing in their patient numbers, necessitating greater coordination efforts and closer management of daily operations [12].

Various teams are responsible for managing OR staff. The OR charge nurse supervises registered nurses, surgical scrub technicians and unit secretaries. Management of surgical and anesthesia teams involves oversight of attendings, fellows, residents, medical students, physician's assistants, and certified registered nurse anesthetists (CRNAs). Collaboration

Table 34.2 Factors That Contribute to Scheduling and Coordination [12]

Information type	Methods of obtaining information
Patient status	**Information systems**: telephones, pages, house phones, printed documents
Patient room	
Scheduled surgery	
Anesthesia staff status	
Room staff status (e.g., technician, nurse availability)	**Direct observations**: data derived from observations and conversations by nursing managers, anesthesia and surgical staff
Equipment status	
Special needs (equipment/positioning needs)	**Social networks**
Surgeon availability	**OR board**: focal point of collaboration and scheduling efforts.
Pending changes	

amongst all of these teams helps facilitate efficient patient movement within the OR suite [12]. A large part of achieving successful collaborative efforts is the management of human behavior, particularly those of problem physicians, i.e., those with excessive complaints, those who are underproductive and those who are simply difficult to work with.

Data and Decision Making

OR decision making is often based on incomplete or sporadic information. Inappropriate command of information may result in repercussions that propagate inefficiencies throughout the system. As mentioned in "Coordination Challenges in Operating-Room Management: An In-Depth Field Study," the investigators examined an OR suite and determined that several factors contribute to scheduling and coordination, as seen in Table 34.2. In addition, they identified specific components of the OR system and the issues underlying inefficient systems (Table 34.3).

OR Operations

There are multiple goals, listed in Table 34.4, that managers have in regards to OR operations. Aside from these metrics, OR managers must also take care of day-to-day operations, including running the board, making daily staff schedules, and managing acute scheduling changes (e.g., cancellations, add-ons,

Table 34.3 Components of the OR System [12]

Component	Problem areas	Underlying cause
Equipment	Lack of availability; special needs not addressed	Under equipped facility; unaffordability of needed equipment
Information	Inaccuracies in patient status, location or scheduling	Fluctuation in patient status due to illness; unpredictability of scheduling changes
Staff/ satisfaction	Availability/various personality conflicts, political issues	Fixed staffing/ harsh political climate, human nature issues, unprofessional behavior
Scheduling	Unexpected changes to patient status, admissions/ cancellations, case lengths	Unpredictability of medicine.

late starts). Outside of the OR, the manager must also be aware of, and be able to handle, issues surrounding ICU bottlenecks, PACU delays, and non-operating room anesthesia demands (e.g., cardiac catheterization lab), a growing surgical entity.

Accounting/Financial Know-How

When it comes to financial and accounting statements, anesthesiologists need to know what to look for and how to potentially fix any issues [4]. These statements come into play when working with hospital administrators to make decisions regarding the financial needs of the OR. Having basic financial and accounting acumen (e.g., understanding past financial statements, questioning future projections) places anesthesiologists in a unique position. Here, anesthesiologists can give financial input and balance the clinical and safety needs of the patients directly affected by these decisions. See Table 34.5.

Addressing the Knowledge Gap Currently in Place

Comparing ACGME requirements to the practical skills required for administrators, it is apparent that many of the responsibilities OR managers undertake are not addressed during residency training. While residents may be exposed to a certain, usually clinical, components of OR management, such as running the board, a true understanding of the complexities of that role may not be within the purview of their experiences.

A recent survey revealed that residents felt they had adequate exposure in quality management and OR scheduling; however, they did not feel comfortable with concepts related to actual practice management. A few management specific training programs exist across the country (e.g., Stanford, MGH, UCI); but they are at the fellowship level. This curriculum would need to include not only basic OR scheduling but also basic business concepts, such as leadership skills, OR logistics, finance and accounting, organizational development and effective communication across specialties [5]. Obtaining such a skillset differs radically from the didactic programs that are currently the norm.

The goals actually accomplished during training versus what residents will likely need upon entering the workforce are outlined in Table 34.6. Most anesthesiologists are capable of mastering this body of knowledge but additional education and experience are needed to become fully competent in these areas. As a professional society, anesthesiologists should recognize that an inefficient perioperative process can limit the care a hospital can provide and ultimately, endanger the financial viability of an institution [5]. Moving forward, residency directors and hospital administrators should recognize the value anesthesiologists bring to the table.

Teaching the New Curriculum

Our suggestion for bridging this gap is to incorporate a management curriculum into residency training programs. A dedicated didactic series, management rotation, simulation lab to test leadership skills and triage, journal clubs, specific readings, and guest lecturers are all ways to incorporate management framework into established residency teaching. Table 34.7 is a summary of lecture topics that can be incorporated into any residency program. In addition, encouraging resident participation in continuing medical education (CME) courses on management or attending management conferences can also further their exposure and education on the topic.

Online learning modules can supplement lectures and readings. For example, the ABA and American College of Healthcare Executives websites and *Harvard*

Table 34.4 OR Operational Goals [13]

Goal	Description	Method
Reduce cost of supplies	Cost analysis by surgeon and procedure; comparison to national benchmarks and average costs at an institution can help identify areas of improvement	Cost transparency: label supplies with pricing information to increase staff awareness
Efficient block time use	Overall goal is to decrease over- and underutilization	Make adjustments based on surgeon history, case mix, staffing availability and hospital goals for subspecialty practices (BK CHP); release of block time may eliminate underutilization and increase schedule flexibility
Avoid equipment issues	Equipment malfunction or simultaneous scheduling of cases that require the same equipment can lead to delays and disgruntled staff	Regular meetings and scrutiny of the schedule can help uncover scheduling conflicts in regard to equipment use
First case start times	Any delays can hold back the entire schedule in that OR; per Dr. Macario at Stanford SOM, well-functioning ORs should have less than 45 min delay total over an 8-h period	Ensure all pertinent patient information is readily available to practitioners; ensure patients follow preoperative instructions; ongoing communication with OR staff to ensure OR will be ready to receive patient on time
Turnover times	Time between cases used to clean the room and set up for next case; shorter than delays, but lengthy turnovers can create delays	Decreasing turnover times must not outdo time needed for adequate patient care and OR setup (Macario article)

Table 34.5 Different Types of Accounting Statements [14]

Statement	Description
Statement of operations	Describes all revenues, expenses and net profit for a given time
Cash flow	Presents operating, investing, and financing activities, basically summarizing cash receipts and payments for a company at a given time
Statement of changes	Net assets pinpoints the reasons for which changes in a company's value may occur
Balance statement	• Revenue: from patients, research, investments • Expenses: Salaries/benefits, overhead • Operating gain/loss: income earned after expenses paid (i.e., the bottom line) • Excess of revenue over expense: money actually earned from all parts of business or OR

Business Review are potential sources for management articles, cases studies and lecture topics [1].

Fletcher et al. identified an anesthetist's nonclinical technical skills (ANTS), which are imperative to being an effective leader and manager [15]. Yee et al. tested the ANTS system using simulation lab sessions with 27 volunteers. They identified some limitations with this system, in that a participant's assertiveness, assuredness and management of a patient is largely influenced by underlying medical knowledge (see Table 34.8).

They showed that simulation lab evaluations are a reliable and usable measure of nontechnical skills ability [16]. Thus, simulation is another tool of learning and assessment that may be used for management training.

Implementation and Assessment of Curriculum

Implementation

A management rotation designed to introduce this new set of knowledge and ANTS into residency programs would be ideal. A dedicated time for lectures, clinical experience, and learning assessments would allow for the best exposure to the material. However, implementing such a rotation into an already tightly packed training schedule may be difficult. Taking a resident out of the OR for four weeks may create shortfalls when it comes to ACGME-mandated case numbers and conflicts with ensuring case numbers

Table 34.6 Comparison of Current OR Management Teaching to What Is Required in the Workplace

Goals currently accomplished [5]	Workplace duties actually required [5]
Daily management of OR schedule	Oversee management of perioperative services, coordinate, facilitate and manage changes
Planning for patients in pre, intra and postoperative stages of surgery	Collect and analyze data related to quality, performance or cost improvement projects
Strong work ethic to ensure effective and appropriate use of OR resources	Use of conflict resolution techniques as a leader of a multidisciplinary team
Management and oversight of PACU patients	Performance evaluations of perioperative personnel
Work in preoperative clinics	Ensure staff, equipment and supplies are available
	Convey the mission of the organization

and overall OR experience. Integrating specialty rotations with management teaching is another alternative; yet, this may interfere with the already limited subspecialty exposure that is currently required for training completion by the ACGME.

As a compromise, a combination rotation may offer a more viable solution. In this model, residents would partake in a general OR/management rotation wherein there are dedicated OR days and dedicated management days each week. Time outside the OR would be filled with lectures; participation in OR committees; attendance at departmental quality improvement meetings; assistance with tactical or operational scheduling issues; and management of the preoperative clinics and PACUs [1]. This time could also be utilized for resident driven management projects. In reference to the ANTS study discussed earlier, simulation lab sessions can also be utilized to teach leadership, communication, and teamwork.

Implementation of any specialty-specific rotation is not without its financial and structural barriers. Removing a resident from the OR will result in less staffing capacity and a tighter daily schedule [1]. In addition, some attending anesthesiologists may perceive this as an imposed workday or a loss of already limited administrative time. Staff must also be willing participants in giving lectures and serving as mentors to residents while they work on assignments and

projects. Alternatively, a web-based tutorial could serve as a platform to build an OR management rotation for academic programs without the local faculty expertise (Tsai et al.). In short, the whole department must come together in cooperation and support. In fact, a multi-disciplinary effort with the collaboration from nurses and surgeons is required. For instance, if surgeons and nurses are aware that a resident manager exists, then they will be more likely to use that individual as a resource when addressing daily OR scheduling issues. Such exposure will not only provide residents with a better work experience, but will also give the perioperative staff a different management perspective.

Finally, residency directors should recognize that a perioperative management experience shouldn't necessarily be a separate distinct rotation. The leadership concepts and management frameworks can be co-opted into other clinical rotations. For instance, at the University of Vermont Larner College of Medicine, the Department of Anesthesiology redesigned the PACU rotation. At the beginning of the first week, the resident works with the PACU nurses recovering inpatients and outpatients. As the week progresses, the resident assumes clinical responsibilities for all the patients. In the second week, the resident works with the charge PACU nurse staffing and triaging all surgical patients and continues with their clinical oversight (Farhang et al., SEA presentation).

Overall, it is imperative that residents are not seen as just another "pair of hands." While helping start cases, place IVs, give breaks or perform preoperative assessments is important to maintain OR workflow and should always be part of the purview of an effective OR leader, the primary role of the resident should be of a manager [17]. Performing these tasks, then, should not compromise a resident's ability to execute their management responsibilities.

Assessment

Determining learning progress can be accomplished by establishing a set of milestones [11, 18] using ACGME guided standards and benchmarks, for OR management knowledge and skills [19, 20]. Evaluating resident learning styles and empowering them to create their own learning objectives can help facilitate teaching [21]. For example, some trainees may prefer independent learning versus those that are drawn to group projects and collaborative efforts. Assessments can be done in the form of pre- and post-tests using both multiple choice and essay questions. In addition,

Table 34.7 Breakdown and Description of Lecture Topics by Subject Matter [1]

Topic breakdown			Brief description
Management	Basic principles	Definitions	Key terms
		Management vs. leadership	Differences and qualities of each
	OR responsibilities	OR scheduling	Nursing/ancillary/anesthesia shifts
			Surgeon block times
		Daily OR assignments	
		Running the board	Accommodating emergencies and add-ons; adapting to last-minute changes
	OR efficiency	Turnover and first case start times	Methods of measurement and why it's important
		Block time utilizations	Raw vs adjusted
			Over vs under
			Preventing overutilization
	Leadership	Qualities of a good leader	Coordinating with the entire perioperative team; motivating team members
		Effective methods of communication	
		Being a team player	
OR/hospital operations	Workflow	Workflow processes	
		Process redesign, reengineering	
	LEAN	Definition	Understanding of LEAN mindset and culture
	Six Sigma		Definition and understanding
Human resources	Managing human behavior		Maintaining workplace morale, correcting toxic behavior; managing staff across generational gaps; the process of hiring/firing individuals
Finance	Costs versus charges	Different reimbursement/ payment schemes	Medicare/Medicaid; private payers, bundled payments
		Anesthesia billing practices	Importance of accurate charting
			Charge per anesthesia billing unit
		Hospital costs and charges	Cost per minute in OR
			Cost of staffing/overtime
			Medications; anesthesia supplies; surgical equipment
			Cost of unanticipated PACU admissions
			Cost of case cancellations
	Revenue streams	Patient revenue	
		Research revenue	
		Academic revenue	
		Other	
Accounting	Worksheets	Balance sheet	Read statements and make decisions from information available; learn how to use Excel
		Income statement	
		Cash flow statement	

(continued)

Table 34.7 *(Cont.)*

Topic breakdown			Brief description
IT	Data gathering	Advantages	What is possible and what is not regarding data gathering and analysis
		Limitations	
Legal	Contracts	What is negotiable	
		Pitfalls/what to watch out for	
	Insurance coverage	Malpractice	What appropriate coverage should include
		Disability	
Perioperative care	Preoperative clinics	Clinic management	Nursing/ancillary staff; MD staffing; communication across disciplines
		Care pathways	Development and implementation
	PACU	Scheduling	Staffing issues
		Delays	Bed availability; Bottlenecks
	Perioperative surgical home		
	Offsite Care	Endo/IR/cath/MRI	Specific issues related to anesthesia delivery and management outside of the OR
	QA/QI		Importance and function of committees

Clinical responsibilities

- Work with the anesthesiologist in charge
- Assist with acutely evolving clinical situations where requested
- Determine acuity of unplanned/emergency case add-ons
- Make daily OR assignments for the following day – i.e., which resident/attending CRNA is assigned to which cases
- Hold PACU phone, help manage PACU patients
- Help maintain OR flow
- Facilitate patient transitions from preop to OR
- Assist where needed with preop evaluations, IV placements, etc.
- Journal Club readings; assigned articles and book chapters
- Work on a project, namely pertaining to a management process that may be improved and propose a method of implementation.
- Encourage and support attendance at national anesthesia management meetings if trainee shows interest

Table 34.8 ANTS Required for Effective Leadership and Management

Skill category	Category elements
Task management	Planning, preparation, prioritizing, appropriate utilization of resources
Team building	Coordinating teams, communication and exchange of information, assigning tasks according to team member capabilities, team support
Situational awareness	Gathering information, identifying issues and accurately anticipating changes etc.
Decision making	Identifying options, making risk–benefit evaluations decisions

specific assignments can be given to residents to test decision-making processes, (e.g., having residents read actual accounting or financial statements and identify any issues and devise solutions).

Further evaluation of resident management learning can occur in much the same way clinical evaluations occur each day through conversations, the application of the OR management literature, and directed questions. In addition, specific Internet resources geared towards management learning can be used, e.g., the National Patient Safety Foundation provides online certification on patient safety [1]. Resident projects, such as grand rounds presentations and quality improvement projects, can also help facilitate resident learning and also assessment by faculty members. See Table 34.9.

Table 34.9 Summary of Implementation and Assessment [1]

Methods of Implementation		Methods of Assessment	
Didactics	Online modules; Power point presentations	Pre- and post-tests	Before and after rotation or individual lectures
Journal club	Exploration of different management topics in a group discussion setting	Practical assignments	Accounting or finance worksheets – problem solving/decision making
One-on-one teaching	Practical day-to-day learning based on active, ongoing issues	Daily assessment	Assessing daily learning based improvement by anesthesia scheduler
Simulation lab	Leadership training exercises with discussion and feedback afterward	Online certifications	Online exams assessing specific management learning

Results of a Management Curriculum

Many residents may not have any interest in pursuing a career or undertaking an administrative position involving the business aspects of medicine. In much the same way, many residents also are not interested in careers in pediatrics, obstetrics, pain management, or cardiothoracic anesthesia. Yet, the exposure to those clinical and medical concepts is essential to becoming a well-rounded physician anesthesiologist demands that trainees have exposure to these topics. With a rapidly changing healthcare environment, a new line of work is presenting itself to anesthesiologists: perioperative management. In keeping up with this change, residents will also need exposure to this vital aspect of OR.

Even without a focused career in management, residents will need to communicate intelligently and develop rudimentary tactical and operational plans with their colleagues and hospital administrators. Anesthesiologists are already deeply involved with every aspect of a patient's perioperative care. As a result, they are poised to take over management of these areas. Training in the management arena should start early on, namely during residency. Implementing a specific, standardized OR management curriculum would provide a means of preparing residents for the future practice of our specialty.

This chapter is presented from the perspective of an anesthesiologist; however, the majority of managers in a hospital system are not physicians, and, therefore, have very little, if any, understanding of the clinical, operational, and logistical training that future anesthesiologists undergo during residency. After residency, many anesthesiologists find themselves in a dynamic, stressful, different environment, adjusting to new hospital policies, adhering to rules that seemingly have no benefit, and struggling to adapt to the economic changes affecting healthcare. More and more, anesthesiologists are finding it challenging to maintain quality patient care while remaining efficient and abiding by the regulations, and many are at a loss as to what many of these changes mean. The business understanding and management know-how, for many, is simply not there; the knowledge gap is very real. Although few physicians have the time to develop real-world experience, we believe that an OR management curriculum that exposes anesthesiologists in training to a basic knowledge and business concepts is vital. Coupled with the systems-based education of the perioperative process, future anesthesiologists should be invaluable to hospital systems.

References

1. Vig S, Boggs S, Kaye A, Tsai M, Urman R. Creating a standardized operating room management curriculum for anesthesia trainees. *Journal of Medical Practice Management*. 2016.

2. Zambouri A. Preoperative evaluation and preparation for anesthesia and surgery. *Hippokratia*. 2007;11(1):13–21.

3. Whinney C. Perioperative evaluation. January 2009. www.clevelandclinicmeded.com/medicalpubs/diseasemanagement/preventive-medicine/perioperative-evaluation/

4. Carroll C, Juers M, Kent S. *Improving the scheduling of operating rooms at UMass Memorial Medical Center*. Worcester Polytechnic Institute, 2014. https://web.wpi.edu/Pubs/E-project/Available/E-project-030614-144337/unrestricted/Final_OR_Paper.pdf

5. Boggs S, Frost E, Feinleib J. Anesthesiologists as operating room directors: Results of a survey. *International Journal of Anesthetics and Anesthesiology*. 2016;3(1).

6. DiCanio M. Waking up to the consolidating anesthesia marketplace. October 22, 2014. www.beckershospitalreview.com/hospital-management-administration/waking-up-to-the-consolidating-anesthesia-marketplace.html

7. Vaidya A. Frenetic consolidation: The anesthesia market today & where ASCs fit in. February 5, 2016. www.beckersasc.com/anesthesia/frenetic-consolidation-the-anesthesia-market-today-where-ascs-fit-in.html

8. Girotto JA, Koltz PF, Drugas G. Optimizing your operating room: Or, why large, traditional hospitals don't work. *International Journal of Surgery.* 2010;8(5):359–67.

9. Vetter TR, Goeddel LA, Boudreaux AM, Hunt TR, Jones KA, Pittet J-F. The perioperative surgical home: How can it make the case so everyone wins? *BMC Anesthesiology.* 2013;13(1).

10. Dexter F, Wachtel RE. Strategies for net cost reductions with the expanded role and expertise of anesthesiologists in the perioperative surgical home. *Anesthesia & Analgesia.* 2014;118(5):1062–71.

11. www.acgme.org/Portals/0/PFAssets/ProgramRequirements/040_anesthesiology_2016.pdf. February 9, 2015.

12. Plasters CL, Seagull FJ, Xiao Y. Coordination challenges in operating-room management: An in-depth field study. *AMIA Annual Symposium Proceedings.* 2003;2003:524–8.

13. Gamble M. Six cornerstones of operating room efficiency: Best practices for each. January 18, 2013. www.beckershospitalreview.com/or-efficiencies/6-cornerstones-of-operating-room-efficiency-best-practices-for-each.html

14. Bragg S. *Budgeting: The comprehensive guide.* 3rd ed. Accounting Tools, 2014.

15. Fletcher G, Flin R, McGeorge P, Glavin R, Maran N, Patty R. Anaesthetists' non-technical skills (ANTS): Evaluation of a behavioural marker system dagger. *British Journal of Anaesthesia.* 2003;90(5):580–8.

16. Yee B, Naik VN, Joo HS, et al. Nontechnical skills in anesthesia crisis management with repeated exposure to simulation-based education. *Anesthesiology.* 2005;103(2):241–8.

17. Cole DC, Giordano CR, Vasilopoulos T, Fahy BG. Resident physicians improve nontechnical skills when on operating room management and leadership rotation. *Anesth Analg.* 2017 Jan;124(1):300–7.

18. Wachtel RE, Dexter F. Curriculum providing cognitive knowledge and problem-solving skills for anesthesia systems-based practice. *Journal of Graduate Medical Education.* 2010;2(4):624–32.

19. Swing SR, Clyman SG, Holmboe ES, Williams RG. Advancing resident assessment in graduate medical education. *Journal of Graduate Medical Education.* 2009;1(2):278–86.

20. Smith DT, Kohlwes RJ. Teaching strategies used by internal medicine residents on the wards. *Medical Teacher.* 2011;33(12):e697–e703.

21. Marjamaa R, Vakkuri A, Kirvelä O. Operating room management: Why, how and by whom? *Acta Anaesthesiologica Scandinavica.* 2008;52(5):596–600.

Further Reading

Gabriel RA, Gimlich R, Ehrenfeld JM, Urman RD. Operating room metrics score card – Creating a prototype for individualized feedback. *Journal of Medical Systems.* 2014;38(11):144.

Kodali BS, Kim KD, Flanagan H, Ehrenfeld JM, Urman RD. Variability of subspecialty-specific anesthesia-controlled times at two academic institutions. *Journal of Medical Systems.* 2014;38(2):11.

Kodali BS, Kim D, Bleday R, Flanagan H, Urman RD. Successful strategies for the reduction of operating room turnover times in a tertiary care academic medical center. *Journal of Surgical Research.* 2014;187(2):403–11.

Malapero RJ, Gabriel RA, Gimlich R, et al. An anesthesia medication cost scorecard – Concepts for individualized feedback. *Journal of Medical Systems.* 2015;39(5):48.

Peccora CD, Gimlich R, Cornell RP, Vacanti CA, Ehrenfeld JM, Urman RD. Anesthesia report card – A customizable tool for performance improvement. *Journal of Medical Systems.* 2014;38(9):105.

Organizations Dedicated to and Current Overview of Enhanced Recovery After Surgery

Bret D. Alvis, Adam B. King, Matthew D. McEvoy, and Jesse M. Ehrenfeld

Contents

Introduction

Overview of Enhanced Recovery After Surgery

Enhanced Recovery After Surgery (ERAS) protocols were first developed by the ERAS study group to emphasize the quality of recovery patients experienced after surgery [2]. These protocols emphasized a multidisciplinary team working together with the patient at the center using a multicomponent approach to eliminate delays in recovery by focusing on applying evidence-based care and continuous audits of this patient-centered care model [2]. In Europe and the UK, the concept and principles of ERAS have become a large part of their surgical care, including support from the National Health System [3]. In the United States, the American Society for Enhanced Recovery (ASER) and the Evidence-Based Perioperative Medicine society partnered to incorporate ERAS into a larger field of perioperative medicine [3].

Rational for ERAS

Bringing standardized practice with minimal physiologic disruption is the key rationale for implementing ERAS pathways throughout the perioperative care arc. Each component of the care pathway is evaluated with the goal of bringing evidence-based practice to the outpatient clinic, preoperative unit, operating room (OR), postoperative recovery unit, hospital ward, and finally to the discharge destination of home/care center. Agreement on the end points of management should be reach prior to implementation, as

this is critical to program success [2]. In Europe and the UK, each surgical ward gets its own unique focus, personnel, and specialists. While not an original goal of ERAS in its initial development by the ERAS study group, reduction in a patient's length of hospitalization (LOS) in an important goal and well published result of ERAS protocol implementations [1–5]. There are several case–control studies that demonstrate a 3-day reduction in LOS after the initiation of ERAS pathways for various surgical procedures [6–18] Two day hospital stays after sigmoid resections [2], a 1 to 2 day reduction in length of stay after elective colorectal procedures [4, 19, 20], a 1-day reduction after liver surgery [21], and 4-day reductions in LOS after gynecologic surgery have been reported [13]. All are examples of the LOS benefits that have been demonstrated with the implementation of ERAS pathways. In addition to reductions in LOS, Sarin et al. demonstrated a 30-day all-cause readmission rate decrease of 11.6 percent [19]. Reductions in LOS and readmissions rates may be due to decreases in perioperative complications rates associated with implementation of ERAS pathways. There is strong evidence that the reduction in complication rates can be up to 50 percent when ERAS principles are utilized with colorectal surgery [2].

Adherence to the ERAS protocols is very important to the effectiveness of the protocol at reducing these complications [2]. It is not surprising that the literature suggests that higher compliance to a developed ERAS protocol is strongly associated with lower complication rates, LOS, readmission rates, and mortality [22, 23]. Gustafsson et al. in 2016 demonstrated that when the colorectal ERAS protocol had a 70 percent compliance, mortality fell by 42 percent when compared to patients for whom compliance fell below 70 percent, even after the data was adjusted for several possible confounders [24]. In an era of healthcare cost containment, an additional benefit of ERAS implementation is savings in healthcare costs. Ljungqvist et al. described results from Alberta, Canada after implementation of a colorectal ERAS pathway at two hospitals, reporting a 1.5-day reduction in LOS, a 1 percent reduction in complication rates, 8 percent fewer readmissions, and short length of stay when readmitted. This led to a combined savings of $2,800–5,900 per patient [2, 25]. McEvoy et al. demonstrated a 17 percent reduction in median cost per patient for 544 patients after establishing a colorectal ERAS protocol [4, 5]. Kalogera et al. demonstrated a median cost per patient reduction of 18.8 percent after reviewing 241 cases after gynecologic surgery [13]. Thiele et al. demonstrated a $7,129 reduction in direct costs per patient that corresponded with a net savings of $777,061 after the implantation of a colorectal ERAS pathway [26]. A recent report summarized much of these cost savings by using existing publications to model of net financial costs. This report demonstrated a range of $830–3,100 per day cost reduction which totals a net first year annual savings up to $395,717 (estimated an implementation coast of $552,783 versus total first year savings of $948,500) [1].

Despite multiple studies showing the benefits of ERAS implementation, the longer-term benefits are not as well known [2]. Interestingly, Savaridas et al. recently demonstrated a significantly lower 2-year mortality rate (2.7% vs. 3.8%) after the introduction ERAS principles for of hip and knee replacement surgery [27]. They concluded there to be a significant survival benefit with the routine use of an enhanced recovery program for hip and knee arthroplasty. While this is encouraging, many questions still remain to be explored in this area of inquiry.

Background of ERAS

Colorectal surgery was the starting nexus for the development of ERAS and the current literature is predominately in this surgical arena [2]. However, there is a growing body of evidence showing consistent findings with the institution of ERAS protocols with liver resections, pancreatic surgery, gastric surgery, esophageal surgery, thoracic surgery, major urologic surgery, gynecologic surgery, orthopedic surgery

and even emergency general surgery [2]. "Enhanced Recovery" (ER) was first proposed by Kehlet [28]. The ER mentality came about because there was doubt that traditional perioperative management practices such as fasting, liberal fluid administration, nasogastric tubes, and opioid-centric pain management strategies in the postoperative period, were up to date and it was believed that these practices deserved some reevaluation [29]. ERAS pathways have now been employed for over a two decades in Europe.

Despite success in Europe, there was continued resistance to implementation in the United States. However, due to concerns about healthcare quality, the Institute for Healthcare Improvement (IHI) issued a triple aim [30]. The goal of this triple aim was to improve the individual experience, improve the health of a defined surgical population and reduce the per capita cost of surgical care [5]. This call to action by the IHI, along with a consistent messages of the need to improve the value of healthcare, were instrumental in leading to some early adoption of ERAS concepts in the United States [5]. Then, because of the initial successes in colorectal surgery, ERAS pathways have begun to spread to other surgical populations in the United States. Overall, these pathways have been developed using interventions that demonstrated outcome benefits for colorectal surgery patients and continue to be successfully applied to many other surgical specialties such as urology, orthopedics, and gynecology (Box 35.1) [31].

Box 35.1. ERAS Pathways Promoted by International Consensus – ERAS® Society (http://erassociety.org), American Society for Enhanced Recovery (http://aserhq.org), and Evidence-Based Perioperative Medicine (http://www.ebpom.org)

1. Colorectal surgery [35]
2. Major head and neck cancer [37]
3. Liver surgery [36]
4. Cystectomy [40]
5. Gastrointestinal [41]
6. Bariatric surgery [42]
7. Rectal/pelvic surgery [31]
8. Pancreaticoduodenectomy [43]
9. Gastrectomy [44]
10. Gynecologic/oncology [45]
11. Breast reconstruction [46]

Key Components of an ERAS Pathway

There are numerous patient interventions that result in a successful ERAS pathway (Table 35.1). With the overall goal being cohesiveness in the perioperative period, communication between the patient and the caregivers during each phase is a critical component to success. There are 20 to 25 key interventions that have been described and that require consistent effort to ensure execution in any ERAS pathway (Table 35.2) [2]. A few of the more critical interventions are discussed below briefly.

Drinking

Preoperative clear liquid intake up to 2 h prior to surgery, whether it be water or carbohydrate solutions, have demonstrated a reduction of insulin resistance, improved well-being, and possibly faster recovery [2, 32].

Eating

Preoperative nutritional screening and support is an imperative component of an ERAS pathway to help reduce complications [2]. The administration of solids prior to surgery still requires the 6-h cessation per the practice guidelines for preoperative fasting [33]. However, early intake of oral fluids and solids in the postoperative period is key to support energy, protein supply, reduce starvation-induced insulin resistance, and improve length of stay [2]. This is recommended to start as soon as possible after surgery.

Fluid Management

Traditional fluid management strategies are of particular important, especially for colorectal surgery [18]. "Fluid responsiveness," an extension from Shoemaker and colleagues' concept of goal-directed fluid therapy [34], promotes the use of dynamic indicators of a patient's volume status to guide fluid therapy to maintain an optimal preload [29]. Normovolemic (e.g., zero-balance) fluid regimens in major surgery have led to more favorable outcomes when compared to excessive fluid regimens [35].

Analgesia

A consensus for an avoidance of long-acting opioids exists [2]. A multimodal approach to opioid-sparing pain control is an important aspect of all ERAS pathways [2, 5]. This approach includes a regional anesthetic plan whenever possible. Whether this means a neuraxial technique or a regional approach is dependent on the patient and the surgical approach (laparoscopic vs. open) in an ERAS pathway. However, overall open abdominal approaches to tend to support the need for a neuraxial analgesic approach [2].

Mobilization

Continued postoperative bed rest is associated with multiple documented deleterious effects – muscle atrophy, thromboembolic disease and insulin resistence [36]. Early mobilization and minimized time in bed except for sleep is a key feature to an ERAS pathway.

Organizations

European

In 2001 a group gathered in London produced an ERAS protocol based on published evidence for patients undergoing colonic surgery [2]. This group consisted of contributors from the University of Edinburgh, Karolinksa Institutet and Ersta Hospital Stockholm, University of Copenhagen and Hvidovre Hospital, University of Northern Norway and Tromso Hospital, and University of Maastricht. The motivation for this came from several surveys that confirmed varying grades of perioperative care across Northern Europe with minimal adoption of evidence-based practices [2]. The ERAS Society (www.erassociety.org) was founded to focus and consolidate progress not only through research and education but also develop models that will aid in the implementation of best perioperative practices [2].

American

Despite the evidence supporting their implantation, few centers in the United States have successfully adopted ERAS pathways into their routine practice [19] One concern that tends to cause hesitation is the cost of such a program [1]. However, Stone et al. reported that despite initial implementation costs, a successful program can lead to substantial savings even in its first year of implementation [1]. These initial successes have led to the formation of ASER. The society was developed to establish collaborative relationships between ERAS centers in the United States and to provide outreach education for those interested in development of new programs.

Table 35.1 Key Patient Interventions for a Successful ERAS Pathway

Care element by perioperative phase	Goal of care element
Preadmission	
Cessation of smoking and excessive intake of alcohol	Reduce complications, particularly pulmonary and wound healing
Preoperative nutritional screening and, as needed, assessment and nutritional support	Properly assess nutritional status and frailty state and reduce overall complications
Medical optimization of chronic disease	Reduce complications, particularly risk of delirium, MACE, PPC, AKI, and glycemic control issues
Preoperative	
Structured preoperative education with engagement of the patient and relative or caretakers in perioperative goals of care discussion and expectations for functional recovery, analgesia, and length of stay	Reduce anxiety, involve the patient in order to improve compliance with protocol
Preoperative complex carbohydrate loading and oral hydration	Reduce insulin resistance, improve well-being and patient comfort in preoperative period; faster recovery?
Thromboprophylaxis	Reduce DVT and PE
Risk-based PONV prophylaxis	Minimize PONV
Intraoperative	
Minimally-invasive surgical techniques when indicated	Reduce surgical stress, complications, and pain for faster recovery
Standardized maximodal nonopioid analgesia and avoidance of long-acting opioids with epidural for open surgery	Avoid or reduce postoperative ileus and promote optimal analgesia – functional recovery with fewest side effects from medications; reduce stress response and insulin resistance
Goal-directed fluid therapy per current evidence	Avoid hypovolemia or hypervolemia complications of ischemia or volume overload
Restrictive use of surgical site drains	Support mobilization, reduce pain and discomfort, no proven benefit of use
Removal of nasogastric tubes before reversal of anesthesia; no standard postoperative use	Reduce the risk of pneumonia, support oral intake of solids, reduce patient discomfort
Control of body temperature using warm air flow blankets and warmed intravenous infusions	Reduce complications, specifically surgical site infection
Postoperative	
Early ambulation – DOS and at least QID thereafter	Encourage functional recovery; support return to normal movement
Early intake of oral fluids and solids (offered the DOS), including protein and energy-rich choices	Support positive nitrogen balance, reduce insulin resistance
Early removal of urinary catheters and intravenous fluids (POD1)	Support ambulation and mobilization; reduce risk of UTI
Use of chewing gums and laxatives and peripheral opioid-blocking agents (when using moderate to high-dose opioids)	Support return of gut function
Maximodal approach to achieving optimal analgesia with opioid avoidance	Optimal analgesia – defined as fastest functional recovery and optimized patient comfort with fewest medication side effects (not necessarily lowest pain score)
Multimodal approach to control of nausea and vomiting	Minimize postoperative nausea and vomiting and support energy and protein intake
Prepare for early discharge	Avoid unnecessary delays in discharge
Audit of outcomes and process in a multiprofessional, multidisciplinary team on a regular basis	Control of practice (a key to improve outcomes)

Based on [22;30–33].
MACE, major adverse cardiac events; PPC, postoperative pulmonary complications; AKI, acute kidney injury; DVT, deep vein thrombosis; PE, pulmonary embolus; PONV, postoperative nausea and vomiting; DOS, day of surgery; QID, four times each day.

Table 35.2 Key Components of any ERAS Pathway [2, 41]

Preoperative	Intraoperative	Postoperative
Smoking cessation	Minimal invasive surgical approaches if applicable	Early mobilization
Nutritional screening +/− nutritional support	Avoidance of long-acting opioids	Early intake of oral fluids and solids
Medical optimization of disease processes	Standardized anesthesia practice	Early cessation of urinary catheters
Structured preoperative information	Maintenance of fluid balance – avoiding over- or underhydration	Early cessation of intravenous fluids
Carbohydrate/water treatment	Epidural anesthesia for open procedures, if applicable	Early initiation of bowel regimens
Venous thrombosis prophylaxis	Minimize use of surgical drains, if applicable	Opioid-sparing pain control with a multimodal pain treatment plan
Infection prophylaxis	Nasogastric tube removed prior to cessation of anesthesia	Early initiation of discharge plan
Nausea and vomiting prophylaxis	Body temperature control with warm fluids and warm air flow blankets	Regular audit of ERAS pathway and outcomes

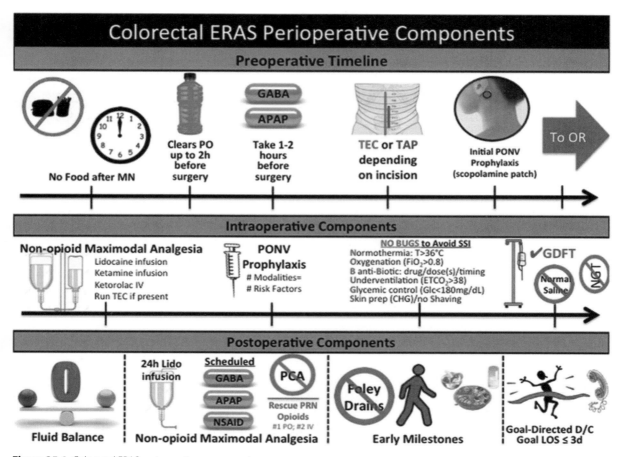

Figure 35.1 Colorectal ERAS perioperative components.

Start Time	Surgeon Room	MRN	Procedure	Labs	Anti-coag meds	Allergies
03-28 11:00	VOR3 RM 30	▇	LAPAROSCOPIC GASTRIC BYPASS (43644)			NKDA
03-28 07:30	VOR3 RM 26	▇	CYSTECTOMY W/ILEAL CONDUIT (51595); FLAP CLOSURE; ABDOMEN/TRUNK (15734); FLAP CLOSURE; EXTREMITY (15738); PELVIC EXENTERATION (45126)	Plt 158 (2017-02-15)		NKDA
03-28 07:30	VOR3 RM 29	▇	WHIPPLE PROCEDURE (48153)	INR 1.1 (2017-02-24) Plt 127 (2017-02-24) PTT 24.8 (2017-02-23)		Tape
03-28 08:00	VOR3 RM 03	▇	EXPLORATORY LAPAROTOMY (49000); ILEOSTOMY (44310)	INR 1.1 (2017-03-18) Plt 376 (2017-03-19) PTT 27.7 (2017-03-18)		NKDA
03-28 10:00	VOR3 RM 35	▇	ORIF BIMALLEOLAR ANKLE FX (27814)			
03-28 07:30	VOR3 RM 22	▇	COLECTOMY (44155)	INR 1.1 (2015-08-12) Plt 484 (2017-02-08) PTT 34.1 (2015-08-12)		Adhesive tape Adhesive tapes
03-28 07:30	VOR3 RM 30	▇	LAPAROSCOPIC GASTRIC BYPASS (43644)	Plt 258 (2016-08-12)		Augmentin

Figure 35.2 Example of OR schedule.

Here are your clinical assignments for **Monday 2017-03-27**. 1 case with a perioperative pathway.

3 case(s) in VOR3 RM 22 with ▇

07:30 42yo F for laparoscopic cholecystectomy w/wo ioc (47563); laparoscopic partial bowel resection (44205) ▇ Surgeon)

Preop (2017-03-23), Intraop (2017-03-13)

→ CEBA guideline for colorectal surgery attached

PONV: 2 intervention(s) recommended

13:00 50yo F for egd w/peg or pej placement (49451) ▇ (Surgeon)

Preop (2016-12-23), Intraop (2016-11-22)

Acute Lung Injury Risk: Consider 390-520 mL TV with PEEP*

PONV: 3 intervention(s) recommended

14:30 51yo M for laparoscopic partial bowel resection (44205) ▇ (Surgeon)

No preop for MRN 41627464 , No intraop for MRN ▇

PONV: 2 intervention(s) recommended

*(6-8 mL/kg ideal body weight)

*IBW: ideal body weight

Figure 35.3 Example of clinical cases.

Conclusions

ERAS programs have been successfully developed in Europe and the United States. Implementation of these programs has led to reductions not only in hospital LOS but also in perioperative morbidity and mortality [2, 37–39]. For those looking to start a new ERAS program, there are European and American Societies dedicated to the practice of enhanced recovery and numerous published protocols published for a variety of surgical populations to help guide you and your perioperative systems through development. Due to changes in healthcare finance in the United States, implementation of ERAS programs may be an important component of improving the quality of perioperative care and cost reduction moving forward.

References

1. Stone AB, Grant MC, Pio Roda C, et al. Implementation costs of an enhanced recovery after surgery program in the United States: A financial model and sensitivity analysis based on experiences at a quaternary academic medical center. *J Am Coll Surg* 2016; 222: 219–25.

2. Ljungqvist O, Scott M, Fearon KC. Enhanced Recovery After Surgery: A review. *JAMA Surg* 2017; 152: 292–8.

3. King AB, Alvis BD, McEvoy MD. Enhanced Recovery After Surgery, perioperative medicine, and the perioperative surgical home: Current state and future implications for education and training. *Curr Opin Anaesthesiol* 2016; 29: 727–32.

4. King AB, Geiger T, Tiwari V, Sandberg WS, McEvoy MD. *Effect of ongoing process improvement on an Enhanced Recovery After Surgery pathway for colorectal surgery patients.* San Diego, CA: American Society of Anesthesiologists, 2015.

5. McEvoy MD, Wanderer JP, King AB, et al. A perioperative consult service results in reduction in cost and length of stay for colorectal surgical patients: Evidence from a healthcare redesign project. *Perioper Med* 2016; 5: 3.

6. Vanounou T, Pratt W, Fischer JE, Vollmer CM, Jr., Callery MP. Deviation-based cost modeling: A novel model to evaluate the clinical and economic impact of clinical pathways. *J Am Coll Surg* 2007; 204: 570–9.

7. Tang J, Humes DJ, Gemmil E, Welch NT, Parsons SL, Catton JA. Reduction in length of stay for patients undergoing oesophageal and gastric resections with implementation of enhanced recovery packages. *Ann R Coll Surg Engl* 2013; 95: 323–8.

8. Reismann M, Dingemann J, Wolters M, Laupichler B, Suempelmann R, Ure BM. Fast-track concepts in routine pediatric surgery: A prospective study in 436 infants and children. *Langenbecks Arch Surg* 2009; 394: 529–33.

9. Porter GA, Pisters PW, Mansyur C, et al. Cost and utilization impact of a clinical pathway for patients undergoing pancreaticoduodenectomy. *Ann Surg Oncol* 2000; 7: 484–9.

10. Khreiss W, Huebner M, Cima RR, et al. Improving conventional recovery with enhanced recovery in

11. Kennedy EP, Rosato EL, Sauter PK, et al. Initiation of a critical pathway for pancreaticoduodenectomy at an academic institution: The first step in multidisciplinary team building. *J Am Coll Surg* 2007; 204: 917–23; discussion 23–4.

12. Kennedy EP, Grenda TR, Sauter PK, et al. Implementation of a critical pathway for distal pancreatectomy at an academic institution. *J Gastrointest Surg* 2009; 13: 938–44.

13. Kalogera E, Bakkum-Gamez JN, Jankowski CJ, et al. Enhanced recovery in gynecologic surgery. *Obstet Gynecol* 2013; 122: 319–28.

14. di Sebastiano P, Festa L, De Bonis A, et al. A modified fast-track program for pancreatic surgery: A prospective single-center experience. *Langenbecks Arch Surg* 2011; 396: 345–51.

15. Daneshmand S, Ahmadi H, Schuckman AK, et al. Enhanced recovery protocol after radical cystectomy for bladder cancer. *J Urol* 2014; 192: 50–5.

16. Connor S, Cross A, Sakowska M, Linscott D, Woods J. Effects of introducing an Enhanced Recovery After Surgery programme for patients undergoing open hepatic resection. *HPB (Oxford)* 2013; 15: 294–301.

17. Blom RL, van Heijl M, Bemelman WA, et al. Initial experiences of an enhanced recovery protocol in esophageal surgery. *World J Surg* 2013; 37: 2372–8.

18. Balzano G, Zerbi A, Braga M, Rocchetti S, Beneduce AA, Di Carlo V. Fast-track recovery programme after pancreatico-duodenectomy reduces delayed gastric emptying. *Br J Surg* 2008; 95: 1387–93.

19. Sarin ALE, Naidu R, Yost CS, Varma MG, Chen LL. Successful implementation of an Enhanced Recovery After Surgery program shortens length of stay and improves postoperative pain, and bowel and bladder function after colorectal surgery. *BMC Anesthesiology* 2016; 16: 55

20. Miller TE, Thacker JK, White WD, et al. Reduced length of hospital stay in colorectal surgery after implementation of an enhanced recovery protocol. *Anesth Analg* 2014; 118: 1052–61.

21. Day RW, Cleeland CS, Wang XS, et al. Patient-reported outcomes accurately measure the value of an enhanced recovery program in liver surgery. *J Am Coll Surgeons* 2015; 221: 1023.

22. Gustafsson UO, Hausel J, Thorell A, et al. Adherence to the Enhanced Recovery After Surgery protocol and outcomes after colorectal cancer surgery. *Arch Surg* 2011; 146: 571–7.

23. Group EC. The impact of enhanced recovery protocol compliance on elective colorectal cancer

resection: Results from international registry. *Ann Surg* 2015; 261: 1153–9.

24. Gustafsson UO, Oppelstrup H, Thorell A, Nygren J, Ljungqvist O. Adherence to the ERAS protocol is associated with 5-year survival after colorectal cancer surgery: A retrospective cohort study. *World J Surg* 2016; 40: 1741–7.

25. Nelson G, Kiyang LN, Crumley ET, et al. Implementation of Enhanced Recovery After Surgery (ERAS) across a provincial healthcare system: The ERAS Alberta colorectal surgery experience. *World J Surg* 2016; 40: 1092–103.

26. Thiele RH, Rea KM, Turrentine FE, et al. Standardization of care: Impact of an enhanced recovery protocol on length of stay, complications, and direct costs after colorectal surgery. *J Am Coll Surgeons* 2015; 220: 986.

27. Savaridas T, Serrano-Pedraza I, Khan SK, Martin K, Malviya A, Reed MR. Reduced medium-term mortality following primary total hip and knee arthroplasty with an enhanced recovery program. A study of 4,500 consecutive procedures. *Acta Orthop* 2013; 84: 40–3.

28. Kehlet H. Multimodal approach to control postoperative pathophysiology and rehabilitation. *Br J Anaesth* 1997; 78: 606–17.

29. Thiele RH, Rea KM, Turrentine FE, et al. Standardization of care: Impact of an enhanced recovery protocol on length of stay, complications, and direct costs after colorectal surgery. *J Am Coll Surgeons* 2015; 220: 430–43.

30. Berwick DM, Nolan TW, Whittington J. The triple aim: Care, health, and cost. *Health Aff (Millwood)* 2008; 27: 759–69.

31. Nygren J, Thacker J, Carli F, et al. Guidelines for perioperative care in elective rectal/pelvic surgery: Enhanced Recovery After Surgery (ERAS(R)) Society recommendations. *Clin Nutr* 2012; 31: 801–16.

32. Amer MA, Smith MD, Herbison GP, Plank LD, McCall JL. Network meta-analysis of the effect of preoperative carbohydrate loading on recovery after elective surgery. *Br J Surg* 2017; 104: 187–97.

33. Anesthesiologists tASo. Practice guidelines for preoperative fasting and the use of pharmacologic agents to reduce the risk of pulmonary aspiration: Application to healthy patients undergoing elective procedures. *Anesthesiology* 2011; 114: 495–511.

34 Shoemaker WC, Appel PL, Kram HB, Waxman K, Lee TS. Prospective trial of supranormal values of survivors as therapeutic goals in high-risk surgical patients. *Chest* 1988; 94: 1176–86.

35. Lassen K, Soop M, Nygren J, et al. Consensus review of optimal perioperative care in colorectal surgery: Enhanced Recovery After Surgery (ERAS) Group recommendations. *Arch Surg-Chicago* 2009; 144: 961–9.

36. Melloul E, Jubner M, Scott M, et al. Guidelines for perioperative care for liver surgery: Enhanced Recovery After Surgery (ERAS) Society recommendations. *World J Surg* 2016; 40: 2065.

37. Dort JC, Farwell DG, Findlay M, et al. Optimal perioperative care in major head and neck cancer surgery with free flap reconstruction: A consensus review and recommendations from the Enhanced Recovery After Surgery Society. *JAMA Otolaryngol Head Neck Surg* 2017; 143: 292–303.

38. Fearon KCH, Ljungqvist O, Von Meyenfeldt M, et al. Enhanced Recovery After Surgery: A consensus review of clinical care for patients undergoing colonic resection. *Clin Nutr* 2005; 24: 466–77.

39. Kolarczyk LM, Hance LM, Bednar P, Kim HJ, Isaak R. Implementation of an Enhanced Recovery After Surgery (ERAS) clinical pathway using Lean Six Sigma principles: A framework for ongoing quality improvement. *SDRP J Anesth Surg* 2016; 1: 1.

40. Cerantola Y, Valerio M, Persson B, et al. Guidelines for perioperative care after radical cystectomy for bladder cancer: Enhanced Recovery After Surgery (ERAS((R))) Society recommendations. *Clin Nutr* 2013; 32: 879–87.

41. Feldheiser A, Aziz O, Baldini G, et al. Enhanced Recovery After Surgery (ERAS) for gastrointestinal surgery, part 2: Consensus statement for anaesthesia practice. *Acta Anaesthesiol Scand* 2016; 60: 289–334.

42. Thorell A, MacCormick AD, Awad S, et al. Guidelines for perioperative care in bariatric surgery: Enhanced Recovery After Surgery (ERAS) Society recommendations. *World J Surg* 2016; 40: 2065–83.

43. Lassen K, Coolsen MM, Slim K, et al. Guidelines for perioperative care for pancreaticoduodenectomy: Enhanced Recovery After Surgery (ERAS(R)) Society recommendations. *Clin Nutr* 2012; 31: 817–30.

44. Mortensen K, Nilsson M, Slim K, et al. Consensus guidelines for enhanced recovery after gastrectomy: Enhanced Recovery After Surgery (ERAS(R)) Society recommendations. *Br J Surg* 2014; 101: 1209–29.

45. Nelson G, Altman AD, Nick A, et al. Guidelines for postoperative care in gynecologic/oncology surgery: Enhanced Recovery After Surgery (ERAS(R)) Society recommendations—Part II. *Gynecol Oncol* 2016; 140: 323–32.

46. Arsalani-Zadeh R, ElFadl D, Yassin N, MacFie J. Evidence-based review of enhancing postoperative recovery after breast surgery. *Br J Surg* 2011; 98: 181–96.

Chapter 36

Checklist Utility in the Perioperative Care Environment

Blas Catalani and Ezekiel B. Tayler

Contents

Introduction

The use of checklists to improve efficiency, maintain quality, and sustain performance in process/task completion is not a new concept. The application of well established, validated data management processes developed in nonhealthcare industries to perioperative patient management however, is a concept that is encountered with growing frequency in the healthcare setting. Expertise from other industries that utilize checklist-based protocols such as automotive manufacturing (Six Sigma), Formula One car racing, and aviation training facilities has been extrapolated and successfully incorporated into efforts to improve patient safety and quality of care in the perioperative setting [1, 2]. Systematic reviews and meta-analyses suggest a relationship between checklist use in surgery and fewer postoperative complications [3].

TJC "Universal Protocol"

Implemented in 2004, The Joint Commission (TJC) "Universal Protocol" is a longitudinal protocol aimed at prevention of wrong site, wrong procedure, wrong person surgical errors [4]. While not a checklist by itself, the use of standardized checklists is encouraged by TJC to ensure comprehensive protocol compliance. The three components of the TJC "Universal Protocol" include: (1) preprocedure verification process, (2) marking of the procedure site, and (3) intraoperative time-out prior to initiation of the procedure. Patient involvement/participation is encouraged during the first two steps of this Universal Protocol.

WHO "Safe Surgery Checklist"

Created in 2008 by the WHO, the Safe Surgery Checklist is limited only to the operative environment and identifies three phases of an operation, each corresponding to a specific period in the normal perioperative workflow: (1) before the induction of anesthesia ("sign in"), (2) before the incision of the skin ("time out"), and (3) before the patient leaves the operating room (OR) ("sign out") [5]. A checklist is used at each phase and must be completed prior to proceeding with the operative procedure [6]. Further information on the WHO checklist and the associated implementation manual is available from the WHO directly, with specific recommendation to add to and modify the checklist to fit local practice.

SURgical PAtient Safety System, aka "SURPASS"

Published in 2008 and created in the Netherlands by de Vries and colleagues [7], the SURPASS checklist is a multidisciplinary checklist that accompanies patients throughout their hospital stay. While it is less specific than the WHO checklist, the SURPASS checklist addresses a broader scope of patient care beginning with admission to the hospital, continuing through the perioperative and operative encounters, and ending with patient discharge.

Among the reported benefits of SURPASS implementation are optimization of antibiotic dosing for surgical site infection prophylaxis [8] as well as the assertion that nearly 33 percent of surgical malpractice claims in the Netherlands might have been intercepted and the associated physical/financial damage prevented with SURPASS checklist use [9].

In the perioperative setting, when compared to other validated surgical safety checklists, the SURPASS instrument lacks specific mention of any of the following intraoperative-oriented criteria: pulse oximetry, difficult airway, risk of blood loss (although blood product availability is addressed), team introductions, and anticipation of critical events [10]. The developers of the SURPASS checklist also openly acknowledge its limited utility as a sole checklist tool for the intraoperative environment [11], highlighting that an outcome comparison between SURPASS and single intraoperative checklist remains a subject for future study.

Preoperative Phase of Care

Preanesthesia Checkouts

In an effort to address the ever-evolving presence of advancing technology and the resultant changes in anesthetic equipment, the American Society of Anesthesiologists (ASA) published guidelines in 2008, which served as an update/revision of the original 1993 "Preanesthesia Checkout" (PAC) recommendations. Instead of providing a specific checklist for all circumstances, this update to the PAC guidelines provides a framework to facilitate *development* of PACs that are appropriate for a specific setting in which an anesthetic will be delivered. Accordingly, these ASA guidelines address three primary objectives: (1) outline essential items that need to be available and functioning properly prior to delivering every anesthetic, (2) identify the frequency with which each of the items needs to be checked, and (3) suggest which items may be checked by a qualified anesthesia/biomedical/manufacturer-certified technician [12]. The inclusion of the recommendation to split (where possible) responsibility for components of the preanesthesia checkout procedures between the anesthesia provider and a properly trained anesthesia/biomedical technician is of critical importance. The goal of this division in responsibility is to improve compliance with the PAC requirements for a given institution. These guidelines also delineate the requirements for the safe delivery of anesthesia care to include:

- Reliable delivery of oxygen at any appropriate concentration up to 100 percent

- Reliable means of positive pressure ventilation
- Backup ventilation equipment available and functioning
- Controlled release of positive pressure from the breathing circuit
- Anesthesia vapor delivery (if intended as part of the anesthetic plan)
- Adequate suction
- Means to conform to standards for patient monitoring as defined in the ASA 2005 monitoring guidelines [13]

Additional Preanesthetic Items

While the ASA PAC guidelines establish a means to consistently evaluate the integrity of a provider's anesthetic delivery equipment, additional checklists are used to ensure all other equipment is accounted for and assessed as it pertains to the surgical procedure at hand. An informal, yet effective example of this is "MSMAIDS" in which:

M =	Machine (addressed in PAC guidelines) + functioning electronic health record (EHR)/computer interface
S =	Suction (addressed in PAC guidelines)
M =	Monitors (addressed in PAC guidelines)
A =	Airway: mask, oral/nasal airways, laryngoscope, endotracheal tube (including cuff inflation check), stylette, ambu bag, gum elastic bougie, means for securing ETT (tube holder, tape, etc.), bite block, backup O_2 E-cylinder (>1000 psi) with regulator
I =	IV: necessary equipment for establishing and securing IV access
D =	Drugs: IV fluids (and primed IV tubing), case-pertinent drugs (induction, maintenance, emergence), emergency drugs
S =	"Special Equipment": fluid warmer, forced-air warming blanket, blood products, any case-specific needs (e.g., central venous/arterial line kits, pressure transducers, double-lumen ETT, fiber optic/video laryngoscopes, etc.)

The occurrence of the preoperative, anesthesia-specific "time-out" procedure (WHO "sign-in") varies by institution with regard to precise timing and location; however, the act has been validated by the WHO and serves as a valuable final check of patient information (often involving the patient directly) prior to entering the often intimidating OR environment.

Intraoperative Phase of Care

Intraoperative checklist usage largely revolves around ensuring that communication of pertinent information occurs while simultaneously attempting to prevent miscommunication as well. Emphasis on facilitating clear, unobstructed communication is important given that miscommunication can lead to hospital sentinel events and may lead to adverse events [14]. Examples include (but are not limited to):

- Preincision "surgical time out" criteria of the TJC Universal Protocol;
- Antibiotic administration prior to incision TJC Surgical Care Improvement Project versus the SURPASS checklist, which emphasizes antibiotic administration prior to induction of anesthesia
- Blood product cross check and two-person "check-in" confirmation of blood products prior to their administration

Handoff of Patient Care in the OR

Errors related to the historically informal, unstructured, "unstandardardized" nature of handoffs in the hospital setting has been implicated by TJC in up to 70 to 80 percent of sentinel events [15, 16], leading to the provision by TJC of SHARE guidelines to inform the development of intervention tools (i.e., checklists and protocols) to facilitate handoff events that include:

S = Standardization of critical content (patient details involved in information transfer)

H = Hardwiring within the hospital system through use of standardized tools and methods (e.g., checklists)

A = Allow opportunities to ask questions

R = Reinforce quality and measurement through incorporation into clinical governance and ongoing audit

E = Educate and coach in the conduct of successful handovers

Communication quality suffers across the continuum of care provision in the hospital setting. In the perioperative setting, particularly during an operative procedure, providers' interactions with each other (as a team) and with their environment (as a system) are critical determinants of error, suggesting that successful reduction of communication breakdowns can substantially improve patient safety and reduce errors [16]. No more evident is such potential for reduction in compromises of patient safety than that which resides with intraoperative anesthesia provider handoffs. Anesthesia providers are responsible for such a broad scope of patient management, that there is a distinct probability of unintentional omission of key information during an intraoperative handoff between providers. This probability compounds with subsequent handoffs within the same case, as does the potential for associated adverse events resulting from such omissions (e.g., antibiotic redosing intervals/time points during prolonged procedures).

Postoperative Phase of Care

Handoff of Patient Care in the PACU

Handoff events occurring in the PACU setting are fraught with similar challenges to intraoperative handoffs. When delivering a patient to the PACU, a focused handoff report from the anesthesia provider to the PACU nurse/care team is expected. In many institutions, postoperative care handoffs are often incomplete, increasing risk of a negative impact on patient safety [17, 18]. Utilization of a standardized checklist has been shown to dramatically improve the quality and reliability of handoffs delivered in the PACU setting [19] while simple instruction of providers regarding important handoff information (without implementation of a written checklist) does not increase the amount of information handed over between providers in the PACU [20]. While specific checklists vary between institutions and patient populations, the information given in a PACU handoff should at the very least include:

- Patient name
- Age
- Surgery/procedure that patient has just undergone
- Relevant past medical history (e.g., hypertension, diabetes, prior CABG, smoker, etc.)
- Intraoperative medications: benzodiazepines, opioids (including last dose time), antiemetics, antihypertensives, infusions, etc.
- I/O: IV fluids/blood products given; estimated blood loss/urine output
- Lines/drains: IV access, and catheters in place
- Complications (if applicable)

It is important to also acknowledge that patients may not always recover in the PACU, even if PACU recovery was part of the original anesthetic plan. Initially unforeseen ICU admission, for whatever reason, necessitates a more detailed discussion of the patient's preoperative and intraoperative course as well as pertinent patient medical history.

Handoff of Patient Care in the ICU

The ICU houses a multitude of disease states in various stages of development. In order to acquire the necessary data to safely take a patient to the OR and deliver anesthesia, one must have a basic understanding of how an intensive care physician manages a patient. A systems-based approach is a very standardized and common technique to evaluating a patient's status in the ICU. By using a systems approach, one can readily ascertain a patient's stability, or lack thereof, and make an informed decision on whether to proceed to the OR, wait, or gather more material. Such an approach will also help the anesthesiologist formulate the most appropriate anesthetic plan should the patient be cleared for the operative procedure in question.

Simple examination of the patient, such as personal inspection of the various infusions, can provide a substantial amount of information; however, some information will need to be taken either from the supporting nurse and/or physician as they are intimately familiar with the patient's hemodynamic profile and clinical course. The value of standardized checklist use in the ICU setting has been validated repeatedly, leading to effective consideration and implementation of ICU best care practices [21].

In many ways, an anesthesiologist should be able to approach all patients in such a fashion, regardless of context (ICU/burn/trauma, obstetrics, ambulatory/outpatient, elective/inpatient) so as not to miss any important details; however, the preoperative considerations of the ICU patient should include at least cursory review of the following details:

- Neurological
  - Mental status and any recent changes from baseline (avoidance of benzodiazepines)
  - Duration of immobility (ICU patients are usually poor candidates for succinylcholine)
  - Sedation/pain/psychiatric medication regimen
  - Current indwelling catheters for pain control (epidural, paravertebral, perineural, etc.)
  - Any preexisting nerve damage (positioning considerations)
  - Note presence of intracranial pressure monitors and current preoperative values

- Cardiovascular
  - Complete cardiac history including interventions (previous MI, placement of PCI/stents, CABG, valve replacement, AICD/PM, etc.)
  - Recent cardiac imaging (echocardiogram)
  - Note use, duration and dosage of any vasoactive substances
  - Cardiac medications
- Pulmonary
  - Oxygen requirements
  - Recent thoracic imaging
  - If intubated, determine details of intubation (indication, duration, intubation difficulty)
  - Current ventilator settings
  - Pulmonary medications
- Renal
  - Presence/absence of Foley catheter
  - Hourly urine output (if less than 0.5 cc/kg/h, is patient being managed for ARF or is this a chronic condition?)
  - Character of urine (concentrated, bloody, cloudy)
  - If on extracorporeal support such as CRRT, CVVH or Hemodialysis, determine reason for intervention, timing of last session (especially how much volume removed, how much blood returned, and any antibiotics given during session)
- Infectious disease
  - Microbiology history (especially if patient is septic)
  - Current antibiotic regimen (dosage/timing)
  - Contact/isolation precautions
- Hematology
  - Review CBC and coagulation profile
  - Determine blood product availability
  - Recent transfusions (determine appropriate transfusion threshold)
  - Deep vein thrombosis prophylaxis (dosage, interval, and timing of last dose)
- Fluids/electrolytes/nutrition
  - Type/rate of IVF
  - Review available electrolyte panels (especially K, Cr, glucose)
  - NPO status (if tube fed, where is tube: stomach vs. postpyloric, and how long have feeds been held?)

- Determine fluid status (may include visualizing IVC with ultrasound)
- Endocrine
  - Endocrine disorders (diabetes, hypothyroidism)
  - Current endocrine medications (timing and dosage)
  - Steroid use (drug, dosage and timing)
- Musculoskeletal
  - Skin integrity
  - Presence and stage of ulcers (positioning considerations)
  - Movement restrictions (fractures, restraints)
- Tubes/lines/drains:
  - Location and duration of intravenous/arterial lines
  - Drain locations and output

It is important to note that a patient arriving to the ICU postoperatively may be new to the ICU team. This can occur for a number of reasons, such as the patient is an altogether new ICU admission (not ICU status preoperatively), or the ICU care team has changed shifts while the patient was in the OR. Even if the patient was ICU status prior to surgery, use of a standardized checklist to guide transfer of care from the OR to the ICU can reduce the risk of missed information and improve satisfaction among perioperative providers [22]. Upon arrival to the ICU, use of a checklist to guide a similar systems-based approach to transferring information about the patient's operative course can be used to include the following information:

- Neurological
  - Timing of last paralytic dosage (presence/absence of twitches, reversal given)
  - Emergence estimation (to estimate urgency of sedation needs if patient has remained intubated or there is residual paralytic effect)
  - Total amount of pain medications (including last dosing)
- Cardiovascular
  - Evidence of a cardiac event (reason if known)
  - Any changes in rhythm from preoperative baseline
  - New imaging results if available (TTE, TEE, EKG)
  - Cardiac medications given intraoperatively

- Pulmonary
  - Current oxygen requirements
  - Evidence of pulmonary event (reason if known)
  - ABG results and interpretation (if available)
  - New imaging results if available (CXR, CT)
  - Ventilator setting recommendations
- Renal
  - Intraoperative urine output (diuretics if given)
  - Character of urine (concentrated, bloody, cloudy)
- Infectious disease
  - Antibiotics given and timing
- Hematology
  - Blood loss (expected or unexpected)
  - Current CBC if known
  - Amount and types of blood products given
- Fluids/electrolytes/nutrition
  - Total and types of IVF given
  - Note any electrolyte abnormalities if known (were they replete if necessary?)
  - Estimate fluid status (was the patient responsive to IVF intraop)
- Endocrine
  - Total amount of medications given (insulin bolus/infusion)
  - Steroid use (stress or routine dosing)
- Tubes/lines/drains
  - Additional venous/arterial access placed

"Signing out" a patient or transferring information from one provider to another is an extremely important process. There has to be a balance between giving just the right amount of information to safely take care of patient, and giving too much or too little data. It is important to make sure the receiving provider feels comfortable with the information provided before leaving the patient and that an opportunity to ask questions has been provided to ensure key information is not omitted at the time of care transfer.

Challenges to Successful Checklist Implementation

While the published literature reflects significant improvements in surgical outcomes attributed to the use of surgical safety checklists [3] and has led to their worldwide adoption, the effect of mandatory implementation of such checklists is unclear

345

and in some institutions has not been associated with significant reductions in operative mortality or complications [23]. Accordingly, while the SHARE guidelines provided by TJC establishes a framework for developing instruments and protocols to improve care, without effective strategies for implementation, reinforcement, and education, such protocols risk the possibility of becoming an ineffective "box-checking" exercise [15]. Worse still, unilateral, uniformed implementation of safety checklists in surgery risks engendering resistance within an organization such that the checklist becomes a negative, rather than positive, change [24].

Checklists offer clear advantages in multiple healthcare settings, the most frequent of which involves patient care handoff between providers at all levels of responsibility within and amongst the healthcare team(s). Handoff quality is influenced by a number of factors, including information transferred, shared understanding between providers involved in the handoff, and the working atmosphere in which the handoff is delivered, emphasizing the presence of distraction and/or multitasking [25, 26].

Until validated in a new environment, when implementing checklists in the perioperative setting, it is important to remember the simple adage, "What works for you, 'works for YOU.'" It is important to acknowledge that successful checklist usage requires equally that there be high provider compliance rates AND that the checklist tool be appropriate for the environment in which it is implemented. All checklists must be developed, modified and refined to fit the context of patient care being addressed as well as the features unique to the institution/environment in which it is being utilized. Often, careful refinement of a protocol based on end-user input can lead to the production of a successful, validated instrument [27]. For instance, a checklist used in the surgical ICU of "Hospital A" may not function effectively (or at all) in the medical ICU of the same hospital, let alone be effective with verbatim implementation in the surgical ICU of "Hospital B." For this very reason, organizations such as the WHO specifically recommend addition and modification of their checklist templates and protocols to fit local practice. Further, compliance with checklist use is crucial to successful implementation as evidenced during the initial validation of the SURPASS checklist, where the extent of improvement in surgical complications was associated with greater checklist compliance in hospitals with a preexisting high standard of care [10, 28]. Even the most attentively designed, validated checklist tool will fail to improve outcomes without consistent provider/team member compliance with its appropriate use during the events for which it was designed.

Another concern in design and implementation of checklist instruments, whether written or electronic, is the risk of "Checklist Fatigue" on the part of the intended participants. If the very people using the checklists are overwhelmed or frustrated with using the instrument(s), then compliance will suffer. In addition, if there are so many checklists encountered by a care provider over the course of perioperative patient care, the providers can become indifferent to delivery of quality information or desensitized the importance of thorough checklist completion.

The modern EHR provides an interesting and often perplexing challenge for effective checklist implementation. Use of an EHR checklist has been shown to improve relay and retention of critical patient information and anesthesia provider communication at intraoperative handoff of care [29]; however, if the checklist is incomplete or conversely overly burdensome, the integrity of the handoff is compromised, as is patient safety. When designing an EHR-based checklist, careful consideration of the needs and planned use of the instrument must be made in order to avoid creating an instrument that impedes efficient transition of care between members of the healthcare team.

References

1. Catchpole KR, et al. (2007). Patient handover from surgery to intensive care: Using Formula 1 pit-stop and aviation models to improve safety and quality. *Paediatr Anaesth*, 17 (5), 470–8.

2. Parker BM, et al. (2007). Six Sigma methodology can be used to improve adherence for antibiotic prophylaxis in patients undergoing noncardiac surgery. *Anesth Analg*, 104 (1), 140–6.

3. Gillespie BM, et al. (2014). Effect of using a safety checklist on patient complications after surgery: A systematic review and meta-analysis. *Anesthesiology*, 120 (6), 1380–9.

4. www.jointcommission.org/standards_information/up.aspx (accessed November 25, 2016).

5. www.who.int/patientsafety/safesurgery/ss_checklist/en/ (accessed November 25, 2016).

6. World Alliance for Patient Safety. (2009). *WHO Surgical Safety Checklist*. World Health Organization.

http://apps.who.int/iris/bitstream/10665/44186/2/9789241598590_eng_Checklist.pdf (accessed November 25, 2016).

7. de Vries EN, et al. (2009). Development and validation of the SURgical PAtient Safety System (SURPASS) checklist. *Qual Saf Health Care*, 18(2), 121–6.

8. de Vries EN, et al. (2010). The SURgical PAtient Safety System (SURPASS) checklist optimizes timing of antibiotic prophylaxis. *Patient Saf Surg*, 4(1), 6.

9. deVries EN, et al. (2011). Prevention of surgical malpractice claims by use of a surgical safety checklist. *Ann Surg*, 253(3), 624–8.

10. Treadwell JR, Lucas S. Preoperative checklists and anesthesia checklists. In: *Making Health Care Safer II: An Updated Critical Analysis of the Evidence for Patient Safety Practices.* Rockville, MD: Agency for Healthcare Research and Quality, 2013. www.ncbi.nlm.nih.gov/books/NBK133353/ (accessed November 25, 2016).

11. de Vries EN, et al. (2012). Nature and timing of incidents intercepted by the SURPASS checklist in surgical patients. *BMJ Qual Saf.*, 21(6), 503–8.

12. ASA Committee on Equipment and Facilities. *2008 Recommendations for Pre-anesthesia Checkout Procedures.* Park Ridge, IL: American Society of Anesthesiologists, 2008. www.asahq.org/resources/clinical-information/2008-asa-recommendations-for-pre-anesthesia-checkout (accessed November 25, 2016).

13. American Society of Anesthesiologists. Standards for basic anesthetic monitoring. October 25, 2005. www.asahq.org/publicationsAndServices/standards/02.pdf (accessed November 25, 2016).

14. Piekarski F, et al. (2015). Quality of handover in a pediatric postanesthesia care unit. *Paediatr Anaesth*, 25(7), 746–52.

15. Pucher PH, et al. (2015). Effectiveness of interventions to improve patient handover in surgery: A systematic review. *Surgery*, 158(1), 85–95.

16. Greenberg CC, et al. (2007). Patterns of communication breakdowns resulting in injury to surgical patients. *J Am Coll Surg*, 204(4), 533–40.

17. Milby A, et al. (2014). Quality of post-operative patient handover in the post-anaesthesia care unit: A prospective analysis. *Acta Anaesthesiol Scand*, 58(2), 192–7.

18. Segall N, et al. (2012). Can we make postoperative patient handovers safer? A systematic review of the literature. *Anesth Analg*, 115(1), 102–15.

19. Boat AC, et al. (2013). Handoff checklists improve the reliability of patient handoffs in the operating room and postanesthesia care unit. *Paediatr Anaesth*, 23(7), 647–54.

20. Salzwedel C, et al. (2013). The effect of a checklist on the quality of post-anaesthesia patient handover: A randomized controlled trial. *Int J Qual Health Care*, 25(2), 176–81.

21. Byrnes MC, et al. (2009). Implementation of a mandatory checklist of protocols and objectives improves compliance with a wide range of evidence-based intensive care unit practices. *Crit Care Med*, 37(10), 2775–81.

22. Petrovic MA, et al. (2012). Pilot implementation of a perioperative protocol to guide operating room-to-intensive care unit patient handoffs. *J Cardiothorac Vasc Anesth*, 26(1), 11–6.

23. Urbach DR, et al. (2014). Introduction of surgical safety checklists in Ontario, Canada. *N Engl J Med*, 370(11), 1029–38.

24. Borchard A, et al. (2012). A systematic review of the effectiveness, compliance, and critical factors for implementation of safety checklists in surgery. *Ann Surg*, 256(6), 925–33.

25. Manser T, et al. (2010). Assessing the quality of patient handoffs at care transitions. *Qual Saf Health Care*, 19(6), e44.

26. van Rensen EL, et al. (2012). Multitasking during patient handover in the recovery room. *Anesth Analg*, 115(5), 1183–7.

27. Nagpal K, et al. (2010). Postoperative handover: Problems, pitfalls, and prevention of error. *Ann Surg*, 252(2), 171–6.

28. de Vries EN, et al. (2010). Effect of a comprehensive surgical safety system on patient outcomes. *N Enl J Med*, 363(20), 1928–37.

29. Agawala AV, et al. (2015). An electronic checklist improves transfer and retention of critical information at intraoperative handoff of care. *Anesth Analg*, 120(1), 96–104.

Chapter

37

Anesthesiology Disaster Management and Emergency Preparedness

Ezekiel B. Tayler, Blas Catalani, Jill Cooley, and Chris Sharp

Few, if any, hospitals in America today could handle 100 patients suddenly demanding care. There is no metropolitan area, no geographically contiguous area, that could handle 1,000 people suddenly needing advanced medical care in this country right now.

– U.S. Congress, Senate, Committee on Government Affairs. FEMA's Role in Managing Bioterriost Attacks and the Impact of Public Health Concerns on Bioterrorism Preparedness. 107th Cong. 1st sess. July 23, 2001. Testimony of Tara J. O'Toole, M.D., M.P.H., Johns Hopkins Center for Civilian Biodefense Studies

Introduction

Whether the above statement still holds true is open for debate; however, there is no question that mass casualties will continue to occur in this country and around the world. A mass casualty event (MCE) can be defined as an incident that has produced more casualties than a customary response assignment can handle [1]. There are a number of oversight agencies responsible for informing the public and medical community about MCEs [2–4]. Hospital administrators and individual departments also have a duty to prepare and train their staff to be able to respond at an MCE and work with other facilities in the region. The department of anesthesiology is not limited to the operating room (OR) and should be a leader when it comes to planning and coordinating for emergency situations.

MCEs are often intimidating because of the uncertainty involved. Patients are not the only victims during a disaster as hospital employees also have a duty to their own family members who may also be in harm's way. With proper education and planning, a department can quickly and efficiently mobilize to aid in patient care and also tend to individual responsibilities outside of the hospital. It is the purpose of this chapter to outline how both a hospital and an anesthesiology department can effectively respond to an MCE and collaborate with other departments in the process.

MCEs of modern historical importance include the Oklahoma City bombing, 2001 World Trade Center attack, 2004 Indian Ocean tsunami, Hurricane Katrina, 2015 Philadelphia Amtrak train derailment, and the 2016 Florida night club shooting – the list goes on and on. In all of these situations, the results were large number of victims that often overwhelmed the resources of the community's healthcare system. In some of the aforementioned circumstances, healthcare facilities and workers were also debilitated, causing a tremendous surge in demand for their services. Lack of power, destroyed or damaged equipment, medication shortages and security issues can fuel an already volatile situation. In the immediate aftermath of an MCE, it is important to quickly allocate resources and make decisions to save as many lives as possible. Making such decisions could have a large impact in an institution's ability to function and could save thousands of lives in the process.

MCE can be separated into two categories: (1) those that result in an immediate or sudden impact (see Figure 37.1) and (2) those that result in a developing or sustained impact (see Figure 37.2) [5]. Examples of the first category include detonation of bombs, mass transit crashes, or natural disasters. The initial impact can cause an influx of wounded patients but then generally tapers off. The second MCE category could consist of massive exposure to anthrax or an influenza pandemic. There is a gradual increase in the number of people affected; however, the numbers of patients could eventually overwhelm the healthcare system. There could be an initial decline in patient numbers secondary to treatment; however, reinfection might cause another rapid increase in casualties. The second type of MCE would be expected to last a longer and necessitate prolonged planning for resource allocation. It is worthy to note that the first type of MCE is more unpredictable as a sudden impact requires triage and temporizing measures. With regard to a developing MCE, some of the circumstances could be considered predictable and public education would help in preventing the spread of more disease and loss of life. Regardless of the type of MCE, preparation is the key to keeping a hospital system functional. Looking to the leadership of a hospital will help with guidance during an emergency and allow one to be an integral part of the process.

Hospital Preparedness

An *all-hazards* approach to key actions provided by a hospital during any disaster event is a model used by the WHO [6] and Federal Emergency Management Agency [7]. The goal is to provide institutional organization in chaotic and disorganized circumstances.

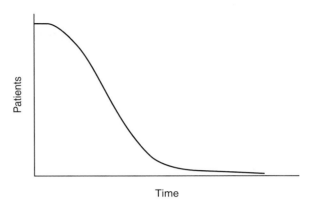

Explosions, Airplane or Train Crashes Due to Bombings (e.g., Madrid Train Bombings), Earthquakes

Figure 37.1 Immediate (sudden peak) impact.

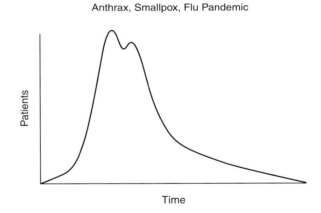

Anthrax, Smallpox, Flu Pandemic

Figure 37.2 Developing (sustained) impact.

A hospital emergency response checklist developed by WHO contains nine key components in order to achieve (1) continuity of essential services, (2) well-coordinated implementation of hospital operations at every level, (3) clear and accurate internal and external communication, (4) swift adaptation to increased demands, (5) the effective use of scarce resources, and (6) a safe environment for healthcare workers.

Command and Control

A hospital should establish a committee or command group responsible for directing hospital-based emergency management operations. The goal of the command group is to act as the central command station where all information flows to and from in order to coordinate care. Representatives from all departments should be involved in development of the command group including but not limited to hospital administration, security, surgical and medical department chairs, engineering, nursing administration, pharmacy, infection control, and waste management. During an emergency, the command group should set up a location where operations can be organized and disseminated effectively. The location should be equipped with appropriate technology to also be able to communicate with other institutions in the surrounding area and country [8].

Communication

The hospital has a responsibility to communicate with its staff, surrounding community and, potentially, public officials to ensure informed decision making. Without clear communication, deterioration of trust could occur and worsen a stressful situation. A spokesperson from the command group should be appointed to act as such a liaison. Hospital staff should be briefed on their roles and responsibilities within the incident action plan. If media is still available, key messages should be drafted on a regular basis and distributed to departments within the hospital and community [9, 10]. Back-up communication systems should be sought (e.g., satellite phones, pagers, two-way radios) if loss of electricity occurs. Contact lists should be kept up to date and preserve as much documentation throughout the incident.

Safety and Security

Civil unrest is not uncommon in situations where access to food, water and healthcare becomes cut off or difficult to acquire. Demands on law enforcement will undoubtedly be overwhelmed so it is important to have a series of actions to ensure hospital staff and patient protection during an emergency. A hospital security team should be established to identify areas of vulnerability and coordinate an increased presence in these areas (e.g., ED entrance, entry/exits, food/water access points, pharmaceutical stockpiles). A reliable method of identifying authorized personnel, patients, and visitors along with transport mechanisms should be implemented. Areas for radioactive, biological and chemical decontamination and isolation should also be developed if warranted [11]. The security team should be prepared to call on outside law enforcement

teams and military operations in situations where order cannot be preserved.

Triage

There are many ethical dilemmas to deciding who will receive more care than others. The World Medical Association has stated, "It is unethical for a physician to persist, at all costs, at maintaining the life of a patient beyond hope, thereby wasting to no avail scarce resources needed elsewhere" [12]. It is important to have patient triage clinicians with training in an MCE. A team consisting of an emergency department (ED) physician, emergency nurse, surgeon, and anesthesiologist should be more than adequate to quickly assign patients into varying levels of care. A safe area for triage should be established and an internationally accepted protocol used with clear labeling tags [13]. There is a paucity of literature when it comes to the best tool for triaging patients during a disaster situation. Healthcare workers are generally very accurate at assigning triage levels in the ED on a daily basis [5]; however, to what degree this is true in a disaster has not yet been proven. If possible, multiple triage teams should be available if an MCE were to overwhelm the capacity of a small number of providers.

Surge Capacity

Surge capacity is defined as the ability to expand beyond normal capacity to meet increased demand for clinical care [4]. During an MCE, the most critically ill patients often become the standard of care. Elective cases in the OR should cease and discharge criteria be modified for those who do not need hospital care. Additional sites outside of the hospital should be sought out in case the hospital becomes too full to function (e.g., hotels, schools). Transport services and post mortem care should also be addressed [14].

Continuity of Essential Services

Access to water, food and human waste removal are basic services that should be maintained even in an MCE. Maternal and childcare in tandem with urgent operations must also be accessible in the capacity that a hospital operated before an emergency. Plans to address evacuation strategies and the necessary equipment to carry them out must constantly be addressed. If there aren't enough transport ventilators or medications for critically ill patients, the hospital should reach out to the community and attempt to ensure availability of these resources [6, 15].

Human Resources

A well run human resources department can effectively manage hospital staffing and address legal issues with credentialing for nonhospital workers. It may be necessary to work outside the scope of practice for a large number of clinicians and allow those who have no formal training to engage in life saving procedures (e.g., voluntary medical personnel, retired staff, medical students). Temporary credentialing, when appropriate, can be employed so long as state laws are followed [16]. Healthcare workers will likely be taxed to exhaustion, so it is important for the human resources department to keep track of hours logged in order to give necessary breaks to prevent burnout. Social workers, interpreters and clergy for families or staff should be made available [17]. Leave policies and maintaining an updated staff list allow for better workforce management and communication with the command personnel.

Logistics and Supply Management

Ensuring a continuous supply of materials to take care of a large number of patients is a daunting task. Agreements may need to be made with suppliers to forgo payment in order to ensure necessary materials for wound care, OR procedures and waste disposal. Additional protection of supply stores from theft and maintaining an updated inventory of all equipment, supplies and medications should be enacted. An alert system when stores get low can be put in place so a restocking process occurs automatically with appropriate suppliers [18].

Postdisaster Recovery

When delivering a general anesthetic, planning should occur not just for induction but also for maintenance and emergence phases. After an initial disaster and management period, so too is there a recovery phase. Planning for recovery should be begin at the onset of the event. Breaking down parts of the facility and returning it to its original purpose may take the same if not more time than it did to erect its alternative function. A successful treatment of a large number of patients may still necessitate an evacuation to a larger or multiple smaller facilities, and strategies should be made ahead of time if possible. Debriefing of staff, allowing for mental health needs and recognizing extraordinary efforts will help with the healing process and allow for normalization to occur [19, 20].

Anesthesiology Department Preparedness

Anesthesiology touches many areas of the hospital system, so it is important to realize how integral a role it plays during an MCE. Leadership will be needed in obstetrics, ORs, critical care units, and pain management systems. Liaisons will likely be established in various parts of the hospital and report back to the chair or other leader of the anesthesia department so as to better allocate resources. It is essential to have these roles setup prior to an emergency and practice through simulation to ensure proper execution when necessary.

There is a deficiency of literature with regard to intradepartmental planning for an MCE. Most studies focus on resuscitative efforts or humanitarian disaster relief operations [21, 22], but little on management and prospective organization skills. It is rarely possible to estimate the severity of a disaster or even the predictability of an event occurring. The Joint Commission requests an institution perform a Hazard Vulnerability Analysis (HVA) for organizations to determine the focus of their emergency planning, though there is no specific tool nor method deemed the gold standard. An HVA is defined as the identification of potential emergencies and the direct and indirect effects these emergencies may have on the staffing firm's operation and demand for its services [23]. Whatever plan for dealing with mass casualties is agreed upon, it should allow for flexibility and be well organized.

Once a chain of command has been established, priorities should be sent out to the appropriate staff. Box 37.1 shows a management strategy for the OR during mass casualty. It addresses staffing issues, communication responsibilities, blood bank availability and ensuring adequate supply chains. A well carried out disaster management system should have multiple arms of activity and closed loop communication to aid in weakened areas of the coordination effort.

Personal Protective Equipment

Hazards may be encountered in a disaster that one may not have had exposure to in the past. If structural

---

Box 37.1. OR Procedures for Mass Casualty Management

☐ Refer to facility's operations manual
Open up appropriate annex

☐ Activate call-in tree
Assign an individual to activate. Use clerical personnel or automatic paging system, if available

☐ Assess status of ORs
Determine staffing of ORs 0–2, 2–12 and 12–24 h. Hold elective cases.

☐ Alert current ORs
Finish current surgical procedures as soon as possible and prepare to receive trauma

☐ Assign staff
Set up for trauma/emergency cases

☐ Anesthesia Coordinator should become OR medical director
Work with OR nursing manager to facilitate communication and coordination of staff and facilities

☐ Report OR status to Hospital Command Center (HCC)
Enter telephone, email address of HCC

☐ Ensure adequate supplies
Coordinate with anesthesia techs/supply personnel to ensure adequate supplies of fluids, medications, disposables, other

☐ Contact PACU
Accelerate transfer of patients to floors/ICUs in preparation for high volume of cases

☐ Anesthesiologist should act as liaison in ED
Send an experienced practitioner to the ED to act as a liaison (your eyes and ears) and keep communications open to Anesthesia Coordinator

☐ Consider assembly of Stat Teams
Combination of anesthesia, surgical, nursing, respiratory personnel to triage, as needed

☐ HAZMET/WMD event
Review special personal protective procedures, such as DECON and isolation techniques. Consider if part of the OR or hallways should be considered "hot" or should have ventilation altered. Good resources include CHEMM/REMM websites

☐ Coordinate with blood bank
Verify blood availability

☐ Coordinate with other patient care areas
ICUs, OB, Peds, etc. to ensure continuity of care for new and existing patients

Developed by the Committee on Trauma and Emergency Preparedness, American Society of Anesthesiologists. Available at: www.asahq.org/resources/resources-from-asa-committees/committee-on-trauma-and-emergency-preparedness

---

damage occurred to the OR, one might be delivering an anesthetic wearing a hard hat. It is important to know what types of personal protective equipment (PPE) is available, ensure adequate supply, understand how to use them, and potentially purchase additional tools.

The Occupational Safety and Health Administration (OSHA) issues regulations for workplace health and safety and the CDC issues recommendations for when and what PPE should be used to prevent exposure to infectious diseases. There are four major components to the hierarchy of safety for healthcare workers [24]: (1) training in isolation policies and procedures, and procedures for recognizing patients with a communicable disease before they expose workers; (2) engineering controls like negative pressure rooms for patients

Table 37.1 Healthcare Providers Working in Predecontamination (Triage) and Decontamination Areas [26]

Hazard	Level of PPE*	Note
Radiation	Level C PPE should be worn until risk characterization determines that level D PPE provides sufficient protection	In all cases where radiation is suspected, first receivers should also wear a personal radiation dosimeter to monitor their radiation absorbed dose
Organophosphates, e.g. cyclohexyl sarin	Level A PPE should worn until risk characterization determines exposure levels	There are no current OSHA permissible exposure limits (PELs) for exposure to nerve agents.
Blister agents, e.g., sulfur/nitrogen mustard	Level A PPE should worn until risk characterization determines exposure levels	There are no current OSHA PELs for exposure to blister agents
Measles	Level D PPE	

* Level of PPE based on first receivers delivering care to victims more likely to be externally contaminated.

with airborne diseases such as tuberculosis; (3) work practice controls such as not recapping needles; and (4) personal protective equipment. There are two civilian classification systems within the United States with regard to PPE [25] – one described by OSHA/ Environmental Protection Agency and the other by the National Fire Protection Association. The former will be described although both have a four-tier system going from the most protective to least protective.

Level A is the most protective of the PPE systems. It includes a positive-pressure full-face piece self-contained breathing apparatus, totally encapsulating chemical and vapor-protective suit, inner and outer chemical-resistant gloves, and chemical-resistant boots, with steel toe and shank. Advantages of this level is maximum available skin, respiratory, and eye protection; however, duration of use may be limited secondary to heat, other physical and psychological stressors, limited air supply, and need for advanced training.

Level B PPE elements include positive-pressure, full-face piece self-contained breathing apparatus, hooded chemical-resistant clothing, inner and outer chemical-resistant gloves and chemical-resistant boots with steel toe and shank. The benefit of level B PPE is less restriction of mobility than level A; however, the same level of training may be needed.

Level C PPE elements include full-face or half-mask, negative-pressure air-purifying respirator, hooded chemical-resistant clothing, inner and outer chemical-resistant gloves, and chemical-resistant boots with steel toe and shank. Level C has increased mobility as compared to level A or level B PPE with much less physical and psychological stress involved with extended operation. No fit testing is required for hooded respirators.

Level D PPE elements include escape masks (N95), water-repellent surgical gowns, safety glasses, face shield or goggles, surgical gloves and waterproof shoe covers. Level D provides a sufficient level of protection when work operations preclude splashes, immersion, or potential for unexpected inhalation or contact with hazardous levels of chemicals and is equivalent to everyday uniforms worn by first receivers (Table 37.1).

Communication

In the event loss of electricity occurs, transmission of basic intel can grind to a halt. Back-up messaging systems should be planned for in order to carry out vital tasks. If written messages are needed, the documents should be signed, dated and filed upon receipt. Text pagers can be utilized so long as there is a functional network. Two-way radios can be used up to a point; however, eventually the system can become overloaded. Key leaders may only have access to a radio in which case written messages should be the secondary transport mechanism.

An alternative to internal communication is to outsource to an external provider. The Hospital Disaster Support Communications System (HDSCS) is a group of about 80 amateur radio operators who volunteer to provide backup internal and external communications for critical medical facilities all over the country whenever normal communications are interrupted for any reason [27]. The HDSCS can provide voice, text, and video communications through their equipment to the hospital and to the surrounding area. A well-run simulation could tie in the aforementioned resources and make a true emergency response less problematic.

Delivery of Anesthesia

Anesthesiologists are inherently masters at adaptability. Loss of electricity, absence of shelter, loss of central supply gases, or not having the necessary tools to intubate are just some of many different scenarios one might face in an emergency. Total intravenous anesthesia would be necessary if electricity was lost and batteries ran out. Those efficient in regional techniques would become invaluable if delivery of volatile anesthetics became unavailable. Knowledge of available resources becomes imperative when deciding how to approach an anesthetic in any situation. A representative from the department should work with logistics and supply management to become aware of medication and equipment availability. If supplies become low, it may be necessary to withhold treatment until only the direst situations. Monitoring vital signs without electricity would require an increased dependence on visual and tactile responses from patients.

In the event of a staffing shortage, it may become necessary to teach basic anesthesia skills to medical students or volunteers. Having someone bag mask an intubated patient for a prolonged period of time can be quickly taught to a willing participant. A postanesthesia recovery unit could be staffed by a lead nurse and a number of novice providers taught to recognize key postoperative complications. It is important to consider that although an anesthesiologist's role is ultimately to deliver anesthesia, if other tasks become necessary in the interim, it should be done willingly to help with the overall cause. A surgeon may need someone to hold traction, an obstetrician might need some assistance with a delivery or a nurse could be struggling to console a scared patient. Whatever the task, it should be approached with flexibility and efficiency.

Evaluation of Plan

Repetition is the key to mastery and the ideal process to evaluate a mass casualty response plan. A carefully crafted document outlining roles, regulations and contingency plans should be created and updated on a regular basis. Through role playing and interactions between departments, the process can be optimized in preparation for a true emergency. Understanding the limitations of a department and participating in a collaborative effort is important as well as remembering that responding to an MCE cannot be done alone.

Reaching out to other institutions may be appropriate in order to conserve resources and assist in the provision of key services not routinely offered at your institution. Staying up-to-date on the most recent literature on MCE and engaging with the hospital administration and community will help ensure a safe and quality response during a time of crisis.

Summary

Anesthesiologists have the benefit of interacting with many different specialities across the medical spectrum. We are expected to be able to walk out of an obstetric ward having just placed a spinal for a cesarean section to emergently intubate a patient in the trauma bay, regardless of patient age. Such fluidity makes the specialty unique in its ability to "wear many hats" but also places an increased responsibility for observation of quality care and process management. Mass casualty events have the potential to touch all medical specialties at once, so who better than an anesthesiologist to be present as a leader during such times of crisis? While an MCE management plan may not begin with any single department, it is important for anesthesiologists to be at the forefront during its development in order to help guide the institution as well as enrich those involved.

References

1. Thomas J. Mass casualty incident. www
   .emsconedonline.com/pdfs/EMT-Mass%20
   Casualty%20Incident-an%20overview-Trauma.pdf

2. National Center for Injury Prevention and Control. *Interim planning guidance for preparedness and response to a mass casualty event resulting from terrorist use of explosives.* Centers for Disease Control and Prevention, 2010.

3. American Hospital Association. *Hospital preparedness for mass casualties. Summary of an invitational forum convened on March 8–9, 2000 by the American Hospital Association with the support of the Office of Emergency Preparedness.* U.S. Department of Health and Human Services.

4. World Health Organization. *Mass casualty management systems. Strategies and guidelines for building health sector capacity.* World Health Organization, 2007

5. Phillips SJ, Knebel A, eds. *Mass Medical Care with Scarce Resources: A Community Planning Guide.* Prepared by Health Systems Research, Inc., an Altarum company, under contract No. 290-04-0010. AHRQ Publication No. 07-0001. Rockville, MD: Agency for Healthcare Research and Quality 2007

6. *Hospital emergency response checklist. An all-hazards tool for hospital administrators and emergency managers.* World Health Organization, 2011.

7. *SLG 101: Guide for all-hazard emergency operations planning.* Federal Emergency Management Agency, September 1996.

8. *Establishing a mass casualty management system.* Pan American Health Organization, 1995. http://publications.paho.org/product.php?productid=644 (accessed August 17, 2016).

9. *Creating a communication strategy for pandemic influenza.* Pan American Health Organization, 2009. www.paho.org/English/AD/PAHO_CommStrategy_Eng.pdf (accessed August 17, 2016).

10. *Effective media communication during public health emergencies: A WHO wall chart.* World Health Organization, 2005. www.who.int/entity/csr/resources/publications/WHO%20MEDIA%20HANDBOOK%20WALL%20CHART.pdf (accessed August 17, 2016).

11. *Guidelines for vulnerability reduction in the design of new health facilities.* Pan American Health Organization, 2004. www.paho.org/english/dd/ped/vulnerabilidad.htm (accessed August 17, 2016).

12. World Medical Association. Statement on medical ethics in the event of disasters. www.wma.net/en/30publications/10policies/d7/index.html (accessed August 17, 2016).

13. *Emergency triage assessment and treatment (ETAT). Manual for participants.* World Health Organization, 2005. http://whqlibdoc.who.int/publications/2005/9241546875_eng.pdf (accessed August 17, 2016).

14. *Hospital surge model.* U.S. Department of Health and Human Services' Agency for Healthcare Research and Quality, 2010. www.ahrq.gov/prep/hospsurgemodel (accessed August 17, 2016).

15. Wisner B, Adams J, eds. *Environmental health in emergencies and disasters: A practical guide.* World Health Organization, 2003. www.who.int/water_sanitation_health/hygiene/emergencies/emergencies2002/en/ (accessed August 17, 2016).

16. *Adapting standards of care under extreme conditions. Guidance for professionals during disasters, pandemics, and other extreme emergencies.* American Nurse Association, March 2008.

17. *Mental health in emergencies.* World Health Organization, 2003. www.who.int/mental_health/media/en/640.pdf (accessed August 17, 2016).

18. *Humanitarian supply management and logistics in the health sector.* Pan American Health Organization, 2001. www.paho.org/English/Ped/supplies.htm (accessed August 17, 2016).

19. *Hospital assessment and recovery guide.* U.S. Department of Health and Human Services' Agency for Healthcare Research and Quality, 2010. www.ahrq.gov/prep/hosprecovery/hosprec2.htm (accessed August 17, 2016).

20. *Guidance for health sector assessment to support the post-disaster recovery process. Version 2.2.* World Health Organization, 2010. www.who.int/hac/techguidance/tools/manuals/pdna_health_sector_guidance/en/index.html (accessed August 17, 2016).

21. Rossler B, et al. Preparedness of anesthesiologists working in humanitarian disasters. *Disaster Med Public Health Prep.*, 2013; 7(4): 408–12.

22. Dobkin, AB, et al. The anaesthetist in the management of a disaster. *Canad M A J.*, 1957; 76: 763–70.

23. www.jointcommission.org/standards_information/jcfaqdetails.aspx?StandardsFAQId=893&StandardsFAQChapterId=63&ProgramId=0&ChapterId=0&IsFeatured=False&IsNew=False&Keyword=hazard (accessed August 19, 2016).

24. Guidance for the selection and use of personal protective equipment (PPE) in healthcare settings. www.cdc.gov/HAI/pdfs/ppe/PPEslides6-29-04.pdf (accessed August 19, 2016).

25. General description and discussion of the levels of protection and protective gear. Regulations (Standards – 29 CFR) 1910.120 App B. www.osha.gov/pls/oshaweb/owadisp.show_document?p_table=STANDARDS&p_id=9767

26. OSHA best practices for hospital-based first receivers of victims from mass casualty incidents involving the release of hazardous substances. www.osha.gov/dts/osta/bestpractices/html/hospital_firstreceivers.html

27. http://hdscs.org/

Chapter

38

Novel Technology for Patient Engagement

Matthew B. Novitch, Peter A. Gold, Aiden Feng, and Mark R. Jones

Contents

Introduction

Patient preparation in advance of interventions is an essential dimension of operative management, serving to reduce risk, increase both perioperative and postoperative safety, and enhance recovery. Perioperative risk and unacceptable patient outcomes continue to burden healthcare systems globally [1–3]. Timely, accessible patient education and engagement are critical to achieve the quality outcomes desired and successfully transition to value-based care. Ensuring patient safety and compliance throughout the preoperative preparation cycle, however, remains a significant barrier. To this end, evidence has shown that patients who actively manage their own healthcare demonstrate improved clinical outcomes over those who passively receive care [4–7]. Accomplishing these goals will require effective patient engagement and education [8].

While several modalities in practice have intended to mediate this goal, up to 80 percent of information conveyed to patients remains unretained, leading to $115–190 billion in preventable expenditures annually [9]. Given the recent history of reduced healthcare funding, enhanced efficiency in healthcare services is more necessary now than ever [10]. Gastroenterology in particular may benefit from improved patient engagement. Colonoscopy, a foundational procedure of the specialty, is the gold standard screening test for the early detection and prevention of colorectal cancer; 40 percent of all colorectal cancers may be prevented by regular screening [11,12]. Problematically, an estimated 12 percent of patients scheduled for colonoscopy do not show upto their appointment due to

miscommunication or noncompliance [13]. Of those who do attend their appointment, up to 25 percent are inadequately prepared, resulting in unclean bowel that reduces adenoma detection rate and prolongs procedure time.

These episodes of noncompliance result in a net loss of $1.5–2.25 billion to the US healthcare system annually [14]. Failed preparation and no-shows cost hospitals between $1,300 and $1,500 in net losses per patient [14], totaling up to $3 million in costs per year for one hospital alone [15–17]. Without question, improving the success rates of a routine procedure such as colonoscopy would drastically reduce healthcare costs. Figures 38.1a and 38.1b detail the large swath of US procedures represented by colonoscopy alone, and the percentages of colonoscopies affected by inadequate patient engagement.

A wide array of methods has already been applied in an attempt to improve patient education and adherence. Examples include full-time patient educators, dedicated teams that call patients at home to review instructions, video lessons to help standardize information, and education companies dedicated solely to facilitating patient access to healthcare information. Such services have been criticized for insufficient accessibility, the omission of critical disease processes and populations, and the lack of customization for individual conditions or situations. Universal access is further hindered by the fact that only 12% of US adults are sufficiently health literate, rendering these methods cumbersome and ineffective [18].

Certainly, effective systems to reduce healthcare costs in the context of specific, anticipated interventions for the preoperative patient remain

Total Annual Volume of Procedures in the U.S

Figure 38.1a [9,13–17] Total annual volume of colonoscopy procedures in the US.

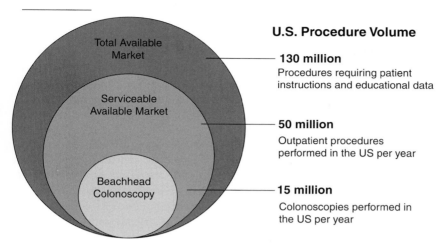

U.S. Procedure Volume

- Total Available Market
- Serviceable Available Market
- Beachhead Colonoscopy

130 million
Procedures requiring patient instructions and educational data

50 million
Outpatient procedures performed in the US per year

15 million
Colonoscopies performed in the US per year

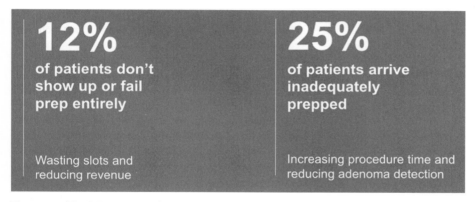

12%
of patients don't show up or fail prep entirely

Wasting slots and reducing revenue

25%
of patients arrive inadequately prepped

Increasing procedure time and reducing adenoma detection

Figure 38.1b[13] Percentages of colonoscopies affected by inadequate patient engagement.

elusive. Streamlined operative management mandates competent patient engagement strategies; outcomes, length of procedure and of hospital stay, as well as overall cost are highly dependent on this often overlooked aspect. This chapter aims to provide information on the present state of software and technology available for engaging patients, novel modalities currently in development, and techniques designed to improve patient engagement and risk stratification.

Engagement

As stated earlier, actively involved patients experience more positive clinical outcomes than those passively receiving care [4–7]. Indeed, successfully engaging patients is fast becoming requisite for high-quality, safe patient care [19]. Graffigna et al. describe patient engagement as a multidimensional psychosocial process resulting from the conjoint cognitive, emotional, and behavioral enactment of individuals toward their health condition and management [20]. Before patients can actively engage in their own care, however, several concepts must be considered. Adherence, compliance, empowerment, and activation are interconnected elements of engagement, each rooted in individualized patient behaviors and their causal interactivity within the healthcare system [21–23]. To fully engage a patient, these key ideas must be reinforced. The result instills in the patient a sense of subjective control and direct responsibility over their disease and outcome [20,24–26].

A burgeoning sphere in the patient engagement dilemma is found in the world of eHealth, which is a term to describe healthcare practice supported by electronic processes and communication. Rapidly evolving technological advancements have allowed a boon in healthcare interventions, and together represent tremendous potential for accelerated patient engagement. Promoting integrated, sustainable, and patient-centered services using eHealth modalities will stimulate effective exchanges among members of the healthcare team and the patient [27]. The majority of eHealth focuses on internet-related technologies to support and educate patients on their healthcare process [28]. Several of these novel technologies have shown moderate effectiveness, including patient education encyclopedias such as Krames (staywell.com); Healthloop, an app which actively engages patients at home daily before and after discharge to continuously monitor their progress; UpToDate, which employs handouts and digital brochures; and Emmi, which enroll patients in 30-min online courses. To maximize impact, however, patient engagement will require not only efficiency and simplicity on the patients' side, but an ease of transition into the already well-established and strictly regulated realm of healthcare. The technologies mentioned above are yet to adequately bridge the gap between the two.

One recently emerged technology, Medumo, provides a marked improvement on the world of eHealth-driven patient engagement. Medumo is a an interactive patient platform built on proprietary algorithms that deliver content in an adaptive and personalized manner based on the patient's health literacy level, among other variables. Medumo uses CareTours, customizable provider-driven education pathways that guide patients throughout their treatment procedure and discharge via SMS text messaging and email. This enables institutions to produce or license clinically validated and patient-reviewed programs via the platform itself. This dynamic technology veers away from fixed digital classes that frontload information and require frequent patient logins. CareTours do not require an app download or log in, which numerous studies have shown to be major barriers to adoption for low-income, minority, and elderly communities [29]. In addition, Medumo monitors user engagement and notifies providers when a user is at risk for specific scenarios. Medumo works without costly electronic medical records integrations or clinician outflow adjustments, and without two-way messaging channels that require management by care providers. Workflow is unchanged by integration of the software within an existing healthcare system, and is available for deployment in less than 2 weeks.

Medumo represents a major step forward in uniting the complexity of modern healthcare with the universality of access necessary to maximize patient engagement. Figures 38.2a and 38.2b highlight the currently available technologies and their respective leaning towards provider or patient preference, and features of Medumo that increase the efficacy of patient engagement in comparison to other existing technologies.

Technology

The majority of engagement between patient and provider has, until recently, consisted primarily of verbal instructions and educational pamphlets. These methods have long been ineffective, as evidenced by the high rates of noncompliance in colonoscopies. Fortunately, the advent of cellular and internet technology has ushered in several new methods. As mentioned previously, SMS text messaging and email are employed by platforms such as Medumo in an effort to increase patient engagement. A randomized controlled trial published in Endoscopy in 2015 demonstrated that phone call and text message reminders achieved significantly higher bowel preparation quality score [30]. While there was no significant difference between phone call reminders compared to text message reminders, phone reminders did require more time for staff members to manage. In practice, text message programs interfere with clinical workflow because physicians and staff need to design, preprogram, and send the messages to patients at the appropriate time. This process is difficult to manage when there are hundreds of patients to engage on a daily basis for an average-sized practice.

The automaticity of Medumo's aforementioned CareTour pathways allows for patient education and instruction without the need for implementation or management by medical staff. These self-automated CareTour pathways encompass patient engagement day-by-day to reduce scheduling leakage, preoperative noncompliance, no-shows, and attrition. Automation allows for the implementation of unique custom protocols in a time-sensitive manner tailored to each patient's preoperative schedule. Messaging is adaptable to patient compliance and noncompliance, as well as evaluation of patient outcomes based on individual engagement. Instead of one-time, front-loaded, verbal, paper, or video-based instructions that represent the pretechnology practices of today, automation is more digestible, accompanying the patients throughout their healthcare journey.

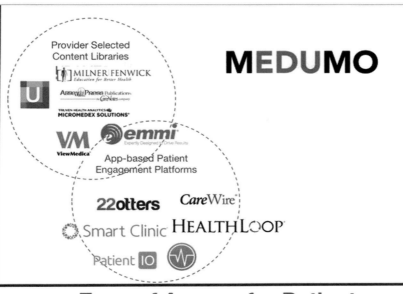

Figure 38.2a Currently available technologies and their respective leaning towards provider or patient preference.

	MEDUMO	HEALTHLOOP	*Care*Wire	emmi
No app download / portal / search	●	○	●	○
No workflow changes for staff	●	○	○	○
Deployment under 2 weeks	●	○	○	○
Message personalization	●	●	●	○
Multi-site clinical validation	●	●	○	○

Figure 38.2b Features of Medumo that increase the efficacy of patient engagement in comparison to other existing technologies.

Fully automated systems will be equipped with programmable message timing, check-in feedback loops, real time data collection capabilities, and adaptive content delivery algorithms. The overall experience increases patient awareness and responsibility without adding extra burden to the workflow of the medical staff. In fact, as the automated systems better learn patient behavior, medical staff workflow will experience new innovative patient-centered improvements. Figure 38.3 demonstrates a typical series of automated multimedia communication delivered to the patient in preparation for a procedure.

With the widespread adoption of smartphone technology, some native smartphone applications have also been developed to assist patients with colonoscopy preparation. For instance, Geisinger Health System Gastroenterology created the Easy Prep: Colonoscopy mobile app that is free to download with preparation instructions, calendars and helpful tips. Other similar examples include Medivo's Colonoscopy Prep Assistant, L.A.E.C. Colonoscopy Helper, and SmartClinic app. Unfortunately, these programs have not been validated in clinical research. Moreover, they require patients to find and download an application from an "app store" which, as discussed, has proven to be a significant barrier to adoption. A recent Accenture report found that hospitals have

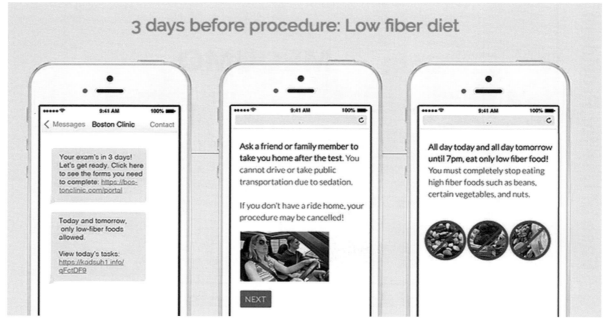

Figure 38.3a A typical series of automated multimedia communication delivered to the patient in preparation for a procedure, 3 days before procedure.

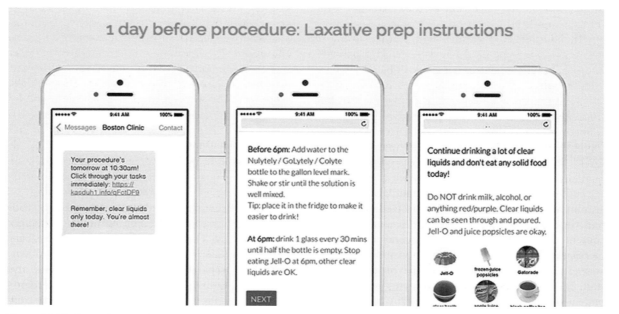

Figure 38.3b A typical series of automated multimedia communication delivered to the patient in preparation for a procedure, 1 day before procedure.

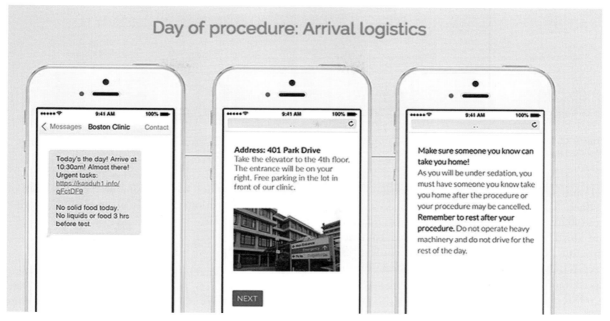

Figure 38.3c A typical series of automated multimedia communication delivered to the patient in preparation for a procedure, on the day of procedure.

engaged less than 2 percent of their patients using mobile apps [31].

In addition to text messaging, other forms of multimedia may be used to further engage patients. Clinical practices have in recent years begun to share videos online with patients to aid in explaining the preparation process. Research has in fact shown that online video-based education improves patient colonoscopy preparation quality [32]. However, many videos are long, inconvenient to access, and are given to patients long before the instructions are actually needed. In a peer-reviewed study investigating instructional videos on YouTube, Ajumobi et al. found that 59 percent of the videos were "low-content" videos with insufficient instructions and many contained unempirical, non–research-based information [33]. Medumo has leveraged the information gleaned from such clinical research to create a set of high-quality videos that can serve as the standard of care going forward.

Clearly, patient engagement and education may be enhanced through multiple forms of technology, e.g., text messaging, email, or multimedia instructional material such as videos. As stated, each method has demonstrated efficacy, albeit separately from others. Medumo combines each system in an automated,

simple to integrate platform. Furthermore, Medumo utilizes adaptive learning to augment the combined effectiveness of each tool. Adaptive learning is a proven educational method focused on computers as interactive instructional tools to deliver resources based on the unique needs of each learner. This modality arose from the work on cognitive psychology of B.F. Skinner in the 1950s, and expanded through the artificial intelligence research of late. It has since been more widely adopted by the education industry. The US Department of Education has endorsed the use of adaptive learning for its ability to simultaneously teach and assess for continuous improvement [35]. Medumo's technology leverages automated, precisely timed text message and email reminders with links to videos and check-in questions that are entirely adaptive to individual patients.

Medumo's solution entails both content and software components. The text and email reminder messages contain content that is adaptive to individual patient needs. This content is delivered through images, videos, and written reminders and supplemented with surveys and other interactive elements to further drive active patient engagement. All content is loaded into the software and delivered automatically, so that a patient consistently receives

43.4%	**41.8%**	**40.5%**	**9.1/10**
reduction in no shows & late cancels	reduction in no shows & same-day cancels	reduction in poor prep quality	average patient satisfaction
$921,000	**$384,000**	**80.6%**	**150+**
in annual savings	in annual savings	engagement	active daily patients

Figure 38.4 Over 40 percent reductions in no-shows, late cancellations, and poor preparation quality have resulted in annual savings nearing a million dollars for a single institution.

relevant information based on their date of procedure. The entire system is hosted on a HIPAA-compliant server with high security standards that are third party verified. The message content and timeline are generated based on clinical expert recommendations and further validated by expert consultants. Using patient responses and engagement level, the software adapts in real time to determine risk of inadequate procedure preparation, failure, and no-show. Medumo checks in with patients at critical intervals, prompting the software to segment patients and deliver customized content accordingly. Patients will receive varying responses and additional automated reminders based on their needs, guiding them through preparation challenges. The program tracks patient engagement, defined as open rates and click-through rates of messages, and survey answers at multiple time points to determine each patient's probability of showing up or completing the preparation. Data from these analyses can be consolidated and sent back to providers and clinic staff to further intervene and prevent poor clinical outcomes.

Outcomes

Medumo has been successfully implemented in several large, tertiary academic medical centers. The most advanced programs are concentrated in gastroenterology departments for colonoscopy. Statistically and clinically significant reductions in inadequate bowel preparation and cancelled procedures were seen following implementation. As highlighted in Figure 38.4, over 40 percent reductions in no-shows, late cancellations, and poor preparation quality have resulted in annual savings nearing a million dollars for a single institution [35]. Another site has seen an overall increase in completed case volume of nearly 2 percent following introduction of Medumo CareTours. Perhaps most encouragingly, the average

patient satisfaction score has maintained at 9.1 out of 10 for all institutions currently using Medumo, with a peak score of 9.6.

Summary

Patient engagement has rapidly become an essential aspect of safe, high-quality healthcare. Actively involved patients experience more positive outcomes than passive patients. Advances in technology have fostered an environment wherein providers and patients may now interact seamlessly without burdening either party, but coordinating the most efficacious methods of patient engagement within the strict realm of HIPAA-compliant modern medicine has remained elusive. Medumo, an interactive patient platform that utilizes instructional videos, critically timed text and email reminder messages, check-in questions, and adaptive instructional guidance has begun to bridge the gap between patient and provider needs, allowing for more effective patient engagement, safer and more reliable procedures, and reductions in healthcare expenditures.

References

1. G. Graffigna, S. Barello, and G. Riva, "How to Make Health Information Technology Effective: The Challenge of Patient Engagement," *Arch. Phys. Med. Rehabil.*, vol. 94, no. 10, pp. 2034–2035, Oct. 2013.

2. J. Gruman, M. H. Rovner, M. E. French, et al., "From Patient Education to Patient Engagement: Implications for the Field of Patient Education," *Patient Educ. Couns.*, vol. 78, no. 3, pp. 350–356, Mar. 2010.

3. R. M. Epstein, K. Fiscella, C. S. Lesser, and K. C. Stange, "Why the Nation Needs a Policy Push on Patient-Centered Health Care," *Health Aff.*, vol. 29, no. 8, pp. 1489–1495, Aug. 2010.

4. D. L. Frosch and G. Elwyn, "I Believe, Therefore I Do," *J. Gen. Intern. Med.*, vol. 26, no. 1, pp. 2–4, Jan. 2011.

5. J. H. Hibbard, E. R. Mahoney, R. Stock, and M. Tusler, "Do Increases in Patient Activation Result in Improved Self-Management Behaviors?," *Health Serv. Res.*, vol. 42, no. 4, pp. 1443–1463, Aug. 2007.

6. J. Greene and J. H. Hibbard, "Why Does Patient Activation Matter? An Examination of the Relationships between Patient Activation and Health-Related Outcomes," *J. Gen. Intern. Med.*, vol. 27, no. 5, pp. 520–526, May 2012.

7. S. Barello, G. Graffigna, E. Vegni, M. Savarese, F. Lombardi, and A. C. Bosio, " 'Engage Me in Taking Care of My Heart': A Grounded Theory Study on Patient-Cardiologist Relationship in the Hospital Management of Heart Failure," *BMJ Open*, vol. 5, no. 3, p. e005582, Mar. 2015.

8. D. L. B. Schwappach, "Review: Engaging Patients as Vigilant Partners in Safety," *Med. Care Res. Rev.*, vol. 67, no. 2, pp. 119–148, Apr. 2010.

9. R. P. C. Kessels, "Patients' Memory for Medical Information," *J. R. Soc. Med.*, vol. 96, no. 5, pp. 219–222, May 2003.

10. M. Elf, P. Fröst, G. Lindahl, and H. Wijk, "Shared Decision Making in Designing New Healthcare Environments: Time to Begin Improving Quality," *BMC Health Serv. Res.*, vol. 15, p. 114, Mar. 2015.

11. K. Feldscher, "40% Prevention Rate for Colorectal Cancers | Harvard Gazette," *Harvard Gazette*, 2013. Available: http://news.harvard.edu/gazette/story/2013/09/40-prevention-rate-for-colorectal-cancers/ (accessed Aug. 24, 2017).

12. D. A. Joseph, R. G. S. Meester, A. G. Zauber, et al., "Colorectal Cancer Screening: Estimated Future Colonoscopy Need and Current Volume and Capacity," *Cancer*, vol. 122, no. 16, pp. 2479–2486, Aug. 2016.

13. S. Gupta, C. Ahn, C. S. Skinner, et al., "Measurement of Colorectal Cancer Test Use with Medical Claims Data in a Safety-Net Health System," *Am. J. Med. Sci.*, vol. 345, no. 2, pp. 99–103, Feb. 2013.

14. U. Hayat, P. J. W. Lee, R. Lopez, J. J. Vargo, and M. K. Rizk, "Online Educational Video Improves Bowel Preparation and Reduces the Need for Repeat Colonoscopy within Three Years," *Am. J. Med.*, vol. 129, no. 11, p. 1219.e1–1219.e9, Nov. 2016.

15. R. M. Goffman, S. L. Harris, J. H. May, et al., "Modeling Patient No-Show History and Predicting Future Outpatient Appointment Behavior in the Veterans Health Administration," *Mil. Med.*, vol. 182, no. 5, pp. e1708–e1714, May 2017.

16. J. T. Chang, J. L. Sewell, and L. W. Day, "Prevalence and Predictors of Patient No-Shows to Outpatient Endoscopic Procedures Scheduled with Anesthesia," *BMC Gastroenterol.*, vol. 15, no. 1, p. 123, Dec. 2015.

17. B. P. Berg, M. Murr, D. Chermak, et al., "Estimating the Cost of No-Shows and Evaluating the Effects of Mitigation Strategies," *Med. Decis. Mak.*, vol. 33, no. 8, pp. 976–985, Nov. 2013.

18. H. K. Koh and R. E. Rudd, "The Arc of Health Literacy," *JAMA*, vol. 314, no. 12, p. 1225, Sep. 2015.

19. D. L. B. Schwappach, "Review: Engaging Patients as Vigilant Partners in Safety," *Med. Care Res. Rev.*, vol. 67, no. 2, pp. 119–148, Apr. 2010.

20. G. Graffigna, S. Barello, A. Bonanomi, and E. Lozza, "Measuring Patient Engagement: Development and Psychometric Properties of the Patient Health Engagement (PHE) Scale," *Front. Psychol.*, vol. 6, p. 274, Mar. 2015.

21. J. R. Vest and T. R. Miller, "The Association between Health Information Exchange and Measures of Patient Satisfaction," *Appl. Clin. Inform.*, vol. 2, no. 4, pp. 447–459, 2011.

22. I. Aujoulat, W. d'Hoore, and A. Deccache, "Patient Empowerment in Theory and Practice: Polysemy or Cacophony?," *Patient Educ. Couns.*, vol. 66, no. 1, pp. 13–20, Apr. 2007.

23. E. Guadagnoli and P. Ward, "Patient Participation in Decision-Making," *Soc. Sci. Med.*, vol. 47, no. 3, pp. 329–339, Aug. 1998.

24. J. H. Hibbard, J. Stockard, E. R. Mahoney, and M. Tusler, "Development of the Patient Activation Measure (PAM): Conceptualizing and Measuring Activation in Patients and Consumers," *Health Serv. Res.*, vol. 39, no. 4 Pt 1, pp. 1005–1026, Aug. 2004.

25. J. Gruman, M. H. Rovner, M. E. French, et al., "From Patient Education to Patient Engagement: Implications for the Field of Patient Education," *Patient Educ. Couns.*, vol. 78, no. 3, pp. 350–356, Mar. 2010.

26. K. L. Carman, P. Dardess, M. Maurer, et al., "Patient and Family Engagement: A Framework for Understanding the Elements and Developing Interventions and Policies," *Health Aff.*, vol. 32, no. 2, pp. 223–231, Feb. 2013.

27. G. Eysenbach, "What Is E-health?," *J. Med. Internet Res.*, vol. 3, no. 2, p. E20, 2001.

28. S. Barello, S. Triberti, G. Graffigna, et al., "eHealth for Patient Engagement: A Systematic Review," *Front. Psychol.*, vol. 6, p. 2013, 2015.

29. K. G. M. Volpp and N. S. M. Mohta, "Patient Engagement Survey: Technology Tools Gain Support But Cost Is a Hurdle," July 10, 2017. Available: http://catalyst.nejm.org/patient-engagement-technology-toolsgain-support/ (accessed Aug. 28, 2017).

30. J. Park, T.-O. Kim, N.-Y. Lee, et al. "The Effectiveness of Short Message Service to Assure the Preparation-to-Colonoscopy Interval before Bowel Preparation for Colonoscopy," *Gastroenterol. Res. Pract.* doi:10.1155/2015/628049

31. Accenture. "Why Healthcare Providers Need to Up Their Mobile Game," 2015. Available: www.accenture.com/us-en/insight-health-losing-patience (accessed August 28, 2017).

32. U. Hayet, P. J. Lee, R. Lopez, J. J. Vargo, and M. K. Rizk. "Online Educational Video Improves Bowel Preparation and Reduces the Need for Repeat Colonoscopy within Three Years,"*Am, J. Med.*, vol. 129, no. 11, pp. 1219.e1–1219.e9, 2016.

33. A. B. Ajumobi, M. Malakouti, A. Bullen, H. Ahaneku, and T. N. Lunsford, "YouTube™ as a Source of Instructional Videos on Bowel Preparation: A Content Analysis." *J. Cancer Educ.* doi:10.1007/s13187-015-0888-y

34. Department of Education. "National Education Technology Plan – Office of Educational Technology," December 2015. Available: https://tech.ed.gov/netp/ (accessed Aug. 28, 2017).

35. J. Nayor, A. Feng, T. Qazi, and J. R. Saltzman, "Improved Patient Preparedness for Colonoscopy Using Automated Time-Released Reminders," abstract submitted to ACG Annual Meeting, Orlando, FL, October 17, 2017.

Index